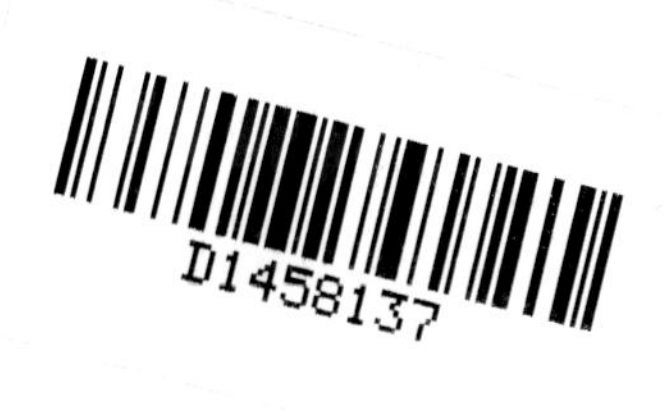

Surgery of the Eyelids, Lacrimal System, and Orbit

Ophthalmology Monographs

A series published by Oxford University Press in cooperation with the American Academy of Ophthalmology

Series Editor: Richard K. Parrish, II, MD, Bascom Palmer Eye Institute

American Academy of Ophthalmology Clinical Education Secretariat:
Louis B. Cantor, MD, Indiana University School of Medicine
Gregory L. Skuta, MD, Dean A. McGee Eye Institute

1. *Retinal Detachment: Principles and Practices*, third edition
   Daniel A. Brinton, MD, and Charles P. Wilkinson, MD
2. *Electrophysiologic Testing in Disorders of the Retina, Optic Nerve, and Visual Pathway*, second edition
   Gerald Allen Fishman, MD, David G. Birch, MD, Graham E. Holder, MD, and Mitchell G. Brigell, MD
3. *Visual Fields: Examination and Interpretation*, third edition
   Edited by Thomas J. Walsh, MD
4. *Glaucoma Surgery: Principles and Techniques*, second edition
   Edited by Robert N. Weinreb, MD and Richard P. Mills, MD
5. *Fluorescein and Indocyanine Green Angiography: Technique and Interpretation*, second edition
   Joseph W. Berkow, MD, Robert W. Flower, David H. Orth, MD, and James S. Kelley, MD
6. *Neuroimaging in Ophthalmology*, second edition
   Michael C. Johnson, MD, FRCSC, Bruno A. Policeni, MD, Andrew G. Lee, MD, and Wendy R.K. Smoker, MD, FACR
   [First edition published as *Magnetic Resonance Imaging and Computed Tomography: Clinical Neuro-Orbital Anatomy*, by Jonathan D. Wirtschafter, MD, Eric L. Berman, MD, and Carolyn S. McDonald, MD]
7. *Cataract Surgery and Intraocular Lenses: A 21st-Century Perspective*, second edition
   Edited by Jerry G. Ford, MD, and Carol L. Karp, MD
8. *Surgery of the Eyelids, Lacrimal System, and Orbit*, second edition
   Edited by Michael T. Yen, MD
   [First edition published as *Surgery of the Eyelid, Orbit, and Lacrimal System,* volumes 1, 2, and 3, edited by William B. Stewart, MD]
9. *Surgical Anatomy of the Ocular Adnexa: A Clinical Approach*
   David R. Jordan, MD, and Richard R. Anderson, MD
10. *Optic Nerve Disorders*, second edition
    Edited by Lanning B. Klein, MD, and Rod Foroozan, MD
11. *Laser Photocoagulation of the Retina and Choroid* [with slide set]
    James C. Folk, MD, and José S. Pulido, MD
12. *Low Vision Rehabilitation: Caring for the Whole Person*
    Edited by Donald C. Fletcher, MD
13. *Glaucoma Medical Therapy: Principles and Management*, second edition
    Edited by Peter A. Netland, MD, PhD
14. *Diabetes and Ocular Disease: Past, Present, and Future Therapies*, second edition
    Edited by Ingrid U. Scott, MD, MPH, Harry W. Flynn, Jr., MD, and William E. Smiddy, MD
15. *HIV/AIDS and the Eye: A Global Perspective*
    Emmett T. Cunningham, Jr., MD, and Rubens Belfort, Jr.
16. *Corneal Dystrophies and Degenerations: A Molecular Genetics Approach* [with CD]
    Edited by Ming X. Wang, MD, PhD
17. *Strabismus Surgery: Basic and Advanced Techniques*
    Edited by David A. Plager, MD; written by Edward G. Buckley, MD, David A. Plager, MD, Michael X. Repka, MD, and M. Edward Wilson, MD; contributions by Marshall M. Parks, MD and Gunter K. von Noorden, MD
    www.oup.com/us/aao/plager/strabismus
18. *A Compendium of Inherited Disorders and the Eye*
    Elias I. Traboulsi, MD
    www.oup.com/us/aao/traboulsi/genetic

SURGERY OF THE EYELIDS, LACRIMAL SYSTEM, AND ORBIT

Second Edition

Edited by
Michael T. Yen, MD

Published by Oxford University Press
in cooperation with
the American Academy of Ophthalmology

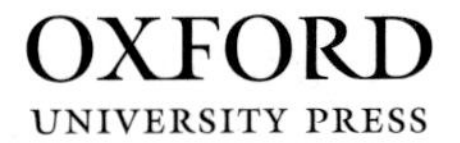

OXFORD
UNIVERSITY PRESS

Oxford University Press, Inc., publishes works that further
Oxford University's objective of excellence
in research, scholarship, and education.

Oxford New York
Auckland Cape Town Dar es Salaam Hong Kong Karachi
Kuala Lumpur Madrid Melbourne Mexico City Nairobi
New Delhi Shanghai Taipei Toronto

With offices in
Argentina Austria Brazil Chile Czech Republic France Greece
Guatemala Hungary Italy Japan Poland Portugal Singapore
South Korea Switzerland Thailand Turkey Ukraine Vietnam

Published by Oxford University Press, Inc.
198 Madison Avenue, New York, New York 10016
www.oup.com

Oxford is a registered trademark of Oxford University Press

Library of Congress Cataloging-in-Publication Data

Surgery of the eyelids, lacrimal system, and orbit / Edited by Michael T. Yen, MD. — Second edition.
p. ; cm. — (Ophthalmology monographs ; 8)
Includes bibliographical references.
ISBN 978-0-19-534021-1 (hardback : alk. paper) 1. Eyelids—Surgery. I. Yen, Michael T., editor.
II. American Academy of Ophthalmology, issuing body. III. Surgery of the eyelid, orbit, and lacrimal system.
IV. Series: Ophthalmology monographs ; 8.
[DNLM: 1. Eyelids—surgery. 2. Eye Diseases—surgery. 3. Lacrimal Apparatus—surgery. 4. Orbit—surgery.
5. Reconstructive Surgical Procedures—methods. W1 OP372L v.8 2011 / WW 205]
RE80.S843 2011
617.7'71059—dc22
2010051246

1 3 5 7 9 8 6 4 2

Printed in China

Legal Notice

The American Academy of Ophthalmology provides the opportunity for material to be presented for educational purposes only. The material represents the approach, ideas, statements, or opinion of the authors, not necessarily the only or best method or procedure in every case, nor the position of the Academy. Unless specifically stated otherwise, the opinions expressed and statements made by various authors in this monograph reflect the authors' observations and do not imply endorsement by the Academy. The material is not intended to replace a physician's own judgment or to give specific advice for case management. The Academy does not endorse any of the products or companies, if any, mentioned in this monograph.

Some material on recent developments may include information on drug or device applications that are not considered community standard, that reflect indications not included in approved FDA labeling, or that are approved for use only in restricted research settings. This information is provided as education only so physicians may be aware of alternative methods of the practice of medicine, and should not be considered endorsement, promotion, or in any way encouragement to use such applications. The FDA has stated that it is the responsibility of the physician to determine the FDA status of each drug or device he or she wishes to use in clinical practice, and to use these products with appropriate patient consent and in compliance with applicable law.

The Academy and Oxford University Press (OUP) do not make any warranties as to the accuracy, adequacy, or completeness of any material presented here, which is provided on an "as is" basis. The Academy and OUP are not liable to anyone for any errors, inaccuracies, or omissions obtained here. The Academy specifically disclaims any and all liability for injury or other damages of any kind for any and all claims that may arise out of the use of any practice, technique, or drug described in any material by any author, whether such claims are asserted by a physician or any other person.

DISCLOSURE STATEMENT

Each author states below any significant financial interest or other relationship with the manufacturer of any commercial product discussed in the chapters that he or she contributed to this publication or with the manufacturer of any competing commercial product.

The following authors state that they have no significant financial interest or other relationship to disclose:

Chrisfouad Alabiad
Richard L. Anderson
Christine C. Annunziata
C. Robert Bernardino
Mauricio R. Chavez
Peter Dolman
Raymond S. Douglas
Bita Esmaeli
Robert Goldberg
Adam Hassan
David E. Holck
Jennifer I. Hui
Adam Hsu
Catherine J. Hwang
Thomas N. Hwang
Thomas E. Johnson
David R. Jordan
Marsha C. Kavanagh
Robert C. Kersten
Don O. Kikkawa
Stephen R. Klapper
Bobby Korn
H.B. Harold Lee
Craig Lewis
Mark Lucarelli
Douglas P. Marx
Timothy J. McCulley
Lisa Mihora
William R. Nunery
Matthew P. Ohr
D.J. John Park
J.D. Perry
Jed Poll
Ashvini K. Reddy
Geoffrey E. Rose

Bryan Seiff
Stuart Seiff
Heeral Shah
Erin M. Shriver
Alexander Taich
Nicolas Uzcategui
M. Reza Vagefi
David H. Verity
Ralph Wesley
Chun Cheng Lin Yang
Kimberly G. Yen
Michael T. Yen

The following authors disclosed their interests or relationships:

Roger Dailey receives unrestricted educational grants from Allergan, Inc.

Jill A. Foster is a consultant with Allergan, Inc. and Medicis.

Andrew Harrison is a consultant for Menz Pharmaceuticals.

John B. Holds is a consultant with QLT Phototherapeutics.

John McCann is the owner of McCann Medical Matrix and is on the Speaker Bureau for Allergan, Inc.

J. Justin Older has received honoraria from Ellman International for lectures he gave.

Contents

Contributors

Chrisfouad Alabiad, MD
University of Miami Miller School of Medicine
Miami, Florida

Richard L. Anderson, MD, FACS
Center for Facial Appearances
Salt Lake City, Utah

Christine C. Annunziata, MD
University of California San Diego
La Jolla, California

Carlo Rob Bernardino, MD, FACS
Oculoplastics and Aesthetic Surgery
Vantage Eye Center
Monterey, California

Mauricio R. Chavez, MD
Oregon Health & Sciences Center
Portland, Oregon

J. Richard O. Collin, MA, FRCS, FRCOphth, DO
Moorfields Eye Hospital
London, England

Roger A. Dailey, MD, FACS
Oregon Health & Sciences University
Portland, Oregon

Peter J. Dolman, MD
University of British Columbia
Vancouver, British Columbia, Canada

Raymond S. Douglas, MD
University of Michigan Medical School
Ann Arbor, Michigan

Bita Esmaeli, MD
MD Anderson Cancer Center
Houston, Texas

Jill A. Foster, MD
Ohio State University
Columbus, Ohio

Robert A. Goldberg, MD
University of California Los Angeles
Los Angeles, California

Andrew Harrison, MD
University of Minnesota
Minneapolis, Minnesota

Adam S. Hassan, MD
Eye Plastic & Facial Cosmetic Surgery
Grand Rapids, Michigan

David E. E. Holck, MD
Wilford Hall Medical Center
San Antonio, Texas

John B. Holds, MD
Saint Louis University
St. Louis, Missouri

Adam Hsu, MD
MD Anderson Cancer Center
Houston, Texas

Jennifer I. Hui, MD
University of Miami Miller School of Medicine
Miami, Florida

Catherine J. Hwang, MD
University of California Los Angeles
Los Angeles, California

Thomas N. Hwang, MD, PhD
University of California San Francisco
San Francisco, California

Thomas E. Johnson, MD
University of Miami Miller School of Medicine
Miami, Florida

David R. Jordan, MD
University of Ottawa School of Medicine
Ottawa, Ontario, Canada

Marsha C. Kavanagh, MD
Ohio State University
Columbus, Ohio

Robert C. Kersten, MD
University of California San Francisco
San Francisco, California

Don O. Kikkawa, MD
University of California San Diego
La Jolla, California

Stephen R. Klapper, MD
Klapper Eyelid and Facial Plastic Surgery
Carmel, Indiana

Joel Kopelman, MD
Wilford Hall Medical Center
San Antonio, Texas

Bobby Korn, MD, PhD
University of California San Diego
La Jolla, California

H.B. Harold Lee, MD
Oculofacial Plastic & Orbital Surgery
Indianapolis, Indiana

Craig Lewis, MD
Cleveland Clinic Foundation
Cleveland, Ohio

John V. Linberg, MD
West Virginia University
Morgantown, West Virginia

Mark J. Lucarelli, MD, FACS
University of Wisconsin School of Medicine
Madison, Wisconsin

Douglas P. Marx, MD
Baylor College of Medicine
Houston, Texas

John D. McCann, MD, PhD
Center for Facial Appearances
Salt Lake City, Utah

Timothy J. McCulley, MD
The Wilmer Eye Institute
Johns Hopkins School of Medicine

Director of Oculoplastic Surgery
King Khaled Eye Specialist Hospital
Riyadh, Saudi Arabia

Lisa Mihora, MD
Wilford Hall Medical Center
San Antonio, Texas

William R. Nunery, MD
Oculofacial Plastic & Orbital Surgery
Indianapolis, Indiana

Matthew P. Ohr, MD
Ohio State University
Columbus, Ohio

J. Justin Older, MD
University of South Florida College of Medicine
Tampa, Florida

D.J. John Park, MD
University of Minnesota
Minneapolis, Minnesota

J.D. Perry, MD
Cleveland Clinic Foundation
Cleveland, Ohio

Jed Poll, MD
Mount Ogden Eye Center
Ogden, Utah

Ashvini K. Reddy, MD
Baylor College of Medicine
Houston, Texas

Geoffrey E. Rose, BSc, MS, MRCP, FRCS, FRCOphth, DSc
Moorfields Eye Hospital
London, England

Bryan Seiff, MD
Delaware Eye Institute
Rehoboth Beach, Delaware

Stuart Seiff, MD
Pacific Eye Associates
San Francisco, California

Heeral Shah, MD
Baylor College of Medicine
Houston, Texas

Alexander Taich, MD
University of Michigan Medical School
Ann Arbor, Michigan

Nicolas Uzcategui, MD
Eye Consultants of Syracuse
Syracuse, New York

M. Reza Vagefi, MD
Scheie Eye Institute, University of Pennsylvania
Philadelphia, Pennsylvania

David H. Verity, MA, MD, FRCOphth
Moorfields Eye Hospital
London, England

Ralph E. Wesley, MD
Wesley & Klippenstein
Nashville, Tennessee

Chun Cheng Lin Yang, MD, MSc
Costa Rica Oculoplastics Inc.
Hospital CIMA San José
San José, Costa Rica

Kimberly G. Yen, MD
Baylor College of Medicine
Houston, Texas

Michael T. Yen, MD
Baylor College of Medicine
Houston, Texas

I

Eyelid Reconstruction

1

Eyelid Lacerations and Acute Adnexal Trauma

NICOLAS UZCATEGUI, MD

When evaluating a patient who has sustained any type of trauma, life-threatening injuries should be addressed or ruled out before proceeding with assessment for ocular and adnexal trauma. In the setting of trauma the practitioner must never forget the basics of life support and systemic trauma assessments. The first goals are to maintain a patent airway and to provide respiratory support. Adequate circulation and perfusion need to be reestablished once an airway has been established. The nature of the accident should alert the practitioner as to the possibility of a cervical spine injury. In accidents that are unwitnessed, that produce loss of consciousness, and/or that are produced by high-velocity impacts to the head, face, and neck, the patient should have C-collar stabilization/immobilization until the cervical spine can be cleared both radiologically and clinically. Only then should ocular and adnexal injuries be assessed.

Adnexal trauma is addressed only after the integrity of the globe and intraocular contents has been confirmed by a complete eye examination. A dilated funduscopic examination can be deferred for a reasonable amount of time if a neurologic injury and central nervous system compromise is suspected, since the use of mydriatic agents is a relative contraindication in these circumstances. If a facial nerve injury is not present and/or a ruptured globe has been excluded, the extent of the eyelid and adnexal injuries can be safely determined. Complex lacerations of the eyelid often include extensive wounds involving the eyelid margin, canaliculi, and lateral canthus; these can be associated with tissue loss and can be caused either by sharp objects or bite injuries. In general it is preferable to repair soft tissue injuries within hours of their occurrence; nevertheless, special considerations can delay the primary repair in exceptional circumstances such as severe tissue edema, active infection at the wound site, or extensive hematomas. Intermittent ice compresses, drainage of hematomas, and systemic steroids and/or antibiotics can be instituted prior to repair if swelling or infections limit the possibility of reconstruction. Local wound care and sometimes topical antibiotics are a cornerstone of management in adnexal injury. Tetanus prophylaxis when indicated, wound irrigation when possible, and antibiotic prophylaxis should be the initial steps in isolated ocular adnexal trauma.

1-1 GENERAL PRINCIPLES

From the ophthalmologic standpoint, the assessment and preservation of ocular function is the first priority when treating an already stabilized trauma victim. Visual acuity testing should be done and pupillary response to light and globe integrity need to be determined when possible prior to soft tissue adnexal repair. If vision cannot be assessed (i.e., unconscious, nonverbal, uncooperative patients or preverbal children), examination under sedation or anesthesia is warranted to determine globe integrity. As a general guideline, the information in Table 1-1 can help prioritize the workflow when confronted with a patient with adnexal trauma in need of soft tissue repair.

Surgical repair must be conceptualized prior to execution. The mechanism of injury should determine the initial evaluation of adnexal injuries. Blunt injuries are usually self-limited to the area of impact, while penetrating and high-speed trauma tend to produce significantly more damage, including damage to areas remote from the point of impact. Wounds and injuries require thorough examination to determine the extent of damage. The examiner should inspect not only for anatomic or structural damage, but also for functional integrity. A complete assessment should not miss the status of the medial and lateral canthus, lid margin, canaliculi, levator excursion and integrity, and soft tissue loss.

Since penetrating orbit trauma can occur with retained foreign bodies with minimal to no ocular findings, it could lead to misdiagnosis. MRI and CT imaging fails to identify the retained organic material in approximately 50% of the cases.

Table 1-1 Priorities in the Treatment of Adnexal Repair

1. Patient stabilization
2. Problem-focused history and physical examination
3. Assessment of visual function and system
4. Assessment of soft tissue injuries
5. Radiologic assessment
6. Wound care
7. Establish treatment plan (consider consults with other disciplines)
8. Photographic documentation of injury (especially in cases with potential medicolegal implications)
9. Reassessment and follow-up

Organic matter, wood in particular, can be isodense with air and/or fat and virtually unrecognizable to imaging modalities (Fig. 1-1). When an organic foreign body is suspected and CT imaging or MRI can identify the object producing the injury, it can also help identify concomitant intracranial involvement; this is of particular importance since penetrating orbitocranial injuries carry a worse prognosis due to their higher complication and mortality rate. The orbital septum serves as a landmark to divide the eyelid from the orbit. The presence of air after penetrating injury in the orbit is an almost unequivocal sign that the orbital septum has been breached, and the practitioner should have a high index of suspicion for associated injury to the orbit contents (i.e., neurovascular structures) when examining these patients. Orbit emphysema can be seen as a complication of fractures of the orbit walls involving trauma to the adjacent sinuses.

Wound care should include cleaning of tissues and placement of temporary dressings when appropriate. A bulb syringe used with normal saline solution for copious irrigation, while exerting low pressure, is very useful to remove loose dirt

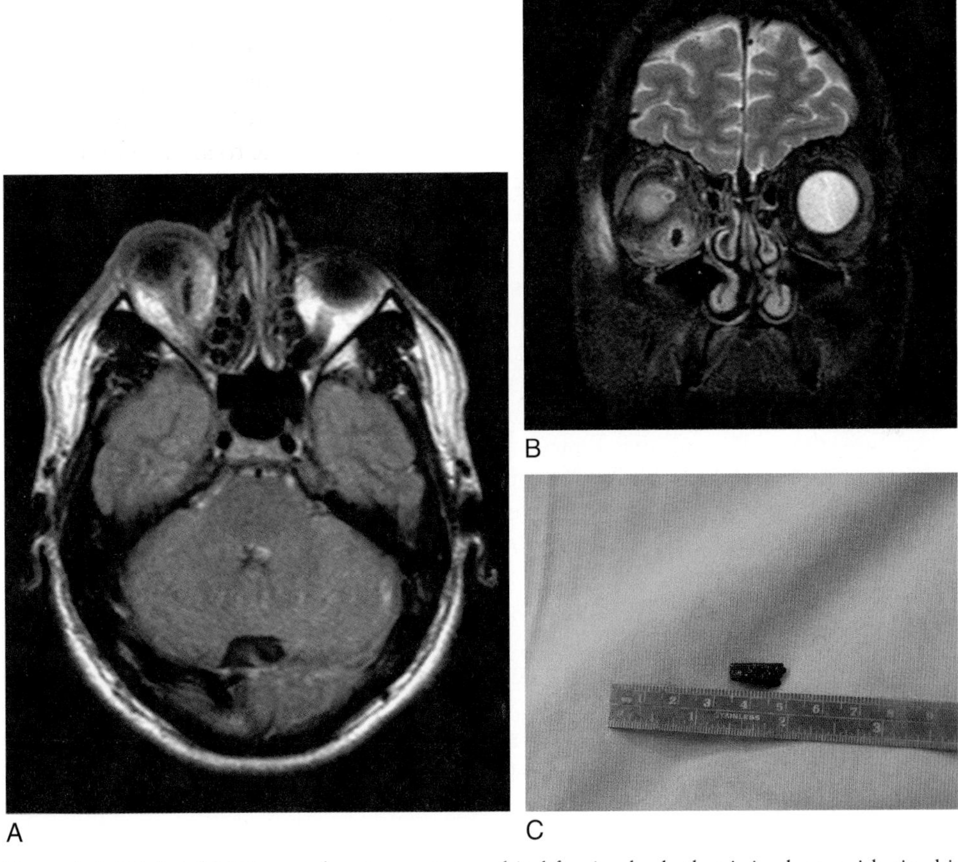

Figure 1-1 (A) Axial MRI scan showing an intraorbital foreign body that is isodense with air; this is highly suggestive of an organic material such as wood. (B) Coronal MRI scan demonstrating the same foreign body with surrounding orbital inflammation. (C) The organic material removed from the orbit was a broken-off piece of a tree branch. (Images courtesy of Michael T. Yen, MD)

and debride superficial necrotic material and is an adjunct to hemostasis. "Floating" the wound edges can assist with tissue identification and help determine whether tissue loss is present.

Photographic documentation of injuries serves multiple purposes. It can demonstrate postoperative improvement, and it can also be useful when explaining to the patient and family the technical limitations that the surgeon faces when performing the repair. This is especially the case if there has been tissue loss that was not salvaged at the scene to be used as a composite tissue graft during repair. Photographic documentation can also be useful for documenting findings should any medicolegal inquiry arise in the future.

1-2 REPAIR OF EYELID INJURIES

The eyelid is empirically divided in two layers: the anterior and posterior lamellae. In a simplified form, each of them contains two layers of tissue, thus forming a four-layer structure. The anterior lamella contains the skin and orbicularis muscle, while the posterior lamella contains the tarsus and lid retractors, and the conjunctiva. The involvement of the lamella in each case will determine the surgical technique to be used in reconstructive planning. When dealing with forces that breach the integrity of the eyelid, an organized planning sequence should be followed for evaluation and management of eyelid reconstruction/repair:

1. Preliminary wound evaluation by inspection: Try to determine which lamellae of the eyelid and other anatomic structures are involved.
2. Radiological studies, if indicated.
3. Tetanus toxoid booster, if indicated and not done by primary responders.
4. Anesthesia by local infiltration: The use of a product combined with epinephrine (1:100,000 or 1:200,000) can facilitate hemostasis, which could be helpful for the identification of anatomic structures. Consider general anesthesia if extensive injuries can be visualized (usually involving the lid margin, canaliculi, levator palpebrae superioris complex), if tissue loss is suspected, if there is extensive associated "degloving" injuries, or when adequate repair can be compromised due to lack of patient cooperation or other circumstances.
5. Cleansing of the wound and gentle debridement: Remove all foreign material.
6. Protect the globe with a rigid scleral shell or "contact" lens prior to adnexal manipulation.
7. Complete wound exploration with careful attention to the integrity of the canaliculi, canthal tendons, and levator aponeurosis, when possible by verifying its excursion.
8. Careful control of hemostasis, by pressure or using light bipolar or monopolar cautery.
9. Remove devitalized tissue only if you are certain it is not salvageable.
10. Open reduction and internal fixation of fractures should, in general, precede reconstruction of soft tissues.

11. Repair the canthal structures, canaliculi, and levator aponeurosis prior to other myocutaneous defects.
12. Perform synthesis by layers of eyelid structures, with good wound edge eversion, without suturing the orbital septum, to avoid late retraction/scarring.

Failure to adhere to these principles can lead to complications when attempting to repair eyelid lacerations. Some of the more common mistakes are:

Excessive wound margin debridement
Failure to remove foreign bodies from the wound bed
Inappropriate tissue handling, excessive pressure and/or tension
Failure to recognize damage to specialized eyelid structures (canaliculi, levator aponeurosis complex)
Poor reapproximation of tissues: misaligned anatomic structures (i.e., lid margin, canthi, etc.) or inadequate tension on sutures
Improper suture removal (too early or too late)

1-2-1 *Simple Lacerations.* When a laceration produces a clean, linear wound that is not under tension, it can be reapproximated primarily with the use of adhesives or cyanoacrylate tissue glue. Commercial products like Steri-Stips® (3M) are readily available and useful when selecting this synthesis method. Cyanoacrylate is a polymer capable of reapproximating tissues, maintaining its tensile strength for several days. It has become more popular in wound closure, but its utility is limited due to its cost, the need to have a dry surface for the polymer to bond to the underlying skin, and the difficulty in handling the liquid glue before it polymerizes, making it difficult to maintain eversion of the skin at the wound edge. When there is gaping of the wound and exploration determines that there has not been any tissue loss and primary reapproximation of the wound is feasible, either absorbable or nonabsorbable 6-0 or 7-0 sutures can be used. Wound retraction, more evident at the wound edges, is a common problem, especially in wounds that have been open for some time or if the direction of the wound is against the relaxed skin tension lines. Nonabsorbable sutures should be removed in 5 to 7 days; early removal improves scar prognosis. Epithelialization of the wound suture tract can occur with delayed suture removal. The clinician should remember that small penetrating wounds can also be associated with globe injury.

1-2-2 *Deep Lacerations.* When eyelid lacerations are deeper, it is important to evaluate the eyelid excursion and to determine whether there has been functional compromise of the levator aponeurosis or the levator itself. Prolapsed fat through the wound is a clear sign of violation of the orbit septum and will require layer-by-layer inspection to assess the integrity not only of the levator, but also of the extraocular muscles and globe itself.

In a patient with a laceration with compromised levator excursion, the reconstruction strategy should attempt to identify the levator muscle and proceed to its reattachment. The septum must be recognized as a landmark during repair, and all structures, both anterior and posterior to the septum, that have been breached need to be reapproximated with simple interrupted sutures. The orbit fat can be repositioned and in certain circumstances small portions can be excised carefully if the surgeon cannot completely reposition the protruding fat pads and they interfere with proper wound closure. The septum must not be sutured to the skin, orbicularis muscle, levator aponeurosis, or conjunctiva, since postoperatively the retraction that will occur will create cicatricial eyelid retraction and lagophthalmos could develop. The key elements that will ensure successful repair, and that apply to any reconstruction situation, can be summarized as: (1) minimal to no excision of tissue to revitalize the wound edges, (2) closure by layers except for the reapproximation of the orbital septum, (3) avoiding wound tension and dead space, and (4) meticulous hemostasis.

1-2-3 *Eyelid Margin Lacerations.* Regardless of the extent of the injury, superficial or deep, associated with an isolated small eyelid laceration or an extensive complex large eyelid or facial wound, lid margin lacerations are repaired using the same technique. To achieve a successful repair the examiner must identify the landmarks of the eyelid margin.

A good cosmetic and functional result will depend on precise direct reapproximation of the eyelid margin structures and the lack of tarsal irregularities on the edges of the wound. The tarsal plate needs to be identified and its borders should be regularized so that the borders of the laceration form an angle perpendicular to the sagittal plane of the eyelid; this can be done with a #15 Bard-Parker® blade. Only the minimal amount of tissue that is necessary to achieve a "square edge" on the tarsus should be removed. Resections of the tarsal irregularities must span the compete length of the tarsal plate on its vertical dimension. The now-vertical edges of the tarsal place can be sutured together with either 7-0 or 6-0 polyglactin (Vicryl®) sutures. The first suture prior to suturing the tarsus should be placed over the eyelid margin through the meibomian gland orifices; this can be done with a simple bite or a mattress suture, 1 to 2 mm from the wound edge, penetrating 1 to 2 mm deep on both sides of the wound. Once this suture is in place traction can be applied. Vicryl®, braided nylon, and silk are suitable materials for this first traction suture. It should be left loose with long ends until the end of the repair and tied when the traction is no longer needed. Vicryl® is the suture of choice to repair the tarsal plate with two or three interrupted stitches. Tarsal sutures are passed partial thickness through the tarsus to avoid erosive suture keratopathy, especially when repairing the upper eyelid (Fig. 1-2).

Once the tarsus has been reapproximated, the rest of the eyelid margin can be aligned with sutures anterior to the gray line and through the mucocutaneous border to precisely align the eyelashes. Achieving eyelid margin eversion is necessary to prevent "notching" of the eyelid after repair. The skin and orbicularis closure can be done with other absorbable and/or permanent sutures. After tying the lid margin sutures that were left long, these are bundled and reflected over the eyelid margin, where there are secured with a separate anchoring suture to the skin and orbicularis to prevent them from rubbing on the corneal surface. Lid margin sutures and nonabsorbable sutures need to be removed in 7 to 10 days.

1-2-4 *Blunt Injuries.* Contusion injuries caused by blunt objects exerting pressure that exceeds the elasticity of the tissues, followed by a certain degree of pressure

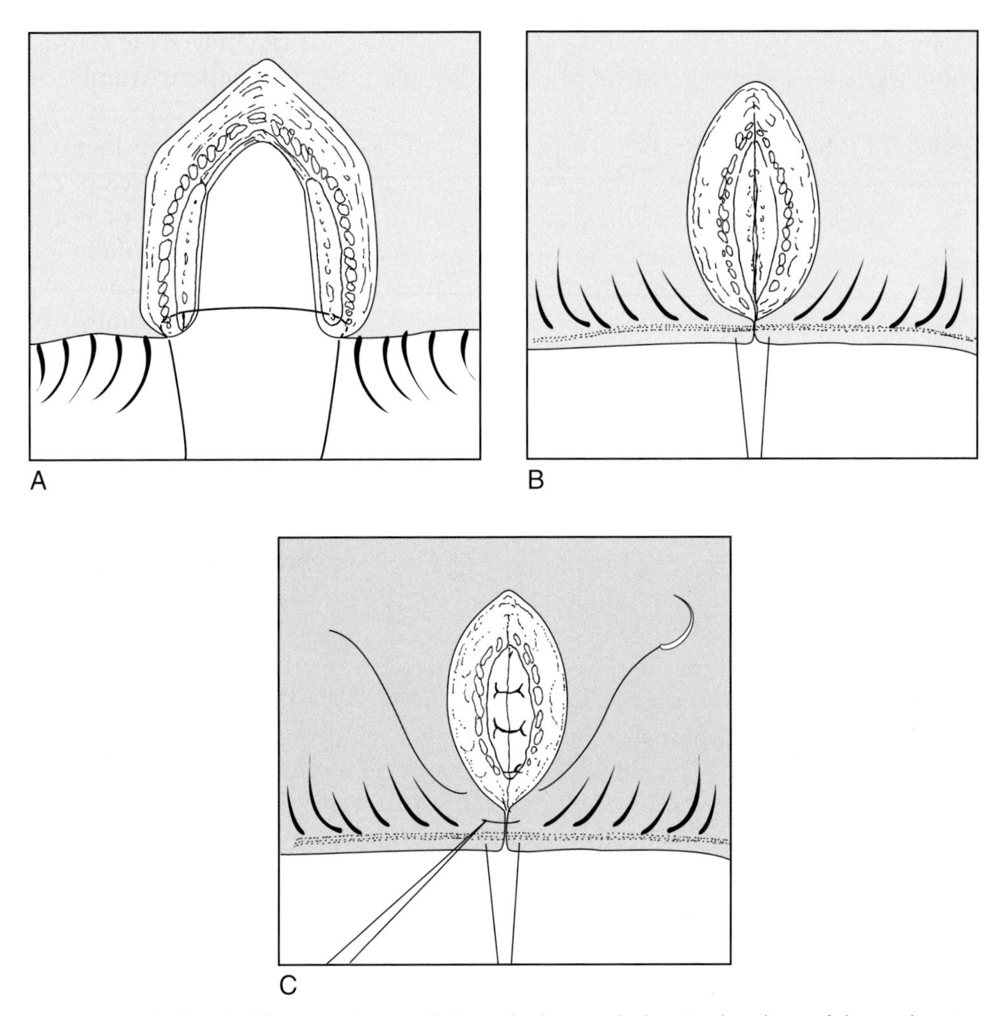

Figure 1-2 (A) A 6-0 silk suture is passed through the tarsal plate in the plane of the meibomian gland openings. (B) The marginal suture placement must align the tarsal segments. Absorbable sutures may then be placed in a lamellar fashion through the tarsus. (C) Additional cutaneous sutures are passed to align the eyelashes. The skin–muscle layer is closed next. The marginal sutures are anchored under the skin sutures to prevent ocular surface irritation.

necrosis, can produce significant distortion of the eyelid tissues. The eyelid compromise is variable and can range from partial to complete avulsion with various degrees of tissue devitalization. Shearing forces on the tissue can disrupt the canthal tendons, canaliculi, levator aponeurosis, and skin and orbicularis, sometimes requiring extensive debridement prior to finding wound edges that are suitable for reapproximation.

1-2-5 *Tissue Loss.* When dealing with avulsion-type injuries of the eyelids, the goal of repair and reconstruction should be preservation of the globe and eyelid function. With these injuries it is common to find the retracted tissue "rolled into" the wound, and careful manipulation can reveal that meticulous anatomic repair by primary reapproximation is often possible. However, if there is true loss of eyelid tissue, efforts should be made to recover the segment of tissue missing, since reimplantation of the segment is often successful. If there has been tissue loss and the segment of eyelid tissue is available, every attempt should be made to preserve it. The composite portion of the eyelid might be incorporated in the wound repair even if the tissue appears ischemic. The avulsed tissues used as a composite graft during repair can offer variable success depending on their degree of viability at the time of repair. If there is true tissue loss and the tissue is not available, eyelid reconstruction is performed either with a combination of procedures and or in a planned staged fashion. Both the anterior lamella and the posterior lamella will need to be reconstructed.

The success of the reconstruction is largely dependent on the ability to use a vascular supply that will adequately support either the anterior or posterior lamellar graft, whichever the surgeon decides to use. The lost posterior lamella needs to be repaired with a mucosalized surface: homologous tarsus, hard palate, nasal cartilage, and ear cartilage grafts are suitable alternatives for this repair. When tarsus is used it can be done as a free graft or as a pedicle flap from the superior eyelid, a lid-sharing procedure. Loss of the anterior lamella of the eyelids can be covered with a myocutaneous flap. This is obtained in most cases by advancing lateral eyelid tissue medially after a canthotomy and cantholysis, but infrequently it requires additional full-thickness skin-grafting procedures. The surgeon should remember the high failure rate of grafts when they are not placed over an adequately vascularized bed. It is impossible to provide a single algorithm for eyelid repair with tissue loss; the multiple reconstructive options will depend not only on the amount of missing tissue, but also on the age and therefore the amount of tissue laxity of the patient, as well as other individual variations.

Tissue advancement when necessary is determined on an empiric basis. Semicircular flaps, originally described by Mustarde and modified by Tenzel, permit substantial tissue mobilization into eyelid defects. In general the tissue advancement is achieved by a skin muscle incision at the level of the lateral canthal angle of approximately 5 to 7 mm that is prolonged in a curvilinear fashion. The upward or downward direction of the semicircle will be determined if the lower or the upper eyelid will be mobilized, respectively. The diameter of the semicircle will be determined by the extent of the defect or desired tissue mobilization. The skin and muscle are dissected from the sub-orbicularis oculi fascia, providing the necessary mobilization of the tissue into the defect. The lateral orbit attachments to the rim as well as the orbito-malar ligament can be released to release the tension if necessary. Once the tarsus and the eyelid margin have been reapproximated with the technique described above, the posterior lamella can be reconstructed with a free mucosalized graft or by simply mobilizing the conjunctiva into the posterior surface of the skin–muscle flap using 6-0 or 7-0 plain or chromic gut sutures. The lateral canthal angle can then be reformed by fixing the skin muscle flap into the periosteum of the orbit rim, at the level of the lateral orbit tubercle, using 4-0 Vicryl® or (polydioxanone) PDS® sutures 3 to 5 mm superior to the level of the medial eyelid raphe. This overcorrection is necessary to counter the effect of gravity and scarring in the postoperative period. The myocutaneous flap is then anchored to the periosteum of the anterior zygoma with the same sutures to also prevent cicatricial lid retraction and secondary lagophthalmos from scarring. The skin can be sutured according to the surgeon's preference with either absorbable or nonabsorbable sutures. In the immediate postoperative period the patient should be closely monitored for evidence of wound necrosis or infection. Other techniques, such as the Hughes tarsoconjunctival flap or the Cutler Beard procedures, described in the eyelid reconstruction section when dealing with excision and reconstruction following the resection of eyelid lesions, could be useful adjuncts when confronted with extensive full-thickness eyelid tissue defects.

1-3 CANTHAL INJURIES

Displacement or rounding of the canthal angles after trauma can suggest injury to the canthal tendons. Failure to identify canthal injuries and disruptions can lead to lid globe distraction. This condition leads, in the medial eyelid, to ectropion and epiphora; at the level of the lateral cantus it can produce ectropion, lid retraction, and lagophthalmos, as well as problems with blinking.

The medial canthal tendon measures an average 6 mm long (4 to 8 mm range) in the adult and is approximately 3 mm wide. It attaches the anterior aspect of the tarsal plate to the anterior lacrimal crest, located in the ascending process of the maxilla anterior to the nasolacrimal sac fossa. Posteriorly the tarsus is attached to the posterior lacrimal crest by Hoerner's muscle, which is nothing more than the lacrimal portion of the orbicularis oculi. Lacerations of the deep head of the medial canthal ligament can cause telecanthus, unlike lacerations of the superficial head of the canthal ligament. Lacerations of the medial canthal tendon often coexist with canalicular injury, so it is important to identify canalicular injury prior to medial canthal tendon repair.

The lateral canthal tendon also has an anterior (superficial) and a posterior (deep) attachment to the orbit at the level of the lateral rim. The lateral canthal tendon measures approximately 6 mm long and 2 mm wide; it lies posterior to the orbicularis oculi muscle and attaches anteriorly to the periosteum of the zygomatic arch. Posteriorly it attaches to the lateral orbit tubercle approximately 5 mm posterior to the orbit rim, approximately 10 mm below the frontozygomatic suture.

1-3-1 *Lateral Canthal Disruption*. Injury to the lateral canthal tendon is not uncommon. Lateral canthal reattachment can be deferred if there is marked proptosis and orbital compartment syndrome is a concern. In lateral canthal injuries, when possible the lateral canthal tendon or its remnant should be placed slightly posterior to the lateral orbital rim and reattached to the periosteum of the lateral orbit wall. A double-armed 4-0 Vicryl® or 4-0 polyester suture can be used, passing the arms through the medial cut edge of the tendon or lateral edge of the tarsus. The use of half-circle needles facilitates this task. The lateral edge of the tarsus is reattached with deep bites through the periosteum of the inner aspect of the lateral orbital rim.

When the periosteum is damaged or there is dehiscence of the tissues after placing tension on the sutures, several options are available. The first and easiest would be the use of a Mitek® Screw (Ethicon/Johnson & Johnson Company, DePuy Mitek,

Inc. 325 Paramount Drive, Raynham, MA 02767A) or a cantilevered plate to establish a point of fixation in the bone. Any of these are drilled into the bone at the desired point in height and place of fixation. With the Mitek® Screw the attached sutures to the fixation screw can then be passed through the tarsus and tied to each other, completing the tarsal attachment. When a cantilevered plate is used the suture is passed through one of the "eyelets" of the plate and then the needle portion is used to pass a firm bite through the tarsus. The surgeon must ensure that the tension placed on the suture is enough to reattach the tissue but not enough to cut the suture against the metal plate. When cantilevered plates or Mitek®-type suture screws are not available, two small holes with a 1- or 1.5-mm burr can be drilled full thickness through the zygomatic bone in the lateral orbit wall at the level of Whitnall's tubercle. Both holes are drilled in the same plane to 3 mm apart. The holes may or not taper into a common aperture inside the orbit wall. It is critical to maintain the structural integrity of the channels that are being drilled into the orbit wall. Once the holes and channels have been completed, a separate suture is connected to the tarsus, the needles can be cut, and each end of the suture is threaded through the bone tunnel; a small 30-gauge wire loop can be used for this task. Once the sutures have been passed through the tunnels and have exited on the outer aspect of the orbit rim they can be tied to each other, completing that canthal repair. The lateral commissure can be reformed using a 6-0 chromic suture, realigning the gray lines of the upper and lower lids, and suture by layers of the muscular and cutaneous portions of the wound is completed as described above, following the same general principles of basic eyelid repair.

1-3-2 *Medial Canthal Disruption/Canalicular Involvement.* The medial canthal tendon is made up of an anterior and posterior limb, but it is the posterior limb placement that determines the canthal position and cosmesis of the eyelid. The anterior limb of the medial canthal tendon can be repaired using a simple interrupted absorbable suture stitch. If both limbs are severed, the primary goal is to reattach the posterior limb. Posterior canthal tendon limb repair can be done with a double-armed 5-0 Vicryl® suture. Each arm can be passed through the cut ends of the tendon and then through the periosteum of the posterior lacrimal crest, aiming to overcorrect posteriorly and medially. Usually when there is an injury to the posterior limb of the medial canthal tendon there is a concomitant injury to the canalicular system.

If there is concomitant canalicular injury, posterior tendon repair should precede lacrimal repair, but canalicular intubation is easier to perform prior to the tendon repair. In more complicated cases, the deep head of the medial canthal tendon can also be reattached to the posterior lacrimal crest or medial orbit with a microscrew or plating system as described before. The anatomic placement of the periosteal sutures from the tarsi to the posterior lacrimal crest should be determined by the height of the contralateral medial canthus, if uninjured. The use of half-circle needles is highly recommended (e.g., P-2 [Ethicon] or ME 2 [Davis and Geck, Inc.]) due to the limited space and exposure of the anatomic region. The knot should be placed posterior to the lacrimal sac to achieve adequate alignment and to avoid postoperative scarring, which could further compromise the lacrimal passages. When this is not possible, transnasal wiring may be required. When there is concomitant injury to the medial and lateral canthal tendons, the medial canthal tendon should be repaired first. This is particularly important when dealing with naso-ethmoid fracture or dehiscence of the periosteum over the posterior lacrimal crest. Comminuted fractures can be stabilized with microplates to fixate the bone fragments and provide support to the medial canthal tendon. Prophylactic intubation of the canaliculi and nasolacrimal duct system is advocated in extensive midface injuries.

1-4 SPECIAL CONSIDERATIONS: DOG BITES

According to the Centers for Disease Control nearly 800,000 Americans seek medical attention for dog bites; half of these are children. Of those injured, 386,000 require treatment in an emergency department and about a dozen of these injuries are fatal. The highest rate of dog-bite injury occurs in children between ages 5 and 9 years, and the rate decreases as children get older. Almost two-thirds of injuries among children ages 4 years and younger are to the head or neck region. A recent study reports that a majority of documented dog attacks involve a known animal; 87% of the cases involve dogs belonging to the family or friends of the victims. Eyelid dog bites are therefore common facial injuries that often involve the lacrimal canaliculi (Fig. 1-3).

Although the incidence of infection following repair of these lacerations is low, prophylactic antibiotics should be administered to all patients. Antibiotics are directed at common canine oral bacterial flora. Cases of facial or wound infection are very rare and no systemic infection secondary to a dog bite has ever been reported.

The incidence of canalicular lacerations secondary to eyelid dog bites is reported in the literature to be as high as 70%. Good function and appearance of repaired

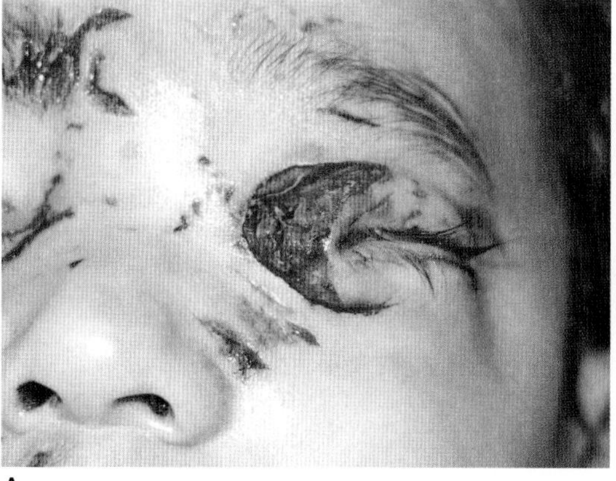
A

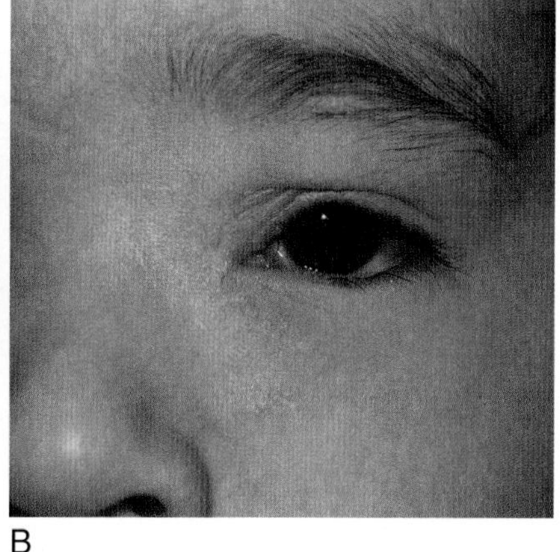
B

Figure 1-3 (A) A dog-bite injury involving laceration of the left upper and lower eyelids, canaliculus, medial canthal tendon, and nasolacrimal sac. (B) After primary repair and reconstruction, the patient has a patent nasolacrimal system and mild residual scarring of the eyelids. (Images courtesy of Michael T. Yen, MD)

eyelid dog bites is achieved with appropriate surgical management; these wounds heal nicely, leaving minor scarring and no infection. However, in some cases eyelid deformities are left and might require further reconstructive surgery.

SUGGESTED READINGS

Beadles KA, Lessner AM. Management of traumatic eyelid lacerations. *Semin Ophthalmol.* 1994;9(3):145–151.

Chang EL, Rubin PA. Management of complex eyelid lacerations. *Int Ophthalmol Clin.* 2002;42(3):187–201.

Dunya IM, Rubin PA, Shore JW. Penetrating orbital trauma. *Int Ophthalmol Clin.* 1995;35:25–26.

Hartstein ME, Fink SR. Traumatic eyelid injuries. *Int Ophthalmol Clin*. 2002;42(2):123–134.

Leone CR Jr. Periorbital trauma. *Int Ophthalmol Clin.* 1995;35(1):1–24.

Levin LA. Neuro-ophthalmologic diagnosis and therapy of central nervous system trauma. *Neurosurg Clin North Am.* 1999;10(4):623–630.

Long J, Tann T. Adnexal trauma. *Ophthal Clin North Am.* 2002;15(2):179–184.

Lustrin ES, Brown JH, Novelline R, Weber AL. Radiologic assessment of trauma and foreign bodies of the eye and orbit. *Neuroimaging Clin North Am.* 1996;6(1):219–237.

Nasr AM, Haik BG, Fleming JC, Al-Hussain HM, Karcioglu ZA. Penetrating orbital injury with organic foreign bodies. *Ophthalmology.* 1999;106(3):523–532.

2

Clinical Presentation of Eyelid Lesions

J. JUSTIN OLDER, MD

Appropriate evaluation of an eyelid lesion is necessary before deciding on a course of surgical or nonsurgical treatment. A differential diagnosis is established based on the patient's history and the physical characteristics of the mass. Many eyelid masses have similar physical and behavioral characteristics. In some cases, radiologic examination can be helpful in determining the extent or even the type of tumor. Certain malignant tumors may look benign or have the appearance of other malignancies. Biopsy is required for the definitive diagnosis.

2-1 MALIGNANT TUMORS

When faced with an eyelid lesion, the physician must first determine whether the lesion is benign or malignant. This determination will then dictate the next direction of diagnostic tests. If a mass has been present for several months to years or if there has been a history of bleeding, malignancy must be considered. Pain is usually not a component of malignancy, but some moderate discomfort may be present. Malignant lesions are usually destructive. The skin may be altered by a mass or ulceration. A malignancy located at the eyelid margin usually results in loss of lashes. Small malignancies may be similar in appearance to early inflammations, but as these malignancies grow, destruction of tissue is usually evident.

If malignancy is not suspected, then a decision as to whether the lesion is inflammatory or not should be made. Small inflammatory lesions such as blepharitis may be ulcerative, cause loss of lashes, and simulate eyelid carcinoma. Swelling, redness, and pain are all characteristics of inflammatory masses such as styes or chalazia. Infected glands away from the lid margin can also have these signs. Swelling in the area of the medial canthus could be a lacrimal sac mucocele if there is no evidence of redness, or it could be a lacrimal sac tumor. Benign lesions that are not inflammatory may have swelling but usually not pain. They may be translucent, such as hair follicle cysts. These tumors often transilluminate. They may have a clear fluid that can be easily identified through thin skin, or there may be a yellowish content such as sebaceous material within the cyst. Some benign lesions may be papillomatous or have keratinized ends, such as cutaneous horns. However, cutaneous horns or papillomas may also be low-grade carcinomas.

If the lesion is thought to be inflammatory, medical treatment can be instituted and the lesion observed. If the lesion improves within several weeks, then no further treatment may be necessary. However, if the lesion remains abnormal in appearance, a biopsy or surgical destruction of the lesion might be indicated. If the lesion is highly suggestive of a chalazion that has not responded to medical therapy, surgical treatment is appropriate. Incision and drainage of the lesion through either a conjunctival or a skin approach can be done. Some surgeons send tissue from all chalazia for microscopic diagnosis; others send tissue from only recurrent chalazia to rule out the possibility of malignancy.

A skin abscess of the eyelids that does not respond to medical therapy can also be incised and drained. If the lesion is thought to be benign but not inflammatory, it can be left alone or removed. Cystic lesions can be drained, or the entire cyst can be removed. Small tumors that are thought to be benign can be completely removed and sent for pathologic evaluation.

Preoperative photographs or accurate descriptions of the location of the lesion should be done prior to an excisional biopsy. If the diagnosis of malignancy is returned and if there is no evidence of a scar, the preoperative photo or drawing will help the surgeon excise more tissue in the area where the initial tumor was removed. Occasionally, a tumor that was thought to be benign is removed incompletely, leaving malignant cells that have to be removed at a later date.

If a malignant tumor is suspected, an incisional biopsy should be done to obtain a pathologic diagnosis and still save some of the tumor so that when it is entirely removed the margins can be entirely evaluated. Biopsies of tumors right at the lid margin or the gray line can be done by simply shaving the lesion. Many of these lid-margin tumors are benign and no further treatment will be necessary. If the diagnosis of malignancy is returned, the appropriate medical or surgical therapy will have to be instituted. For a relatively large tumor that is thought to be malignant, the incisional biopsy can be either a wedge, a shave, or a punch.

One of the most valuable diagnostic tools with regard to eyelid lesions is suspicion. Many eyes—even lives—have been lost because a potentially severe malignancy such as a sebaceous cell carcinoma, malignant melanoma, or squamous cell carcinoma has been treated as an inflammation. Rarely occurring malignant eyelid tumors include sweat gland carcinoma, Merkel cell tumor, and rhabdomyosarcoma in a child. Metastatic eyelid carcinoma is rare, but it should be considered in the differential diagnosis.

2-1-1 *Basal Cell Carcinoma.* Basal cell carcinoma is the most common eyelid malignancy, accounting for about 90% of all eyelid cancers. It is most commonly found on the lower eyelid and medial canthal area but occasionally is seen on the upper lid and lateral canthus. The vast majority of patients with this type of tumor are usually in the sixth, seventh, or eighth decade of life, but sometimes a basal cell carcinoma occurs in patients between the ages of 20 and 40. These tumors appear almost exclusively in patients with fair complexions who have been exposed to the sun on an extended basis.

Rarely do these tumors appear in people with deeply pigmented skin. The most common known etiologic association is extended sun exposure. Basal cell carcinomas do not cause pain, but occasionally patients complain of mild discomfort or itching in the area of the tumor.

Although basal cell carcinomas have various appearances, the physical characteristics can be grouped into several categories. The appearance traditionally associated with basal cell carcinoma is an elevated mass with smooth, rounded edges and telangiectasias. The mass is usually firm and may have an ulcerated center. Because bleeding can occur from the ulcerated center, there may be crusting in this area. This nodular type of tumor is the least aggressive, and the subcutaneous borders are similar to the visible extent of the tumor. Occasionally, the nodular tumor is multicentric.

A more aggressive type of basal cell carcinoma, referred to as *morpheaform* or *sclerosing*, typically has cutaneous extensions that are not clinically visible. A morpheaform basal cell carcinoma is often flat and indurated, and it may or may not have ulcerations with bleeding. If this lesion occurs on the lid margin, it can simulate a chronic blepharitis. A small lesion may simply show an area of eyelash loss and mild deformity at the lid margin. Pigmented basal cell carcinomas, which are rare, can occur on the eyelids, and simulate nevi or melanomas (Fig. 2-1).

Basal cell carcinomas tend to grow slowly, with patients having histories of the tumor being present for more than 10 years with little increase in size. In some cases, however, the tumors grow rapidly, with extensive eyelid and adnexal damage done over a period of 1 or 2 years. These tumors rarely metastasize, but they can extend into the adnexal region and by contiguous extension progress to the sinuses and the brain. Although basal cell carcinomas rarely are the cause of death, they can cause significant morbidity in the ocular and adnexal region.

Because basal cell carcinomas do not metastasize, local therapy is effective. Surgical removal of the tumor, using microscopic evaluation of the surgical margins, gives the lowest rate of recurrence. Radiation therapy is also effective in eliminating tumors, and cryotherapy usually results in about a 90% cure rate in selected tumors. Reconstructive techniques in the eyelid area are extremely effective in restoring form and function to the eyelids.

Microscopic evaluation of the margins is essential to achieve the highest cure rate. The technique can be a variation of the method described by Mohs, or it can be what is traditionally known as frozen-section control, in which the tumor is removed and all of the surgical margins are examined under the microscope by the pathologist or the pathologist and the surgeon.

2-1-2 *Squamous Cell Carcinoma.* Squamous cell carcinoma, the second most common primary eyelid malignancy, occurs no more than one tenth as frequently as basal

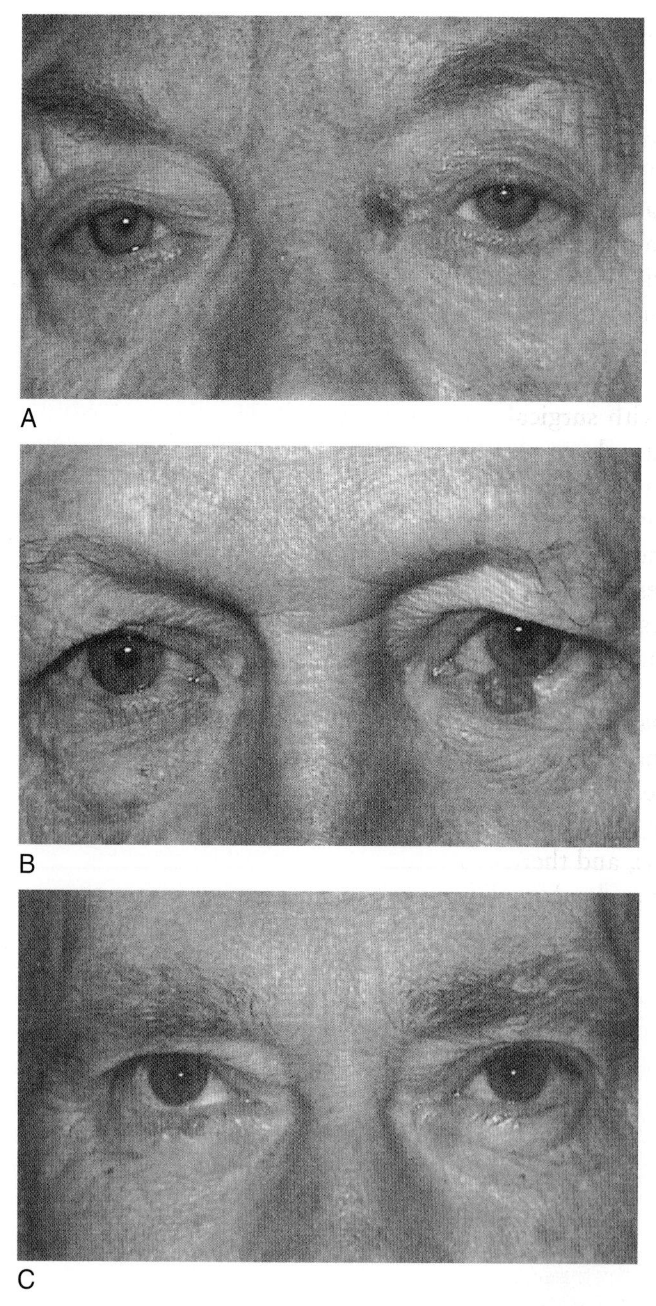

Figure 2-1 Basal cell carcinoma. (A) Left medial canthus. (B) Left lower lid. (C) Right lower lid.

cell carcinoma. This tumor occurs in various degrees of malignancy. It may be present as an intraepidermal carcinoma known as squamous cell carcinoma in situ, or it may be rapidly progressive and spread to the orbit and adjacent sinuses. Lymph nodes in the neck are usually the first place metastases occur. The tumor may present on the conjunctival surface as a flat, white, leukoplakic area. A more malignant conjunctival variety may appear as multiple irregularities with increased vasculature, or it may give a velvety appearance to the tarsal conjunctiva. The lesion may also appear as an ulcerated lesion on the lid margin in which lashes are lost. Squamous cell carcinoma can be nodular or flat. It may be ulcerated, but it usually does not have the round, smooth, pearly-appearing edges of a basal cell carcinoma. Low-grade squamous cell carcinoma can present as a cutaneous horn. In some cases, squamous cell carcinoma occurs along with basal cell carcinoma, and the pathologic diagnosis is referred to as a *basosquamous cell carcinoma*. There is thought to be an etiologic association with sun exposure (Fig. 2-2).

Because squamous cell carcinomas are potentially lethal, aggressive treatment is indicated. Surgical excision, using microscopic evaluation of the margins, gives the best cure rate for squamous cell carcinoma. If metastases are not yet present, the control rate with surgical excision is thought to exceed 90%. Radiation therapy and cryotherapy have also been used for squamous cell carcinoma, but the cure rates are not as good as with basal cell carcinoma when these modalities are used.

In the previous edition of this text, keratoacanthoma was considered benign, but it has since been reclassified as squamous cell carcinoma–keratoacanthoma type. These lesions grow rapidly up until about 6 weeks. They are raised, dome-shaped tumors with distinct borders and a keratin core in the center. As with other types of squamous cell carcinoma, surgical excision is the treatment of choice.

2-1-3 *Sebaceous Gland Carcinoma.* Sebaceous gland carcinoma is the third most common primary eyelid malignancy, reportedly representing approximately 1% of malignant eyelid tumors. Although the tumor can occur as early as the second decade of life, it usually appears in patients over 50. The tumor presents as an enlarging mass, and there is often a history of previous treatment for a chalazion. The tumor can also look like eyelid inflammation, and in some cases the entire

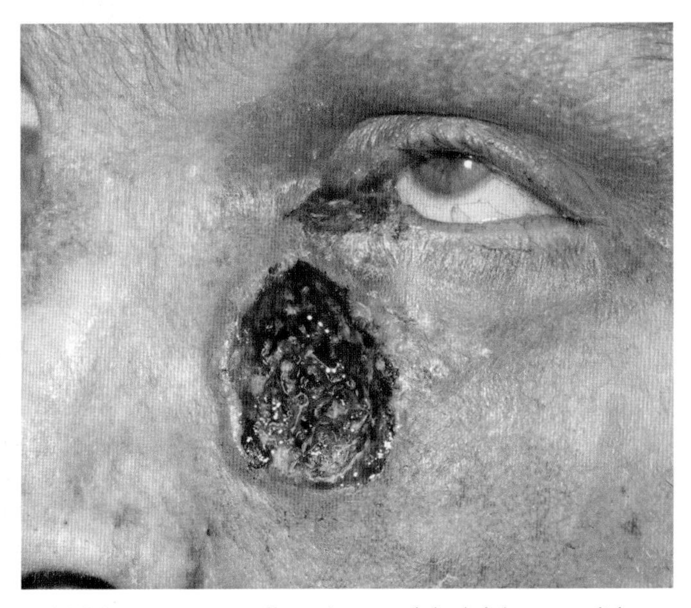

Figure 2-2 Large, invasive squamous cell carcinoma of the left lower eyelid.

bulbar conjunctiva appears inflamed but is actually involved with spreading carcinoma (Fig. 2-3). The pathologic appearance can vary from well differentiated to poorly differentiated, with the poorly differentiated cell type having a more aggressive behavior. If left untreated, these tumors usually spread to regional lymph nodes and to other organs of the body.

The best treatment for sebaceous gland carcinomas is surgical excision. Because spread to adjacent nerves and blood vessels occurs, free margins by microscopic evaluation are essential but not sufficient when excising these tumors: there should be a 5- to 6-mm border of normal tissue on all sides. In cases of ocular involvement, exenteration is the treatment of choice. Radiation therapy and chemotherapy have not proven effective in treating sebaceous gland carcinomas.

2-1-4 *Melanoma.* Primary malignant melanoma can occur on the eyelids. It may arise from the cutaneous or the conjunctival surface. Several types of cutaneous melanomas exist, including lentigo maligna melanoma and nodular melanoma. Lentigo maligna melanoma is less likely to metastasize than nodular melanoma.

A biopsy should be done to verify the diagnosis of malignant melanoma. Wide surgical excision, as with sebaceous gland carcinoma, is the treatment of choice. Metastatic workup should also be done because these tumors often spread to the lymph nodes, liver, or other organs. Sentinel node biopsy has become popular in evaluating the spread of tumor.

2-1-5 *Lymphoma.* A lymphoma may present as a solitary eyelid tumor. Therefore, it should be considered in the differential diagnosis of eyelid tumors. Quite characteristic in appearance, a lymphoma is salmon-colored if it is on the bulbar conjunctiva of the eye but is gray and velvety-appearing if it is in the eyelid.

A biopsy should be taken to verify the diagnosis. Treatment is either radiation or chemotherapy depending on the other systemic involvement, if any.

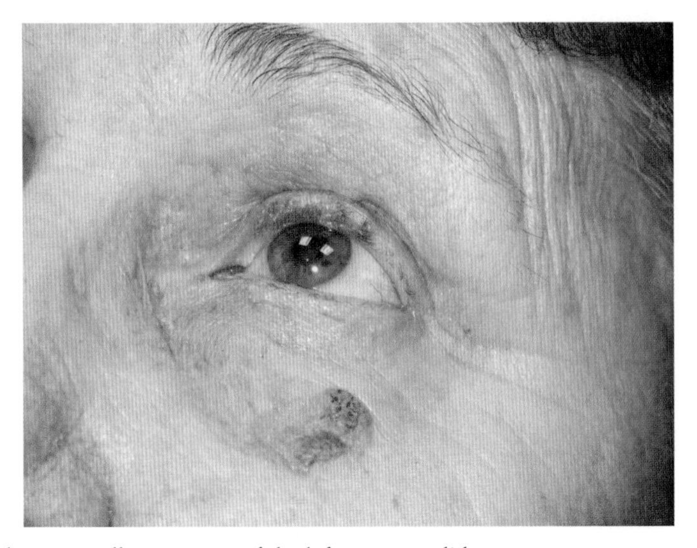

Figure 2-3 Sebaceous cell carcinoma of the left upper eyelid.

2-2 BENIGN TUMORS

Benign tumors often require removal and, therefore, must be considered when discussing the subject of eyelid reconstruction. They also must be understood because they are considered in the differential diagnosis of malignant eyelid tumors.

2-2-1 *Pigmented Lesions.* Pigmented lesions other than malignant melanoma are usually benign, but some have the potential to undergo malignant change. Lentigo maligna is an acquired pigmented lesion that usually occurs in adults over 50. It is brown or black and flat. About one third of these lesions undergo malignant transformation.

The most common types of nevi are junctional, intradermal, and compound. A junctional nevus is usually brown and has little potential for malignant change. The intradermal nevus is often elevated. It is sometimes brown to black, but often is flesh-colored. Intradermal nevi have no malignant potential. The compound nevus is a combination of junctional and dermal components and has a low malignant potential derived from its junctional elements.

Lentigo maligna and compound nevi should be removed because of their malignant potential; intradermal nevi can be removed for cosmetic reasons.

2-2-2 *Benign Epithelial Tumors.* A papilloma is an upward proliferation of skin resulting in an elevated, irregular lesion. It is often pedunculated and is then known as a *skin tag*. Squamous papilloma is benign. However, some premalignant lesions, such as actinic keratosis or cutaneous horn with malignant potential, can have papillomatous-like formations. Seborrheic keratosis is one of the most commonly seen skin lesions on the eyelids. It is usually well circumscribed, raised, and black or brown. It is always benign (Fig. 2-4).

2-2-3 *Precancerous Epithelial Tumors.* Actinic keratosis appears as a flat, scaly lesion that may be papillomatous or project as a cutaneous horn. Actinic keratosis can undergo transformation to squamous cell carcinoma and, therefore, should be excised. Dysplasia of the conjunctival epithelium may appear as leukoplakia. However, this may be precancerous and change to a squamous cell carcinoma.

2-2-4 *Adnexal and Cystic Tumors.* These tumors include sebaceous gland tumors, sebaceous adenomas, tumors of hair follicles, and tumors of sweat glands. Some of

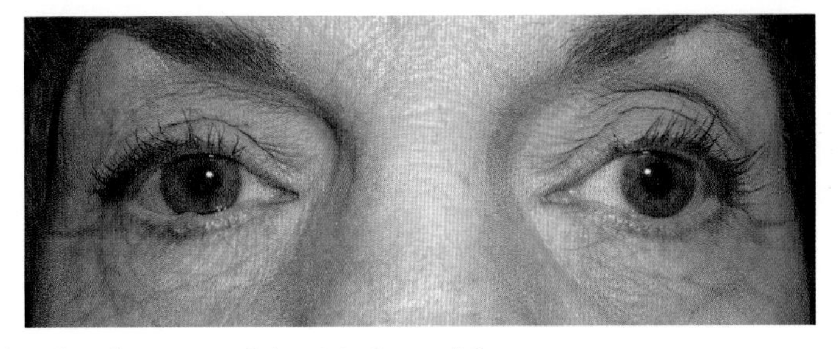

Figure 2-4 Seborrheic keratosis of the right lower lid.

these tumors are cystic, such as an eccrine hydrocystoma, which is usually a small cystic lesion on the eyelids but can enlarge to 1 cm and be subcutaneous. Cystic lesions are usually clearly identified because they transilluminate easily. They often occur on the lid margins. Sudoriferous cysts arise from the ducts of the glands of Moll, sebaceous cysts arise from the sebaceous glands, and epidermal inclusion cysts are usually caused by implantation of epidermis in the dermis following trauma. Patients may want these lesions removed for cosmetic reasons or because they fear cancer may result from them.

2-2-5 *Xanthelasma*. Xanthelasma is a benign lipid deposition that occurs in middle-aged or elderly people. It is usually found in the inner aspect of the upper or lower eyelid. Patients with xanthelasma often have increased serum cholesterol, and it is the role of the ophthalmologist to be sure that patients presenting with xanthelasma have an evaluation for serum cholesterol and lipids. These benign lesions will continue to grow. Patients often want them removed for cosmetic reasons. Surgical excision is the usual treatment of choice, but the CO_2 laser has been used with some success.

2-2-6 *Chalazion*. A chalazion is an inflammation of the meibomian glands. It may vary in size from several millimeters to more than a centimeter (Fig. 2-5). The gland fills up with granulation material. In many cases they will resolve on their own or with warm compresses, although the warm compresses might have to be continued for several weeks. These may occur on the upper or lower lid. If the chalazion persists, surgical intervention is the treatment of choice. A skin or conjunctival incision is made and the contents are curetted out of the sac. Contents may be sent for pathological examination if there is any suspicion of malignancy. Sebaceous cell carcinoma may clinically resemble a chalazion.

2-2-7 *Viral Inflammations*. Viruses can sometimes cause benign growths of the eyelids. Molluscum contagiosum presents as one or more papules on the eyelids. These lesions may have an ulcerated center and often secrete viruses, resulting in a conjunctivitis that is a toxic reaction to the virus. Verruca vulgaris presents as an elevated, papillomatous growth that may be slow-growing or may enlarge over a period of weeks (Fig. 2-6).

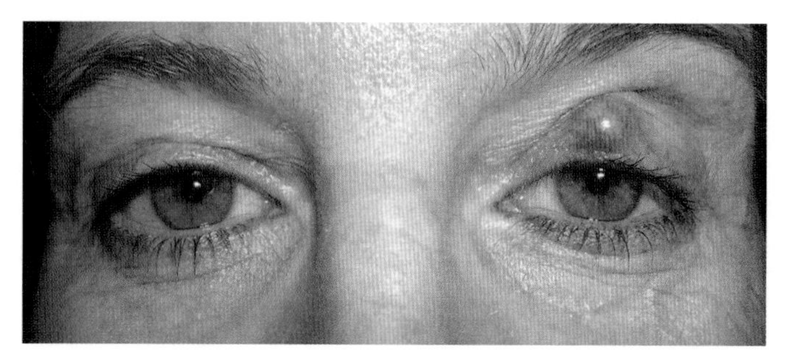

Figure 2-5 Chalazion of the left upper lid.

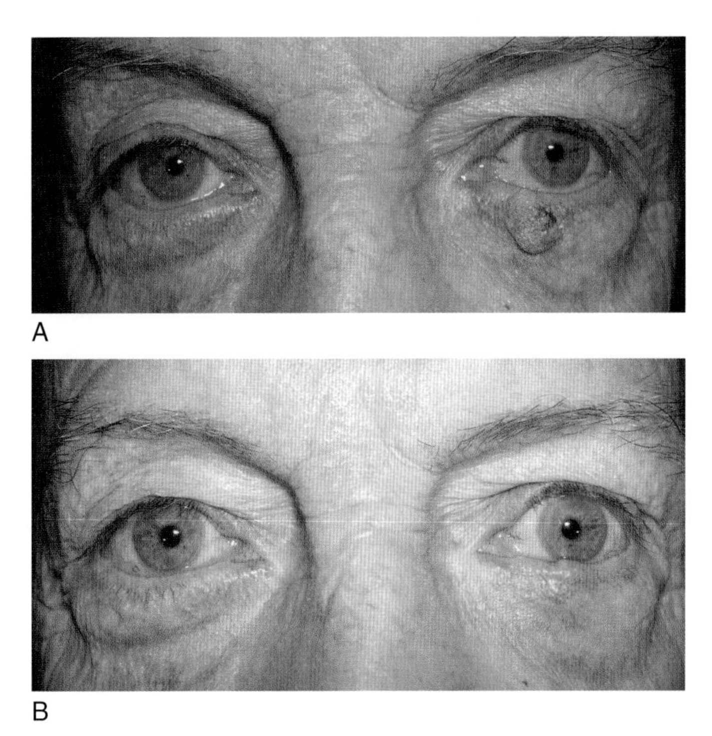

Figure 2-6 (A) Verruca vulgaris of the left lower lid in an elderly man. (B) Same patient after removal and repair with full-thickness retro-auricular skin graft.

SUGGESTED READINGS

Hornblass A. Tumors of the ocular adnexa. In: Hornblass A, ed. *Tumors of the Ocular Adnexa and Orbit.* St Louis: CV Mosby Co., 1979:1–16.

Jakobiec FA, ed. *Ocular and Adnexal Tumors.* Birmingham, AL: Aesculapius Publishing Co., 1978.

Kersten RC, Ewing-Chow D, Kulwin DR, and Gallon M. Accuracy of clinical diagnosis of cutaneous eyelid lesions. *Ophthalmology.* 1997;104:479–484.

Margo CE, Waltz K. Basal cell carcinoma of the eyelid and periocular skin. *Surv Ophthalmol.* 1993;38(2):169–192.

Older JJ. *Eyelid Tumors: Clinical Diagnosis and Surgical Treatment.* 2nd ed. Manson Publishing Ltd., 2003.

Older JJ, Quickert MH, Beard C. Surgical removal of basal cell carcinoma of the eyelids utilizing frozen section control. *Trans Am Acad Ophthalmol Otolaryngol.* 1975;79:658–663.

Perlman GS, Hornblass A. Basal cell carcinoma of the eyelids: a review of patients treated by surgical excision. *Ophthalmic Surg.* 1976;7: 23–27.

Rakofsky SI. The adequacy of the surgical excision of basal cell carcinoma. *Ann Ophthalmol.* 1973; 5:596–600.

Reese AB. *Tumors of the Eye.* 3rd ed. Hagerstown, MD: Harper & Row, 1976.

Shields JA. *Diagnosis and Management of Orbital Tumors.* Philadelphia: WB Saunders Co., 1989:341–350.

Spencer WH, Font RL, Green WR, et al. Eyelids and lacrimal drainage system. In: Spencer WH, ed. *Ophthalmic Pathology: An Atlas and Textbook.* 3rd ed. Philadelphia: WB Saunders Co., 1986:2149–2254.

3

Management of Periocular Neoplasms

ROBERT C. KERSTEN, MD

Epithelial malignancy of the eyelid is a common problem, representing about 14% of skin cancers in the head and neck region.[1] The goals when treating any skin cancer are complete elimination of the tumor and minimal sacrifice of normal adjacent tissues. These concepts are of paramount importance when treating periocular epithelial malignancies because of the complex nature of the periocular tissues and their critical function in protecting the underlying globe, as well as the increased risk that recurrent tumor in this area poses.

Many modalities have been advocated, by a variety of medical practitioners, for the treatment of epithelial malignancies in the periocular region. There are two key considerations in selecting a treatment for skin cancers. The first is that the selected modality must be capable of eradicating all tumor cells to which it is applied. The second is that some mechanism must exist to ensure that it is applied to all the existing tumor cells. Because tumors of the lid margins and canthi often exhibit slender strands and shoots of cancer cells that may infiltrate beyond the clinically apparent borders of the neoplasm, appropriate monitoring to ensure that the treatment modality reaches all of the cancer cells is essential.[2] Numerous studies have demonstrated that clinical judgment of tumor margins is inadequate, significantly underestimating the area of microscopic tumor involvement.[3-9] The introduction of frozen-section control to document adequacy of tumor excision marked a major advancement in the treatment of eyelid malignancies and now represents the standard of care.[10,11] Any treatment modality that does not use microscopic monitoring of tumor margins must instead encompass a wider area of adjacent normal tissue in hopes that any microscopic extensions of tumor will fall within this area. The purpose of this chapter is to explore alternative methods of periocular cancer treatment.

3-1 MOHS MICROGRAPHIC EXCISION

Mohs micrographic technique is a refinement of frozen-section control of tumor borders that, by mapping tumor planes, allows a three-dimensional evaluation of tumor margins rather than the two-dimensional examination provided by routine frozen section. The modality was initiated by Frederick E. Mohs, MD, in 1936.[12] In the Mohs technique, removal is performed by a dermatopathologist with specialized training in tumor excision and mapping of borders. The unique feature of Mohs micrographic surgery is that it removes the skin cancer and adjacent tissue in a sequence of horizontal layers monitored by microscopic examination of horizontal sections through the undersurface of each layer. Careful mapping of residual cancer in each layer is possible, and subsequent horizontal layers are then excised in cancer-bearing areas until cancer-free histologic layers are obtained at the base and on all sides of the skin cancer. This modality has evolved and been modified over the years with the guidance of Mohs and his coworkers.[13-15]

As initially described, the technique relied on in situ fixation of tissues before excision by the application of a zinc chloride paste to facilitate the stepwise excision and sectioning of layers of possible cancer-bearing tissue. Because the zinc chloride fixative tended to penetrate too deeply through the eyelid skin and was found to be toxic to the globe, Mohs omitted in situ chemical fixation and instead excised fresh tissue to be processed with frozen sections in a technique that was otherwise the same as his original method.[16] This fresh-tissue technique has become the preferred technique, and the term *Mohs chemosurgery* has given way to *microscopically controlled surgery* or *micrographic surgery*.[14,17]

3-1-1 *Advantages.* Mohs micrographic excision is an excellent modality that has been shown to give the highest cure rate for skin cancers occurring on various body surfaces.[13,14] In addition to its high cure rate, the technique offers several other advantages. The Mohs technique obviates the need to remove generous margins of clinically normal adjacent tissue by allowing precise layer-by-layer mapping of tumor cells. This is extremely important in the periocular regions because of the specialized nature of the periocular tissues and the challenges in creating ready substitutes that will provide a satisfactory functional and cosmetic result. Because routine frozen-section monitoring of periocular skin cancers in the operating room involves significant downtime while waiting for turnaround of results from the pathologist, Mohs micrographic excision performed in the dermatologist's office allows for more efficient use of operating room time. Although small lesions may be allowed to granulate, excision in the majority of periocular cases is followed by immediate reconstruction, usually by a second surgeon who has expertise in reconstructing periocular defects.[2] Reconstruction can be scheduled immediately following Mohs micrographic excision or on a subsequent day with better prediction of the operating room time required. Taking responsibility for tumor excision out of the hands of the reconstructing surgeon also ensures that concern over the difficulties of reconstruction does not limit aggressive tissue removal where it is required.

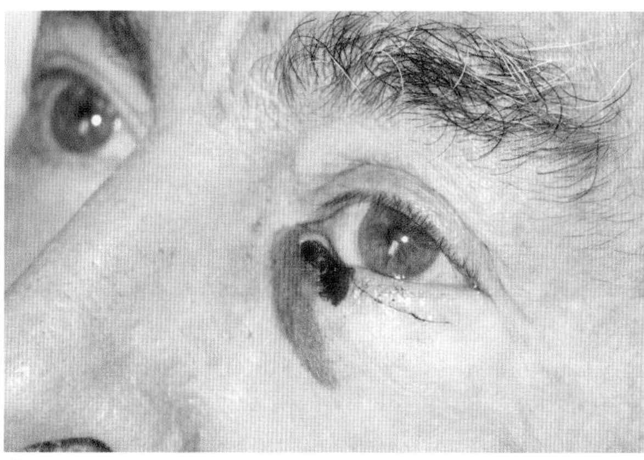

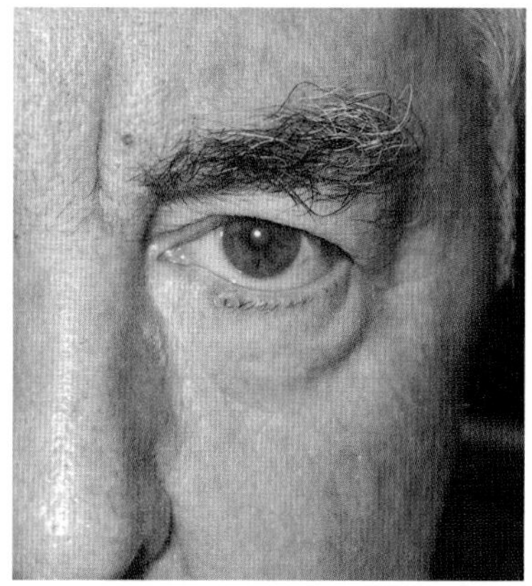

Figure 3-1 Mohs micrographic excision for basal cell carcinoma of the left lower eyelid. (A) Tumor in left lower eyelid. (B) Mohs surgery results in excision of tumor with maximal preservation of eyelid tissue.

Mohs micrographic excision has been shown to provide the most effective treatment for any skin cancer. However, it is particularly recommended for the following types of periocular skin cancers:

1. Skin cancers arising in the medial canthal region, where, because of natural tissue planes, the risk of deeper invasion is greater and where the borders of involved tissue are more difficult to define
2. Recurrent skin cancers
3. Large primary skin cancers of long duration
4. Squamous cell carcinomas
5. Morpheaform or fibrotic basal cell carcinomas
6. Any skin cancers whose clinical borders are not fully demarcated (Fig. 3.1)

3-1-2 *Disadvantages*. Although Mohs micrographic surgery allows for the most precise histologic monitoring, some cancer cells are rarely left behind, and a 2% to 3% long-term recurrence rate has been reported for primary periocular skin cancers.[14] Careful follow-up, searching for early signs of recurrence, remains important. One criticism of Mohs micrographic surgery is that surgical excision and surgical reconstruction are usually divided between two surgeons and often at two different physical sites. Some surgeons and patients find this cumbersome. In addition, Mohs micrographic surgeons are not available in all communities, although there has been a significant increase in the number of surgeons trained in the technique over the past decade so that this has become less of a problem, especially in metropolitan areas.

3-2 IRRADIATION

Historically, irradiation enjoyed significant popularity among a large segment of the medical community for the treatment of epithelial malignancies, and a number of studies reported better than 90% cure rates for periocular basal cell carcinomas.[18,19] More recently, however, investigators have observed that basal cell carcinomas treated by irradiation recur at a higher rate and behave more aggressively than tumors treated by surgical excision.[20,21]

The radiation dose used to treat patients varies depending on the size of the lesion and the estimate of its depth, but averages around 3.5 to 4 mGy. These treatments are usually fractionated over several weeks. Proponents of radiation therapy point to the lack of discomfort with radiation treatment and to the fact that no hospitalization or anesthesia is required. Patients are able to continue to work during the time they are receiving radiation therapy but must interrupt their routine daily to receive the treatment. Although radiation therapy is not recommended as the treatment of choice for periocular cutaneous malignancies, there are occasionally patients who, for various reasons, cannot undergo surgical excision and reconstruction and for whom radiation may be useful. However, it is important to continue to look closely for evidence of recurrence well beyond the 5-year postoperative period routinely used for surgically managed cutaneous malignancies.

3-2-1 *Disadvantages.* It is now generally accepted that basal cell carcinomas recurring after radiation therapy are more difficult to diagnose, present at a more advanced stage, cause more extensive destruction, and are much more difficult to eradicate.[22,23] The greater extent of destruction may be explained by the presence of adjacent radiodermatitis, which may mask underlying tumor recurrence and allow the tumor to grow more extensively before it can be clinically detected.[20]

Additional reasons account for the declining use of irradiation. To be effective, radiation of a cutaneous malignancy depends on an accurate estimate of the depth and extent of the lesion to determine the type, dose, and field of radiation. Because clinical estimates of tumor depth and extent in the periocular region are notoriously unreliable, determining appropriate treatment parameters for irradiation is difficult and uncertain. The damaging effect of radiation on periocular tissues poses another drawback to its use. Irradiation causes dermal and subcutaneous atrophy, resulting in cosmetically unsightly telangiectasia and thinning of the skin as well as depigmentation. Radiation therapy in tumoricidal doses also causes permanent alopecia of eyelashes and brow hairs.[19,24] Furthermore, radiation has a damaging effect on mucous membranes and can cause permanent canalicular stenosis and conjunctival leukoplakia.[19] Cataract formation was a problem historically, but proper shielding of the lens with eye shields placed behind the lids can prevent this complication. Although most surgeons would oppose the use of radiotherapy as the primary modality in treating periocular skin cancers, it is felt to be specifically contraindicated for lesions in the medial canthus, lesions greater than 1 cm, and recurrent tumors.[4,18,20,25]

Although a number of studies reported high success rates with radiation for periocular basal cell carcinomas, many of these studies did not include long-term follow-up. Investigators have now determined that it may take longer for a recurrence of a radiation-treated malignancy to become clinically apparent than for a surgically treated tumor. The average time from initial treatment to recurrence of skin cancer treated by surgical means is 18 months,[26] whereas one study found an average time to recurrence of 5⅓ years following irradiation, with a range of up to 20 years.[20] Thus, earlier studies with shorter follow-up almost certainly underestimated the total recurrence rate following radiation therapy. More recent studies with longer follow-up have reported a recurrence rate between 17% and 20%.[24,27]

The radiation changes induced in surrounding tissue make it more difficult to track recurrent tumors micrographically and render subsequent reconstruction after excision more difficult. It has also been reported that radiation therapy may disturb the protective barrier offered by the periosteum and allow for greater likelihood of bony cancerous involvement with recurrences.[2] A final concern with radiation therapy, which is not shared by other treatment modalities, is the fact that the treatment itself may induce new tumor formation.[20]

3-3 CRYOTHERAPY

Cryosurgery has received wide acceptance for treating skin cancers of the extremities. The technique involves an application of liquid nitrogen to rapidly freeze tumor-containing tissues, followed by a slow thaw. A second and sometimes third cycle of freezing and thawing is necessary to eliminate malignant tissues. The advantage of cryotherapy in treating cutaneous malignancies is that cancer cells are more susceptible to cryogenic damage than are nonmalignant cells, and thus treatment may eliminate the malignant tissue while sparing adjacent normal tissue.

To ensure effective cryodamage within the malignant tissues, it is strongly recommended that thermocouple needles be used to monitor the depth of freezing so that a minimum temperature of –30°C is reached in the deepest levels of the malignancy. In fact, some investigators now recommend that a minimum temperature of –50°C may be desirable for full cancer necrosis.[28,29] Liquid nitrogen is required to develop such low temperatures and is usually administered with a spray apparatus, although a liquid nitrogen cryoprobe can also be used in a "closed system." Cryogens such as carbon dioxide, Freon, and nitrous oxide do not generate the sufficiently low temperatures required for skin cancer treatment.

The one area where cryotherapy has been accepted as the standard of care is in the treatment of conjunctival primary acquired melanosis (PAM) and malignant melanoma.[30] Conjunctival melanoma is associated with PAM with atypia in up to 75% of cases.[31,32] In these cases, any nodular melanoma should be treated with surgical excision but the surrounding PAM can be ablated by cryotherapy.[33] This obviates the need for extensive surgical excision in those cases where the PAM is quite diffuse. If the bulbar conjunctiva is involved by PAM, the conjunctiva is ballooned away from the globe with lidocaine to limit cryogenic damage to the ciliary body and choroid. When a sealed nitrous oxide cryoprobe is used, the conjunctiva is retracted from the globe after adhesion of the probe to the tissues by formation of an ice ball. Usually, after 8 to 10 seconds, the ice ball fuses with the outermost aspect of the sclera and the application is then discontinued. If liquid nitrogen is used as the cryogen, then a 1-second spray application is thought to be sufficient.

In patients presenting with PAM without nodular melanoma, multiple biopsies are recommended to determine whether atypia exists. If atypia is absent, then melanoma is unlikely to develop and residual areas of pigmentation may be observed. If atypical melanocytes are present, then cryotherapy of the PAM is recommended to prevent the development of malignant melanoma.[31]

3-3-1 *Disadvantages.* The use of cryotherapy to treat periocular epithelial malignancies has been quite limited. One drawback is the effort required to thoroughly protect the eyeball from spillover damage due to the sprayed liquid nitrogen.[34] There are also problems with properly monitoring the extent and depth of tumor involvement to ensure that sufficiently low temperatures are achieved in all tumor cells. As in radiation therapy, the lack of precise histologic monitoring of the margins of the tumor requires that an ill-defined area of adjacent normal tissue must also be treated. Postoperative edema and swelling may be alarming and are often followed by a period of intense serous effusion and weeping that may last several weeks. Cancer necrosis caused by the cryosurgery leaves a wound, which then must heal by secondary intention. This is a particular problem in the periocular region, where scar contracture may cause distortion of the loose tissue margins of the eyelids. Re-epithelialization may take 3 to 10 weeks, depending on the size and depth of the wound. Scar remodeling and maturation may take additional months.[35] The final scar from cryosurgery is markedly hypopigmented, and the cryodamage also results in loss of lashes or eyebrow hairs.[36]

For these reasons, cryosurgery of periocular malignancies would rarely be the chosen modality. However, in those rare circumstances in which surgical excision is not possible for whatever reason, cryotherapy does provide an alternative treatment.[37,38] One study has demonstrated that significant expertise by the operating surgeon is required for optimal results and, even then, tumors larger than 1 cm have an unacceptably high recurrence rate.[39]

3-4 PHOTORADIATION

Photoradiation therapy is a new technique that has been investigated for the treatment of a variety of solid malignant tumors. The technique involves systemic administration of hematoporphyrin derivative (HPD), a photosensitizing compound that is preferentially retained by malignant cells. The HPD must be given intravenously 72 hours prior to treatment, at which time a powerful red light (630 nanometers) illuminates the lesion and adjacent tissue for a specified period. The red light induces a chemical reaction in the HPD, which results in the production of cytotoxic compounds. This produces necrosis of the HPD-containing tumor cells and sloughing of the lesion, with healing by secondary intention.[45] Variable success has been reported in the treatment of periocular basal cell carcinoma by photoradiation, and its use at this time is considered largely experimental.[45-47]

3-4-1 *Disadvantages.* As in other nonsurgical methods, the main limitation of HPD therapy is the lack of histologic monitoring of the depth and extent of the epithelial malignancy. In addition, penetration of red light is reduced below the surface, which limits the depth of tumor necrosis. Because the area of tumor necrosis must heal by secondary intention, distortion of the periocular tissue by scar contracture is a risk. Another significant drawback to HPD therapy is the fact that patients remain extremely photosensitive for 30 days after injection of HPD and must remain out of direct sunlight during this time.

3-5 CHEMOTHERAPY

3-5-1 *Topical 5-Fluorouracil.* Topical chemotherapy with 5-fluorouracil (5-FU) is widely used for the treatment of actinic keratosis, a superficial lesion caused by sun damage that may be a precursor of squamous cell carcinoma. Although 5-FU topical therapy is successful in eradicating this superficial premalignant lesion, adequate concentrations of 5-FU do not appear to penetrate deeply enough to destroy malignant cells in the dermis.[40-42] For this reason, it is not recommended as a treatment even of small epithelial malignancies. In fact, several investigators have confirmed that topical 5-FU treatment of basal cell carcinomas and squamous cell carcinomas results in unacceptably high recurrence rates.[43,44]

3-5-2 *Cisplatin.* Several investigators have reported partial response of periocular basal cell carcinomas to cisplatin and doxorubicin chemotherapy, either administered systemically or applied topically in combination with iontophoresis.[48,49] In all these cases, this treatment appears to be palliative rather than curative, although investigators have reported success in reducing the size of extensive periocular tumors so that less radical excisional surgery could subsequently be performed. Patients who refuse surgical excision, are medically unable to undergo surgery, or have failed to respond to previous radiation or other secondary modalities may rarely be considered candidates for this treatment. Significant side effects are associated with intravenous cisplatin chemotherapy, including severe nausea and vomiting, renal insufficiency, ototoxicity, encephalopathy, and various visual disturbances.[50-55]

3-5-3 *Corticosteroids.* Although capillary hemangioma is not a malignant neoplasm, it is a frequent management problem in the periocular region. Capillary hemangiomas represent the most common ocular adnexal tumors of childhood. These vascular hamartomas usually appear during the perinatal period, enlarge rapidly over the next few months, remain stable for a period of several months, and then involute spontaneously. Resolution usually begins in the second year of life and is complete in 60% of cases by 4 years of age and in 76% of cases by 7 years of age.[56,57] Before regressing, however, the hemangioma can distort affected periocular structures and result in visual compromise.[58,59] If vision is compromised, treatment to prevent amblyopia becomes necessary and is usually effected by the administration of local or systemic corticosteroids.[60-62]

Because of the numerous systemic side effects associated with oral corticosteroid use, several authors have advocated intralesional corticosteroid injections.[62] A 50:50 mixture of triamcinolone acetamide 40 mg/mL and betamethasone sodium phosphate 6 mg/mL is used; 1 to 2 mL is injected within the substance of the hemangioma. Use of a 10-cc syringe reduces the hydraulic pressure and thus the likelihood of flow reversal if inadvertent intravascular injection should occur. A 27-gauge needle should be used and aspiration should be carried out prior to injection in an attempt to avoid intravascular injection. The response to the corticosteroid injections is usually visible within 1 to 3 days, and the most rapid involution occurs in the first 1 or 2 weeks after injection. Gradual but slow involution may continue for 6 to 8 weeks. If the first injection results in inadequate involution of the hemangioma, a second injection can be repeated approximately 8 weeks later, with anticipation of additional response. The mechanism of action of intralesional steroid injection is not completely understood, but steroids are thought to enhance or produce vascular constriction within the lesion, facilitating local thrombosis or embolization and capillary closure with resultant local tissue hypoxia.[63]

Although safer than systemic steroid administration, intralesional corticosteroid injection has also been associated with complications. These include visible crystalline deposits subcutaneously, fat atrophy, eyelid necrosis, inadvertent intravascular injection with central retinal artery occlusion, and adrenal suppression. [64-67]

The central retinal artery should be monitored with indirect ophthalmoscopy during injection and a large syringe and small needle should be used. Linear subcutaneous fat atrophy tends to follow the expected course of lymphatic channels to the center of the regional lymph nodes. This has been reported to resolve within 14 months. Adrenal suppression from intralesional injections is thought to be rare but may result in significant growth retardation. There is usually a compensatory increase in growth once suppression resolves, which usually occurs within 5 months.

3-5-4 *Topical Imiquimod.* A recent innovation in the treatment of periocular epithelial malignancies is the application of topical immunotherapy using imiquimod, which is an immune response modifier. This medication has been used for the topical treatment of genital warts, basal cell carcinoma, cutaneous metastases, malignant melanoma, vascular tumors, actinic keratoses, and primary lentigo maligna. Imiquimod is an immune response modifier that produces indirect antitumor activity by stimulating the cell-mediated response and local-sided counterproduction.[68-70] In addition, apoptosis is induced in tumor cells, while the surrounding normal tissues remain relatively unaffected.[71,72]

Imiquimod is applied as a 5% cream, usually twice a day every other day, to the lesion. The treatment is usually continued for 3 months. Imiquimod causes irritation and a significant inflammatory response in a significant subset of patients. This may require decreasing from a twice-daily to a once-daily treatment regimen. In addition, it is important to prevent imiquimod from contacting the conjunctiva, because this will cause a severe inflammatory response.

Recent interest has focused on the use of imiquimod for the treatment of lentigo maligna. Topical therapy is particularly desirable in these patients, who are often older and have extensive involvement of the periocular skin. Imiquimod has also been used in the treatment of keratoacanthoma, but most results are anecdotal. However, it does appear to be a promising new therapeutic modality.

REFERENCES

1. Koplin L, Zarem H. Recurrent basal cell carcinoma: a review concerning the incidence, behavior and management of basal cell carcinoma, with emphasis on the incompletely excised lesion. *Plast Reconstr Surg.* 1980;65:656–664.

2. Anderson RL, Ceilley RI. Multispecialty approach to excision and reconstruction of eyelid tumors. *Ophthalmology*. 1978;85:1150–1163.
3. Einaugler RB, Henkind P. Basal cell epithelioma of the eyelid: apparent incomplete removal. *Am J Ophthalmol*. 1969;67:413–417.
4. Aurora AL, Blodi FC. Reappraisal of basal cell carcinoma of the eyelids. *Am J Ophthalmol*. 1971;70:329–336.
5. Rakofsky SI. The adequacy of the surgical excision of basal cell carcinomas. *Ann Ophthalmol*. 1973;5:596–600.
6. Chalfin J, Putterman AM. Frozen section control in the surgery of basal cell carcinoma of the eyelid. *Am J Ophthalmol*. 1979;87:802–809.
7. Doxanas MT, Green R, Iliff CE. Factors in the successful surgical management of basal cell carcinoma of the eyelids. *Am J Ophthalmol*. 1981:91:726–736.
8. Wilder LW, Smith B. Determination of the tumor margin in the excision of basal cell epitheliomas of the eyelids. *Ann Ophthalmol*. 1970;2:887–888.
9. Francis IC, Benecke PS, Kappagoda MB. A ten-year hospital survey of eyelid cancer. *Aust J Ophthalmol*. 1984; 12:121–127.
10. Cole JG. Histologically controlled excision of eyelid tumors. *Am J Ophthalmol*. 1971;70:240–244.
11. Older JJ, Quickert MH, Beard C. Surgical removal of basal cell carcinoma of the eyelids using frozen section control. *Trans Am Acad Ophthalmol Otolaryngol*. 1975;79:658–662.
12. Mohs FE. Chemosurgery: a microscopically controlled method of cancer excision. *Arch Surg*. 1941;42:279–295.
13. Mohs FE. Chemosurgery for skin cancer: fixed tissue and fresh tissue techniques. *Arch Dermatol*. 1976;112:211–215.
14. Mohs FE. Micrographic surgery of the microscopically controlled excision of eyelid cancers. *Arch Ophthalmol*. 1986; 104:901–909.
15. Robins P, Henkind P, Menn H. Chemosurgery in treatment of cancer of the periorbital area. *Trans Am Acad Ophthalmol Otolaryngol*. 1971;75:1228–1235.
16. Mohs FE. *Chemosurgery: Microscopically Controlled Surgery for Skin Cancer*. Springfield, IL: Charles C. Thomas, 1978.
17. Tromovitch TA, Stegman SJ. Microscopically controlled excision of cutaneous tumors in cancer. *Ophthalmic Surg*. 1978;41:653–658.
18. Fitzpatrick PJ, Jamieson DM, Thompson GA, et al. Tumors of the eyelid and their treatment by radiotherapy. *Radiology*. 1972;104:661–665.
19. Gladstein AH. Radiotherapy of eyelid tumors. In: Jakobiec FA, ed. *Ocular and Adnexal Tumors*. Birmingham, AL: Aesculapius Publishing Co., 1978:508–516.
20. Rodriguez-Sains RS, Robins P, Smith B, Bosniak SL. Radiotherapy of periocular basal cell carcinomas. *Br J Ophthalmol*. 1988;72:134–138.
21. Collin JRO. Basal cell carcinoma in the eyelid region. *Br J Ophthalmol*. 1976;60:806–809.
22. Hirshowitz B, Mahler D. Incurable recurrences of basal cell carcinoma of the mid-face following radiation therapy. *Br J Plast Surg*. 1971;71:205–211.
23. Taylor GA, Barisoni D. Ten years' experience in the surgical treatment of basal-cell carcinoma: a study of factors associated with recurrence. *Br J Surg* 1973;60:522–525.
24. Newell J. Radiation therapy of eyelid lesions. In: Fox SA, ed. *Ophthalmic Plastic Surgery*. 4th ed. New York: Grune & Stratton; 1970:559–566.
25. Gladstein AH, Epics C. Simplicity and safety of x-ray therapy of basal cell carcinomas on periocular skin. *J Dermatol Surg Oncol*. 1978;4:586–593.
26. Robins P. Chemosurgery: my fifteen years of experience. *J Dermatol Surg Oncol*. 1981;7:779–789.
27. Cobbett JR. Recurrence of rodent ulcers after radiotherapy. *Br J Surg*. 1965;52:347–349.

28. Gage AA. What temperature is lethal for cells? *J Dermatol Surg Oncol.* 1979;5:459–460.
29. Stone D, Zacarian SA, Diperi C. Comparative studies of mammalian normal and cancer cells subjected to cryogenic temperatures in vitro. *J Cryosurg.* 1969;2:43–45.
30. Jakobiec FA, Brownstein S, Albert W, et al. The role of cryotherapy in the management of conjunctival melanoma. *Ophthalmology.* 1982;89:502–515.
31. Jakobiec FA, Folberg R, Iwamoto T. Clinicopathologic characteristics of premalignant and malignant melanocytic lesions of the conjunctiva. *Ophthalmology.* 1989;96:147–166.
32. Folberg R, MacLean IW, Zimmerman LE. Conjunctival melanosis in melanoma. *Ophthalmology.* 1984;91:673–678.
33. Jakobiec FA, Rinei FJ, Fraunfelder FT, Brownstein S. Cryotherapy for conjunctival primary acquired melanosis in malignant melanoma. *Ophthalmology.* 1988;95:1058–1070.
34. Zacarian SA, ed. *Cryosurgical Advances in Dermatology and Tumors of the Head and Neck.* Springfield, IL: Charles C. Thomas, 1977:98–149.
35. Elton RF. The course of events following cryosurgery. *J Dermatol Surg Oncol.* 1977;3:448–451.
36. Wingfield DL, Fraunfelder FT. Possible complications secondary to cryotherapy in ophthalmic surgery. *Ophthalmic Surg.* 1979;10:47–55.
37. Kuflik EG. Cryosurgery for basal-cell carcinomas on and around eyelids. *J Dermatol Surg Oncol.* 1978;4:911–913.
38. Biro L, Price E. Basal-cell carcinomas of eyelids: experience with cryosurgery. *J Dermatol Surg Oncol.* 1979;5:397–401.
39. Fraunfelder FT, Zacarian SA, Wingfield DL, Limmer BL. Results of cryotherapy for eyelid malignancies. *Am J Ophthalmol.* 1984;97:184–188.
40. Dillahac J, Jansen GT, Honeycutt WM, Holt GA. Further studies with topical thiofluorouracil. *Arch Dermatol.* 1965;92:410–417.
41. Klostermann GF. Effects of 5-fluorouracil (5-FU) ointment on normal and diseased skin: histological findings and deep section. *Dermatologica.* 1970;140(suppl 1):47–54.
42. Mohs FE, Jones DL, Bloom RF. Tendency of fluorouracil to conceal deep foci of invasive basal cell carcinoma. *Arch Dermatol.* 1978;114:1021–1022.
43. Klein E, Stoll HL Jr, Milgrom H, et al. Tumors of the skin. V. Local administration of anti-tumor agents to multiple superficial basal cell carcinomas. *J Invest Dermatol.* 1965;45:489–495.
44. Goette DK. Topical chemotherapy with 5-fluorouracil: a review. *J Am Acad Dermatol.* 1981;4:633–649.
45. Tse DT, Kersten RC, Anderson RL. Hematoporphyrin derivative photoradiation therapy in managing nevoid basal cell carcinoma syndrome. *Arch Ophthalmol.* 1984;102:990–994.
46. Dougherty TJ. Photoradiation therapy for cutaneous and subcutaneous malignancies. *J Invest Dermatol.* 1981;77:122–124.
47. Dahlman A, Wile AG, Burns RG. Laser photoradiation therapy of cancer. *Cancer Res.* 1983;43:430–434.
48. Luxemberg MN, Guthrie TH. Chemotherapy of basal cell and squamous cell carcinoma of the eyelids and periorbital tissues. *Ophthalmology.* 1986;93:504–510.
49. Morley M, Finger PT, Perlin M, et al. Cisplatinum chemotherapy for ocular basal cellcarcinoma. *Br J Ophthalmol.* 1991;75:407–410.
50. Berman IJ, Mann MP. Seizures in transient cortical blindness associated with cis-platinum therapy in a 30-year-old man. *Cancer.* 1989;45:764–766.
51. Pippitt CH, Muss HB, Homesley HD, Jobson VW. Cisplatin–associated cortical blindness. *Gynecol Oncol.* 1981;12:253–255.

52. Walsh TJ, Clark AW, Parhad IM, Green WR. Neurotoxic effects of cisplatin therapy. *Arch Neurol.* 1982;39:719–720.
53. Bacher R, Schutt P, Oseika R, et al. Peripheral neuropathy in ophthalmic toxicity after treatment with cis-platinum. *J Cancer Res Clin Oncol.* 1990;96:219–221.
54. Coher RJ, Cuneo RA, Cruciger NP, et al. Transient left homonymous hemianopsia and encephalopathy following treatment of testicular carcinoma with cis-platinum, vinblastine and bleomycin. *J Clin Oncol.* 1983;1:392–393.
55. Griffin JD, Garanick MB. Eye toxicity of cancer chemotherapy: a review of the literature. *Cancer.* 1981;48:1539–1549.
56. Bowers RE, Graham EA, Tomlinson KM. The natural history of the strawberry nevus. *Arch Dermatol.* 1960;82:667–671.
57. Margileth AM, Museles M. Cutaneous hemangiomas in children. *J Am Med Assoc.* 1965;194:523–526.
58. Stigmar G, Crawford JS, Ward CM, Thomson HG. Ophthalmic sequelae of infantile hemangiomas of the eyelid and orbit. *Am J Ophthalmol.* 1978;85:806–811.
59. Haik BG, Jakobiec FA, Ellsworth RM, Jones IS. Capillary hemangioma of the lids and orbits: an analysis of the clinical features and therapeutic results in 101 cases. *Ophthalmology.* 1979;86:760–792.
60. Fost NC, Esterly NB. Successful treatment of juvenile hemangiomas with prednisone. *J Pediatr.* 1968;72:351–356.
61. Hiles DA, Pilchard WA. Corticosteroid control of neonatal hemangiomas of the orbit and ocular adnexa. *Am J Ophthalmol.* 1971;71:1003–1008.
62. Kushner BJ. Intralesional corticosteroid injection for infantile adnexal hemangioma. *Am J Ophthalmol.* 1982;93:496–500.
63. Jakobiec FA, Jones LS. Vascular tumors, malformations and degenerations. In: Duane TD, Jaeger EA, eds. *Clinical Ophthalmology.* Philadelphia: JB Lippincott Co., 1982:1.
64. Weiss AH. Adrenal suppression after corticosteroid injection of periocular hemangiomas. *Am J Ophthalmol.* 1989;107:518–522.
65. Droste PJ, Ellis FD, Sondhi N, Helveston EM. Linear subcutaneous fat atrophy after corticosteroid injection of periocular hemangiomas. *Am J Ophthalmol.* 1988;105:65–69.
66. Sutula FC, Glover AT. Eyelid necrosis following intralesional corticosteroid injection for capillary hemangioma. *Ophthalmic Surg.* 1987;18:103–105.
67. Shorr N, Seiff SR. Central retinal artery occlusion associated with periocular corticosteroid injection for juvenile hemangioma. *Ophthalmic Surg.* 1986;17:229–231.
68. Arlette J, Trotter M. Squamous cell carcinoma in situ of the skin: History, presentation, biology and treatment. *Australasian J Dermatol.* 2004;45:1–11.
69. Salasche S, Shumack S. A review of imiquimod 5% cream for the treatment of various dermatological conditions. *Clin Exp Dermatol.* 2003;28:1–3.
70. Schon M, Bong AB, Drewniok C, et al. Tumor-selective induction of apoptosis and the small-molecule immune response modifier imiquimod. *J Nat Cancer Inst.* 2003; 95: 1138–1149.
71. Kossard S. Treament of large facial Bowen's disease: case report. *Clin Exp Dermatol.* 2003;28:13–15.
72. Cotter MA, McKenna JK, Bowen GM. Treatment of lentigo maligna with imiquimod before staged excision. *Dermatol Surg.* 2008;34:147–151.

4

Reconstruction of the Lower Eyelid

D.J. JOHN PARK, MD, AND ANDREW HARRISON, MD

The lower eyelid, tethered medially and laterally by the canthal tendons, is normally suspended at the level of the inferior limbus with the aid of orbicularis tone counterbalanced by the force of the lower eyelid retractors and gravity. The lower eyelid is apposed to the globe because of the posterior position of the canthal tendon insertions relative to the projection of the globe. Disruption of the normal anatomic relationships from trauma or inflammatory disease or as a result of surgical resection of tumors can result in a poorly functioning lower eyelid with poor cosmesis.

The lower eyelid has been conceptualized as consisting of three layers or lamellae. The anterior lamella is composed of skin and orbicularis muscle; the middle lamella is composed of the lower eyelid retractor (capsulopalpebral fascia) and fat; and the posterior lamella is composed of tarsus and conjunctiva. One or more of the lamellae may be disrupted following trauma or tumor resection, and each layer must be addressed in order to reconstruct a normal-appearing and -functioning lower eyelid. Imbalance of tension at the anterior and posterior lamellae, especially in the setting of lower eyelid laxity, can result in malrotation of the eyelid margin, causing entropion or ectropion. For example, inflammation and scarring of the conjunctiva from Stevens-Johnson syndrome or ocular cicatricial pemphigoid will produce entropion, whereas contraction of vertical cutaneous scar or ichthyosis will cause ectropion. A balance of tension of the lamellae must be maintained during reconstruction of the lower eyelid in order to prevent secondary malrotation.

Disruption of normal anatomy as often seen following trauma can be addressed by reapproximation of the disrupted segments to their normal anatomic positions. Only rarely will trauma to the lower eyelid result in loss of tissue. Reconstruction with local flaps or free grafts is occasionally needed in traumatic cases that present in a delayed fashion. Local flaps and free grafts are needed to fill and reconstruct a defect in the lower eyelid, a situation that most often presents following resection of tumor.

Location of the defect or the disruption as well as the extent of involvement along the horizontal extent of the lower eyelid is important as it delineates structures that may be involved and dictates the surgical options for reconstruction. Involvement of the medial-most extent of the lower eyelid will require exploration and possible primary reconstruction of the lacrimal drainage apparatus and medial canthal tendon, whereas defects or disruptions at the lateral-most extent of the eyelid may involve the lateral canthal tendon and require reconstruction of the suspensory element to the lateral lower eyelid.

4-1 PATIENT EVALUATION

Evaluation of any patient should begin with a thorough medical history to identify certain factors that may impede healing and to get a sense of the general health of the patient. Older and more infirm patients, who do not have the constitution to undergo a long surgery, may be better served by reconstructive options that require shorter anesthesia time and can be achieved in one stage, even if it comes at the expense of optimal surgical outcome. Long random local flaps (those with no inherent vascular leash) should be avoided in patients with known wound healing problems, such as chronic smokers and those with collagen vascular disease, as there is an increased risk of flap loss from necrosis in these patients. Cessation of anticoagulants and antiplatelet agents in preparation for surgery should be coordinated with the patient's primary physician or cardiologist. Ophthalmic medical history is also important to consider in surgical planning. For instance, monocular patients would be ill served by a staged procedure in which the seeing eye is obstructed by a flap, such as the Hughes procedure.

Evaluation of the lower eyelid should be done within the context of the complete oculoplastic and ophthalmic examination. Traumatic lacerations or avulsions of the lower eyelid are often found in association with ocular trauma and cannot be overlooked. The mechanism of injury often determines the type of injury to the lower eyelid. Sharp objects are more likely to cause lacerations, whereas blunt ones tend to avulse the lower eyelid, most often at the medial eyelid over the canaliculus where that eyelid is weakest. Severe avulsive injuries of this variety may appear at first glance to be associated with tissue loss. However, the complete disinsertion of the medial aspect of the lower eyelid and retraction laterally gives this appearance; the eyelid can be reconstructed by reapproximation of the edges with cannulation of the lacrimal system.

The type of lesion dictates how it should be managed and affects the dimensions of the resultant defect. Benign lesions with a low rate of local recurrence can be excised with little or no surrounding normal tissue, whereas those that are more locally aggressive, recur frequently, or are malignant necessitate wide local excision with a generous margin of normal tissue. Microscopic control of the margins is crucial to ensure complete excision of lesions. This can be achieved by frozen-section analysis of the margins submitted to the pathologist in addition to the main specimen, which is generally fixed in permanent sections. Alternatively the lesion can be sent for permanent sections after recording the orientation of the specimen. Of course, should a margin turn out to be positive for tumor, further excision of the lesion would be needed. This approach is generally appropriate if there is a low suspicion of malignancy. For large lesions in which the clinical diagnosis is uncertain, an incisional or shave biopsy may be done. For smaller lesions, direct excisional biopsy may be more appropriate. Another option to maintain microscopic control of the margins is to coordinate the surgical care with a Mohs surgeon. Mohs micrographic techniques employ sequential tangential excision of the presumed margins of the lesion with pathologic evaluation of the excised segments. Malignant lesions associated with stigmata of orbital extension, such as fixation to the underlying periosteum or involvement of the forniceal or bulbar conjunctiva, should be evaluated with CT and/or MRI scans.

The location and extent of the defect in the lower eyelid following excision of a lesion should be delineated. Defects in the medial eyelid are likely to involve the lacrimal drainage apparatus. In such cases, care should be taken to identify the remaining structures and any residual medial canthal tissue, as it will dictate the reconstructive options. Defects in the lateral eyelid may have disrupted the lateral canthal tendon and result in rounding of the lateral commissure unless the eyelid is resuspended laterally. The horizontal extent of the defect should be measured. Casual inspection of the defect will invariably result in an overestimation of the defect as the remaining segments retract and shorten. During initial evaluation of the defect the two ends can be pinched toward each other to assess the laxity of the remaining segments and to assess the actual size of the defect. Intraoperatively, this can be more precisely achieved by grasping the two ends with forceps and bringing the ends toward each other.

Defects involving the margin require special attention, as the end result of reconstruction must not cause irritation to the ocular surface, in addition to having a normal or at least unobtrusive appearance. This can best be achieved when the two ends of the margin defects can be brought together primarily. When 25% or less of the horizontal extent of the lower eyelid is missing, then the defect can be reconstructed primarily (Fig. 4-1). In elderly individuals with increased horizontal laxity, up to a 50% defect can be bridged and closed primarily. When primary closure is not feasible, a variety of techniques, many of which will be discussed in the following section, can be employed to reconstruct the eyelid margin.

4-2 SUMMARY OF RECONSTRUCTIVE TECHNIQUES

4-2-1 *Disruption of Anatomy With No Tissue Loss.* Disruption of normal anatomy in the absence of tissue loss occurs as a result of trauma, inflammation, or aging. Although lacerated and avulsed edges may be macerated and irregular in cases of trauma, every attempt should be made to preserve the remaining tissue, and the edges should be reapproximated as is. Changes secondary to aging are associated with stretching or dehiscence of anatomic elements, and reconstruction typically

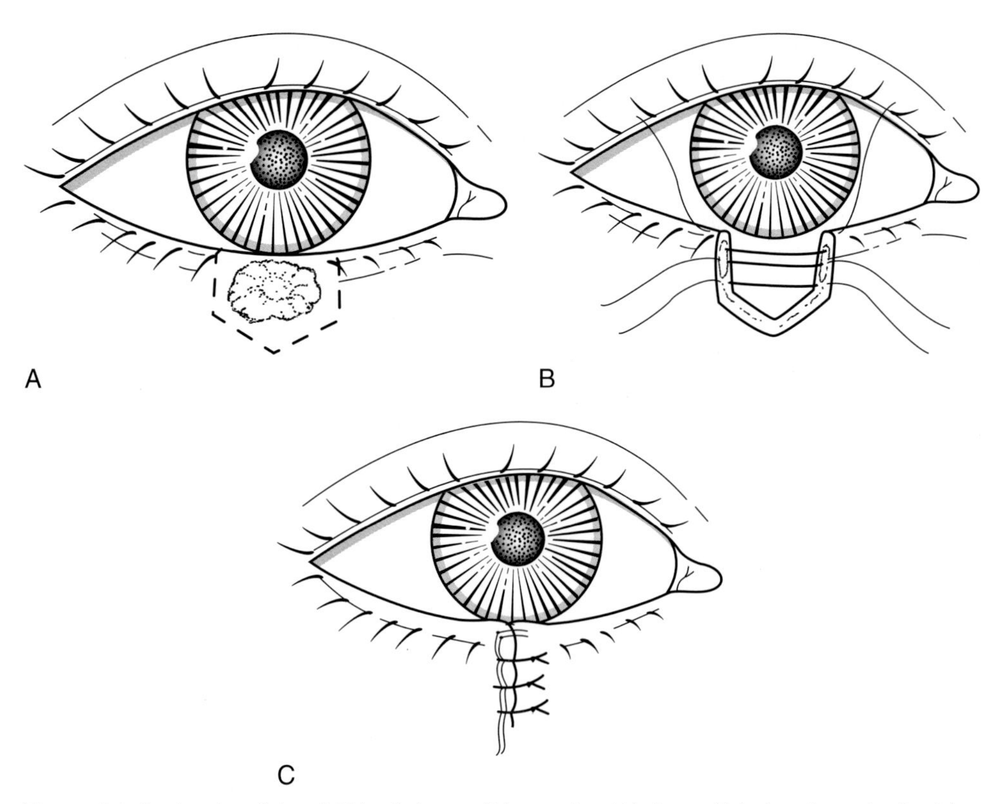

Figure 4-1 Lesion involving 25% of the eyelid margin. (A) A small lesion is excised with a pentagonal wedge excision. (B) 6-0 silk suture is passed through the meibomian gland orifices and 5-0 absorbable polyglactin suture is used to approximate the tarsal edges. (C) Skin closure with inclusion of the eyelid margin suture minimizes ocular surface irritation.

entails plication, resuspension, or reinsertion of the separated elements. For instance, rounding of the lateral commissure and ectropion or entropion occurs in part as a result of disinsertion of the lateral canthal tendon from its bony insertion at the lateral orbital tubercle, and reconstruction consists of resuspension of the lateral eyelid to this area with or without shortening of the eyelid. Inflammation of normal tissue is often associated with scarring and contraction, as in cases of ocular cicatricial pemphigoid, in which the posterior lamella is contracted from chronic inflammation of the conjunctiva, or in cases of Graves ophthalmopathy, in which inflammation and contraction in the middle lamella causes retraction of the lower eyelid. These cases often call for the use of tissue grafts to augment the contracted structures.

Lacerations of the eyelid skin not involving the margin can be closed primarily in a single layer through the skin. This principle holds true even in cases in which the septum may be violated with herniation of orbital fat. Because the eyelid skin is so thin, closure in multiple layers can lead to a raised scar and exaggerated contraction. For lacerations extending into the periorbital area where there is a defined dermis, multilayered closure is appropriate.

Disruption in the eyelid margin from laceration or avulsion requires careful attention. The margin must be reapproximated such that the lash line, the gray line, and the mucocutaneous junction all line up. One method of accomplishing this is with the placement of three interrupted 6-0 silk sutures, one at the gray line and the other two at the anterior and posterior lash line. The ends are kept long and subsequently secured under interrupted cutaneous sutures anteriorly and inferiorly, so as not to irritate the eye. The authors prefer to use two 6-0 chromic sutures placed as a vertical mattress through the gray line and the posterior lash line, with the ends cut very short. When done properly, the ends do not touch the ocular surface, and the mattress sutures produce a subtle eversion and elevation of the edge, which is necessary to avoid secondary notching. Also, the sutures are absorbable, which is a huge advantage, especially in children, who may not be able to cooperate for suture removal. Initially one such suture is placed at the gray line. This is followed by two partial-thickness interrupted 5-0 or 6-0 Vicryl sutures to reapproximate the tarsal edges. This is crucial as the tarsal sutures provide the most tensile support to the closure. A third Vicryl suture can be placed to close the lower eyelid retractors. The overlying skin can be closed with interrupted or running sutures of the surgeon's choice. The authors prefer 6-0 fast-absorbing gut as it does not require subsequent removal and is not associated with increased scarring.

Avulsive injuries involving the margin invariably occur at the canaliculus, the eyelid's weakest point. Small disruptions in this area can be easily overlooked, whereas large avulsions can appear as if a segment of the medial eyelid is missing, as the avulsed segment retracts laterally. Reconstruction of these injuries, whether large or small, is managed in the same fashion. First the proximal and distal ends of the lacerated canaliculus are identified and cannulated with a mono- or bi-canalicular silicone stent. The proximal portion may be difficult to identify, especially when avulsed near the common canaliculus. Following placement of the silicone stents, and using a 6-0 Vicryl suture on a small half-circle needle such as the Ethicon P-2 needle, three interrupted sutures are placed to reapproximate the peri-canalicular orbicularis muscle. The sutures are placed anterior, inferior, and posterior to the canaliculus. All three sutures should be placed and then tied, because it will be impossible to ensure proper placement of subsequent sutures should the first be tied. Even for the most severe avulsions of the medial eyelid, placement of these sutures will reapproximate the eyelid in a natural position. The overlying skin can be closed with 6-0 fast-absorbing gut in a running fashion. No sutures are placed over the skin of the canaliculus.

4-2-2 *Defects of the Central Eyelid Margin*

4-2-2-1 *Defects Less Than 25% of the Central Eyelid Margin.* Defects involving less than 25% of the eyelid margin can be closed primarily. In the instance of preexisting horizontal laxity, up to a 50% defect in the eyelid margin can be closed primarily. Care should be taken to ensure that the edges of the margin are sharp and perfectly perpendicular; otherwise, this may result in a notch if the angle between the margin and the cut edge is too obtuse, or a bump if the angle is too acute. In cases that have undergone Mohs resection, often the margin has to be recut to produce the sharp, perpendicular edge needed at the margin. This can best be achieved with a #15 Bard-Parker blade, taking care to cut away from the globe. The final shape of the defect should be a pentagon, or more precisely the shape of an inverted house, with the walls of the house perpendicular to the margin. The triangular extension inferiorly can be extended further inferiorly or biased laterally to excise any residual Burow's triangle, or dog-ear deformity. The method of closure is identical to that described above for traumatic lacerations of the eyelid margin.

4-2-2-2 *Defects up to 50% of the Eyelid Margin.* With defects involving up to 50% of the central lower eyelid margin that cannot be closed primarily, a variety of approaches can be taken to provide additional length to allow closure of the defect.

Lateral canthotomy and cantholysis can provide as much as 25% additional horizontal length. A slightly superiorly inclined incision is made from the lateral commissure laterally about 5 to 8 mm long through the orbicularis. Traction on the lower eyelid then produces a V-shaped defect in the lower lid lateral canthus, with one arm of the V composed of the skin and orbicularis, the other by the conjunctiva, and the apex by the disinserted lateral commissure. Although the canthotomy in isolation may yield a few millimeters of length, it is the cantholysis that provides the most release. This is done by placing one blade of tenotomy or Stevens scissors under the conjunctiva and the other between the orbicularis and the lateral canthal tendon and severing the connection. Alternatively, this can be done with monopolar cautery. The resulting defect in the lateral canthus can be closed with 6-0 fast-absorbing gut sutures.

Defects of up to 50% of the horizontal extent of the eyelid that cannot be bridged by canthotomy and cantholysis alone can be closed with a Tenzel flap (Fig. 4-2), or semicircular flap. The flap should be designed in such as fashion as to extend superiorly from the lateral commissure, then curving inferiorly. The diameter of the arc should be roughly twice the extent of the defect. The flap should be undermined beneath the orbicularis. Over the zygomatic process of the maxilla, the periosteum and the pre-periosteal tissue should be left undisturbed. More laterally, the superficial temporoparietal fascia should be undisturbed so as to prevent injury to the frontal branch of the facial nerve. The flap should be sufficiently undermined to allow rotation medially. This maneuver must be done in conjunction with lateral canthotomy/cantholysis to complete release of the eyelid. Once the flap is rotated medially to provide horizontal length to the lower eyelid, the curvilinear incision will straighten out with a Burow's triangle at its end, which can be excised in the usual fashion. The final incision is in line with the rhytids of the orbicularis (crow's feet). The marginal defect can then be closed as described above. Several deep interrupted absorbable sutures with 5-0 Vicryl are needed to secure the rotated flap in its new position. The lateral canthus of the upper eyelid can then be secured to the flap to reconstruct the lateral commissure. There must be sufficient tension in the final reconstructed eyelid to maintain apposition to the globe and prevent laxity. In some instances in which the flap appears markedly thinner than the native eyelid, a periosteal flap (described below) can be elevated and secured to the posterior aspect of the Tenzel flap to provide additional bulk. The conjunctival defect is allowed to re-epithelialize and heal by secondary intent.

4-2-2-3 *Defects Greater Than 50% of the Eyelid Margin.* Large defects of the lower eyelid margin require reconstruction of the anterior and posterior lamellae of the eyelid.

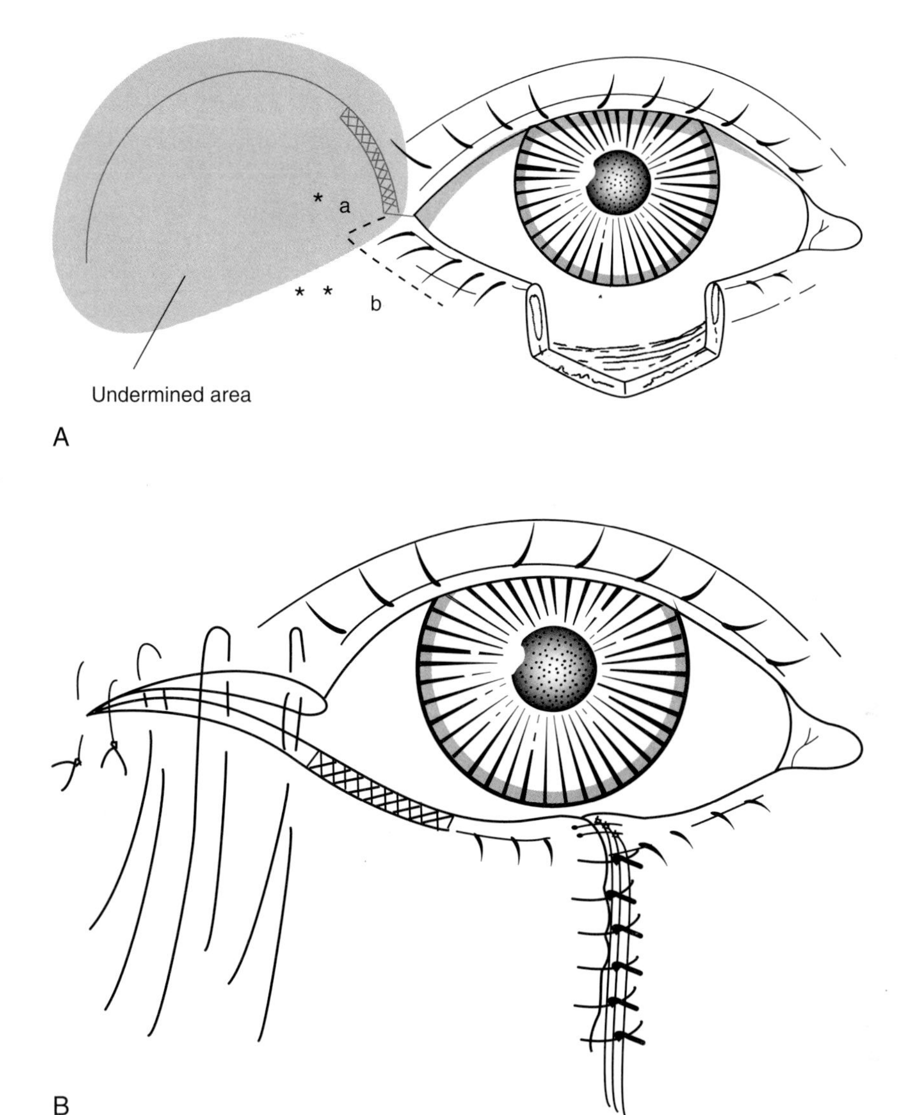

Figure 4-2 Tenzel semicircular flap. (A) Formation of semicircular flap at lateral canthus after pentagonal excision. Flap is incised and undermined subcutaneously to allow closure. Inferior limb of lateral canthal tendon and septum is lysed (*dashed lines*). If needed, lower lid retractors and septum may be incised for further relaxation. Shaded portion of flap becomes part of lid margin. (B) Repair of lateral canthal angle and resuspension of eyelid.

This is generally accomplished by the use of two separate flaps, a tarsoconjunctival flap to reform the posterior lamella and a full-thickness skin graft or myocutaneous advancement flap to reconstruct the anterior lamella. To prevent necrosis, at least one of the flaps must bring a vascular supply with it to support the other flap. In other words, only one of the lamellae can be reconstructed as a free graft; the other has to be a local flap tethered at its base to the vascular supply.

The upper eyelid tarsoconjunctival flap (Hughes flap) is an advancement flap composed of a portion of the upper eyelid tarsus and palpebral conjunctiva (Fig. 4-3).

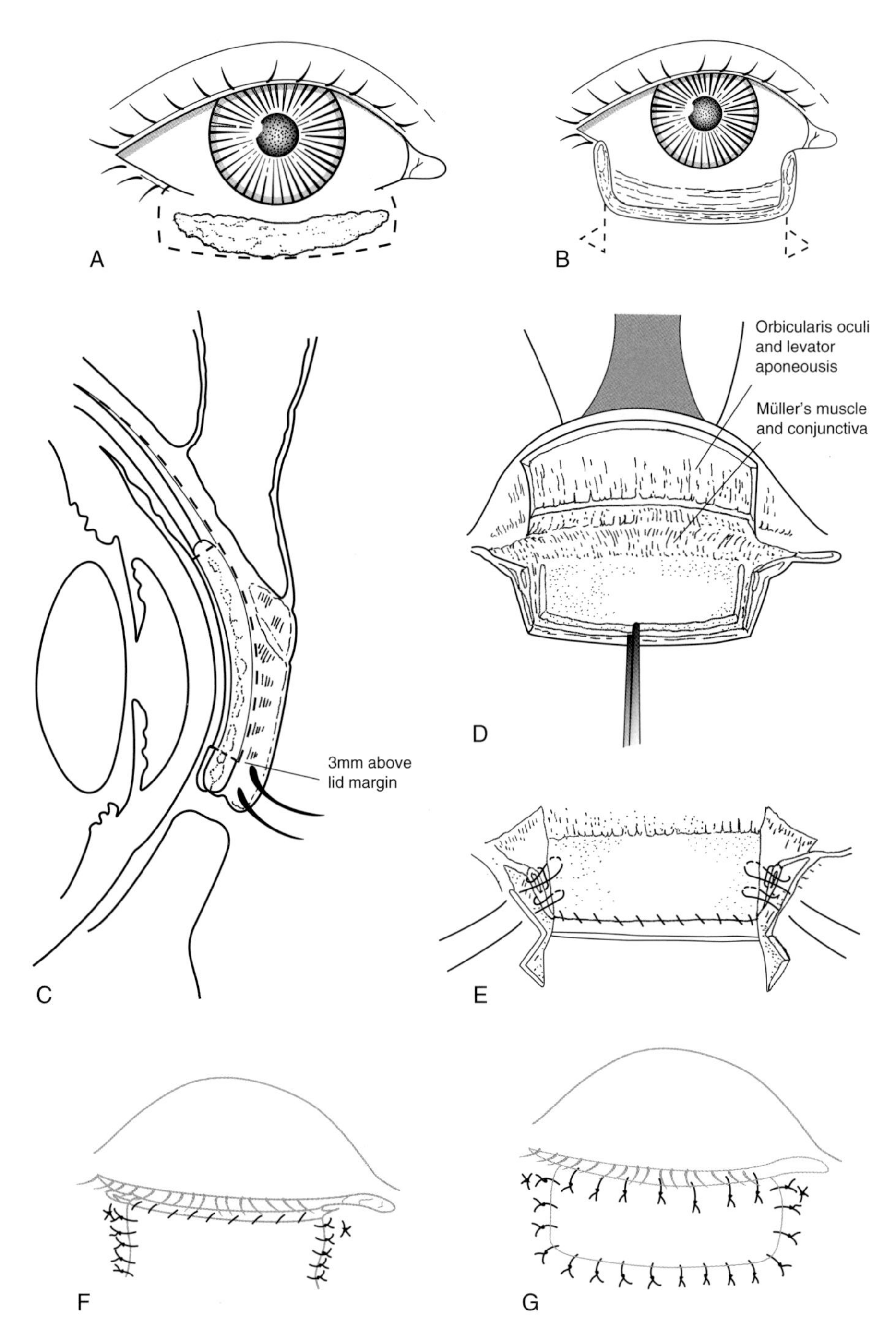

Figure 4-3 Hughes tarsoconjunctival flap. (A) Lesion requiring excision of 75% or more of lower lid. (B) Excision of full-thickness, rectangular section of lower lid. (*Dashed lines* show planned relaxing incisions for advancement of cheek flap.) (C) Splitting of upper lid 3 mm above lid border and formation of tarsoconjunctival flap. (D) Upper lid is everted on Desmarres retractor, and tarso-conjunctival flap from upper lid is advanced. (E) Suturing of tarsus of upper lid to lower lid as tongue-in-groove with sutures nasally and temporally. Absorbable suture is used to secure tarsus to conjunctiva of inferior cul de sac. Advancement cheek flap is incised, undermined, and advanced. (F) Advancement of skin flap from remaining lower lid and cheek mobilized superiorly and sutured to remaining skin of lower lid and tarsoconjunctival flap from upper lid. (G) Alternatively, suturing of free full-thickness skin graft over advanced tarsoconjunctival flap will reconstruct anterior lamella.

It is connected at its base to the forniceal conjunctiva, where it gets its blood supply. Once advanced inferiorly, the flap provides conjunctiva and tarsus to fill the lower lid defect, but the bridge of conjunctiva occludes the visual axis. After 6 to 12 weeks, once collateral circulation has been allowed to develop, this conjunctival bridge can be severed in a second-stage operation. Because of its inherent vasculature, a full-thickness skin graft can be used to reconstruct the anterior lamella.

The horizontal dimension of the Hughes flap can be determined by measuring the residual defect once the two marginal edges are drawn together. A 4-0 silk traction suture is placed at the gray line of the upper lid and the eyelid is everted over a Desmarres retractor. The exposed tarsal conjunctiva is dried and a transverse mark is made parallel to the margin, 4 mm superior to it. At least 3 to 4 mm of tarsus must be left undisturbed so as to avoid notching and other contour abnormalities. The transverse incision is made just through the tarsus, slightly shorter than the measured horizontal defect, and over the central aspect of the tarsus, where it is tallest. Once vertical incisions are made at the flanking ends of the transverse incision, the tarsal flap can be elevated sharply. Dissection is then carried superiorly to separate the conjunctiva from the Müller's muscle. Because the Müller's muscle is vascular and very adherent to the conjunctiva with no inherent intervening plane, this can be technically challenging. The authors have found that gentle hydrodissection with local anesthetic with epinephrine on a 30G needle between the conjunctiva and Müller's muscle makes this process significantly easier. As the dissection is carried superiorly, relaxing vertical incisions in the conjunctiva should be made to the fornix. These incisions should splay outward slightly, such that the base is wider than the end of the flap.

The tarsal component of the Hughes flap can then be secured to fill the lower eyelid defect. The vertical edges of the Hughes flap are sutured to the edges of the marginal defect with partial-thickness 5-0 or 6-0 Vicryl sutures through both the donor and recipient tarsus. The inferior edge of the tarsoconjunctival flap is secured to the edge of the residual conjunctiva of the lower eyelid with running 6-0 plain gut, thereby completing reconstruction of the posterior lamella. The anterior lamellar defect can be filled with a full-thickness skin graft or a small vertical myocutaneous advancement flap, if the vertical extent of the skin defect is minimal.

To construct this myocutaneous flap, vertical incisions from the base of the skin defect are made inferiorly at the two ends of the skin defect. The rectangular myocutaneous advancement flap is undermined just above the septum and advanced superiorly to fill the defect. The superior edge of this flap is secured just slightly inferior to the superior edge of the Hughes flap, and the two Burow's triangles at the inferior aspect of the vertical incisions are excised in the usual fashion. This flap under normal circumstances is less than ideal, as it exerts a downward force on the lower eyelid and will produce secondary retraction. In this situation, however, the Hughes flap provides a counterbalancing superiorly directed force. For this reason, the Hughes flap should be left intact for a longer time until the myocutaneous advancement has healed sufficiently.

The bridging flap of conjunctiva can be severed postoperatively at 6 to 12 weeks. This is done by sliding a grooved director or the handle end of a Desmarres retractor under the flap to protect the globe. A #15 Bard-Parker blade is used to incise the flap, slightly higher than the lower lid margin and beveled anteriorly, such that the conjunctiva can be draped anteriorly and the new mucocutaneous junction recreated away from the globe. The residual conjunctival tissue on the upper lid can be amputated at its base, so as not to irritate the ocular surface.

Free tarsoconjunctival grafts can be used in conjunction with myocutaneous flaps to reconstruct large lower eyelid defects involving the margin. The free tarsal graft is harvested in a fashion very similar to that described above for the Hughes flap, but rather than carrying the dissection superiorly between the conjunctiva and Müller's muscle, the tarsus is amputated at its superior margin. Because this graft is avascular, it depends on perfusion provided by a myocutaneous flap. The above-described vertical myocutaneous advancement flap should not be used in conjunction with the free tarsoconjunctival flap unless the skin defect is very small or a Frost suture is placed to apply vertical traction to the lower eyelid. Of course a Frost suture would negate the principal advantage of this flap versus a Hughes flap, namely the preclusion of obstruction of the visual axis. For this reason, myocutaneous flaps that apply horizontal vector forces, such as a Tenzel flap or laterally based horizontal transposition flap from the upper eyelid, are preferable.

4-2-3 *Lateral Eyelid and Commissure Defects.* Reconstruction of defects of the lateral lower eyelid in which there is a total absence of native eyelid elements laterally requires resuspension of the lateral eyelid, either by direct apposition of the edge of the marginal defect to the periosteum over the lateral tubercle, or by a bridging flap based or secured to this area. If the defect is relatively small and there is sufficient horizontal laxity to allow direct closure, a tarsal strip can be fashioned, and the defect can be closed primarily.

When the defect in the lateral eyelid is too large to preclude primary closure, a bridge of tissue is necessary to fill the residual gap. As described above, the same principles of composite reconstruction of the layers of the eyelid, including the need for at least one well-perfused flap, apply here. Reconstruction can be based on a pedicled flap providing the posterior elements of the eyelid, with a free graft for the anterior lamella, or less preferably, a myocutaneous flap with a free tarsoconjunctival graft.

The periosteal flap is a robust and versatile flap that can provide a strong pedicle of tissue to reconstruct the posterior lamella of the lateral eyelid. Because the periosteum over the zygomatic process of the maxilla is dense and very adherent to the arcus marginalis, the flap is strong with a rigid base and has good tensile strength, and therefore resists secondary rounding of the reconstructed lateral commissure. It has the added advantage of being able to simultaneously provide tissue for both the upper and lower lateral eyelid. The main disadvantage is that the flap is not associated with mucous membrane (the conjunctiva has to re-epithelialize over the periosteum) and the length of the flap is limited to about 10 mm (the horizontal extent of the zygomatic process of the maxilla).

The skin and orbicularis over the zygomatic process of the maxilla should be undermined to expose the underlying pre-periosteal tissue and periosteum. A horizontal relaxing incision can be made. Debulking of the pre-periosteal tissue should be deferred until the flap has been elevated. The proposed level of the new lateral commissure should be marked on the lateral orbital rim; this also marks the inferior edge of the periosteal flap. A second mark is made 4 to 5 mm superior to this mark, and both marks are extended laterally and slightly superiorly to create the lines of a rectangular flap to be based at the lateral orbital rim. The periosteum is incised cleanly and decisively with a #15 Bard-Parker blade, so as not to have frayed edges. The flap is then elevated with a periosteal elevator. The hinged flap can then be flipped over medially to fill the lateral defect and secured to the tarsus at the edge of the defect with partial-thickness interrupted 5-0 or 6-0 Vicryl sutures. Then the posterior lamella, now reconstructed with a vascular pedicled flap, can be covered with a full-thickness skin graft or myocutaneous flap. Defects involving the upper lateral eyelid are closed in a similar fashion, except the periosteal flap is just inferior to the proposed level of the new lateral commissure and extends laterally and slightly inferiorly. For defects involving the lateral aspects of both the upper and lower eyelid, both periosteal flaps can be elevated and the upper flap (destined for the lower lid) crossed over the lower flap (destined for the upper lid).

For horizontal defects larger than 10 mm in the lateral-most aspect of the lower eyelid that cannot be closed with a periosteal flap, or in cases with a high risk of flap necrosis, a tarsoconjunctival transposition flap from the upper lid can be used in place of the periosteal flap. Although the periosteal flap itself has a fairly robust blood supply to feed itself, it tends to support overlying skin grafts relatively poorly because the graft lies in apposition to the undersurface of the periosteum (the more avascular portion of the flap). In contradistinction, the tarsoconjunctival transposition flap, or Hewes flap, is a true axial flap with a discrete artery extending the length of the flap, and therefore provides excellent vascular support, both for itself and any overlying free graft.

The Hewes flap consists of a strip of upper eyelid tarsus with the superior palpebral vascular arcade and is based laterally. The flap is transposed to the lateral lower eyelid for reconstruction of the posterior lamella. Although this flap can bridge larger defects than the periosteal flap and provides a more vigorous vascular supply, it tends to create some irregularities at the reconstructed lateral commissure, as the flap tends to bunch up at its base as it rotates inferiorly. Furthermore, its lateral base has no tarsal elements and is not securely attached to the lateral orbital rim, and therefore provides little support for the newly constructed lateral commissure. For these reasons, and in contradiction to the original description of this flap, the authors have found that these cases occasionally require secondary lateral canthoplasty.

The Hewes flap is marked over an everted upper eyelid. The horizontal extent needed should be measured in a fashion identical to that described for the Hughes flap. The vertical limit of the flap should be about 2 mm superior to the upper border of the tarsus centrally in order to ensure inclusion of the superior vascular arcade. As in the Hughes flap, about 4 mm of tarsus should be left in the upper lid to prevent notching. Because the upper tarsus has a dome-shaped superior edge, the lateral aspect of the flap near its base will have little to no tarsus in it. The flap is elevated and dissected laterally, taking care not to disrupt the vascular arcade. Once defined, the flap can then be transposed inferiorly and the edges of the recipient and donor tarsus secured in the usual fashion. The anterior lamella can then be reconstructed with a free skin graft or myocutaneous flap.

4-2-4 *Medial Lid and Commissure Defects.* Reconstruction of the medial canthal area is covered in a separate chapter, so will be discussed in a cursory manner here. Defects of the medial canthal area may pose the most complex reconstructive challenge. The medial-most aspect of the eyelids and the medial canthal area contain the lacrimal drainage system and must be reconstructed either primarily or secondarily. If the medial-most aspect of the eyelid is intact with several millimeters of undisturbed canaliculus in place, a bi-canalicular silicone stent can be inserted in an attempt to preserve natural drainage of tears. Alternatively, a conjunctivo-dacryocystorhinostomy with the insertion of a Jones tube can be done secondarily.

Unlike defects of the lateral-most aspect of the eyelid, similar defects in the medial eyelid should not be closed primarily, even when the defect is small and can be easily bridged by the residual eyelid, because there are no lashes over the skin of the canaliculus. Direct reapproximation would bring lash-bearing lid margin all the way to the medial commissure and would not only be cosmetically unacceptable, but may cause irritation during blinking. One solution is to bring down a small Hughes flap from the upper eyelid to reconstruct this portion of the eyelid. The medial edge of both these tarsoconjunctival flaps should be secured to residual tissue of the inner crus of the medial canthal tendon; otherwise, the medial eyelid will remain distracted from the globe. The flap can then be covered by a skin graft or myocutaneous flap.

Reconstruction of medial canthal defects is further complicated by the presence of a confluence of thin eyelid skin and thick skin of the lateral nasal wall over a concave surface. Defects of the eyelid skin should be reconstructed with full-thickness skin grafts or myocutaneous flaps derived from eyelid skin, whereas defects of the thicker skin of the lateral nasal wall should be reconstructed with local flaps from the lateral nasal wall, glabella, or forehead. These flaps should be securely attached to the bed of the defect in order to recreate the concavity in this area. Alternatively, small defects in this area can be allowed to heal by secondary intent with little ill effect.

4-2-5 *Defects Not Involving Eyelid Margin.* Unlike other areas of the face, where the final scar should be coincident with relaxed skin tension lines, defects of the lower eyelid should be closed perpendicular to these lines. In other words, unless the vertical dimension of the lower eyelid defect is very short, the final scar should lie perpendicular to the margin, not parallel (which would yield a more favorable scar). This is because horizontally inclined wounds exert vertical traction and would cause retraction of the lower eyelid. Vertically inclined wounds, however, exert horizontal traction and are less likely to cause retraction.

These defects can be closed with rectangular myocutaneous advancement flaps based laterally or medially. To create these flaps, two relaxing transverse incisions are made at the superior and inferior extent of the defect and carried laterally in the case of laterally based flaps, and medially for medially based flaps. The rectangular flap is undermined and elevated and advanced into the defect. Several 6-0 Vicryl sutures should be placed in an interrupted fashion to close the orbicularis to take some tension off the cutaneous closure. Burow's triangles at the base of the flap should be excised in the usual manner. For defects that cannot be closed with a single advancement flap, two such flaps can be made, medially and laterally, to close the defect.

Larger defects not involving the eyelid margin and not amenable to closure with myocutaneous advancement flaps can be covered with a full-thickness skin graft from the upper eyelid, post- or pre-auricular skin, or supraclavicular skin.

4-2-6 *Free Tissue Grafts.* Defects in the skin that cannot be covered by a local myocutaneous flap should be covered with a full-thickness skin graft, provided the underlying recipient bed has enough inherent vascularity to support the graft. Split-thickness grafts should be avoided on the eyelid as well as the rest of the face, as they tend to contract significantly more than full-thickness skin grafts, secondarily become hyperpigmented, and have textural irregularities that match poorly with the surrounding skin. The full-thickness skin graft should be harvested from a site that is most likely to produce the best match to the surrounding recipient skin. The upper eyelid provides the best match, but is limited in the size of the graft that can be safely harvested. Post-auricular skin is also an excellent source and has the added advantage that the donor site wound is well concealed. Supraclavicular skin can be harvested, especially when large grafts are needed for reconstruction. The underlying dermal and subcutaneous tissue of the graft should be thinned to better match the lower eyelid skin and to decrease the chances of flap necrosis.

In certain instances, the lower eyelid may be retracted by foreshortening of the posterior or middle lamella, even in the presence of adequate anterior lamellar length. This situation is commonly encountered in Graves ophthalmopathy, in which the middle lamella contracts from inflammation and fibrosis, and in cases of chronic conjunctivitis (herpetic conjunctivitis, ocular cicatricial pemphigoid, or Stevens-Johnson syndrome), in which the posterior lamella is scarred and contracted. These deformities can be corrected by an interposition free graft that augments the posterior and middle layers of the lid. These grafts can be harvested from the mucoperiosteum of the hard palate. It can also be augmented with a dermal homograft, such as Alloderm or DermaMatrix, or dermal allograft, such as Enduragen. When contraction of the middle lamella is associated with loss or deflation of supporting adipose tissue, dermis fat can be used as the interposition graft (Korn B). Severely retracted lower eyelids may require the rigid support provided by an ear cartilage graft.

The lower eyelid is everted over a Desmarres retractor with the aid of a 4-0 silk traction suture. A transverse incision is made just inferior to the inferior edge of the tarsus with cutting monopolar cautery and dissection is carried forward anteriorly and inferiorly to release the insertion of the capsulopalpebral fascia. Application of vertical traction on the lower eyelid will create a defect in the posterior lamella, the dimensions of which should be measured for sizing of the interpositional graft. The graft, once appropriately sized, can be secured with running 6-0 plain gut suture. A Frost suture should be placed to keep the reconstructed lower eyelid in vertical traction for at least 1 week.

4-2-7 *Special Considerations.* Defects encompassing near-total loss of the lower eyelid require a combination of techniques to reconstruct the layers of the eyelid. As one example, a large Hughes flap can be brought down the medial and central portion of the posterior lamella and a periosteal flap can be lifted to reform the posterior lamella. The anterior lamella can then be reconstructed with a full-thickness skin graft, if the vertical dimension of the defect is short, or with a Mustarde rotational cheek flap, if the defect extends inferiorly to encompass a portion of the medial cheek skin.

In essence, the Mustarde flap is an extension of Tenzel semicircular flap. The flap is carried to the pre-auricular crease inferiorly toward the lobule. The superior limit of the flap should be at least to the level of the lateral eyebrow, as rotation of the flap medially into the defect will straighten the final wound and bring it inferiorly. A relaxing back cut can be made at the distal end of the flap near the lobule to facilitate rotation and a large Burow's triangle excised at the junction of the lateral nasal wall to the medial cheek. Because the Mustarde flap is a vascularized rotational flap, it can accommodate a free graft substitute for the tarsoconjunctiva, such as a nasal chondromucosal graft or a hard palate mucoperiosteal graft. Because this flap is atonic, it is prone to cause secondary ectropion and retraction. This can be prevented in some measure by securing the medial extent of the flap to the residual medial canthal tendon with several interrupted PDS sutures.

Defects involving complete loss of the lower eyelid as well as loss of much of the soft tissue of the midface can be reconstructed with a cervico-facial rotational flap. This is in essence a Mustarde flap that is extended further inferiorly behind the angle of the mandible to the lateral neck. Extension distributes the area over which the tissue is borrowed for closure of the large defect. These flaps require an intimate knowledge of head and neck anatomy in order to prevent injury to branches of the facial nerve and the external jugular vein.

SUGGESTED READINGS

Chandler DB, Gausas RE. Lower eyelid reconstruction. *Otolaryngol Clin North Am.* 2005;38(5):1033–1042.

Hewes EH, Sullivan JH, Beard C. Lower eyelid reconstruction by tarsal transposition. *Am J Ophthalmol.* 1976;81:512–514.

Hughes WL. *Reconstructive Surgery of the Eyelids.* 2nd ed. St Louis: CV Mosby Co., 1954.

McNab AA, Martin P, Benger R, O'Donnell B, Kourt G. A prospective randomized study comparing division of the pedicle of modified Hughes flaps at two or four weeks. *Ophthal Plast Reconstr Surg.* 2001;17(5):317–319.

Mustarde JC. *Repair and Reconstruction in the Orbital Region.* Edinburgh and London: E & S Livingstone Ltd., 1966.

Reeh MJ, Wobig JL, Wirtschafter JD. *Ophthalmic Anatomy.* San Francisco: American Academy of Ophthalmology, 1981.

Robbins P. Mohs' surgery. In: Smith BC, ed. *Ophthalmic Plastic and Reconstructive Surgery.* St Louis: CV Mosby Co., 1987;2: 841–845.

Tenzel RR, Stewart WB. Eyelid reconstruction by the semi-circle flap technique. *Ophthalmology.* 1987;85:1164–1169.

Verity DH, Collin JR. Eyelid reconstruction: the state of the art. *Curr Opin Otolaryngol Head Neck Surg.* 2004;12(4):344–348.

5

Reconstruction of the Upper Eyelid

H. B. HAROLD LEE, MD, AND WILLIAM R. NUNERY, MD

Normal physiologic mechanisms of the upper eyelid are essential for preservation of the eye. Normal function and good cosmesis usually go hand in hand, but preservation of function is the more important of the two priorities.

5-1 GENERAL PRINCIPLES

The general considerations in choosing a reconstruction technique include the restoration of:

1. A smooth conjunctival surface to line the eyelid and protect the cornea
2. Structural support of the tarsal plate
3. A smooth, nonabrasive lid margin
4. Normal vertical eyelid movement without ptosis or lagophthalmos
5. Normal horizontal tension with normal medial and lateral canthal tendon positions

To cover small defects, the conjunctival lining may be rotated or advanced. For larger defects, the lining may be replaced with a buccal mucous membrane graft or a contralateral conjunctival graft. The tarsal plate usually requires 4 mm of vertical height to provide adequate eyelid support. If the 4 mm is unavailable, it may be replaced with lower lid tarsus, a free tarsal graft from the opposite lid, a free cartilage graft, a polytetrafluoroethylene graft, or a preserved sclera graft. The eyelid margin must be free of trichiasis or surface epithelium, which might abrade the cornea.

When levator function is preserved following traumatic or surgical defects of the eyelid, ptosis can usually be avoided or corrected. The levator aponeurosis separates the orbital and palpebral portions of the lacrimal gland, and lacrimal tissue should be preserved when dissecting in the lateral canthal, lateral levator, and lateral anterior orbital areas.

Lagophthalmos of the upper eyelid is usually due either to adhesion of the orbital septum to the tarsal plate or to external vertical skin shortage. Proper horizontal tension can be achieved by measuring full-thickness defects while gently pulling the edges of the defect toward each other. Careful measurement reduces the risk of excessive or deficient horizontal length following reconstruction.

Skin grafts in the upper eyelids should be covered with a moderate pressure dressing for 4 to 6 days to prevent buckling or subgraft hematoma. Full-thickness skin grafts are preferred to split-thickness grafts for optimal tissue match and coloration. Upper eyelid sutures may be permanent or absorbable. Most external permanent sutures are 7-0 caliber. Absorbable 6-0 mild chromic suture may also be used. Sutures may be removed in 5 to 7 days. Vascular advancement flaps are usually left in place from 4 to 6 weeks prior to separation. Smoking should be discouraged for at least 2 to 3 weeks preoperatively and postoperatively because smoking contributes to necrosis of reconstructed eyelid tissue; 2 to 3 weeks may be necessary to reverse the effect of nicotine on tissue perfusion.

With these general principles in mind, this chapter discusses common reconstructive techniques that are applicable to most upper eyelid defects.

5-2 PARTIAL-THICKNESS DEFECTS

Skin defects, or partial-thickness defects, in the upper eyelid are more significant when they occur in the nasal third of the eyelid. Little to no excess vertical skin tissue is available nasally for advancement over the defect, while excess vertical skin usually exists centrally and laterally. Small skin defects may be closed horizontally, leaving a vertical scar, to prevent vertical contracture of the tissue (Fig. 5-1).

If horizontal closure of the tissue is not possible, a full-thickness skin graft may be placed over the defect to prevent lagophthalmos. Full-thickness skin grafting is preferable to split-thickness skin grafting to replace the normal color and texture to the upper eyelid, as well as to minimize vertical contracture of the graft. A full-thickness skin graft may be obtained from the lateral aspect of the same upper eyelid by harvesting in a blepharoplasty distribution. The other upper eyelid or postauricular tissue is also an excellent source.

When upper lid partial-thickness defects are being closed, the orbital septum should be avoided to minimize the risk of closed-compartment hemorrhage into the orbit and to avoid incorporation of the septum into the superficial defect. The levator aponeurosis should be repaired primarily only when a clear laceration or dehiscence is apparent. Otherwise, advancement of the levator aponeurosis should be postponed for 2 to 3 months to judge the lid position accurately.

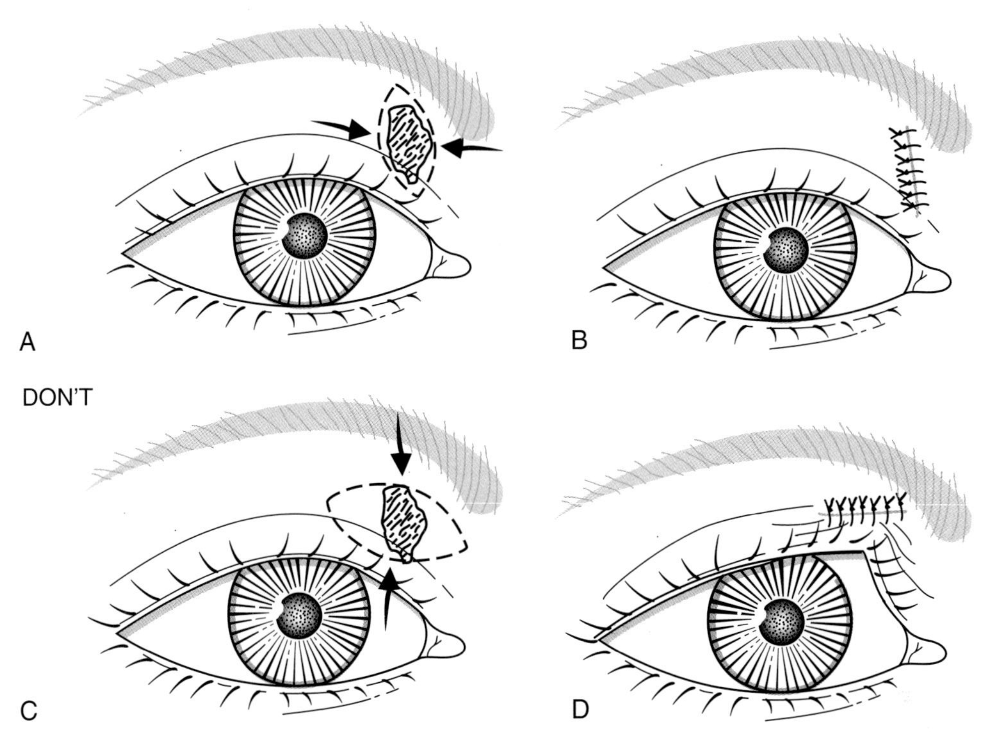

Figure 5-1 Do's and don'ts of closure in partial-thickness defects. (A,B) Correct horizontal closure with vertical scar. (C,D) Incorrect vertical closure with horizontal scar.

5-3 FULL-THICKNESS DEFECTS

5-3-1 *Direct Closure*. Direct closure of a full-thickness upper eyelid laceration through the lid margin is carried out by first reapproximating the eyelash margin with a temporary traction suture. The tarsal plate may then be aligned precisely and closed with partial-thickness permanent 7-0 silk sutures from the anterior surface, to avoid corneal irritation. After closure of the tarsus, the eyelid margin is closed with interrupted 6-0 silk sutures placed at the gray line and lash margin (Fig. 5-2). All eyelashes should be everted and sutured away from the cornea. The ends of the margin sutures are left long and sutured to the external skin tissue to avoid corneal irritation. The skin and orbicularis layers may be closed simultaneously with 7-0 permanent or 6-0 mild chromic sutures. Margin sutures are removed after 7 to 10 days, while skin sutures are removed in 5 to 7 days.

The goal in repairing posttraumatic full-thickness eyelid lacerations is not only to reapproximate normal anatomy, but also to preserve as much tissue as possible. Tissue that is questionably viable should be replaced in its normal location and preserved. Trichiasis or roughness of the lid margin may be repaired secondarily with margin rotation or mucous membrane grafting.

5-3-2 *Wedge Resection*. Wedge resection with primary closure is useful in resecting a lid margin tumor, repairing a coloboma, or removing a small eyelid margin defect.

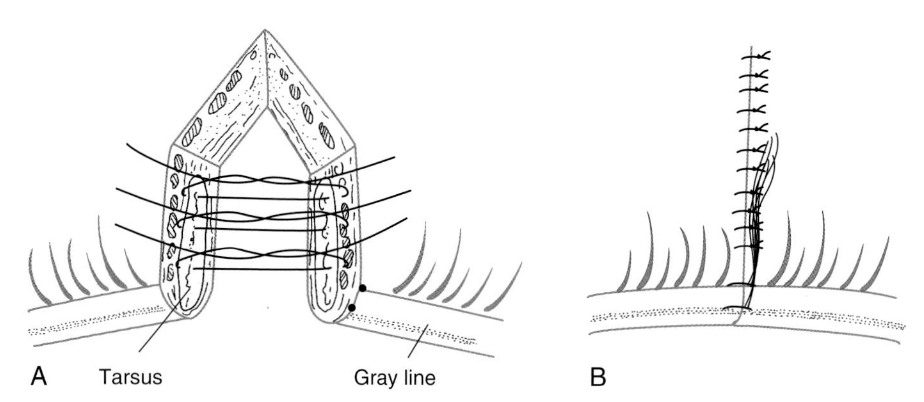

Figure 5-2 Direct closure of upper lid laceration. (A) Location of tarsal and lid margin sutures. (B) Laceration closed, showing margin sutures.

Most lesions can be excised by using a lid-crease incision horizontally and an en bloc, full-thickness, rectangular incision through the lid margin to the lid crease at the superior border of the tarsus (Fig. 5-3A,B,C). A pentagonal excision extending above the lid crease should be avoided because closure of the pentagon creates a vertical scar through the lid crease (Fig. 5-3D,E). A horizontal, relaxing lid-crease incision, however, allows the tarsus to be advanced independently of eyelid tissue above the lid crease and avoids both tissue redundancy above the incision site as well as a vertical scar through the lid crease.

When an en bloc resection of full-thickness tissue is performed, straight scissors are placed in a moderately "toed-in" position to allow straight vertical margins as the remaining tarsus relaxes horizontally. Tarsal incision must continue vertically to the superior border of the tarsus to allow tarsal advancement and reanastomosis. In defects greater than 25% to 30% of the upper lid margin, the superior ramus of the lateral canthal tendon may be incised to allow greater relaxation and less tension on the horizontal closure.

5-3-3 *Semicircular Flap*. A lateral, inverted, semicircular flap may be combined with direct closure for full-thickness defects of up to two thirds of the eyelid margin (Fig. 5-4A). An inverted semicircle is marked on the skin surface, beginning at the lateral canthus and extending laterally approximately 3 cm. The skin and orbicularis tissue are undermined under the entire flap, and the superior ramus of the lateral canthal tendon is severed. The lateral aspect of the eyelid may then be advanced medially to cover the defect.

The posterior surface of the advanced semicircular flap may be covered by a tarsoconjunctival advancement flap from the lateral aspect of the lower eyelid (Fig. 5-4B). A vertical, full-thickness, lower eyelid incision is made, and the tarsoconjunctival advancement flap is prepared by excising the lower eyelid skin tissue and lash margin from the flap. The tarsus and conjunctiva may then be advanced superiorly into the lateral aspect of the upper eyelid flap. The lower eyelid defect may be repaired primarily, anterior to the tarsoconjunctival flap (Fig. 5-4C). The lateral tarsoconjunctival flap may be released in 4 to 6 weeks. As an alternative to semicircular skin advancement, the advanced lower

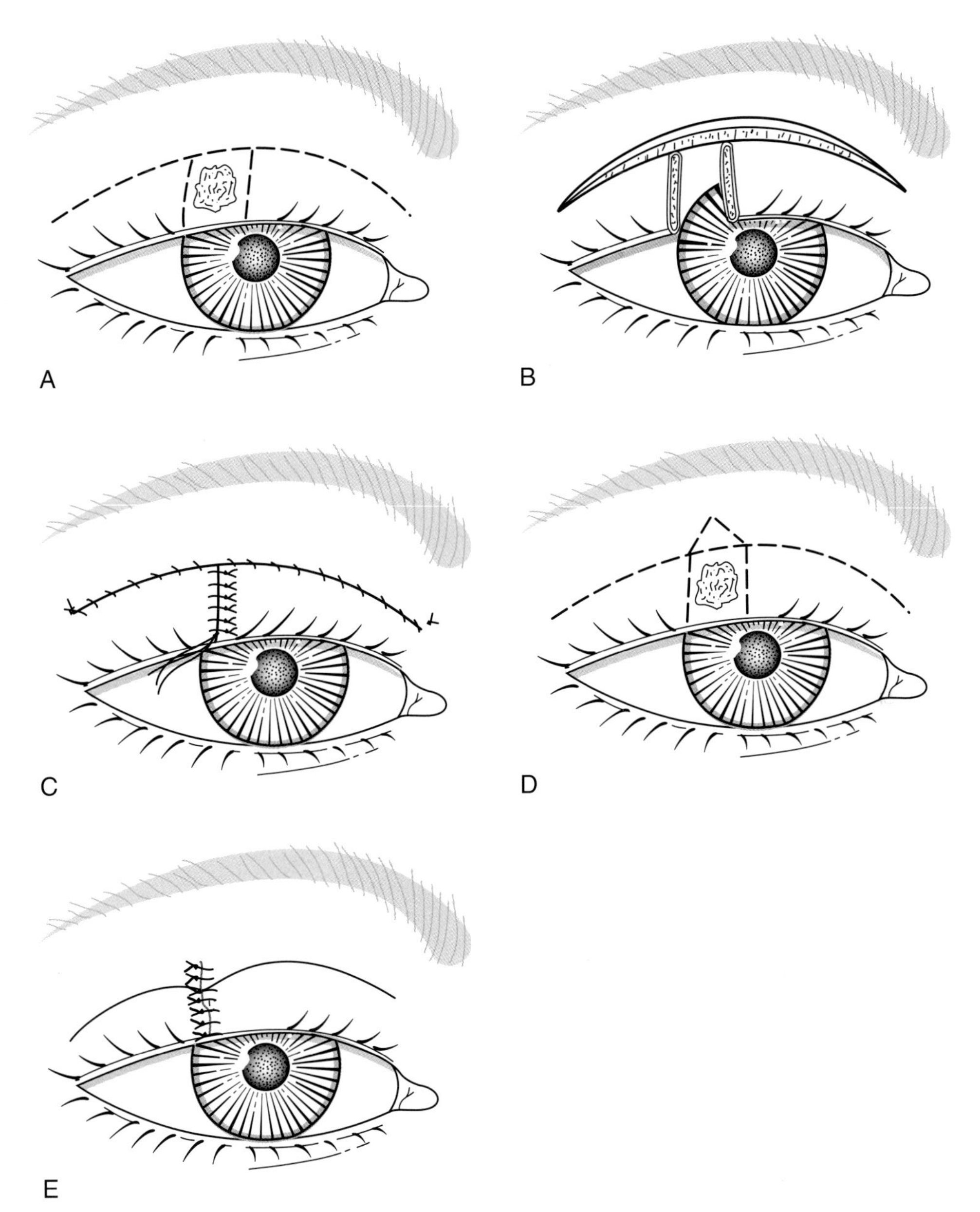

Figure 5-3 Do's and don'ts in wedge resection. (A,B,C) Correct en bloc incision and lid crease relaxation. (D,E) Incorrect pentagonal excision through lid crease.

lid tarsoconjunctival flap may be covered with full-thickness skin tissue rather than a rotated, inverted semicircle.

5-3-4 *Sliding Tarsoconjunctival Flap.* Horizontal advancement of an upper eyelid tarsoconjunctival flap is useful for full-thickness defects of up to two thirds of the upper lid margin (Fig. 5-5A). The residual upper eyelid tarsus is bisected horizontally (Fig. 5-5B). The superior portion of the tarsus is advanced horizontally along with its levator and Müller's muscle attachments. The tarsoconjunctival advancement

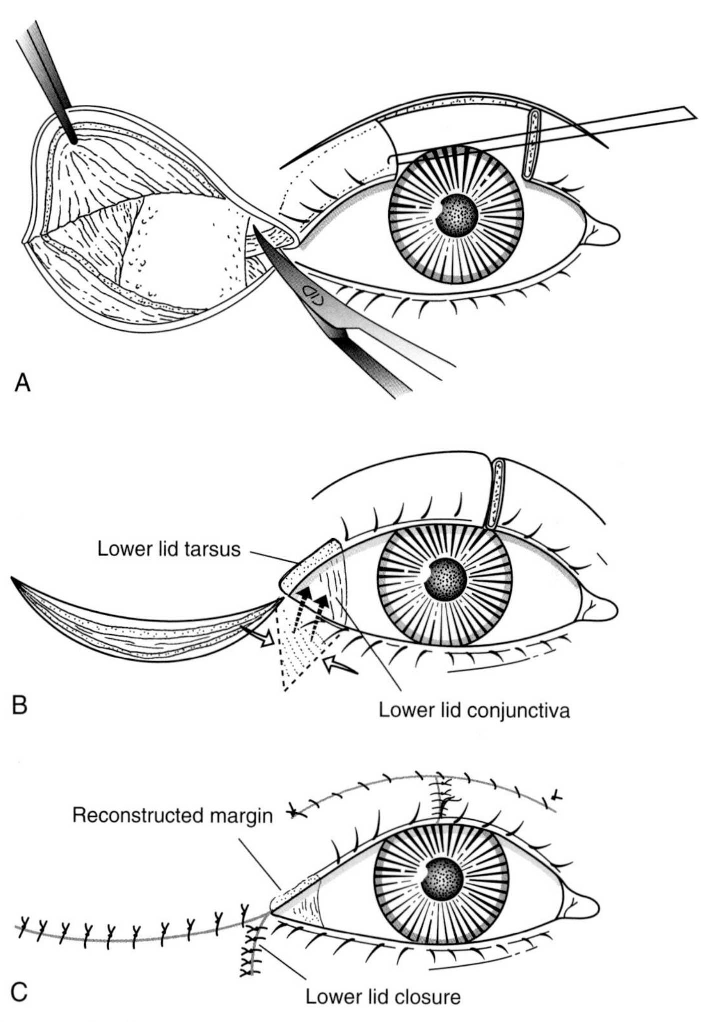

Figure 5-4 Semicircular flap. (A) Lateral, inverted, semicircular flap for full-thickness defect. (B) Posterior surface of advanced semicircular flap covered by tarsoconjunctival advancement flap. (C) Lower lid defect repaired primarily.

flap created is then sutured in a side-to-side fashion to the lower portion of the upper lid tarsus and to the lateral or medial canthal tendon (Fig. 5-5C). The lower portion of the upper lid tarsus remains attached to the orbicularis and skin tissue. After the horizontal tarsoconjunctival advancement, the external skin tissue is rebuilt by using full-thickness skin grafting or semicircular adjacent tissue advancement (Fig. 5-5D, E).

5-3-5 *Cutler-Beard Reconstruction*. A Cutler-Beard reconstruction is useful for upper eyelid defects covering up to 100% of the eyelid margin. A three-sided inverted U-shaped incision is marked on the lower eyelid, beginning below the tarsus (Fig. 5-6A). A full-thickness incision is made through the lower eyelid, horizontally below the tarsus, and extended inferiorly to the lower limits of the inferior fornix. The conjunctiva is then dissected away from the lower lid tissue and advanced into

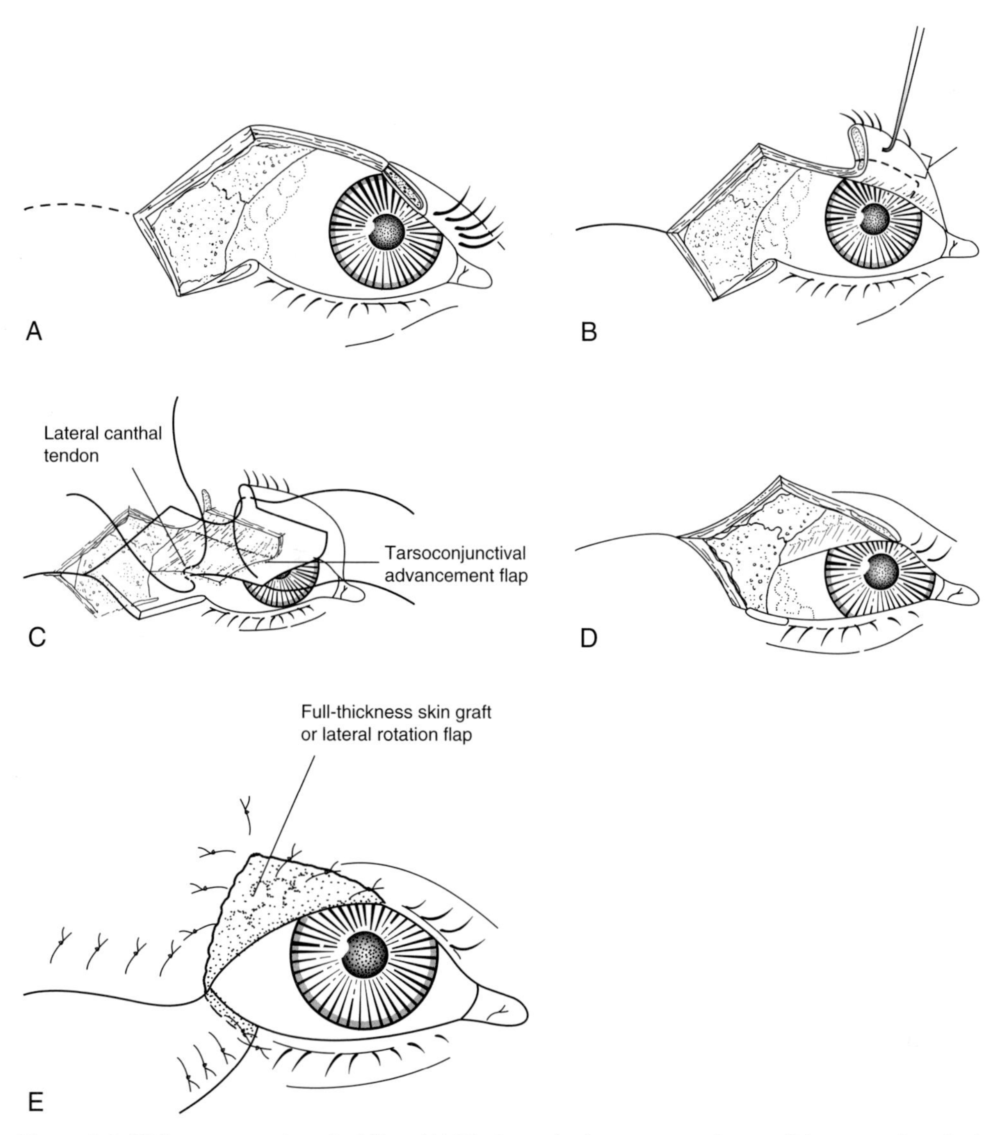

Figure 5-5 Sliding tarsoconjunctival flap. (A) Horizontal advancement of upper lid tarsoconjunctival flap. (B) Residual upper lid tarsus is bisected horizontally. (C) Flap is sutured to lower portion of upper lid tarsus. (D,E) External skin tissue is rebuilt using full-thickness skin graft.

the upper eyelid defect along with its blood supply from the inferior retractor muscle layer (Fig. 5-6B).

After the lower lid conjunctiva has been sutured to the remaining upper eyelid conjunctiva, tarsal support to the upper eyelid is replaced by placing preserved sclera, autogenous cartilage, or synthetic polytetrafluoroethylene anterior to the conjunctival flap (Fig. 5-6C). The lower lid skin-and-muscle flap is then advanced to the upper lid to cover the cartilage, sclera, or polytetrafluoroethylene graft (Fig. 5-6D).

The lower lid tissue is advanced posteriorly to the remaining lower lid tarsal and lid margin bridge. The lower lid skin tissue of the bridge is then sutured to the posterior conjunctiva of the bridge to complete the closure.

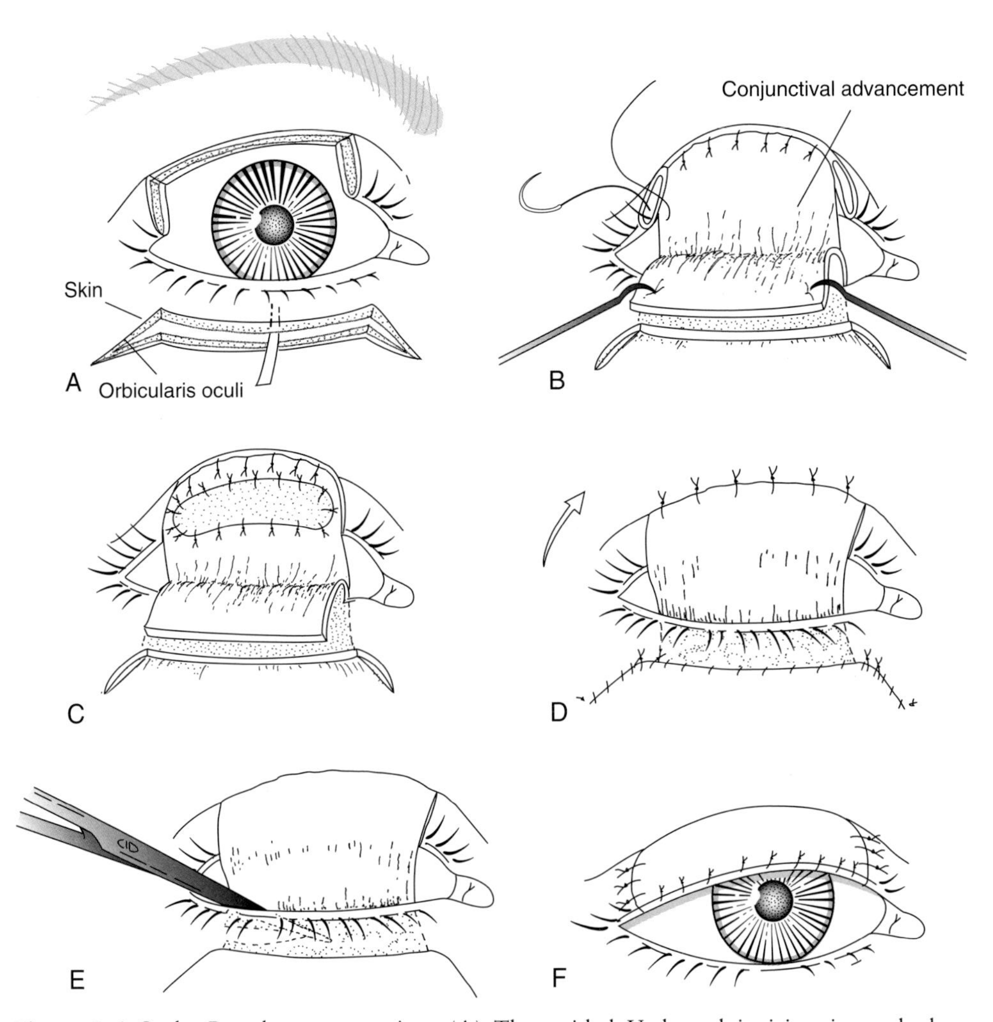

Figure 5-6 Cutler-Beard reconstruction. (A) Three-sided U-shaped incision is marked on lower lid. (B) Conjunctiva is dissected from lower lid tissue and advanced into upper lid defect. (C) Tarsal support is replaced by sclera, cartilage, or polytetrafluoroethylene graft. (D) Lower lid flap is advanced to cover graft. (E) Full-thickness incision is made through flap inferior to lower lid bridge margin. (F) Inferior margins of bridge are reanastomosed to remaining lower lid skin.

The bridge flap is left intact for 8 weeks prior to separation. When the bridge flap is separated, a full-thickness incision should be made through the flap at a position inferior to the lower lid bridge margin (Fig. 5-6E). The conjunctiva and skin are then sutured directly in the newly separated upper eyelid tissue. The inferior margins of the lower lid bridge are freshened and reanastomosed to the remaining lower lid skin and conjunctival layers (Fig. 5-6F).

5-3-6 *Modified Cutler-Beard Reconstruction*. Although the Cutler-Beard technique is versatile and applicable to many large defects, secondary procedures following the separation of the flap are common. These procedures may include correction of lower eyelid ectropion or placement of a mucous membrane graft along the upper eyelid margin to reduce irritation from skin, hair follicles, or scar tissue at the upper eyelid margin. Ectropion following Cutler-Beard reconstruction is usually repaired from the posterior, inferior fornix approach, using advancement of the inferior retractor muscle layer.

A modification of the Cutler-Beard reconstruction may avoid these complications (Fig. 5-7A). The modified Cutler-Beard procedure emphasizes the importance of replacing upper eyelid tarsus using the full vertical height of the lower lid tarsus. The traditional technique preserves lower eyelid tarsus rather than using it for the upper eyelid defect. The modification begins with the excision of the uppermost tip of the external lamella, including the cilia. Next, the external lamella (skin, orbicularis) is separated from the internal lamella (tarsus, conjunctiva) at the remaining lower eyelid margin (Fig. 5-7B). The dissection is carried in a suborbicularis plane down to the inferior fornix. Next, the inferior retractors are released, creating a skin muscle flap and a separate tarsoconjunctival flap. The release of the retractors prevents ectropion of the lower eyelid. The tarsoconjunctival flap is advanced toward the defect of the upper eyelid (Fig. 5-7C). The flap is sutured in the standard method. Finally, the external lamellar defect of the upper eyelid is reconstructed by one of several methods. If enough redundant skin is present in the lower eyelid, the skin muscle flap can be brought superiorly to cover the previous tarsoconjunctival pedicle flap. In addition, an upper eyelid skin and muscle flap can be

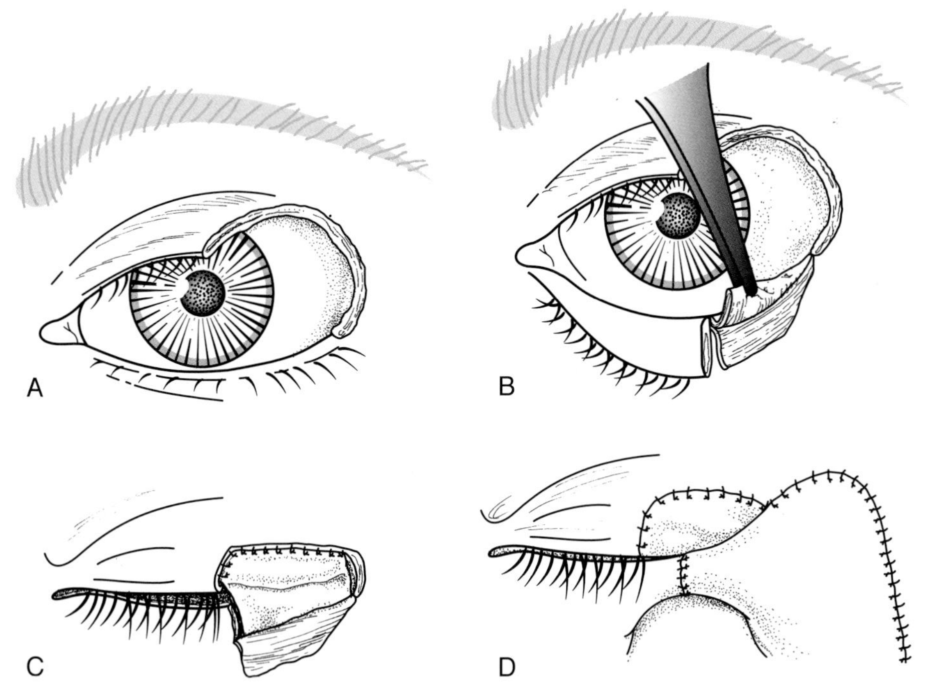

Figure 5-7 Modified Cutler-Beard reconstruction. (A) A partial upper eyelid defect can be reconstructed using the modified Cutler-Beard flap with full height of tarsus. (B) The tarsus and conjunctival flap from the lower eyelid is separated from the skin and orbicularis muscle. (C) The tarsoconjunctival flap is secured into the upper eyelid defect. (D) The lower eyelid defect can be closed over the skin–muscle flap by either primary closure or a Tenzel flap.

advanced and sutured to the lower eyelid tarsoconjunctival flap. This advancement flap can cover any remaining external lamellar defect. Alternatively, a rotational flap or skin graft can be used.

The modified Cutler-Beard procedure can be adjusted to repair partial upper eyelid defects of 50% to 100% (see Fig. 5-7A). The lower eyelid is prepared in the same manner as illustrated above. However, the section of lower eyelid to be recruited for a tarsoconjunctival flap is titrated for the amount of upper eyelid repair. By stretching the lower eyelid flap for the upper eyelid defect, a smaller segment of lower eyelid can be recruited in comparison to the upper lid defect. For example, a partial upper eyelid defect of 50% is repaired with a 30% to 40% lower eyelid tarsoconjunctival flap. With this modification, the lower eyelid defect can be primarily closed, and both upper and lower eyelid tarsus can be preserved.

The lower eyelid defect can be closed over the skin–muscle flap by either primary closure or a Tenzel flap (Fig. 5-7D).

This modification effectively substitutes a lower eyelid defect to reconstruct the original upper eyelid defect. It also uses available lower eyelid tarsus to substitute for the more important upper eyelid tarsus.

Secondary reconstruction for the upper eyelid is performed in a manner similar to a modified Hughes reconstruction in 6 to 8 weeks. The margin and upper portion of the lower eyelid will remain intact. The inferior portion of the lower eyelid is secondarily reconstructed by filling in the remaining defect using the incised pedicle.

5-4 OTHER PROCEDURES

5-4-1 *Full-Thickness Homograft.* A full-thickness en bloc section of tissue from the other upper eyelid may be transplanted into defects of the upper eyelid margin. The resection of the normal eyelid should be performed below the lid crease and should be done only when the remaining normal eyelid can be easily closed with direct closure. This technique is undesirable for patients who smoke, because smokers have a high incidence of graft contracture due to ischemia.

5-4-2 *Rotation of Lower Lid.* Rotation and inversion of the lower lid margin and tarsus into an upper lid defect provides good lid function as well as lashes for the upper eyelid. This procedure is best used, however, for large upper lid defects, and it necessitates complete reconstruction of the lower eyelid margin, using a lateral Mustarde cheek flap reconstruction combined with a hard palate or nasal chondromucosal rebuilding of the lower eyelid tarsus and conjunctiva.

The lower lid margin needed for upper lid reconstruction is outlined laterally, and a horizontal full-thickness incision is made inferiorly in the lower eyelid flap. The lateral aspect of the lower eyelid is then advanced medially through the use of a lateral Mustarde flap. The lower eyelid margin is then inverted and sutured into the upper lid defect. The lower lid rotation is closed medially, and the lateral aspect of the new lower lid margin is backed with a nasal chondromucosal composite graft or a hard palate graft. The bridge adjoining the upper and lower lids is separated after 6 to 8 weeks. Although some surgeons use this technique with success, it is cumbersome and requires both lower eyelid construction and lateral facial advancement.

5-5 FULL-THICKNESS LOSS OF UPPER AND LOWER LIDS

When a full-thickness defect includes the entire upper and lower eyelids, the goal of reconstruction becomes preservation of the globe by complete coverage with mucous membrane and skin tissue. Usually, sufficient conjunctiva is available on the bulbar surface to allow undermining and reflection over the corneal surface. The reflected bulbar conjunctiva inferiorly is sutured to the reflected conjunctiva superiorly. This can then be covered with a full-thickness skin graft or a rotation flap from the lateral face or mid-forehead. After maturation of the tissue, a small opening can be made to permit central corneal vision. Because the upper and lower eyelids are immobile, only a small palpebral fissure should be created to minimize the risk of lagophthalmos and exposure.

If available bulbar conjunctiva is insufficient to cover the globe, full-thickness buccal mucous membrane may be grafted to the posterior surface of the lateral cheek or midline forehead flap to provide a mucosal lining for the globe.

When ample conjunctiva with a good blood supply is available, the reflected mucosal covering may be adequate to support full-thickness skin grafting externally as an alternative to larger flap rotations.

SUGGESTED READINGS

Bergin DJ, McCord CD. Reconstruction of the upper eyelid: major defects. In: Hornblass A, ed: *Oculoplastic, Orbital and Reconstructive Surgery*. Baltimore: Williams & Wilkins, 1988; 1:605–617.

Cahill K, Burns JA. Reconstruction of the upper eyelid: moderate defects. In: Hornblass A, ed: *Oculoplastic, Orbital and Reconstructive Surgery*. Baltimore: Williams & Wilkins, 1988; 1:618–623.

Mauriello JA Jr, Antonacci R. Single tarsoconjunctival flap (lower eyelid) for upper eyelid reconstruction ("reverse" modified Hughes procedure). *Ophthalmic Surg*. 1994;25:374–378.

McCord CD, Wesley R. Reconstruction of the upper eyelid and medial canthus. In: McCord CD, ed: *Oculoplastic Surgery*, 2nd ed. New York: Raven Press, 1986; 8:175–188.

6

Reconstruction of Canthal Defects

C. ROBERT BERNARDINO, MD, FACS

Reconstruction of the medial and lateral canthal region can be quite challenging because in these two regions, soft tissue (canthal tendons) interacts directly with bony tissue to determine the location and function of the eyelids. Poor knowledge of the anatomy in these regions or poor surgical technique and planning can lead to poorly functioning eyelids in both opening and closing as well as associated lacrimal drainage and pump deficiency and aesthetic asymmetry.

Tissue loss in these regions can be from many causes, including trauma, inflammation, and neoplasia. When dealing with malignant neoplasia, it is particularly important to ensure that surgical margins are free of tumor prior to reconstruction. Particularly in the medial canthus, incompletely excised lesions can spread deep into the orbit, into the periocular sinuses (ethmoid and maxillary), and down the nasolacrimal system. Therefore, excision with margin control (Mohs, frozen, or permanent sections) is warranted. When a tumor is heading toward the orbit, this author recommends margin control with permanent fixed tissue to ensure proper diagnosis. When tumor cannot be cleared with this technique an exenteration is offered.

Repair of the canthal regions involves first repairing deep structures and any bony defects with autologous or synthetic materials, followed by resuspending eyelid structures to a location analogous to their native location. If remnants of the canthal tendon are present, it can be sutured to periosteum, or sutured or wired to bone through drilled pilot holes. Other techniques may involve using titanium miniplates to fixate the soft tissue to bone. If canthal tendon is not present, periosteum of the orbital rim can be fashioned into a flap simulating a canthal tendon, or the tarsus of the eyelid can be split with one arm forming a new canthal tendon. No matter what technique is used, care must be taken to ensure the tendon or tendon substitute

Table 6-1 Different Reconstruction Modalities

Type	Advantage	Disadvantage
Secondary Intention	No surgery Can fill thick defects	Contraction may cause dystopia
Split-thickness skin graft	Low donor morbidity Can monitor recurrence	High contraction rate
Full-thickness skin graft	Good skin match	Donor site needs closure Thick grafts can necrose
Myocutaneous flap	Best skin match	Requires proper construction
Vascularized flap	Good for irradiated areas	May require secondary surgery to release flap

is fixed into the orbit, deeper than the orbital rim; failure to do so will cause the eyelids to function poorly.

Once deeper structures are restored, repair of the soft tissue must be undertaken. There are many different approaches to restoring soft tissue defects, from allowing defects to heal by secondary intention, to skin grafts, to skin–muscle flaps. These options are summarized in Table 6-1. Before deciding on a repair technique, there are many different things to consider. For example, can the patient tolerate additional surgeries? For patients who cannot, one might consider allowing the wound to granulate or repair with a skin graft, as flaps often require secondary procedures to release or thin flaps out. If the patient requires adjuvant radiotherapy, nonvascularized repairs such as skin grafts may fail. If there is a significant risk for recurrence, then thin grafts/flaps may be more appropriate since recurrences can be monitored below the new tissue; in these circumstances the author often uses split-thickness skin grafts so that any recurrence can be readily seen beneath the graft.

6-1 HEALING BY SECONDARY INTENTION

For canthal soft tissue defects, healing by secondary intention or granulation tissue is a reasonable solution. Healing takes multiple weeks but can often close a defect without any further intervention. It can also be used to close a large defect into a size that is much more manageable. Medial canthal defects often respond better than lateral canthal defects due to the concavity of the region. If canthal tendons are missing, this technique can also be used and has been coined the "laissez-faire method" by Fox and Beard. As scar contracts, it will pull the eyelids into the defect. However, eyelids can often misdirect during the contracture. The author recommends allowing contracture to occur until the eyelids become misdirected, then intervening with scar excision and reconstruction with a skin graft or flap. With this technique, a defect will close significantly, allowing for smaller follow-up surgery. However, adjuvant radiotherapy, if needed, must be delayed. Also, keratoconjunctivitis from exposure must be guarded against during the healing period.

6-2 SKIN GRAFTING

Split-thickness and full-thickness skin grafts work well in soft tissue reconstruction of both the medial and lateral canthi. Donor tissue should be selected based on color, texture, and thickness match. However, thickness of graft should also be considered in terms of both its ability to "take" and its ability to resist contraction, which are two opposing characteristics. Skin grafts revascularize mainly from their base; thinner grafts revascularize faster than thicker ones. However, thinner grafts often contract more than thicker ones. Fortunately at the canthi it is less of an issue. Contracture mostly causes horizontal displacement of the eyelids rather than vertical displacement at the canthi. However, some considerations must be taken into account when using a skin graft for reconstruction. As mentioned above, thin grafts such as split-thickness grafts are useful if the defect is at significant risk of recurrence. On the other hand, if postsurgical radiotherapy is anticipated, a skin graft is less than desirable. Good donor sites for full-thickness skin grafts include upper eyelids (upper blepharoplasty-type incision), retroauricular, supraclavicular, or inner arm. Grafts can be secured with sutures or tissue adhesive like fibrin glue. However, it is important to immobilize the grafts during the initial healing period (pressure dressings, Frost suturing of eyelids, and bolsters through the graft). This is especially important at the medial canthus, where the graft needs to be secured to the concave surface.

6-3 MYOCUTANEOUS FLAPS

Skin–muscle flaps have many advantages over skin grafts. They often have better tone, texture, and thickness match than skin grafts. Furthermore, since they have intrinsic vascular supply, the risk of failure and contracture is much less. However, flaps require careful construction, particularly when dealing with the canthi. To repair a defect with a flap, one must determine whether the flap will originate from adjacent tissue, as in an advancement or rotational flap, or from tissue more distant, and whether the flap will be based on an arterial supply such as the supraorbital, angular, or temporal artery. Basing the flap on a robust vascular supply allows for transposition of tissue to a distant location such as the contralateral side. It also most resists contracture and remains viable after postoperative radiotherapy. Finally, with advanced techniques, the bridging tissue for a distant flap can be left exposed for future splitting (usually 4 to 6 weeks after initial surgery), or tunneled beneath the skin surface.

6-4 MEDIAL CANTHAL RECONSTRUCTION

If the anterior limb of the medial canthal tendon is missing but the posterior limb is intact, usually soft tissue repair of the overlying tissue is sufficient. No additional reconstruction specific to the canthal tendon is necessary. However, if both limbs are missing, medial canthal reconstruction is necessary. Unlike the lateral canthal tendon, if a superior or inferior limb is present, the other eyelid cannot be sewn to the present limb; such wound closure would cause medial webbing or essentially a tarsorrhaphy.

6-4-1 *Laissez-Faire Method.* As mentioned above, healing by secondary intention is an acceptable alternative to surgical repair of a medial canthal defect. Granulation tissue forms in the base of the defect, often replacing lost tissue volume that skin grafting or other techniques do not address properly. The wound edges also contract circumferentially, which can be advantageous, as the loose ends of the eyelids will be drawn back toward the medial canthus. However, misdirected contracture can cause canthal dystopia with displacement of the canthus upward or downward or anterior. If this occurs, scar tissue should be excised and surgical resuspension of tissue performed.

6-4-2 *Tarsal Rotation/Replacement.* If the posterior limb of the tarsus is absent, one option is to create a tarsal flap to approximate to the posterior lacrimal crest. A vertical incision is made along the medial edge of the tarsus, leaving the eyelid margin intact. This tissue is rotated medially and used to replace the tendon. If not enough tarsus is present, sutures can be passed from the medial tarsus edge to the posterior lacrimal crest, and scar tissue should form along this pathway. A free tarsal graft can also bridge the graft. In this instance, the author prefers to release the lateral canthal tendon and slide the eyelids medially to address the tissue deficit (Fig. 6-1). Another option for lateral defects is to release the lid margin from one

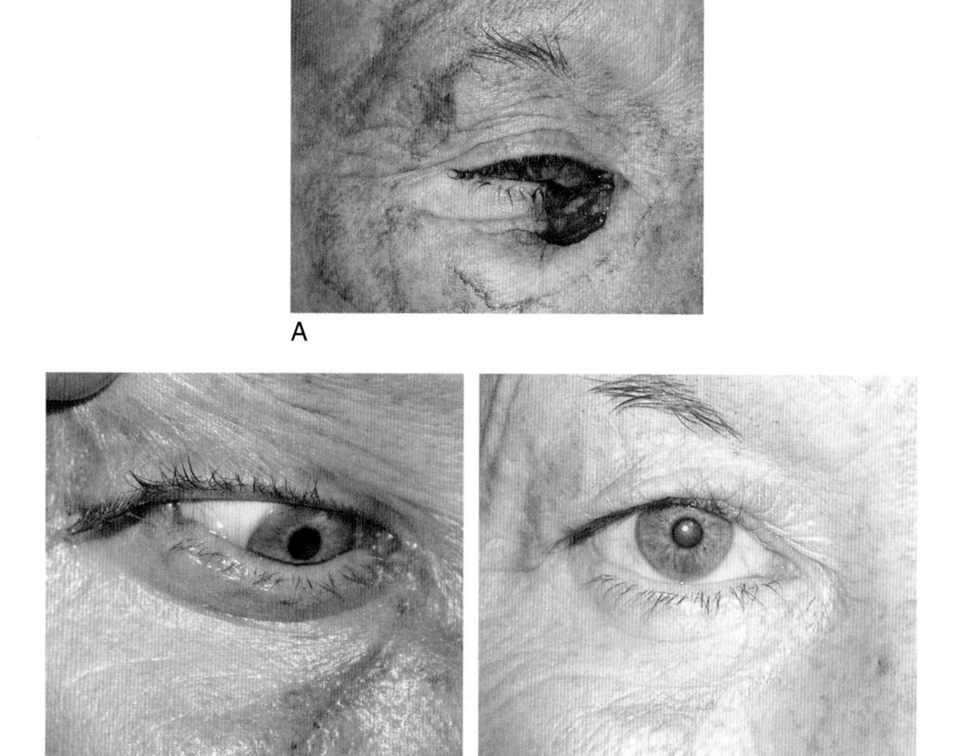

Figure 6-1 (A) Lower eyelid medial canthal defect after Mohs surgery. (B) One week after surgery; release of the lateral canthus to allow the eyelid to be advanced medially. New lateral defect repaired with a tarsoconjunctival flap from the upper eyelid. (C) Three months after surgery.

eyelid and rotate it into the defect of the other eyelid. Once they heal, the lids are split, forming a new lateral commissure and canthus (Fig. 6-2).

6-4-3 *Local Myocutaneous Flaps*. Flaps take tissue from one location and transpose it to another. Localized flaps have the advantage of taking nearby tissue that has similar thickness, color, and texture characteristics to repair a defect. There are many classic techniques that work well around the medial canthus. A V-Y plasty can recruit tissue medially and transpose it more laterally, or superiorly based glabellar tissue can be transposed inferiorly into a defect. Z-plasty and rhomboid flaps can recruit tissue inferiorly. However, these elegant flaps usually address only small defects. For larger defects cheek rotation flaps like the Mustarde can recruit larger amounts of tissue to repair larger defects (Fig. 6-3). However, since these are cheek-based, they can address only defects inferior to the medical canthus. Other bi-lobed or tri-lobed flaps can be fashioned to repair more superior defects. Other rotational flaps can even work across the nasal bridge.

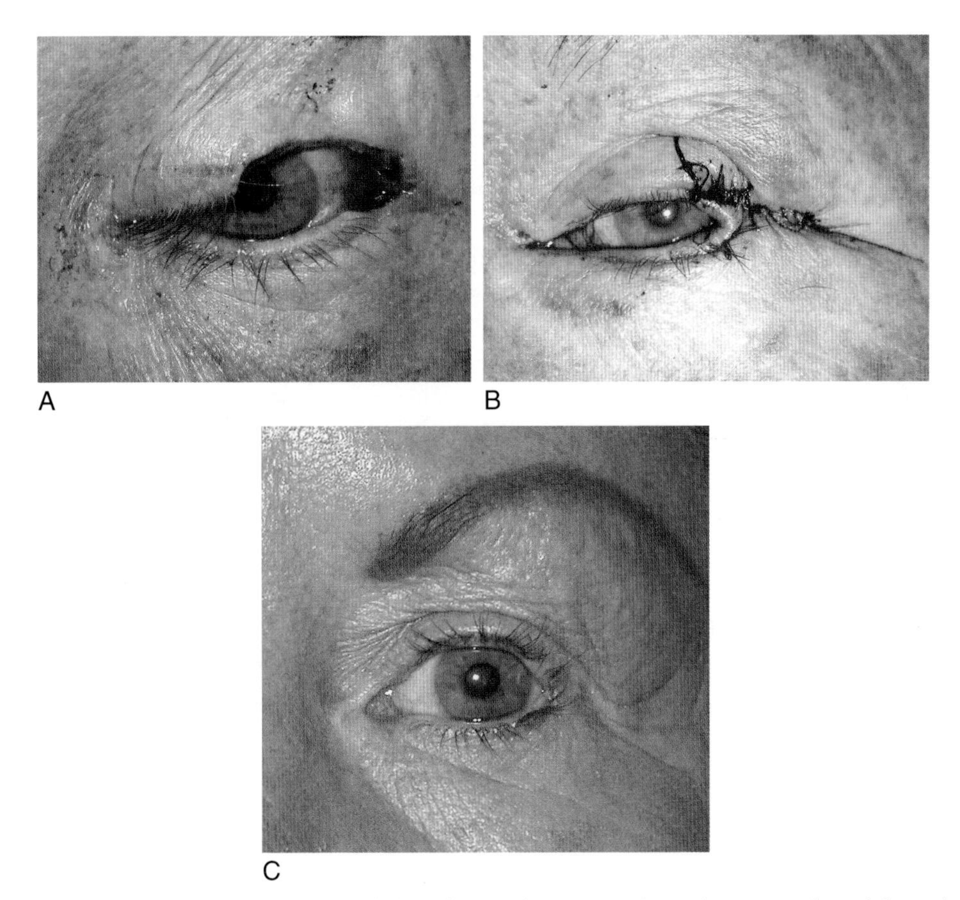

Figure 6-2 (A) Lateral upper eyelid defect after Mohs surgery. (B) Lid margin released from the lower eyelid rotated into the upper eyelid defect. (C) Three months after release of bridge between the eyelids and reformation of lateral commissure.

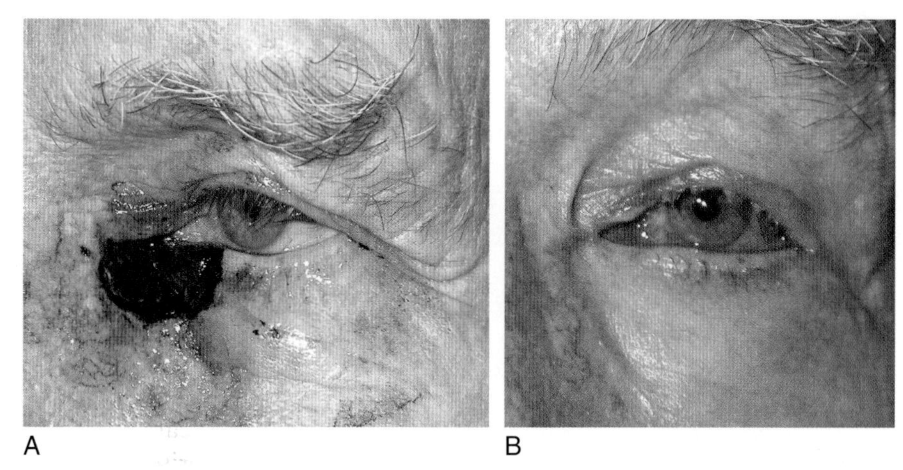

Figure 6-3 (A) Lower eyelid and medial canthal defect after Mohs surgery. (B) Three months after cheek rotational flap (Mustarde).

6-4-4 *Distant Myocutaneous Flaps.* Distant myocutaneous flaps can recruit tissue from nonadjacent tissue and transpose it to the defect. These flaps can be constructed based on a vascular supply or can rely on the intrinsic vasculature of the muscle layer of the flap. Non-vascular-based flaps commonly used in this area include upper eyelid (blepharoplasty), suprabrow, glabellar, and mid-forehead flaps. Care must be taken to keep the proximal portion of the flap as wide as the distal portion since the blood supply is supplied through the body of the flap as opposed to a defined blood vessel. Also, the flap must be kept thick for similar reasons; it may be thinned secondarily 4 to 6 weeks after the initial surgery.

Other flaps can be fashioned based on vascular supply. The most common is the supraorbital, although other vessels such as the angular or temporal arteries can be used. A vascularized flap can be transposed externally, in which case its bridge is bisected at a later date (Fig. 6-4), or tunneled subcutaneously, in which case it need not be bisected at all (Fig. 6-5). When dissecting the flap, the surgeon must guard against damaging the feeder vessel. However, with a robust vascular supply, it is the most appropriate for reconstruction of an irradiated site.

6-4-5 *Lacrimal Reconstruction.* Loss of tissue in the medial canthus will often involve the lacrimal drainage system. If possible, remnant tissue should be identified prior to reconstruction. If the canaliculi are intact, it is worthwhile to canulate and stent it with silicone tubing. However, if canalicular tissue is not present, dacryocystorhinostomy or other lacrimal drainage reconstructive procedures should be withheld for at least a year to ensure no recurrence of malignancy. Such surgery could lead to recurrent tumor invading the adjacent nasal cavity.

6-5 LATERAL CANTHAL RECONSTRUCTION

The lateral canthal region is defined by the lateral canthal tendon, which has two arms or crura, the superior and inferior. These arms, which originate in the eyelids,

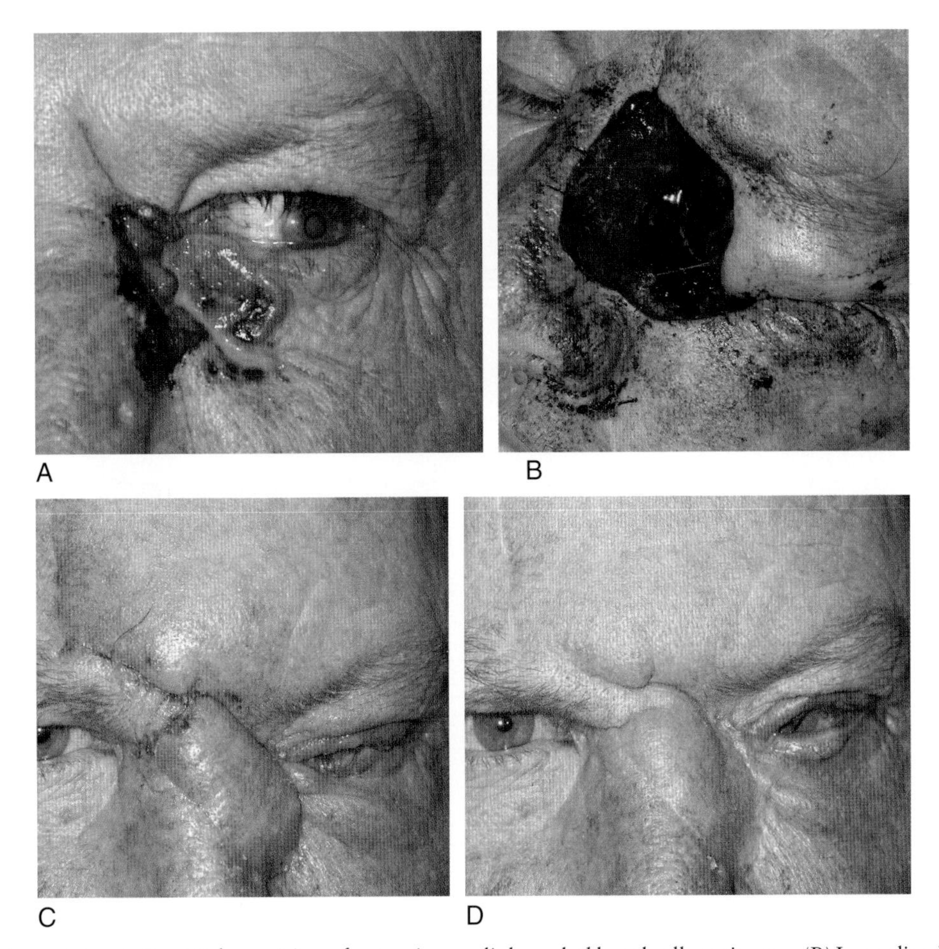

Figure 6-4 (A) Pre-Mohs excision of extensive medial canthal basal cell carcinoma. (B) Immediately after Mohs excision of large medial canthal tumor. (C) One week after right supraorbital forehead flap rotated into the left medial canthal region. (D) Three months after thinning of flap.

coalesce, forming the lateral commissure, which gives the lateral palpebral fissure its "almond" shape. The unified canthal tendon inserts posterior to the orbital rim on Whitnall's tubercle. The lateral canthal tendon is also superiorly displaced a few millimeters compared to the medial canthus.

6-5-1 *Laissez-Faire Method*. Healing by secondary intention is an option in this region. As the tissue contracts, the edges are often drawn into the canthal region. However, misdirection of the eyelid can happen if the contraction is misdirected; once this occurs, the scar should be excised and reconstruction with skin graft or flap should be performed.

6-5-2 *Tarsal Rotation/Replacement*. If the tarsus is missing laterally, tarsal rotation as described above can be employed to replace the posterior lamella and reconstruct the lateral canthal tendon. Another option is a free tarsal graft. For lower eyelid defects, a tarsoconjunctival or Hughes flap works well, although the flap requires a secondary surgery to release the vascularized conjunctival bridge. Another option

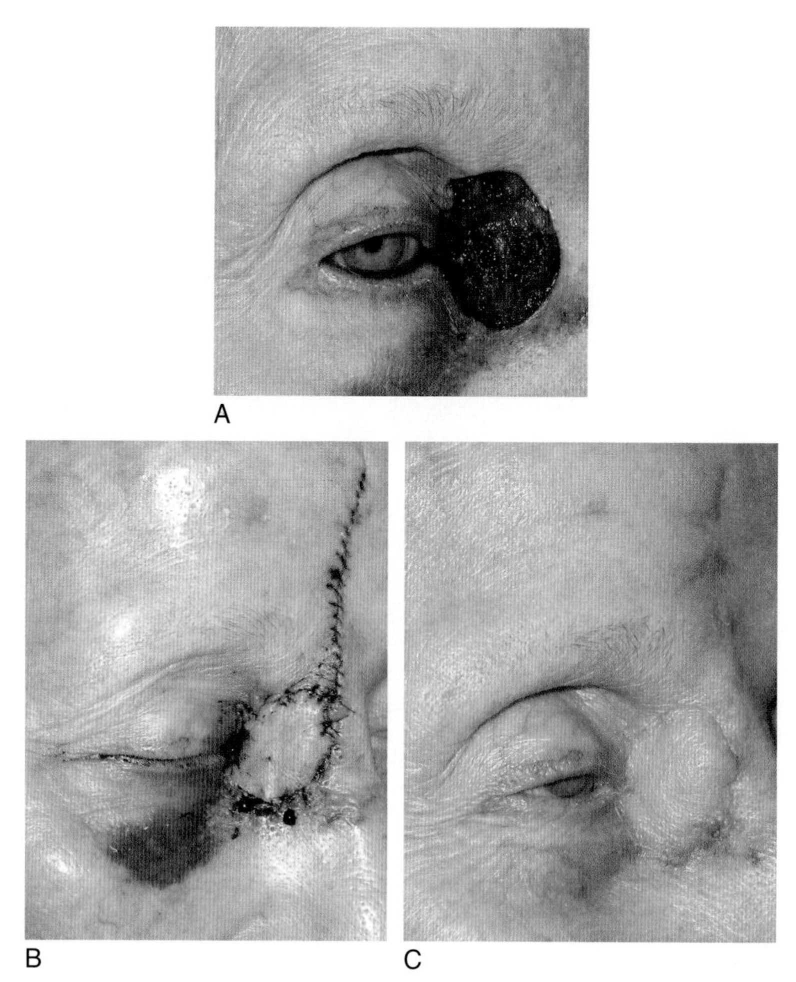

Figure 6-5 (A) Large medial canthal defect after Mohs excision. (B) Immediately after surgery, after island flap from mid-forehead. (C) One week after island flap to medial canthal defect.

is just to repair the anterior lamellar defect, and the posterior aspect of the tissue will re-epithelialize with conjunctiva. However, this sometimes leads to symblepharon. No matter what approach is taken, unlike the medial canthal tendon, the lateral commissure must be reformed by sewing the lateral portion of the lower eyelid to the upper.

6-5-3 *Local Myocutaneous Flaps*. Localized flaps work well here. Abundant tissue from the lateral cheek and forehead can serve as a donor site to the repair. Furthermore, scars from the flaps can often be hidden in naturally occurring wrinkles in the lateral rhytids. Classic rotational flaps include the Tenzel and the Mustarde in this region.

6-5-4 *Distant Myocutaneous Flaps*. Although localized flaps are usually adequate in this region, occasionally vascularized distant flaps are required, particularly if the region has been irradiated for malignancy. Superficial myocutaneous flaps based on branches of the temporal artery work well. In cases where a vascularized substrate is needed for reconstruction in conjunction with a skin graft, a temporalis fascial flap can be tunneled from the temporalis fossa under the skin into the lateral canthal region. This flap typically requires a coronal-type incision to gain access to the temporalis fascia.

6-5-5 *Late Canthal Reconstruction.* Longstanding medial and lateral canthal dystopia presents unique challenges in restoring normal anatomy. In general, release or removal of scar tissue is required, followed by deep fixation of tissue to periosteum or bone to ensure proper positioning of the overlying soft tissue. Vertically displaced canthal tissue can be repositioned with a Z-type plasty, while webbing is often addressed with a Y-V plasty. Anteriorly displaced canthal tissue requires deep fixation into the inner aspect of the orbital rim to ensure the eyelid has proper approximation to the globe.

6-6 CONCLUSION

Although medial and lateral canthal reconstruction can be challenging, proper preoperative planning can ensure success. Addressing the underlying structure of the canthal region, the tendons and the tarsus serve as the scaffolding for the overlying soft tissue. With these properly constructed, the canthal positioning should heal in correct anatomic position, leading to a good functional and cosmetic result.

SUGGESTED READINGS

Bostwick J 3rd, Vasconez LO, Jurkiewicz MI. Basal cell carcinoma of the medial canthal area. *Plast Reconstr Surg.* 1975 Jun;55(6):667–76.

Shore JW, Rubin PA, Bilyk JR. Repair of telecanthus by anterior fixation of cantilevered miniplates. *Ophthalmology.* 1992 Jul;99(7):1133–8.

Leibsohn JM, Hahn F. Medial canthal tendon recostruction with nasal periosteum. *Ophthal Plast Reconstr Surg.* 1992;8(1):35–40.

Fox SA, Beard C. Spontaneous lid repair. *Am J Ophthalmol.* 1964;58:947–952.

Leibovitch I, Huilgol SC, Hsuan JD, Selva D. Incidence of host site complications in periocular full thickness skin grafts. *Br J Ophthalmol.* 2005 Feb;89(2):219–22

Kersten RC, Anderson RL, Tse DT. Tarsal rotation flap for upper eyelid reconstruction. *Arch Ophthalmol.* 1986;104:918–922.

Moretti EA, Gomez Garcia F. Myocutaneous flap (V-Y design) from the nasal bridge for medial canthal reconstruction. *Ophthal Plast Reconstr Surg.* 1998 Jul; 14(4):298–301.

Sullivan TJ, Bray LC. The bilobed flap in medial canthal reconstruction. *Aust N Z J Ophthalmol.* 1995 Feb;23(1):42–8.

Custer PL. Trans-nasal flap for medial canthal reconstruction. *Ophthalmic Surg.* 1994 Sep-Oct;25(9):601–3.

Kilinc H, Bilen BT. Supraorbital artery island flap for periorbital defects. *J Craniofac Surg.* 2007 Sep;18(5):1114-9.

Field LM. The midline forehead island flap. *J Dermatol Surg Oncol.* 1987 Mar;13(3):243-6.

II

Eyelid Malpositions

7

Management of Entropion and Trichiasis

DAVID H. VERITY, MD, MA, FRCOPHTH;
GEOFFREY E. ROSE, BSC, MS, MRCP, FRCS, FRCOPHTH, DSC;
AND J. RICHARD O. COLLIN, MA, FRCS, FRCOPHTH, DO

Entropion is a posterior rotation of the upper or lower lid margin against the globe; the causes include involutional changes within the eyelid tissues or cicatricial shortening of the posterior lamella of the eyelid. Congenital lower lid entropion is rare and results from an excess of skin and orbicularis oculi muscle being only loosely attached to the eyelid retractors.

The symptoms of entropion—which include ocular irritation, lid spasm, pain, redness, and watering—are worse in the presence of a keratinized lid margin (occurring in cicatricial disease) and where the ocular surface is compromised. Discomfort may lead to secondary blepharospasm, which exacerbates the entropion by causing the preseptal part of the orbicularis muscle to override the pretarsal component.

7-1 MECHANISMS AND ASSESSMENT OF ENTROPION

The eyelids and globe should be examined to identify underlying causative factors—in particular the degree and position of tissue laxity, the position of the eyelid margin and lashes, and the thickness of the tarsus. Any secondary effects of entropion, both within the lid and on the ocular surface, should also be noted.

7-1-1 *Tissue Laxity.* Aging of collagen and the force of gravity leads to eyelid laxity and an excess of tissues, particularly the anterior lamella of the lid. Stretching of the orbicularis muscle and canthal tendons results in horizontal laxity, and eyelid stability is further compromised by enophthalmos due to age-related fat atrophy.

Where there is a relative dissociation between the anterior and posterior lamellae, the preseptal orbicularis muscle overrides the pretarsal muscle, leading to eyelid inversion, and this effect is exacerbated both by laxity of the lower lid retractors and age-related tarsal atrophy. Tissue laxity in the absence of orbicularis overriding tends to cause ectropion; with complete loss of retractor action, this can result in complete eversion of the tarsus ("shelf ectropion").

Horizontal laxity of the eyelid tissues is assessed by grasping the lid skin and applying gentle traction in the appropriate direction. The overall horizontal laxity is judged by the extent to which the eyelid can be parted from the globe—greater than about 6 mm is abnormal for a lower eyelid—and by the speed with which the retracted lid returns to the surface of the globe (the "spring-back" test). In a normal lid, the lid returns promptly to the globe, but where there is mild laxity, the lid does not return until the eyelid blinks. Weakness of the canthal tendons is manifest as excessive canthal movement, and the position to which the lacrimal puncta may be displaced is an indication of medial canthal tendon integrity; displacement beyond the pupillary line indicates extreme laxity which can only be addressed by plicating or shortening the medial canthal tendon.

Dissociation between the anterior and posterior lamellae is a significant factor in both upper and lower lid involutional entropion, and blepharospasm, resulting from the discomfort of entropion, exacerbates this effect. This relative vertical dissociation is seen as a movement of orbicularis and skin across the underlying tarsal plate and by the tissue crowding that occurs along the palpebral aperture during forced lid closure. The retractor function of both eyelids should be examined by observing the formation of a lower lid skin crease in down gaze and the definition and movement of the upper lid skin crease; significant dermatochalasis may also contribute to upper lid entropion.

7-1-2 *Tissue Scarring*. Cicatricial entropion is caused by scar tissue formation in the posterior (tarso-conjunctival) lamella, with secondary vertical shortening. Trachoma is the most common cause worldwide, but cicatricial entropion may be secondary to trauma (chemical—including drop preservatives—or thermal), chronic conjunctival inflammations (e.g., blepharo-conjunctivitis), and other acute or chronic inflammatory conjunctival diseases, such as Stevens-Johnson syndrome, ocular pemphigoid, or graft-versus-host disease. In all cases, active conjunctival inflammation should be managed medically (which may involve systemic immunosuppression) before surgery is considered.

The tarsus should be examined for subepithelial fibrosis, the degree of tarsal and/or marginal deformation or rotation should be noted, and the vertical height of the upper tarsus should be measured; less than 8 mm suggests significant tarsal shortening. Upper lid retraction should be recorded as the degree of scleral show between the upper corneal limbus and the upper lid margin, in both the primary position of gaze and in down gaze; a position about 1 to 2 mm below the upper limbus is normal.

Posterior lamellar shortening in the lower eyelid manifests as a vertical shortening of the lower fornix and increased inferior scleral show. Tarsal thickness may be assessed by the ease of horizontal deformation of the lid.

7-1-3 *Secondary Changes.* Entropion is associated with conjunctival migration over the eyelid margin—extending as far as, or beyond, the meibomian gland orifices. Other changes include misdirected or missing eyelashes, metaplastic lashes arising from meibomian glands, marginal telangiectases, and the formation of keratin near the eyelid margin. These changes are often secondary to the underlying disease and frequently lead to further compromise of the ocular surface. Examination of the tear film and corneal epithelium is therefore essential in the patient with an eyelid malposition.

7-2 PRINCIPLES OF SURGICAL CORRECTION OF ENTROPION

Surgery to correct an eyelid malposition should address the causative factors. Horizontal laxity, which is particularly common in lower lid entropion, may be corrected with a full-thickness wedge excision or—rather better—by refixation of the lateral canthal tendon to the orbital rim. Laxity of the canthal tendons—commonly associated with *ectropion*—may be corrected by tendon plication, resection, or refixation.

Dissociation between the two lamellae of the lids—a typical feature of entropion—is reduced by promoting scar-tissue formation between the anterior and posterior lamellae; this is achieved by placing transverse or everting lid sutures, or by any surgery that separates and reapposes the two lamellae. Horizontal shortening of the lower eyelid is often combined with placement of everting sutures, direct plication of the retractor fascia to the lower border of tarsus, or a vertical reduction of the anterior lamella (by skin–muscle blepharoplasty). The surgical approach to the upper lid depends upon several factors but usually involves separation and repositioning of the two lamellae, with disinsertion of the retractors to permit the posterior lamella to drop relative to the anterior lamella.

Cicatricial entropion is associated with vertical shortening of the tarso-conjunctiva and, in the upper lid, may lead to severe corneal disease. The secondary changes of entropion, such as keratin formation and metaplastic or misdirected eyelashes, generally affect the eyelid margin and exacerbate ocular surface disease. Conjunctival keratinization resolves, in some cases, with correction of eyelid malposition or with medical therapy, but persistent keratinization may be treated by recession of the posterior lamella or by eversion of the terminal tarsus. Aberrant lashes that are unaddressed by marginal eversion may be treated with cryotherapy or electrolysis, although such techniques cause further posterior lamellar scarring and, indirectly, increase the tendency to cicatricial entropion. Direct excision of lash follicles may be a preferred option.

7-3 CORRECTION OF LOWER LID INVOLUTIONAL ENTROPION

7-3-1 *Transverse Sutures.* Transverse sutures may provide an effective temporary measure—correcting entropion for some months—and are readily placed "at the bedside" in very debilitated patients; such sutures are more effective than nonsurgical methods such as lid-taping or injections of botulinum toxin.

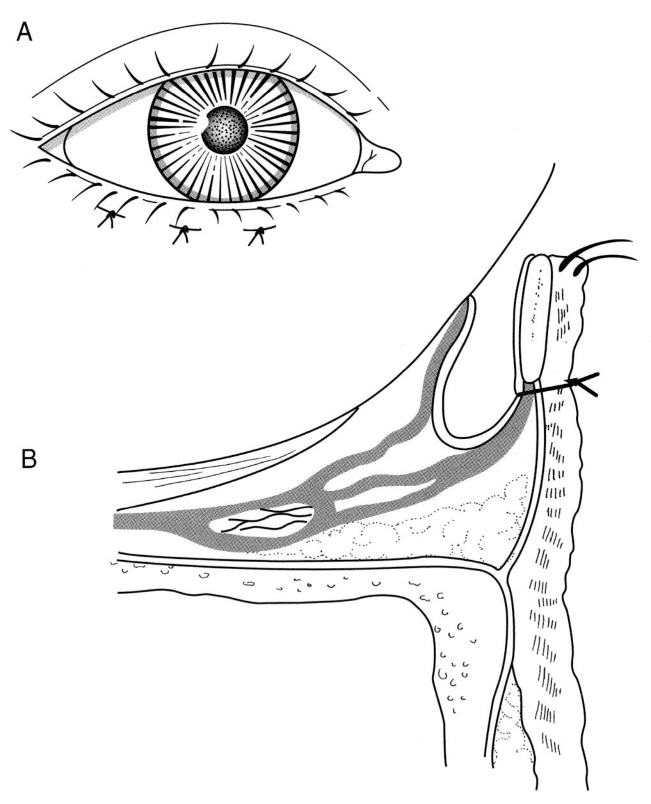

Figure 7-1 Transverse sutures. (A) Placement of transverse sutures. (B) Action of transverse sutures.

Transverse sutures prevent the preseptal orbicularis muscle from overriding the pretarsal component and are particularly indicated when entropion occurs with forced eyelid closure (Fig. 7-1). Three double-armed 4-0 absorbable sutures are passed through the eyelid from the conjunctival surface, just below the tarsus, and brought out through the skin just above the level at which they entered the conjunctiva. These sutures are tied tightly and left in place, although they may be removed if they result in an overcorrection.

Everting sutures are similar to transverse suture but are placed lower in the conjunctival fornix (to pick up the retractor action), then engage the lower border of the tarsal plate, and emerge through the skin closer to the lash line. This pathway through the eyelid causes a greater plication of the retractors and eversion of the lower eyelid, but the sutures are less effective in preventing overriding of the orbicularis muscle. Everting sutures are particularly useful in chronic entropion, where involutional changes are more advanced, and are often placed at the time of lateral canthal tendon refixation.

7-3-2 *Transverse Lid Split with Everting Sutures (Weis Procedure)*. In the Weis procedure, the lid is split transversely and closed with 4-0 absorbable sutures that pass through the conjunctiva, lower lid retractors, and skin (Fig. 7-2). This procedure is associated with a high rate of recurrence as it does not address horizontal laxity of the eyelid.

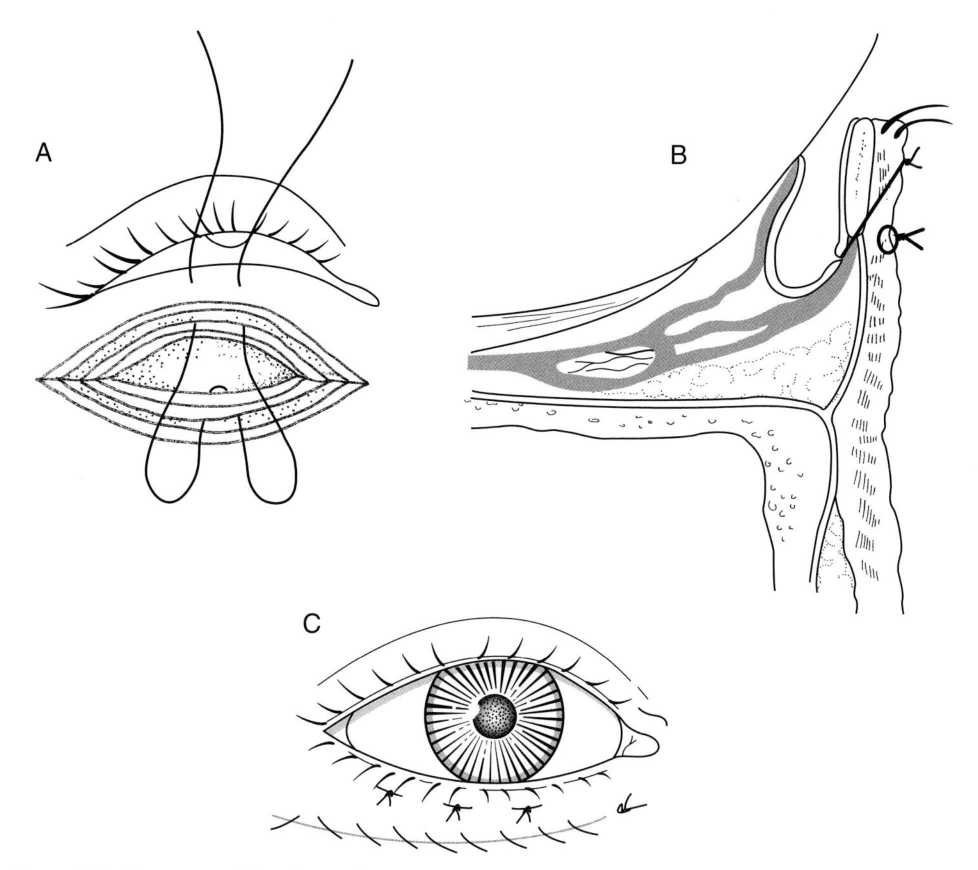

Figure 7-2 Transverse lid split with everting sutures (Weis procedure). (A) Placement of double-armed everting sutures. (B) Action of everting sutures across transverse lid split. (C) Closure with continuous or interrupted sutures.

7-3-3 *Transverse Lid Split, Everting Sutures, and Horizontal Lid Shortening (Quickert Procedure)*. If horizontal tarsal laxity is present but the lateral canthal tendon is intact, lower lid entropion may be corrected by horizontal tarsal shortening, with a transverse lid split and everting sutures (Fig. 7-3). This technique addresses all underlying causative factors, correcting the underlying horizontal laxity, preventing upward movement of the preseptal orbicularis, and stabilizing the tarsus by tightening the lower lid retractors.

A vertical full-thickness eyelid incision is made about 5 mm medial to the lateral canthus and is continued to the lower border of the tarsus. Straight scissors are used to form a horizontal full-thickness cut toward the medial aspect of lid, just below the tarsus, to the level of the lower punctum; a similar horizontal incision is made laterally. The two flaps of eyelid tissue are overlapped, and an appropriate amount of full-thickness eyelid is resected. A standard repair of the tarsus and lid margin is performed and three double-armed absorbable 4-0 everting sutures are placed. The skin should be closed prior to tying the everting sutures so that the final lid position can be adjusted (to a very slight eversion) by the tension in the everting sutures. Where there is excess skin below the horizontal lid incision, the skin incision

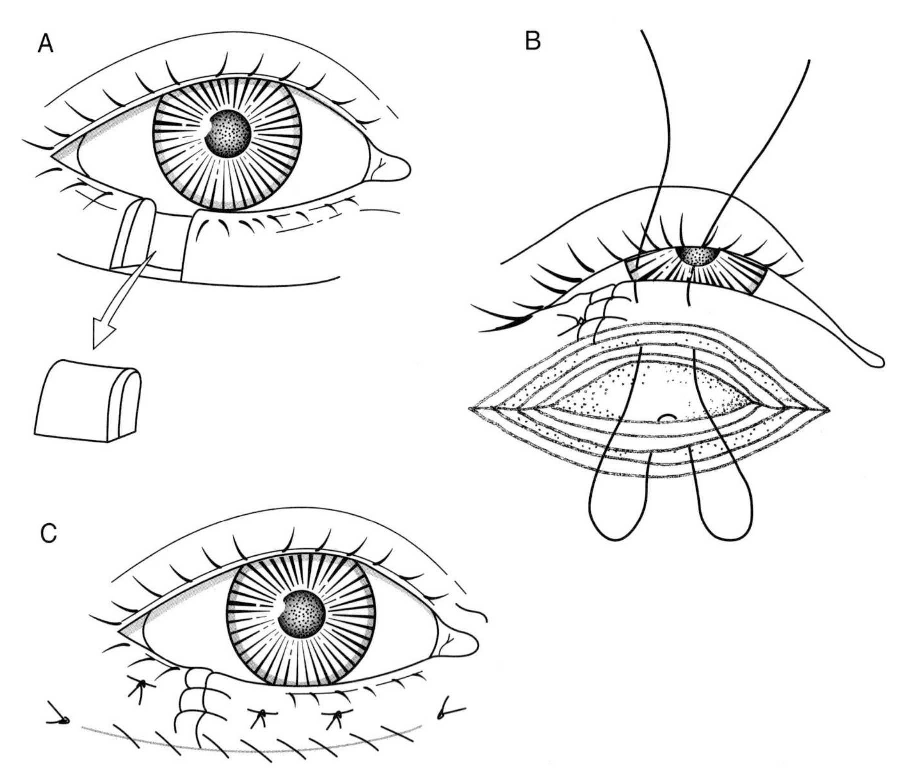

Figure 7-3 Transverse lid split, everting sutures, and horizontal lid shortening. (A) Vertical and horizontal incisions made, lid flaps overlapped, and excess tissue resected. (B) Flaps sutured and everting sutures positioned. (C) The skin of the horizontal lid incision is closed with running or interrupted sutures.

can be extended laterally and the excess skin resected; a subciliary blepharoplasty incision is, however, preferable where a skin excess is identified preoperatively.

7-3-4 *Lateral Canthal Tendon Refixation ("Lateral Canthal Sling," "Lateral Tarsal Strip")*. When there is significant laxity of the lateral canthal tendon, entropion may be corrected by fixing the tendon to the periosteum within the lateral orbital rim, and may also be combined with everting sutures. This procedure is both quick and reliable, does not disrupt the lid margin, and results in practically no scarring, although it occasionally results in distortion of the outer canthus or trichiasis. Care should be taken in patients with prominent globes as overtightening of the lower lid, or a low fixation on the orbital periosteum, may lead to lower lid retraction and inferior scleral show.

The lateral canthal sling requires a slightly oblique lateral canthotomy, together with lower cantholysis to allow sufficient horizontal displacement to correct horizontal lid laxity. An 8-mm strip is fashioned from the lateral tarsus, taking care to remove all adnexal elements, including the lid margin. A 2- to 3-mm gray line split is made in the upper lid to improve elevation of the lower lid. By blunt dissection at a level 2 to 3 mm higher than the lateral tubercle, the periosteum is exposed just inside the lateral orbital rim and a double-armed 5-0 absorbable suture is passed through the periosteum of the inner aspect of the rim; this creates a loop through which the strip is placed, with the needles being passed through the strip on either side of the loop (Fig. 7-4). Traction on both ends of the suture draws the

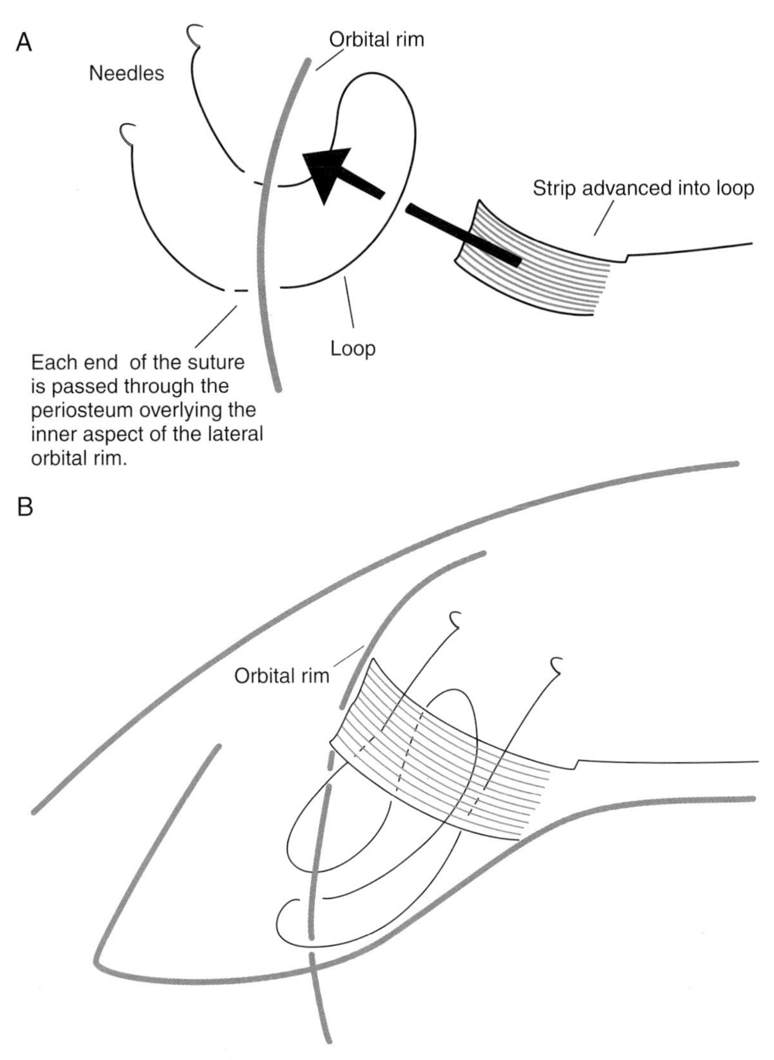

Figure 7-4 Lateral canthal sling. (A) The periosteum is exposed just inside the lateral orbital rim and a double-armed 5-0 absorbable suture is passed through the periosteum of the inner aspect of the rim. (B) This creates a loop through which the strip is placed, with the needles being passed through the strip on either side of the loop.

tarsal strip tightly down onto the periosteum, and the knot binds the loop down onto the tarsal strip. If everting sutures are required, these are most readily placed before tightening the tarsal strip. The lateral canthal angle is then reformed by placing a 6-0 absorbable suture through the gray line of the upper and lower lids, with the knot buried within the incision, and a lash line suture is placed. Any vertical or horizontal excess of the anterior lamella of the lower lid should then be resected (as for standard blepharoplasty), the orbicularis muscle is closed with deep fixation to the free end of the tarsal strip, and the skin is closed with a 6-0 or 7-0 suture.

7-3-5 *Lateral Canthopexy.* When there is a mild degree of lateral canthal or horizontal laxity, the limbs of the lateral canthal tendon may be plicated or reinserted *en bloc* directly into the periosteum of the inner aspect of the lateral orbital wall. This may be achieved via a short horizontal incision immediately lateral to the outer canthus, with the advantage that reformation of the lateral canthus is not required and there is no risk of misdirected lashes at the outer canthus. Everting sutures may also be placed.

7-3-6 *Plication of the Lower Lid Retractors (Jones Procedure)*. Tarsal instability due to poor action of the lower lid retractors may result in recurrent entropion, despite horizontal shortening of the lower eyelid. When such a recurrence occurs, it may be effectively addressed by the Jones procedure (Fig. 7-5), and this cutaneous approach has an important role when a conjunctival approach should be avoided—as with chronic cicatricial conjunctivitides (e.g., ocular pemphigoid).

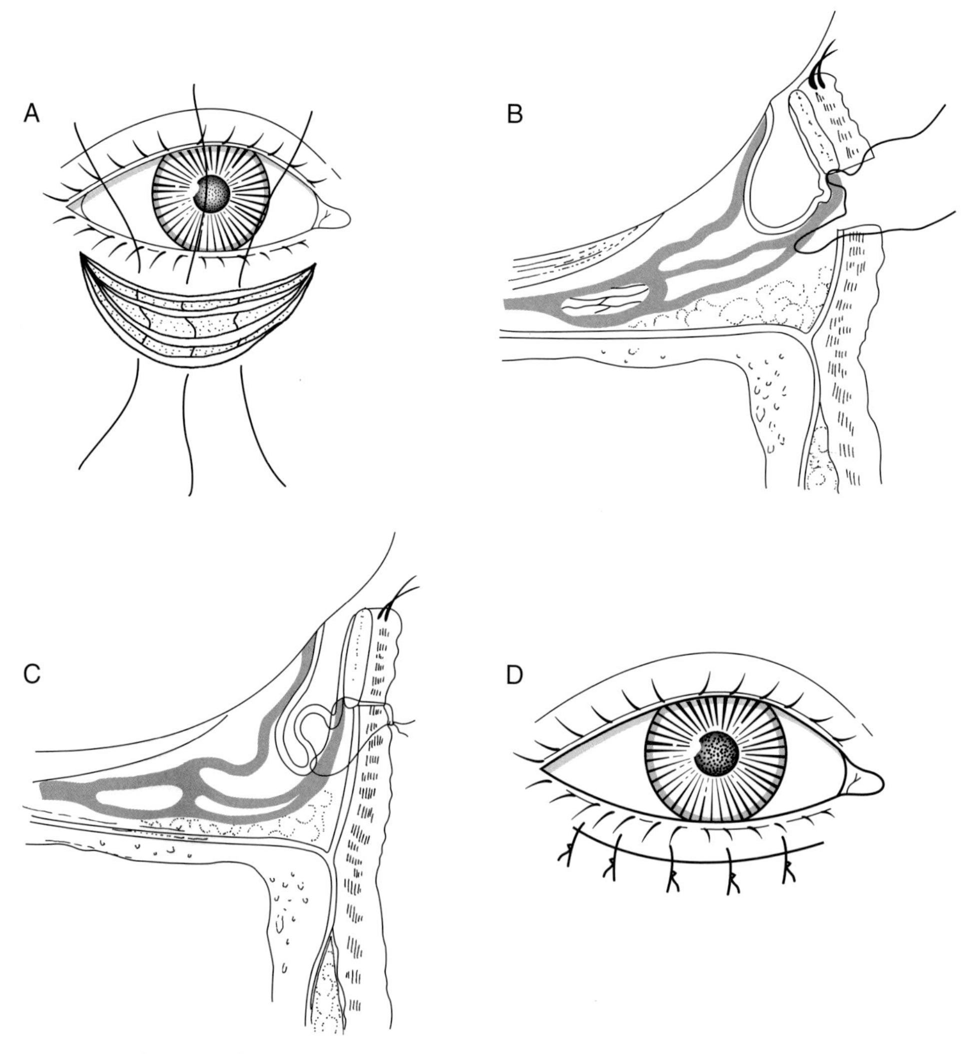

Figure 7-5 Plication of retractors. (A) Placement of plicating sutures. (B) Degree of retractor plication can be graded during surgery. (C) Action of plicating sutures when tightened. (D) Incision is closed.

The lower lid retractors can be approached directly by a horizontal skin–muscle incision 4 mm below the lash line or indirectly through a subciliary blepharoplasty approach. The retractors are exposed by opening the orbital septum beneath the lower lid tarsus and above the lower lid fat pad; the position of the retractor fascia may be confirmed by asking the patient to look up and down.

At the middle of the lid, a 5-0 absorbable suture is passed through the skin edge below the incision, into the lower lid retractors about 8 mm below the tarsus, into the lower border of the tarsal plate, and out through the skin edge above the incision; the suture is tightened to achieve a minor degree of eversion of the eyelid margin. If excessive lower lid eversion or retraction occurs, a smaller plication is performed—that is, the suture is replaced more anteriorly through the retractors. Once the correct position has been achieved, one or more similar sutures are placed on either side of the central suture. These sutures shorten (plicate) the lower lid retractors and also prevent the orbicularis from overriding; they may be removed after 10 to 14 days, or earlier if there is overcorrection or excessive lower lid retraction.

7-4 CORRECTION OF CICATRICIAL ENTROPION OF THE LOWER EYELID

7-4-1 *Tarsal Fracture Procedure*. Tarsal fracture, of value for mild cicatricial entropion of the lower lid, involves a horizontal split in the tarsal plate that permits marginal eversion of the lid, with healing by secondary intention that leads to lengthening of the posterior lamella.

An incision is made horizontally through the posterior aspect of the tarsal plate but not through the overlying orbicularis muscle. A moderate degree of lid retraction is corrected by placing double-armed 5-0 absorbable sutures just below the inferior tarsal fragment; they are brought out just below the lash line. These sutures are tied so as to evert the tarsus margin along this "hinge" and may be removed after 2 to 3 weeks.

7-4-2 *Posterior Lamellar Graft*. Greater degrees of lower lid retraction, as with more than 1.5 mm of inferior scleral show, generally require posterior lamellar grafting; suitable materials include hard palate or buccal mucosa, nasal septal chondromucosa, or ear cartilage. Allogenic grafts include amniotic membrane (which has been used with some success in severe cicatricial conjunctival disease) or acellular human cadaveric dermal matrix. To allow for postoperative contraction, most grafts should be oversized by about 50% in the vertical dimension.

Using a 7-0 absorbable suture, the graft should be fixed between the lower tarsal border and the conjunctival edge; the conjunctiva (fused with the septum and retractors at this point) is dissected free from the overlying orbicularis muscle to allow the graft to settle properly into its host site. Three double-armed 5-0 absorbable sutures are passed through the graft from the conjunctival surface and tied on small cutaneous bolsters. These sutures slightly evert the eyelid margin and also approximate the graft to its vascular bed. The bolstered sutures are removed at 7 to 10 days.

7-4-3 *Gray Line Split and Retractor Repositioning.* This technique is useful when lower lid cicatricial entropion is associated with significant trichiasis. Using a featherblade, a gray line split is made to a depth of 3 mm immediately anterior to the meibomian gland orifices and behind the misdirected eyelashes. A horizontal incision through the skin and orbicularis is made 4 mm beneath the lash line, and the septum is opened to expose the lower lid retractors. The anterior aspect of the tarsus is exposed and three or four double-armed 5-0 absorbable sutures are passed through the retractors and brought out through the pretarsal orbicularis and skin, just beneath the lash line. The sutures are tied to evert the lower lid margin, taking care not to cause eyelid retraction, and the skin incision is closed. The sutures are removed at 2 weeks, or earlier if there is a significant overcorrection.

7-5 CORRECTION OF CONGENITAL LOWER LID ENTROPION

In epiblepharon, which is common among Asian children, there is a medial fold of excess lower lid skin and orbicularis muscle; if this fold causes inversion of the lid margin, a true lower lid congenital entropion results. As epiblepharon usually improves with age, it requires treatment only if there are marked signs of corneal irritation. The excess anterior lamella is excised as a horizontal crescent of skin and muscle, and the repairing skin sutures are attached deeply to the inferior tarsal border and lower lid retractors. To maintain symmetry, bilateral surgery is usually performed.

7-6 CORRECTION OF UPPER LID ENTROPION

Upper lid entropion is typically due to cicatricial changes within the posterior (tarsoconjunctival) lamella, and surgery is therefore directed toward lengthening this lamella, recessing the anterior lamella on the posterior, and eversion of the abnormal eyelid margin.

7-6-1 *Transfixation Sutures.* Transfixation (Pang) sutures provide temporary relief from lash ptosis and minor degrees of upper lid entropion and are of particular value when dermatochalasis is evident. Their placement is analogous to that of lower lid transverse sutures, with double-armed 4-0 absorbable sutures passed from the conjunctival surface, above the upper tarsus, into a predetermined upper lid skin crease.

7-6-2 *Anterior Lamellar Reposition* Mild upper lid entropion, in which the lashes are not abrading the cornea, may be corrected by separating the two lamellae and shifting the anterior lamella upward on the posterior; this is achieved through a skin-crease incision, with separation of the skin and orbicularis muscle from the underlying tarsus, down to the level of the lash roots. The lamellae are reapposed using long-acting 6-0 absorbable sutures, which are passed through the skin immediately above the eyelashes, into the tarsal plate at a higher level, and out through the skin again. In all but the mildest cases, the posterior lamella should also be lengthened by dividing the insertion of the aponeurosis from the anterior tarsal surface, with the extent of retractor disinsertion depending on the severity of the entropion. Greater eversion of the eyelash margin is achieved by splitting the lid margin along the gray line with a feather blade to a depth of 1 to 2 mm before repositioning the anterior lamella. This incision heals very effectively by granulation and should therefore be deep enough at the medial and lateral ends, where entropion is likely to recur. A 2- to 3-mm block of anterior lamella bearing lash follicles may also be excised to reduce the risk of recurrent lash inversion. The small excess of redundant anterior lamella above the skin crease is excised, and the skin is closed with 6-0 or 7-0 absorbable sutures; the crease is reformed at the desired height with inclusion of the aponeurosis in the deep pass of the sutures.

7-6-3 *Tarsal Wedge Resection.* If the entropion is severe and the tarsus is thickened due to scarring, greater eversion may be achieved by excising a horizontal wedge of anterior tarsal plate in addition to an anterior lamellar reposition with gray-line split (Fig. 7-6). Care must be taken not to extend the wedge through to the conjunctival surface. As closure of the tarsal wedge tends to exacerbate posterior lamellar retraction, this is countered by adequate recession of the upper lid retractors. Long-acting absorbable 6-0 sutures are used to close the wedge and evert the lashes, and the skin is closed as described above.

7-6-4 *Lid Split, With or Without Mucous Membrane Graft.* With severe upper lid entropion in the absence of tarsal thickening, the eyelid may be completely separated into two lamellae to permit a radical recession of the anterior lamella (containing in-turning lashes) on the posterior lamella. Care must be taken to separate the two layers *posterior* to all aberrant lashes, and the lamellar division is continued up the anterior surface of the tarsus to its upper border, at which point the Müller's muscle is disinserted. The plane of dissection is continued between Müller's muscle and conjunctiva until the posterior lamella can be freely advanced on the conjunctiva alone. The anterior lamella is recessed to about 4 mm above the posterior lamellar margin, and the two layers are sutured together with double-armed 4-0 absorbable sutures passed through the conjunctiva and tied over the skin at the intended position for the skin crease. The lash-bearing margin of the anterior lamella is sutured to the face of the posterior lamella with absorbable 6-0 or 7-0 sutures; the 4-mm margin of advanced posterior lamella can either be left to granulate or be covered with a graft of conjunctiva or oral mucous membrane (Fig. 7-7).

Any tarsal lashes persisting after lamellar division may be treated by direct excision, or by electrolysis. Cryotherapy may be used but carries the risks of further scar formation or tarsal necrosis.

7-6-5 *Rotation of Terminal Tarsus (Trabut Procedure).* If the lid margin in contact with the globe is keratinized or has a large number of metaplastic lashes, a horizontal bar of terminal tarsus may be rotated anteriorly, away from the globe. A marked loss of eyelashes can occur with this procedure and, as the aesthetic result may be worse than lid-splitting techniques, it should not be undertaken unless specifically indicated.

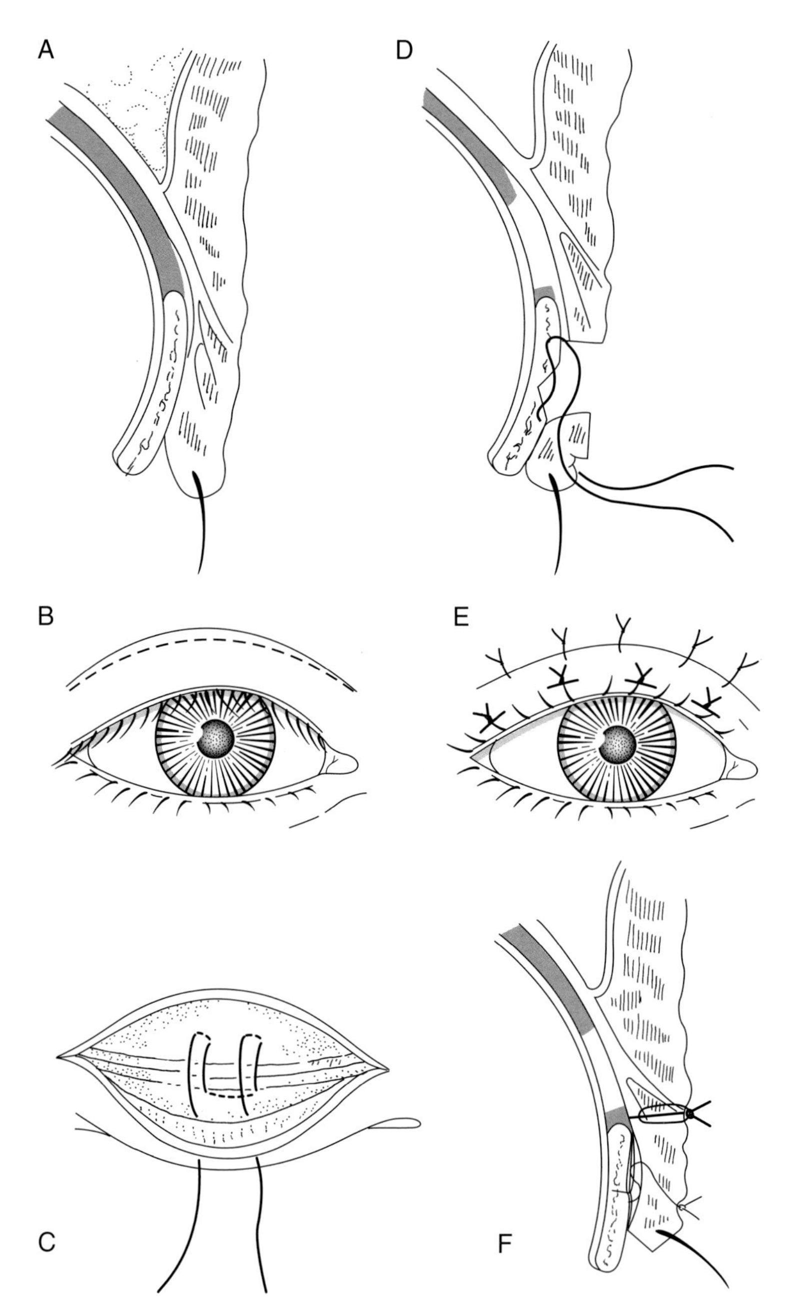

Figure 7-6 Tarsal wedge resection. (A) Side view showing gray-line incision. (B) Skin crease incision, exposing tarsus. (C) Placement of double-armed everting sutures. (D) Side view of everting sutures over tarsal wedge. (E) Action of everting sutures, and incision closure. (F) Side view of closure and everting sutures.

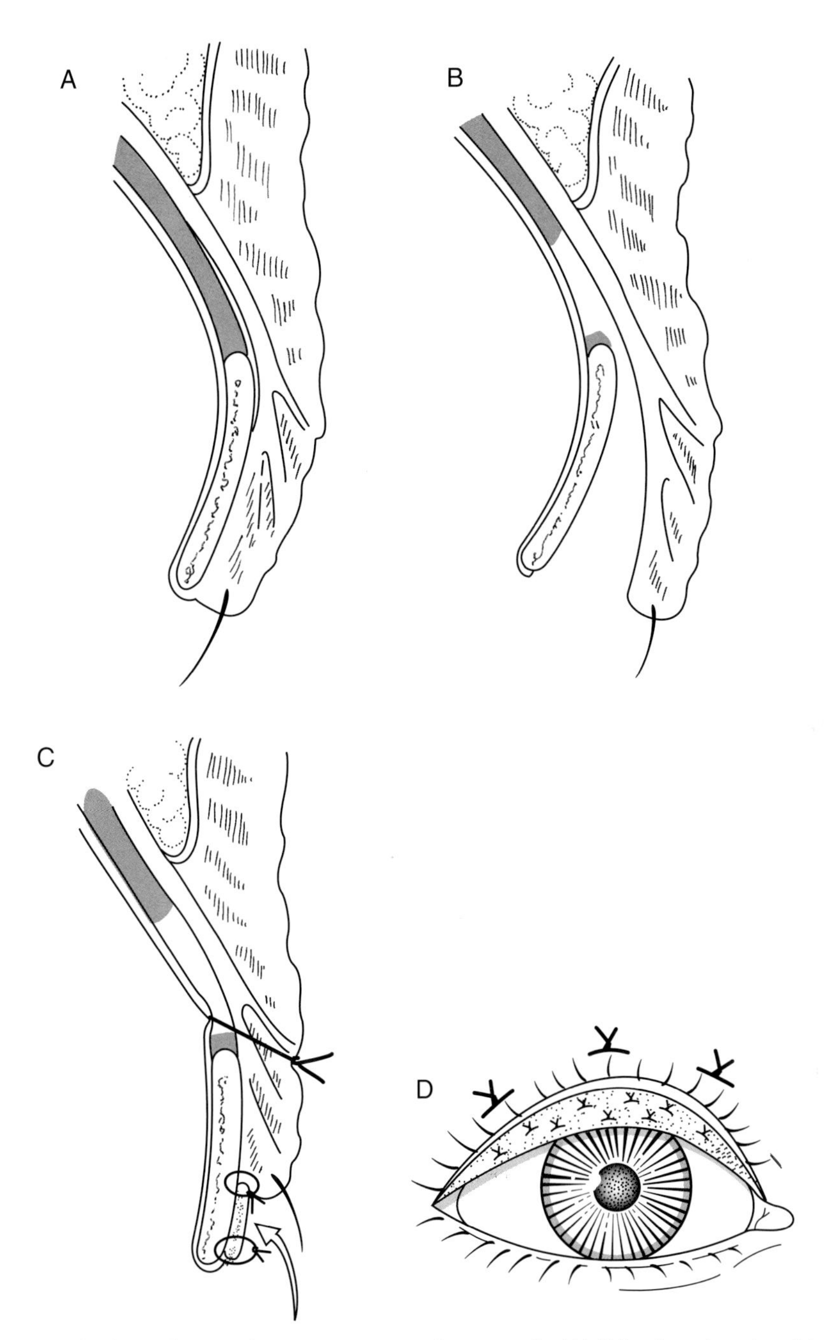

Figure 7-7 Lid split with or without mucous membrane graft. (A) Side view showing thin tarsus. (B) Separation of skin–muscle lamella from tarsal plate, and retractor recession. (C) Anterior lamella fixed in recession on tarsal plate. (D) Anterior view of lamellar fixation sutures, and mucous membrane graft.

The upper eyelid is everted and a tarsal incision is made just above the keratinized conjunctiva; the cut is extended vertically through the lid margin at the lateral canthus and just lateral to the upper punctum, to permit 180-degree eversion of the terminal bar after adequate undermining. The posterior lamella is freely advanced by disinserting the upper lid retractors and separating Müller's muscle from conjunctiva. The two lamellae are then reapposed with three double-armed 4-0 absorbable sutures, which pass through the lid from the conjunctival surface of the superior fornix to the intended skin crease, and the everted terminal fragment of tarsus is sutured to the underlying tarsal plate using interrupted, long-acting 6-0 or 7-0 absorbable sutures.

7-6-6 *Posterior Lamellar Graft*. If upper eyelid retraction is sufficient to cause marked (>5 mm) lagophthalmos on forced eyelid closure, the above measures are unlikely to be adequate and a stiff, mucosal-lined graft may be required to lengthen the posterior lamella.

The upper lid tarsus is everted, incised, and undermined as described above and the tarsal fragment is externally rotated through 180 degrees to evert the lashes. A suitable graft is sutured to the recessed upper eyelid retractors using long-acting 6-0 absorbable sutures. Care is taken to position the knots away from the ocular surface (under the orbicularis muscle), and the graft is pleated to the undersurface of the anterior lamella using 6-0 sutures tied on the skin surface. Suitable graft tissues include hard palate mucosa, or nasal cartilage with muco-perichondrium.

7-7 TREATMENT FOR TRICHIASIS

Trichiasis refers to eyelashes that either originate from an abnormal site (metaplastic lashes or distichiasis) or are directed abnormally. If the eyelid margin is abnormally positioned, this should be corrected, but otherwise a small number of aberrant lashes can be treated with electrolysis. A single area of trichiasis can be managed with a local gray-line split and full-thickness excision of the abnormal anterior lamella, or by a full-thickness pentagon excision of the eyelid; cryotherapy is the treatment of choice for more extensive areas of trichiasis, except with darker skins, where there can be a marked loss of pigmentation.

7-7-1 *Lash Root Exposure and Direct Ablation*. Although time-consuming, direct destruction of the lash follicles is effective if the number of aberrant lashes is small. The lid is everted and a meibomian clamp is placed over the aberrant lash. A partial-thickness vertical incision is made, exposing the lash root, which is destroyed directly with electrolysis or cautery. To allow direct destruction, care should be taken to expose adequately the lash bulb if further tarsal scarring and entropion is to be avoided.

7-7-2 *Cryotherapy*. Lid tissues vary in their sensitivity to cryotherapy: although skin is relatively resistant to tissue freezing, lash and hair follicles are more sensitive than epithelial cells but less sensitive than melanocytes. Cryotherapy carries a risk of permanent depigmentation in dark-skinned individuals, who may therefore be better treated with a combination of electrolysis and entropion surgery.

Abnormal lash follicles may be destroyed by freezing to –20°C; the optimal effect is achieved by rapid freezing, slow thawing, and a repetition of the freeze–thaw cycle. A specially designed cryoprobe should be used and the eye protected with a plastic lid guard. Monitoring of tissue temperatures with a thermocouple is desirable, particularly in pigmented individuals, and complete thawing of the tissues between cycles is important.

7-7-3 *Lid Split and Cryotherapy.* Distichiasis is a rare hereditary condition in which a second row of eyelashes arises from the meibomian gland orifices. In the lower lid, the simplest treatment is to destroy both rows of lashes with cryotherapy. In the upper lid the rows of normal lashes should be saved, if possible. One technique to achieve this is to split the eyelid into the anterior and posterior lamellae and to treat only the posterior lamella with cryotherapy, freezing these abnormal lash follicles to –20°C with a double freeze–thaw cycle. The lamellae are sutured together with three double-armed 4-0 absorbable sutures passed from the conjunctiva and tied in the skin crease, the anterior lamella being recessed about 3 to 4 mm on the posterior lamella. The edge of the anterior lamella is sutured to the face of the posterior, using 6-0 absorbable sutures, and the bare surface is allowed to heal by granulation. The posterior lamella is advanced to allow for contracture after cryotherapy, but any posterior lamella that remains advanced beyond the normal eyelashes after about 6 months can, if necessary, be excised.

SUGGESTED READINGS

Collin JRO. *A Manual of Systematic Eyelid Surgery.* 3rd ed. Philadelphia: Butterworth-Heinemann Elsevier, 2006.

McCord CD Jr, Tannenbaum M. *Oculoplastic Surgery.* 2nd ed. New York: Raven Press, 1987.

8

Management of Ectropion and Floppy Eyelids

DOUGLAS P. MARX, MD, AND MICHAEL T. YEN, MD

Ectropion is defined as an eversion of the upper or lower eyelid away from the globe. Classes of ectropion include involutional, cicatricial, paralytic, and mechanical. Ectropic eyelids develop from horizontal eyelid laxity, medial canthal tendon laxity, vertical skin tightness, neuromuscular dysfunction, and lower eyelid retractor disinsertion. Ocular complications associated with ectropic eyelids include corneal exposure and scarring, conjunctivitis, ocular discomfort, photophobia, epiphora, and decreased vision. The entire face and eye should be carefully examined when a patient presents with ectropion. A systemic approach enables the physician to more fully understand the underlying disease process and best therapeutic approach.

8-1 ECTROPION EVALUATION AND MANAGEMENT

Ectropion can be quantified by pulling the central portion of the lid anteriorly and measuring the number of millimeters from the anterior cornea to the apex of the eyelid. Ectropion etiology can be elucidated by evaluating for horizontal eyelid laxity, orbicularis dysfunction, vertical skin tightness, and lower eyelid retractors disinsertion.

8-2 HORIZONTAL EYELID LAXITY

Horizontal eyelid laxity is typically a result of lateral or medial canthal tendon stretching. Laxity of the canthal tendons produces a redundancy in the eyelid tissues, resulting in ectropion, often referred to as an involutional ectropion. Lateral canthal tendon status can be determined by gently pulling the eyelid nasally. The inferior crus of the tendon can then be palpated to evaluate for dehiscence. The medial canthal tendon can be evaluated by pulling laterally and noting the displacement of the inferior punctum. The severity of canthal tendon laxity should be quantified prior to any surgical intervention.

8-2-1 *Lateral Canthal Tendon Laxity and the Lateral Tarsal Strip Procedure*. Although a variety of methods have been advocated for treatment of lateral canthal tendon laxity, we prefer the lateral tarsal strip, introduced by Anderson. This procedure corrects the underlying anatomic abnormality, does not require reapproximation of the eyelid margin, and is relatively easy to perform (Fig. 8-1).

The lateral canthal region is injected with lidocaine 2% mixed with 1:100,000 epinephrine using a 27- or 30-gauge needle. After ensuring appropriate anesthesia, Stevens scissors are used to create a lateral canthotomy and exposure of the lateral orbital rim. An inferior cantholysis is then performed by incising the inferior crus

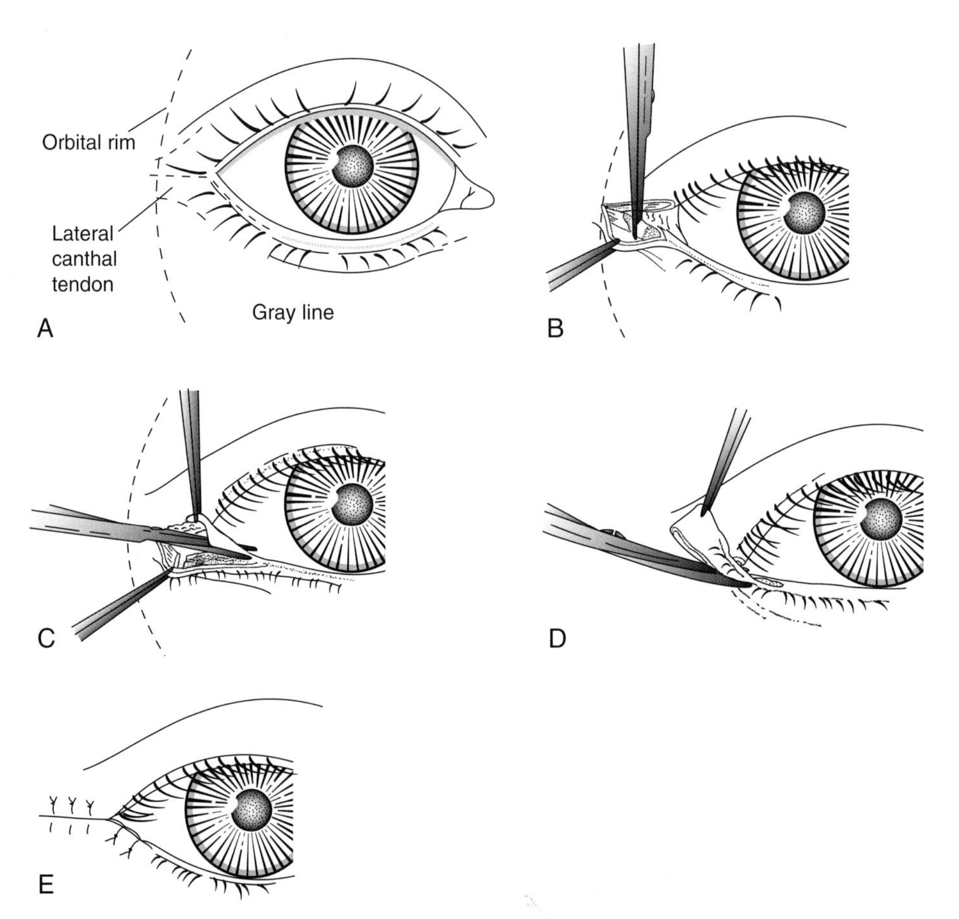

Figure 8-1 Lateral tarsal strip procedure. (A) Lateral canthotomy is performed; lower lateral lid is separated into anterior and posterior lamellae. (B) Lower crus of lateral canthal tendon is vertically incised. (C) Conjunctiva is separated from tarsus at lid margin. After tarsal strip is sutured to periosteum of lateral orbital rim (see Fig. 7-4), (D) excess skin is removed at lid margin. (E) Cutaneous sutures are applied.

portion of the lateral canthal tendon, creating mobility of the entire eyelid. A fine blade or scissors is then used to cut the lateral inferior eyelid at the gray line, separating it into anterior and posterior lamellae. The length of lamellar separation should be individualized to correct the horizontal eyelid laxity. Following customized lamellar separation, scissors are used to create a horizontal incision into the posterior lamella (tarsus and conjunctiva). The length of this incision should be equal to the length of lamellar separation, creating a small strip of tissue. The conjunctiva and epithelial surface should then be removed from the posterior lamellar strip using a #15 Bard-Parker blade. The remaining strip is then pulled laterally until the desired amount of horizontal eyelid laxity is reduced, and the excess tissue is removed using a blade or scissors.

The strip is then fixated to the periosteum of the lateral orbital rim. A 4-0 Vicryl suture with a P2 needle is then passed full thickness through the tarsal strip. The suture is then passed through the periosteum twice; this creates a loop through which the strip is placed. The suture is then passed back through the end of the strip (see Fig. 7-4B and Fig. 8-2A). Traction on both ends of the suture draws the tarsal strip tightly down onto the periosteum and the knot binds the loop down onto the tarsal strip (Fig. 8-2B). To avoid postoperative eyelid laxity and an inferiorly displaced lateral canthus, initial eyelid tightness and lateral canthal elevation should be fashioned slightly above the desired results. Once the tarsal strip has been firmly attached to the underlying periosteum, the redundant anterior lamellar tissue is excised and the lateral canthotomy is closed using 6-0 plain gut sutures in an interrupted fashion.

8-2-2 *Medial Canthal Tendon Laxity.* Medial canthal tendon laxity can be evaluated by pulling the eyelids laterally and noting the displacement of the inferior punctum. The superior and inferior puncta should be aligned vertically. Although a variety of grading scales have been advocated, we prefer to define severe medial canthal tendon laxity as inferior punctum displacement to the medial limbus. Anterior

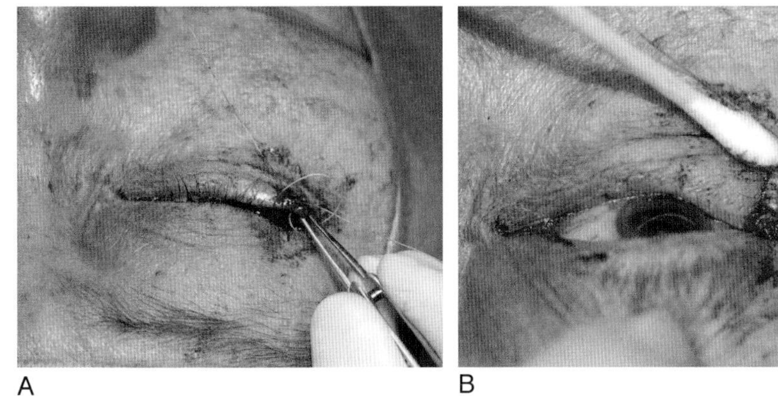
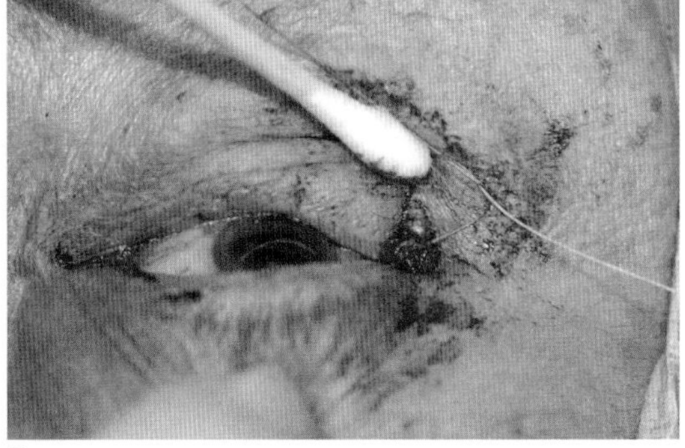

A B

Figure 8-2 (A) The tarsal strip is pulled through the loop of the suture fixating it to the periosteum of the lateral orbital rim. (B) The knot of the suture then fixates the loop in position over the tarsal strip.

punctal displacement can also be found when medial canthal tendon laxity is present. These patients often present with epiphora and foreign body sensation.

When mild to moderate medial canthal tendon laxity is present, a lateral tarsal strip procedure will often correct the associated ectropion without significant displacement of the inferior punctum. Anterior punctual displacement can be addressed simultaneously with a medial spindle procedure. When severe laxity is present, a medial canthal tendon plication can be performed.

8-2-3 *Medial Canthal Tendon Plication*. Medial canthal tendon plication is an excellent method of tightening the inferior limb of the anterior horn of the medial canthal tendon. The canalicular system is intimately associated with the medial canthal tendon and can be significantly damaged during surgical procedures in this region. The canalicular system should be clearly identified during a medial tarsal strip to avoid damaging the canaliculi.

The medial canthal region is injected with lidocaine 2% mixed with 1:100,000 epinephrine using a 27- or 30-gauge needle. After ensuring appropriate anesthesia, an elliptical, vertical incision 1 cm in length is made over the medial canthal tendon approximately 5 mm nasal to the canthus. The inferior portion of the incision should extend a few millimeters inferior to the punctum. A probe is placed into the inferior canaliculus for the duration of the surgery. The orbicularis muscle is then bluntly dissected vertically in the direction of its fibers, exposing the medial canthal tendon using a Freer or cotton applicator. The angular vessels may be in the plane of the dissection and can be retracted or cauterized if necessary. A double-armed 4-0 or 5-0 Merseline suture on an RD 2 needle is passed vertically through the medial canthal tendon near its insertion. The first suture arm is passed through the most nasal portion of the tarsus, exiting through the superior portion of the medial canthal tendon insertion. The second suture is passed in a similar fashion, exiting inferiorly through the medial canthal tendon. Both sutures should travel anterior to the probe to avoid damage to the canalicular system. As the suture is tied, the medial aspect of the eyelid, including the punctum, is pulled toward the canthus and globe. The skin incision over the tendon is closed with interrupted 6-0 absorbable sutures.

8-2-4 *Medial Spindle Procedure*. The medial posterior lamella, including the punctum, is injected with lidocaine 2% mixed with 1:100,000 epinephrine using a 27- or 30-gauge needle. A fusiform, diamond-shaped portion of medial conjunctiva and underlying retractors is excised inferior to the punctum. The vertical and horizontal dimensions of the excised tissue should be adjusted according to the degree of ectropion present. Following excision, two double-armed 5-0 chromic gut mattress sutures are used to close the wound using a horizontal mattress technique. The first suture arm is placed through the lower eyelid retractors at the inferior edge of the incision. The suture is then passed through the upper edge of the wound. The second suture arm is fashioned in the same manner, and both are passed full thickness through the eyelid approximately 10 to 15 mm inferior to the lower eyelid margin. Once both suture arms have been passed through the skin, they are tied and the suture tension is adjusted until the punctum is inverted.

8-3 CICATRICIAL ECTROPION

Cicatricial disease can cause vertical anterior lamellar tightness and associated ectropion. Cicatricial changes can be found in the skin, subcutaneous tissue, orbicularis, and septum. Underlying etiologies include thermal and chemical injuries, trauma, infection, chronic dermatitis, previous skin excisions including blepharoplasties, and drug reactions. Congenital cicatricial ectropion is caused by a shortage of lower eyelid vertical skin, and is present in blepharophimosis syndrome, euryblepharon, and congenital ichthyosis. A thorough history, including medical illnesses, previous surgeries, and medication use, is important for etiology identification. Careful examination of the patient reveals an eyelid that cannot be positioned against the globe and cannot be pulled to the level of the pupil.

If ocular symptoms and irritation can be adequately addressed with lubrication, it is best to wait approximately 6 months following initial cicatrization to allow for scar softening. A lateral tarsorrhaphy may be necessary to protect the globe when significant exposure is present. When minimal cicatrization is present, a Z-plasty procedure provides good results. When extensive cicatrization and ectropion are present, myocutaneous flap advancement and skin grafting are often necessary. If any midface descent is present, a midface lift can be employed as an adjunct procedure.

8-3-1 *Z-Plasty.* A Z-plasty may be performed for a localized vertical scar crossing the skin tension lines (Fig. 8-3). A Z-plasty procedure allows tension to be decreased in one line by transposing the vector forces. The anterior lamella of the ectropic eyelid is injected with lidocaine 2% mixed with 1:100,000 epinephrine using a 27- or 30-gauge needle. A 4-0 silk suture can be placed through the gray line to provide traction intraoperatively and postoperatively. An incision is made along the scar vertically, with another incision at each end of the central line at an angle of approximately 60 degrees, optimizing the eyelid length. The resultant triangular skin flaps are raised, and the subcutaneous scar tissue is freed using Westcott scissors. The skin flaps are undermined until there is no tension, allowing them to transpose easily. As the skin flaps are transposed, the incision will fall within the skin tension lines and the eyelid will be elongated vertically. The skin edges are sutured with interrupted 6-0 plain gut sutures. For lower eyelid repair, the traction suture is taped above the eyebrow. For repair of the upper eyelid, it is taped to the malar region. The traction suture can be removed approximately 1week postoperatively.

8-3-2 *Midface Lift.* Midface descent is a common finding in patients with ectropic eyelids. A variety of successful midface lift techniques have been described. We prefer ectropion repair with associated supraperiosteal midface lift because it is a safe and effective surgical procedure.

Two percent lidocaine with epinephrine is used to infiltrate the lower eyelid, inferior fornix, cheek, and lateral canthus, and to perform an infraorbital nerve block. Using scissors, a transconjunctival incision is created in the inferior fornix of the lower eyelid, inferior to the lower tarsal border. Blunt dissection is then performed

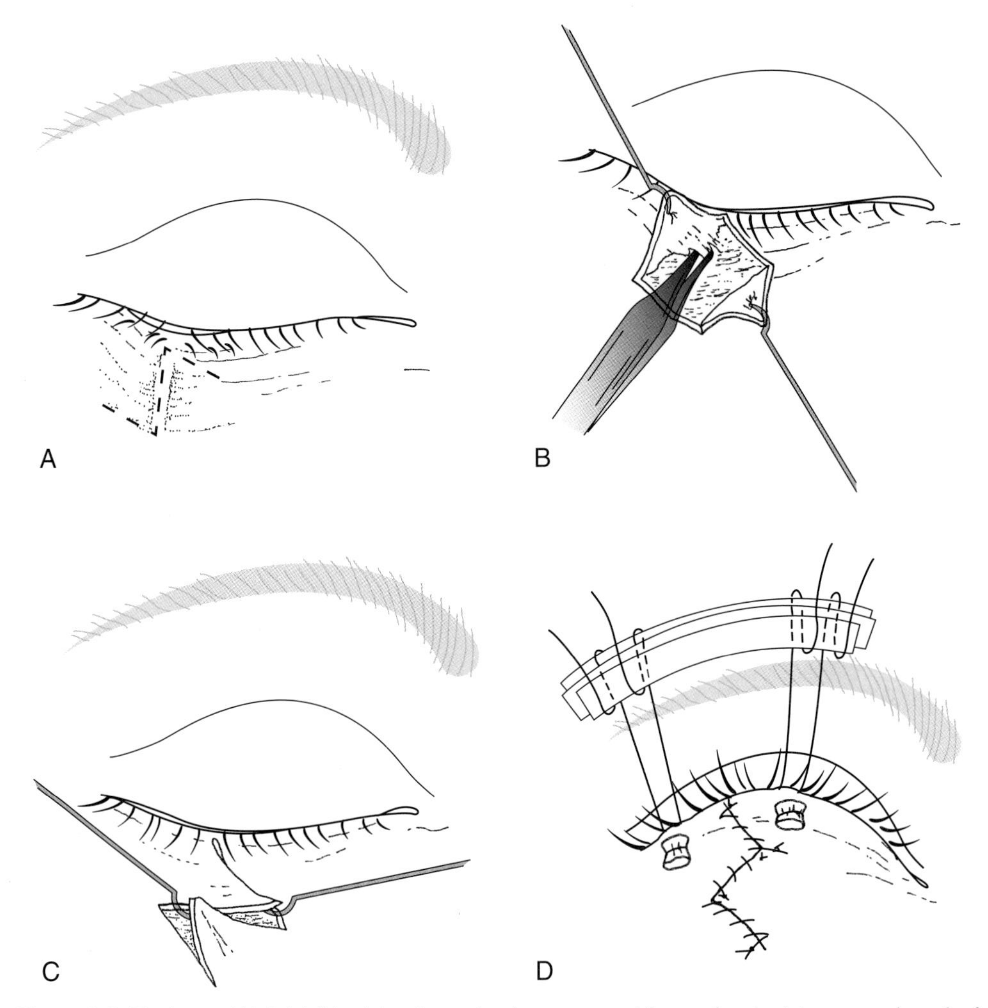

Figure 8-3 Z-plasty. (A) Initial incision is made along scar, with another incision at each end of central line at angle of about 60 degrees. (B) Triangular skin flaps are raised and underlying scar tissue is excised. (C) Skin flaps are transposed, lengthening the lid vertically. (D) Skin is sutured. Traction sutures are inserted to keep lengthened incision stretched.

in the suborbicular fascial plane down to the level of the infraorbital rim. The suborbicularis oculi fat and malar fat pads are extensively undermined in the supraperiosteal plane with a broad elevator down to the nasolabial fold. After creating and elevating the myocutaneous flap, the flap is advanced superiorly to relieve inferior traction and provide additional support to the lower eyelid (Fig. 8-4). The myocutaneous flap is then fixated to the periosteum along the infraorbital rim with several interrupted 4-0 Vicryl sutures. The transconjunctival incision is then closed with a 6-0 plain gut suture.

8-3-3 *Skin Grafts.* Ectropion associated with significant cicatricial changes often require an autogenous skin graft. A full-thickness graft from the retroauricular region is preferred for lower eyelids. Other donor sites include the eyelids, the supraclavicular region, and the inner aspect of the upper arm. A thorough inspection

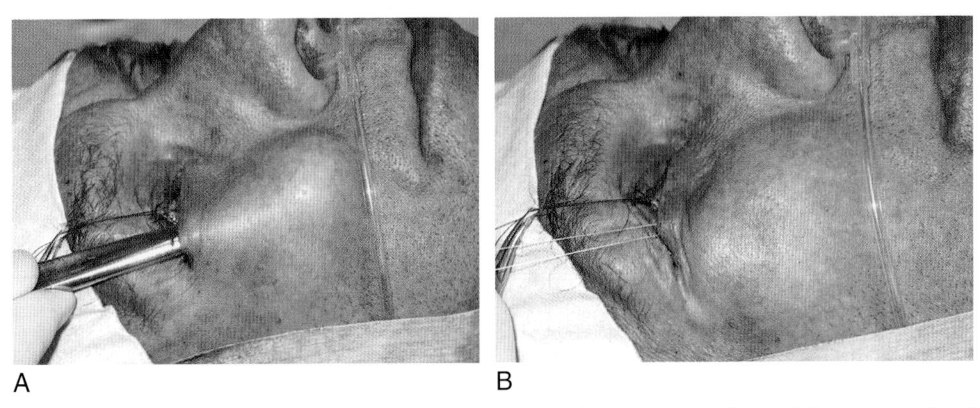

Figure 8-4 Midface lift. (A) Using a broad elevator, the dissection is performed down to the level of the nasolabial fold. (B) After engaging the midface with suture, the midface is elevated superiorly and fixated to the underlying periosteum along the inferior and lateral orbital rim.

of donor sites should be performed prior to any surgical intervention. The donor site tissue availability and the amount of cicatricial changes should be compared.

The donor site and recipient eyelid are injected with lidocaine 2% mixed with 1:100,000 epinephrine using a 27- or 30-gauge needle. After ensuring appropriate anesthesia, 4-0 silk sutures are placed at the medial and lateral eyelid margins of the recipient eyelid to act as traction sutures. Hemostats can then be used to hold the traction sutures superiorly. A sharp blade is used to create a horizontal incision through the anterior lamella of the cicatricial eyelid approximately 2 to 4 mm inferior to the eyelid margin. The length of the horizontal incision is adjusted according to the amount of cicatrization present. The blade is then used to free any remaining scar tissue. The scarred tissue is then removed, exposing the full extent of the defect. Thorough hemostasis is performed using fine cautery to decrease the risk of graft rejection. The eyelid is then placed on stretch to determine the full amount of tissue needed from the donor site. Telfa can then be used to create a template of the required donor tissue. The Telfa template is placed on the donor site, and a marking pen is used to trace around it. The full-thickness skin graft, which should be slightly larger than the defect, is excised as thinly as possible. The donor graft is placed over the recipient bed, and the shapes are compared. Fine scissors are used to trim the donor edges to conform to the recipient bed. The graft is then sutured into the recipient bed using interrupted 6-0 silk sutures. Small drainage holes can be made in the graft to prevent hematomas from forming underneath the graft. Two or three 5-0 nylon sutures are placed at the host–graft junction on both sides of the graft and tied over a Xeroform stent to hold the graft securely against the recipient site. The traction sutures are taped superiorly to provide tension on the recipient eyelid. All donor sites can be closed using interrupted 6-0 absorbable sutures. The Xeroform stent is removed approximately 5 days following surgery. Traction and graft sutures can be removed in 7 to 10 days (Fig. 8-5).

8-3-4 *Flaps and Spacers.* Cicatricial ectropion with a variable amount of tissue loss can result following removal of eyelid malignancies. When up to 50% of the eyelid has been lost, the defect can often be closed with a lateral cantholysis and advancement

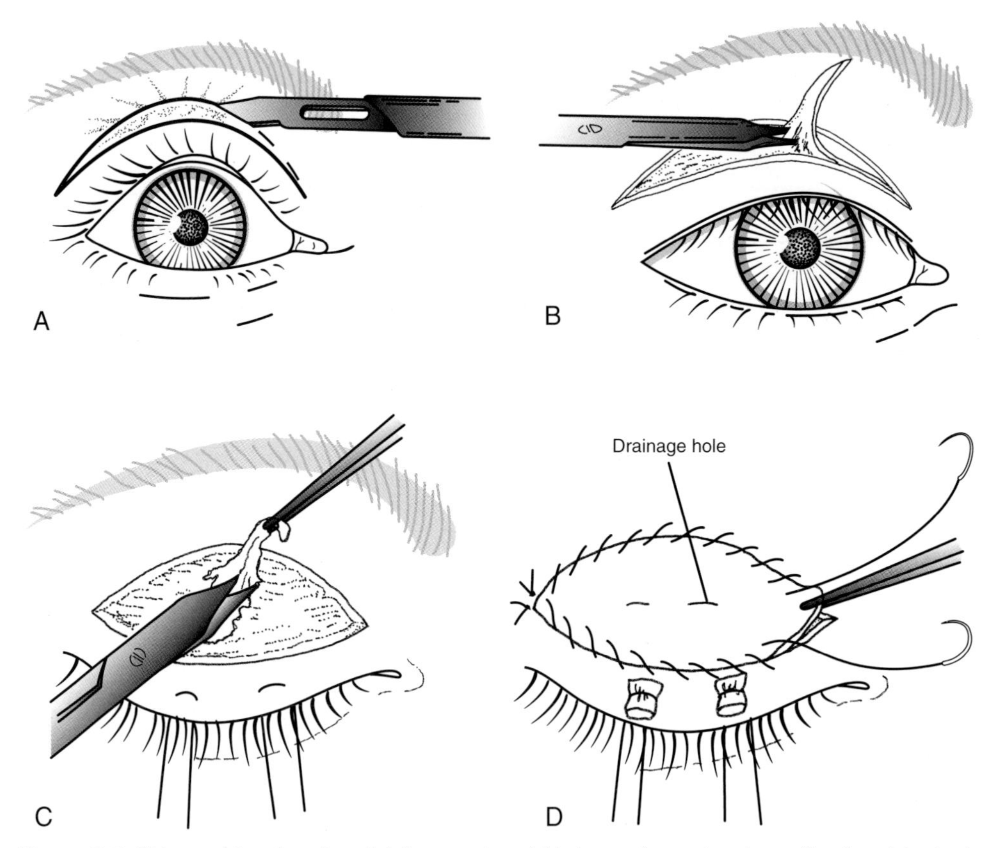

Figure 8-5 Skin grafting for cicatricial ectropion. (A) Area of scarring is outlined and incised. (B) Involved skin and subcutaneous scar tissue are excised. (C) Deep scar tissue is excised. Lid is placed on stretch to determine full extent of defect. (D) Full-thickness skin graft is sutured into position with two running 6-0 nylon sutures.

of the eyelid tissues. Eyelid defects involving 75% of the eyelid can be successfully reconstructed using a tarsoconjunctival flap from the upper eyelid, a myocutaneous rotation flap, or graft. Bipedicle orbicularis oculi muscle flaps have been shown prospectively to provide excellent repair of cicatricial ectropion. A variety of spacer materials, including autogenous hard palate, ear cartilage, and human dermis, have been used in eyelid reconstruction.

8-4 DISINSERTION OF THE LOWER EYELID RECTRACTORS

When the lower lid retractors are totally detached, ectropion or entropion can result. Tse identified four findings in retractor disinsertion, including a deeper inferior fornix, a higher resting lower eyelid position, and diminished lower eyelid excursion on down gaze. Vertical shortening of the posterior eyelid lamella can be performed through a resection of the tarsoconjunctival lower eyelid retractors. Retractor disinsertion can be treated with removal of posterior lamellar tissue combined with suture inversion of the eyelid.

Following adequate anesthesia with 2% lidocaine and 1:100,000 epinephrine, a 4-0 silk suture is placed through the lower eyelid margin to provide traction. Westcott scissors are then used to make a horizontal conjunctival incision inferior to the tarsus. Following the conjunctival incision, the orbicularis muscle is exposed, and the underlying tissue is bluntly and sharply dissected until the inferior orbital rim and orbital fat pads are exposed. Once the orbital fat pads are retracted, the anterior portions of the retractors can be identified. To ensure correct identification of the eyelid retractors, the patient is asked to look down while the retractors are held with forceps. If the retractors have been properly identified, tension will be felt when the patient looks down. Two or three double-armed 5-0 chromic sutures are then used to reattach the eyelid retractors to the inferior portion of the tarsus in an evenly spaced fashion. The sutures are finally tied on the skin surface and allowed to absorb.

8-5 MECHANICAL ECTROPION

Mechanical ectropion is secondary to other ophthalmic or medical conditions. It may be caused by a large tumor of the eyelid that causes the lid margin to roll outward, by acute proptosis of the globe with associated chemosis of the conjunctiva, or by periocular edema, which mechanically pushes the lid margin away from the surface of the globe. Treatment is directed at the primary cause.

8-6 UPPER EYELID EVERSION

Ectropion of the upper eyelids is a rare condition that has been reported in patients with Down syndrome or congenital ichthyosiform dermatitis, and patients with no underlying systemic disease. Although more frequently bilateral, it has been reported unilaterally. The cause is unknown, but abnormalities including overlapping of the lower eyelid margin by the upper eyelid and failure of the septum to fuse with the levator aponeurosis have been described.

Initial treatment consists of aggressive ocular lubrication and hydration of the cornea. When significant corneal epithelial breakdown is present, the eyelids can be sutured into their normal anatomic position using an intermarginal 6-0 black silk suture tied over cotton pegs. When chemotic conjunctiva is the underlying cause of an ectropic eyelid, a double-armed suture can be placed through the fornix conjunctiva and skin with a subconjunctival injection of hyaluronidase. More extensive surgical procedures including full-thickness eyelid shortening and attachment of the orbital septum to the levator aponeurosis have been successfully used.

8-7 FLOPPY EYELID SYNDROME

Floppy eyelid syndrome was first described in obese, middle-aged men who presented with easily everted upper eyelids and papillary conjunctivitis. These patients have a soft, easily folded tarsus, and often present with ocular symptoms including foreign body sensation or ocular irritation from punctuate epithelial erosions and chronic papillary conjunctivitis. Keratoconus, dermatochalasis, blepharochalasis, blepharoptosis, eyelash ptosis, and meibomian gland dysfunction have also been described in patients with floppy eyelid syndrome. Systemic associations such as obstructive sleep apnea, hypertension, and diabetes mellitus have also been described.

Surgical treatments have included pentagonal upper eyelid wedge resection, lateral tarsorrhaphy, and lateral tarsal strip. When lateral canthal tendon laxity is present, a lateral tarsal strip procedure provides excellent symptomatic relief and cosmetic results. When significant medial canthal laxity is present, medial upper eyelid shortening with and without eyelid skin reduction has been successfully used.

SUGGESTED READINGS

Anderson RL, Gordy DD. The tarsal strip procedure. *Arch Ophthalmol.* 1979;97(11):2192–2196.

Anderson RL, Weinstein GS. Full-thickness bipedicle flap for total lower eyelid reconstruction. *Arch Ophthalmol.* 1987;105(4):570–576.

Aristodemou P, Baer R. Reversible cicatricial ectropion precipitated by topical brimonidine eye drops. *Ophthal Plast Reconstr Surg.* 2008;24(1):57–58.

Bentsi-Enchill KO. Congenital total eversion of the upper eyelids. *Br J Ophthalmol.* 1981;65(3):209–213.

Blechman B, Isenberg S. An anatomical etiology of congenital eyelid eversion. *Ophthalmic Surg.* 1984;15(2):111–113.

Chung JE, Yen MT. Midface lifting as an adjunct procedure in ectropion repair. *Ann Plast Surg,* 2007;59(6):635–640.

Culbertson WW, Ostler HB. The floppy eyelid syndrome. *Am J Ophthalmol.* 1981;92(4):568–575.

Dutton JJ. Surgical management of floppy eyelid syndrome. *Am J Ophthalmol.* 1985;99(5):557–560.

Frueh BR, Schoengarth LD. Evaluation and treatment of the patient with ectropion. *Ophthalmology.* 1982;89(9):1049–1054.

Goldberg R, et al. Floppy eyelid syndrome and blepharochalasis. *Am J Ophthalmol.* 1986;102(3):376–381.

Hegde V, et al. Drug-induced ectropion: what is best practice? *Ophthalmology.* 2007;114(2):362–366.

Hove CR, Williams EF 3rd, Rodgers BJ. Z-plasty: a concise review. *Facial Plast Surg.* 2001;17(4):289–294.

Jordan DR, Anderson RL, Thiese SM. The medial tarsal strip. *Arch Ophthalmol.* 1990;108(1):120–124.

Leibovitch I, Selva D. Floppy eyelid syndrome: clinical features and the association with obstructive sleep apnea. *Sleep Med.* 2006;7(2):117–122.

McNab AA. Floppy eyelid syndrome and obstructive sleep apnea. *Ophthal Plast Reconstr Surg.* 1997;13(2):98–114.

Nowinski TS, Anderson RL. The medial spindle procedure for involutional medial ectropion. *Arch Ophthalmol.* 1985;103(11):1750–1753.

O'Donnell BA, et al. Repair of the lax medial canthal tendon. *Br J Ophthalmol.* 2003;87(2):220–224.

Rohrich RJ, Zbar RI. The evolution of the Hughes tarsoconjunctival flap for the lower eyelid reconstruction. *Plast Reconstr Surg.* 1999;104(2):518–526.

Sullivan SA, Dailey RA. Endoscopic subperiosteal midface lift: surgical technique with indications and outcomes. *Ophthal Plast Reconstr Surg*. 2002;18(5):319–330.

Tse DT, ed. Ectropion. *Color Atlas of Ophthalmic Surgery: Oculoplastic Surgery*. Philadelphia: JB Lippincott, 1992.

Uthoff D, Gorney M, Teichmann C. Cicatricial ectropion in ichthyosis: a novel approach to treatment. *Ophthal Plast Reconstr Surg*. 1994;10(2):92–95.

Valenzuela AA, Sullivan TJ. Medial upper eyelid shortening to correct medial eyelid laxity in floppy eyelid syndrome: a new surgical approach. *Ophthal Plast Reconstr Surg*. 2005;21(4):259–263.

Xu JH, Tan WQ, Yao JM. Bipedicle orbicularis oculi flap in the reconstruction of the lower eyelid ectropion. *Aesthetic Plast Surg*. 2007;31(2):161–166.

9

Management of Blepharoptosis

MARK J. LUCARELLI, MD, FACS

9-1 ANATOMY OF UPPER LID

A thorough understanding of upper eyelid anatomy is essential for the ptosis surgeon.

The upper eyelid consists of skin, orbicularis, septum, tarsus, levator, Müller's muscle, and conjunctiva (Fig. 9-1). The skin and orbicularis form the anterior lamella. Conceptually, the orbicularis may be subdivided according to its topography into pretarsal, preseptal, and orbital components (over the orbital rim and extending to the frontalis muscle superiorly). The orbital septum is a fibrous lamellar structure arising from the periosteum over the superior and inferior orbital rims. In the upper eyelid, the orbital septum fuses with the levator aponeurosis approximately 2 to 5 mm above the superior tarsal border in Caucasians. In Asian patients, the septum extends further inferiorly into the eyelid. Preaponeurotic orbital fat is normally located behind the orbital septum in the preaponeurotic space. The preaponeurotic fat is an important landmark for surgeons as it lies immediately anterior to the levator aponeurosis. The tarsus of the upper eyelid is a firm, dense connective-tissue plate that provides rigidity to the eyelid. The upper tarsal plate measures approximately 10 mm vertically in the center of the eyelid. The tarsal plate is usually 1 mm thick.

The levator complex originates from the periorbita of the lesser wing of the sphenoid at the annulus of Zinn. The muscular portion of the levator in adults is approximately 36 mm long, while thc aponeurosis is 14 to 20 mm long. The bony attachments of the aponeurosis are via its horizontal expansions, the medial and lateral horns. The lateral horn, which is much stronger than the medial horn, passes through the lacrimal gland and divides it into the palpebral and orbital lobes. The lateral horn attaches to the periorbita of the orbital tubercle and to the lateral

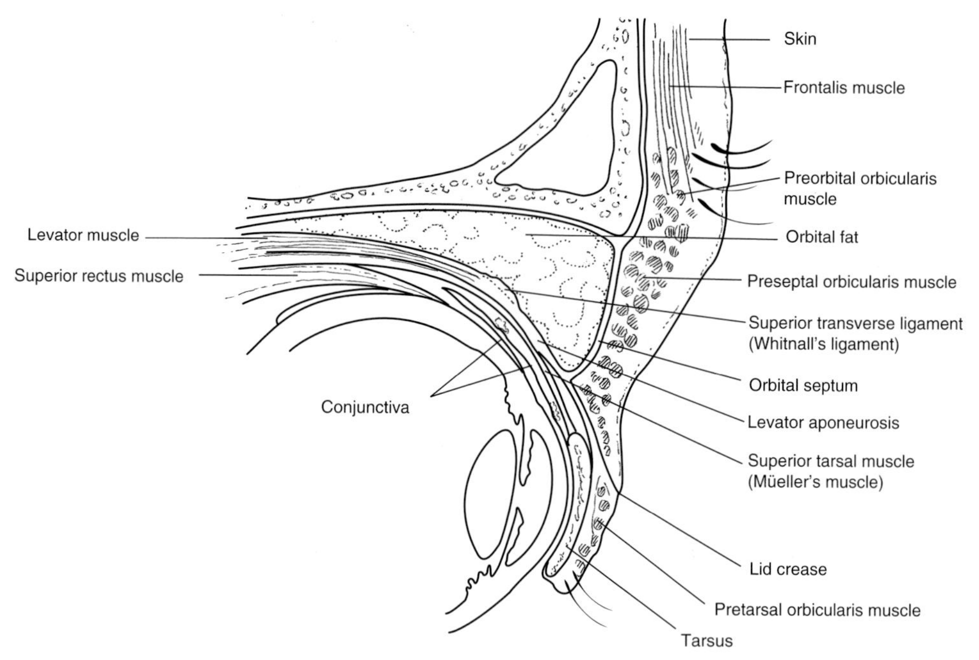

Figure 9-1 Cross-section of upper lid.

canthal tendon. The medial horn is a thin, delicate structure. It attaches loosely with the posterior portion of the medial canthal tendon and curves medially and posteriorly to insert at the posterior lacrimal crest and the adjacent periorbita of the medial orbital wall. Whitnall's superior transverse ligament (Whitnall's ligament) is a condensation of the fascial sheaths of the levator muscle located superior to the area of transition of the levator muscle to the levator aponeurosis (musculoaponeurotic junction). Whitnall's ligament serves as a suspensory sling for the upper eyelid. Medially, Whitnall's ligament attaches to the connective tissue around the trochlea and superior oblique tendon. Laterally, Whitnall's joins the capsule of the lacrimal gland, then arches upward to attach to the periosteum of the lateral orbital wall approximately 10 mm above the lateral orbital tubercle. Fibers from the levator aponeurosis insert onto the inferior 7 to 8 mm of the anterior surface of the tarsus to support the eyelid. Other more superficial fibers of the aponeurosis insert into the pretarsal orbicularis and skin forming the lid crease.

The second retractor of the upper eyelid is Müeller's muscle. It is located between the levator aponeurosis and the conjunctiva. This involuntary smooth muscle is analogous to the inferior tarsal muscle of the lower eyelid. Müeller's muscle begins about 15 mm above the superior tarsal, arising from the underside of the striated levator muscle. It inserts onto the upper border of the tarsal plate. Müeller's muscle is adherent to the conjunctival layer posteriorly and less firmly attached to the aponeurosis anteriorly. The peripheral vascular arcade is found anterior to Müeller's muscle near the superior tarsal border. The conjunctiva forms the most posterior layer of the eyelids and contains the mucin-secreting goblet cells and the accessory lacrimal glands of Krause and Wolfring. These accessory lacrimal glands are found in the subconjunctival tissues mainly in the upper eyelid between the superior tarsal border and the fornix.

9-2 CLASSIFICATION OF PTOSIS

Most cases of ptosis can be classified into one of the following categories: aponeurotic, myogenic, neurogenic, mechanical, or mixed mechanism (Table 9-1). Aponeurotic ptosis results from disinsertion or stretching of the levator aponeurosis and is the most common type of ptosis in adults. Myogenic ptosis may be either congenital or acquired. Acquired forms of myogenic ptosis include myotonic dystrophy, oculopharyngeal dystrophy, and chronic progressive external ophthalmoplegia. It is not uncommon to see involutional changes contributing to the ptosis in such patients. Common examples of neurogenic ptosis include ptosis resulting from third nerve palsy or ptosis from Horner syndrome. Mechanical ptosis is a result of mass effect weighing down the upper lid. This can result from entities such as neurofibromatosis.

9-2-1 *Aponeurotic Ptosis.* Involutional or aponeurotic ptosis is the most frequently encountered type of ptosis. The severity of this type of ptosis ranges from mild to severe. The hallmark on examination is the finding of good levator muscle function. Normal levator function typically ranges from 14 to 16 mm of excursion of the lid margin from extreme down gaze to extreme up gaze, without frontalis recruitment. In aponeurotic ptosis, the upper eyelid crease is often elevated (10 mm or more above the lid margin), and the eyelid tissue may be quite thin. In men, the lid crease typically is found 7 to 8 mm above the upper lid margin. In women the normal position of the crease is usually 8 to 9 mm. In patients of Asian ethnicity, the crease is typically much lower (i.e., 2 to 5 mm).

The pathophysiology of involutional ptosis is disinsertion of the aponeurosis from the tarsus in some cases and attenuation of the aponeurosis in others. The levator aponeurosis may tend to disinsert or stretch with age and tissue degeneration. Eyelid rubbing or stretching, repeated episodes of edema, or chronic ocular inflammation may similarly lead to stretching of the tissue or to disinsertion of the aponeurosis. Blepharochalasis is a rare and often hereditary condition characterized by recurrent attacks of marked eyelid edema. This edema results in stretching and thinning of all eyelid tissues, including the levator aponeurosis. Local blunt trauma can cause ptosis due to a dehiscence of the aponeurosis. Rarely, congenital ptosis with normal levator function can result from birth trauma.

Surgical repair of involutional ptosis is often performed via the external approach. In this approach the disinserted aponeurosis is advanced and sutured to the anterior tarsal surface. If the aponeurosis is attenuated, it can be resected, advanced, and sutured to the anterior tarsal surface. Whenever possible, ptosis procedures are performed under local anesthesia so that an accurate repair can be titrated during the surgery. For mild to moderate degrees of involutional ptosis, conjunctival müllerectomy (Putterman technique) is often an excellent surgical option.

9-2-2 *Levator Maldevelopment Ptosis.* Levator maldevelopment, or congenital myogenic ptosis, results from dysgenesis of the levator muscle. In such cases the levator muscle is infiltrated with fat and often fibrous and inelastic. Such ptosis is usually present at birth. Examination findings include poor levator excursion, lid lag on down gaze, and not infrequently lagophthalmos. The lid crease is often absent or poorly formed.

Table 9-1 Classification of Ptosis

Levator Maldevelopment Ptosis
Simple (defect isolated to levator muscle)
With superior rectus muscle weakness
Blepharophimosis syndrome
Congenital fibrosis of extraocular muscles
Myogenic Ptosis
Oculopharyngeal dystrophy
Chronic progressive external ophthalmoplegia
Muscular dystrophy
Myasthenia gravis
Trauma to levator muscle
Neurogenic Ptosis
Oculomotor nerve palsy
Misdirected oculomotor nerve regeneration
Marcus Gunn jaw-winking ptosis
Horner syndrome
Ophthalmoplegic migraine
Aponeurotic Ptosis
Dehiscent or disinserted aponeurosis secondary to:
Age
Cataract or other ocular surgery
Local blunt trauma
Blepharochalasis
Chronic edema (Graves disease, allergy, etc.)
Mechanical Ptosis
Excessive lid weight (lid or orbital mass)
Scarring
Pseudoptosis
Lack of posterior eyelid support (i.e., enophthalmos, anophthalmos)
Dermatochalasis
Globe malposition

Table 9-2 Levator Muscle Excursion Classified

Levator Function (mm)	Classification
>13 mm	Excellent (normal)
8–12 mm	Good
5–7	Fair
≤4	Poor

Table 9-3 Guidelines for Correction of Levator Maldevelopment Ptosis (in millimeters)-Beard's Table

Degree of Ptosis	Levator Function	Approximate Amount of Levator Resection
Mild (<2)	Good (8–12)	Small (10–13)
	Good (8–12)	Moderate (14–17)
Moderate (3)	Fair (5–7)	Large (18–22)
	Poor (4 or less)	Maximal (23–27)
Severe (4 or more)	Fair (5–7)	Maximal (23–27)
	Poor (4 or less)	Supermaximal (27 or more) Frontalis sling

Levator maldevelopment ptosis has been classified by Beard as (1) mild if the eyelid droops 2 mm or less from its normal level; (2) moderate if the eyelid droops 3 mm; and (3) severe if the eyelid droops 4 mm or more. Pathologic studies of the levator muscle have demonstrated striated muscle fibers to be abundant in ptosis of 2 mm, sparse or absent in ptosis of 3 mm, and absent in ptosis of 4 mm or more. Levator function has been arbitrarily classified by Beard in such cases as (1) poor when the eyelid excursion is 4 mm or less, (2) fair when the eyelid excursion is 5 to 7 mm, and (3) good when the excursion is 8 to 12 mm. Such classification is very useful in a quantitative approach to surgical repair (Tables 9-2 and 9-3).

Surgical correction is generally performed in the preschool age, when accurate measurements of the ptosis and levator action can be obtained. If the ptotic lid covers the visual axis, causes amblyopia, or induces significant astigmatism, a temporizing frontalis sling can be placed until a permanent procedure can be performed. Cases with poor levator function (0 to 4 mm) usually require correction with frontalis suspension. A sling effect can sometimes be created by a "supermaximal" levator resection and advancement. However, many surgeons prefer frontalis suspension when levator excursion is poor. In ptosis cases with fair to excellent levator function, an external levator resection is usually the procedure of choice.

Blepharophimosis syndrome is a rare variant of myogenic ptosis. Blepharophimosis syndrome is characterized by bilateral ptosis with poor levator function, blepharophimosis (narrowed horizontal length of the palpebral fissure), epicanthus inversus, and telecanthus. Other findings such as ectropion of the lateral aspect of the lower eyelids, a flattened glabella and nasal bridge, and low-set "lop ears" are often present. This disorder is transmitted in an autosomal dominant fashion, and mutations have been localized to chromosome 3p. In some cases mental retardation or female infertility has been associated.

9-2-3 *Acquired Myogenic Ptosis.* Acquired myogenic ptosis results from muscular diseases that are often progressive such as myasthenia gravis, chronic progressive external ophthalmoplegia, or oculopharyngeal dystrophy. Ptosis in myasthenia gravis results from dysfunction at the neuromuscular junction and is often fluctuating and is typically significantly worse with fatigue or illness. It may be unilateral or bilateral and may or may not involve the extraocular muscles or other skeletal muscles in the early stages. Diplopia is a common accompanying symptom. Initial treatment is medical, with surgical correction undertaken only after appropriate medical therapy. A Tensilon test for myasthenia gravis may be helpful in the evaluation of suspected myasthenia gravis cases. A small test dose (2 mg) of edrophonium chloride is administered intravenously over a 15- to 30-second period. If the patient experiences no untoward results within 1 minute, the remainder (8 mg) is injected slowly. Resolution or improvement of the ptosis is expected within a few minutes. Occasionally, a cholinergic reaction may occur, and therefore atropine sulfate should always be kept ready for urgent intravenous administration. The ice pack test and acetylcholine receptor antibody testing are sometimes helpful in diagnosing myasthenia gravis as a cause of ptosis.

Chronic progressive external ophthalmoplegia (CPEO) is heterogeneous group of conditions characterized by a gradually progressive bilateral myogenic ptosis accompanied by extraocular muscle paralysis. Autosomal dominant and autosomal recessive inheritance patterns have been described. Mutations of mitochondrial DNA are thought to be implicated in most cases. Usually, the condition progresses until the ptosis is severe and the eyes become fixed in a slightly downward position. Heart block, retinitis pigmentosa, abnormal retinal pigment, and various neurologic signs have been described in association with this syndrome. The Kearns-Sayre variant shows onset before age 20, pigmentary retinopathy, and often cardiac conduction defects. Because the Bell's phenomenon becomes deficient in CPEO, the surgical goal is limited to very conservative correction to raise the lid just above the pupillary axis. In patients whose eyes are fixed in severe downward position, strabismus evaluation may be indicated. If strabismus surgery is to be performed, it should be done prior to ptosis surgery. In elderly patients with myogenic ptosis who have tolerated the ptosis and strabismus for years, surgery is more hazardous because the corneas are more prone to exposure keratitis. Recurrence of ptosis in CPEO and related myopathies is not unexpected as levator function may slowly decline.

Oculopharyngeal dystrophy (OPD) is a myopathy that typically arises in middle age and is associated with difficulty in swallowing. The ptosis and difficulty swallowing usually arise in the fifth decade. OPD can be familial, and autosomal dominant and autosomal recessive patterns of inheritance have been reported. Many of the initially reported cases had French-Canadian ancestry.

Trauma to the levator complex is another category of ptosis. Laceration of the levator muscle by sharp trauma results in immediate ptosis and is best treated as soon as possible after injury. For delayed repairs, the external approach is favored because it allows easier location of the retracted ends of the levator aponeurosis, reapproximation, and adjustment. If possible, local anesthesia with sedation is preferred, as intraoperative adjustment can increase the accuracy of repair. When a case of traumatic ptosis is first evaluated more than several weeks after injury, it is often best to wait several months after trauma before surgical correction. This will allow the tissue reaction to subside and the scar to remodel prior to surgical exploration. Also, traumatic ptosis from blunt trauma may show considerable improvement over the first several months.

9-2-4 *Neurogenic Ptosis.* In oculomotor nerve palsy, ptosis results from congenital abnormality, injury, or lesions of the third cranial nerve. There is usually an associated paresis of the extraocular muscles innervated by the third nerve. Surgery is undertaken only after maximal recovery of oculomotor nerve function has occurred and the status has been stable for several months. Strabismus surgery to align the eye should be performed before ptosis surgery, because correction of the vertical muscle imbalance may change the upper eyelid position. The surgical repair of the ptosis often consists of frontalis suspension. Care should be taken to avoid an exposure keratitis in the postoperative period.

Marcus Gunn jaw-winking ptosis is a synkinetic syndrome caused by an aberrant connection of the oculomotor nerve fibers that innervate the levator muscle and the trigeminal nerve fibers to the muscles of mastication. The ptosis is usually unilateral. In this condition, the ptosis improves when the jaw is moved to the side contralateral to the ptosis. Some of the fifth cranial nerve fibers have been congenitally misdirected into the branch of the third cranial nerve that supplies the levator muscle. Surgical decision making in this disorder (and in general in severe unilateral congenital ptosis) is controversial.

Horner syndrome results from paralysis of the sympathetically innervated Müeller's superior tarsal muscle. The ptosis is associated with miosis, often anhidrosis, and mild lower lid elevation. Congenital cases usually show iris heterochromia. Horner syndrome may be congenital or result from a lesion anywhere along the sympathetic chain. The cause must be investigated by a complete neurologic and medical workup. The ptosis is surgically corrected only after proper neurologic or neuro-ophthalmologic evaluation and management.

9-2-5 *Mechanical Ptosis.* Mechanical ptosis includes those cases of ptosis secondary to increased weight of the eyelid or to scar tissue interfering with the motility of the eyelid. Benign or malignant tumors, such as hemangioma, neurofibroma, rhabdomyosarcoma, dermoids, and even large chalazia, may produce ptosis. Mechanical ptosis may also be secondary to cicatricial changes. Treatment is directed at the mechanical cause.

9-2-6 *Apparent Ptosis or Pseudoptosis.* Pseudoptosis may result from insufficient support of the eyelid by the globe, as seen in phthisis bulbi, microphthalmos, anophthalmos, enophthalmos, and enucleation. Pseudoptosis in these circumstances can usually be relieved by a new prosthesis or a modification of the present prosthesis. If the ptosis persists, it can be treated surgically. Another cause of pseudoptosis is globe malposition. If the eyelids are in a normal position but the globe is mechanically elevated, the resulting pseudoptosis may be objectionable. This may occur with orbital floor or rim trauma, congenital orbital bone asymmetry, fibrous dysplasia of the orbit, orbital inflammatory disease, or inferior orbital tumors. In cases of untreated or overcorrected orbital floor trauma, the globe position can be altered. Hypertropia can also give the appearance of ptosis, as the relationship of the globe and the lid is altered.

9-3 PREOPERATIVE EVALUATION

A detailed history should be obtained from the patient and family members. Critical elements of the history include approximate onset of the ptosis, progression over time, and fluctuation of severity. Possible causative factors such as trauma, contact lens wear, prior ocular inflammatory disease, surgery, or periocular steroid injections should be sought. Possible accompanying symptoms such as diplopia, dysphagia, and generalized weakness should also be considered. The functional significance of the ptosis (i.e., interference with activities such as driving, reading, work, or hobbies) is important to document. It is also important to inquire about dry eye or irritative symptoms, as they may be worsened with surgical elevation of the eyelids.

A complete ophthalmologic examination should be performed if possible. Special attention should be placed on the protective mechanisms of the ocular surface. A careful slit-lamp examination of the ocular surface should look for signs of dry eyes or exposure. The tear meniscus height may be valuable in this regard. The tear breakup time may also be a helpful screening test in this setting. A Schirmer tear secretion test may be valuable if the history or the examination suggests baseline dry eyes. If the tear secretion is below normal, the ocular surface will have to be monitored closely postoperatively. In older patients with marked reduction in tears, an undercorrection of the ptosis may well be indicated.

Attention should also be placed on eyelid components of ocular surface protection. Other eyelid malpositions such as lower lid ectropion or lower lid retraction may require correction prior to or at the same time as ptosis surgery. A subnormal Bell's phenomenon or lagophthalmos should also be identified preoperatively, as these are significant risk factors for postoperative corneal exposure.

The vertical distance from the corneal light reflex to the upper lid margin, marginal reflex distance 1 (MRD-1), is the most accurate way to quantify the upper lid position. MRD should be measured in primary gaze with the patient's forehead relaxed, as chronic frontalis flexion can elevate the upper lids above their true resting position. Normal values for MRD-1 are typically 3.5 to 5 mm. Levator excursion is one of the most important measurements in both children and adults. It is the distance of the eyelid excursion measured from extreme downward gaze to extreme upward gaze, with the frontalis muscle immobilized by the examiner's manually fixing the eyebrow to its normal position (Fig. 9-2). These measurements are taken with a millimeter ruler held in front of the eye centrally. Normal levator excursion is typically 14 to 17 mm. Subnormal levator excursion generally indicates limited function of the levator muscle, suggestive of myogenic ptosis. The position

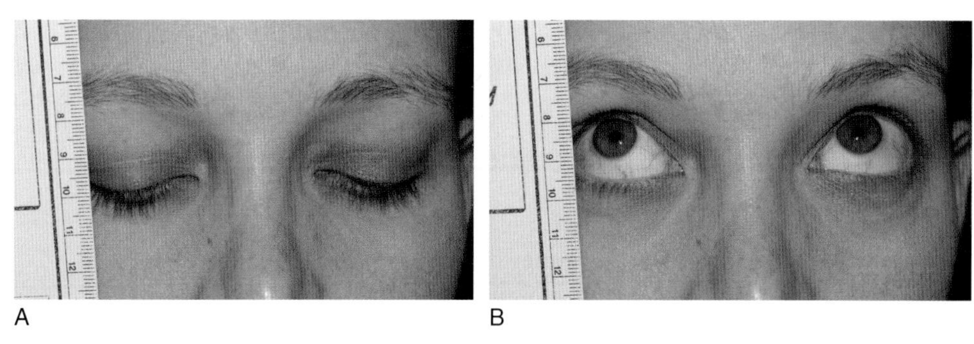

Figure 9-2 Levator function measurements. (A) Distance of upper lid excursion is measured from extreme downward gaze to extreme upward gaze, with frontalis immobilized. (B) Extreme upward gaze.

of the upper lid crease is also an important measurement in the ptosis patient. In Asian patients the lid crease is often found 2 to 5 mm above the lid margin. In other patients, the lid crease typically rests 7 to 9 mm above the margin. The upper eyelid crease is absent or minimal in patients with minimal or no levator function. If the history is vague or inconsistent with examination findings, the patient is asked to bring photographs to corroborate the history and establish the time of onset.

The height and contour of the eyelid crease should be measured and compared to the normal lid if the ptosis is monocular. The eyelid crease is formed by the action of the anterior levator aponeurosis fibers. An abnormally elevated crease indicates a disinsertion or dehiscence of the levator aponeurosis. An absent upper eyelid crease in severe ptosis usually indicates poor levator muscle function.

It is important to note the relative position of the eyelids in down gaze. Some favor making this measurement in the reading position, as that position is relevant to the patient's functional impairment from the ptosis. In severe involutional ptosis, the eyelids not uncommonly block most of the pupils in down gaze. In another variant of involutional ptosis, down gaze ptosis, the patient may have minimal ptosis in primary gaze but severe ptosis in down gaze. In levator maldevelopment ptosis, the fibrotic levator muscle prevents full downward excursion of the eyelid. This retraction in down gaze is referred to as lid lag and is a helpful sign of congenital ptosis.

The presence or absence of Bell's phenomenon should be observed. In patients with myogenic congenital ptosis, presence of Marcus Gunn jaw-winking (aberrant oculomotor nerve innervation) should be assessed by having the patient chew or perform vertical and horizontal jaw movements. These actions can be elicited in infants by observing bottle feeding.

In cases of unilateral ptosis or asymmetric ptosis, the presence or absence of a Hering's effect masking a bilateral ptosis should be determined. This is done by elevating the more ptotic upper lid manually or with 2.5% phenylephrine topically q 5 min × 2. When the more ptotic eyelid is elevated, the contralateral lid will sometimes droop more substantially. The phenylephrine test is also helpful in predicting the result of conjunctival müllerectomy.

Photographs should be taken in primary, up, and down gaze. They give an accurate documentation of the case, are useful for preoperative study, and can be helpful during surgery for intraoperative comparison. Many insurance companies request copies of preoperative photographs and visual field tests as proof of a functional compromise. Photographs may also be important for medicolegal purposes.

9-4 PRINCIPLES OF SURGICAL CORRECTION OF PTOSIS

Selecting the best ptosis procedure for each patient requires a detailed history and a careful clinical examination, tempered by the surgeon's experience and ability. In general, the final result depends on the nature of the ptosis, the type of operation selected, and the skill with which the operation is performed.

In involutional ptosis, external levator repair or conjunctival müllerectomy (Putterman technique) is usually favored. In this scenario, the patient is typically an adult and the procedure is often performed under light sedation. This allows for intraoperative assessment of eyelid height, contour, and symmetry with the patient's cooperation. Some surgeons who are very experienced with ptosis surgery perform this type of ptosis surgery under local anesthesia. Advantages of the anterior approach include familiar anatomic landmarks, adjustability intraoperatively and postoperatively, and versatility in terms of the amount of elevation possible. External levator repair is also combined easily with upper blepharoplasty without additional incisions. The posterior approach of conjunctival müllerectomy also has several advantages. The technique is usually highly predictable (based on the preoperative phenylephrine test). A skin incision is avoided, and the patient need not cooperate intraoperatively for assessment of lid height and symmetry. Also, conjunctival müllerectomy is quicker for most surgeons to perform. Most surgeons reserve conjunctival müllerectomy for ptosis of 2 mm or less or for cases in which the phenylephrine test predicts satisfactory elevation of the lid.

The management of ptosis with limited levator excursion is more complex, more controversial, and beyond the scope of this chapter. Levator maldevelopment ptosis should usually be corrected surgically before the child starts school. The exception is the child with marked ptosis that covers most of the pupil and interferes with normal visual development. Such a patient should be treated for amblyopia, followed closely, and considered for surgery promptly if the amblyopia is not reversible with conservative measures such as occlusion therapy. Other authorities favor early ptosis surgery in patients with significant congenital ptosis, even without detectable amblyopia. The external approach is also recommended in marked ptosis with fair levator function (5 to 7 mm). In levator maldevelopment ptosis surgery, the patient is usually a child or an infant; therefore, general anesthesia is required. A comprehensive description of the management of levator maldevelopment ptosis may be found in *Beard's Ptosis*, 4th ed., by Callahan and Beard (see Suggested Readings section at the end of the chapter).

The degree of levator excursion is the most important parameter in selecting an appropriate surgical plan in the setting of myogenic ptosis. In general, the poorer the levator function, the greater the amount of ptosis. Conversely, the greater the amount of levator function, the smaller the amount of ptosis. If the surgery must be performed under general anesthesia, many surgeons rely on Beard's table (see Table 9-3) to determine the amount of levator resection. This table stratifies the ptosis based on the amount of levator excursion and also the severity of the ptosis. Some surgeons favor use of the Berke table, in which the position of the eyelid relative to the cornea is used as an endpoint at the time of surgery under general anesthesia, but others are critical of this approach as variables that affect eye position (such as depth of anesthesia) are introduced. Others favor a formulaic approach to levator resection surgery in the setting of subnormal levator function.

The management of severe, unilateral myogenic ptosis is particularly complex and controversial. Some surgeons favor unilateral maximal or supermaximal levator resection, and others prefer frontalis suspension. Some authorities, such as Callahan, have suggested placing a sling in the normal lid to improve symmetry, particularly in down gaze. Others, like Beard, have advocated for disabling the levator muscle of the normal lid and performing frontalis suspension bilaterally. Surgeons addressing severe unilateral myogenic ptosis should have an understanding of the wide (and controversial) range of surgical options and the potential difficulties encountered when operating on such patients. In pediatric cases, this complexity necessitates particularly extensive counseling with parents.

Success in ptosis surgery depends as much on making the correct diagnosis and selecting the proper surgical procedure as it does on skillfully performing the surgery.

9-4-1 *External Levator Resection.* The external levator approach is a time-honored method of correcting ptosis (Fig. 9-3). In an adult patient, local anesthesia with or without light intravenous sedation is preferable for this type of surgery. In most adolescent patients, with proper patient selection and preoperative counseling, external levator repair can be done under light sedation.

9-4-1-1 *Technique*

1. With loupe magnification and calipers, the incision site is marked along the intended lid crease as a crescent, with the inferior arc placed at the normal level of the lid crease. The horizontal position of the pupil is marked in each lid with the patient in primary gaze. Topical anesthetic is applied to both ocular surfaces.
2. 1 cc of 1% lidocaine/0.25% bupivacaine solution with 1:100,000 epinephrine is injected subcutaneously along the line of the intended incision.
3. A colored rigid corneal protective contact lens is placed over the eye to protect it during surgery.
4. The skin is incised along the markings. If a crescent has been outlined, the skin–orbicularis blepharoplasty flap is sharply dissected off the underlying septum. A scalpel, electrosurgical unit with microdissection needle, iris scissors, or radiofrequency unit and laser are all suitable methods of skin incision.
5. Meticulous hemostasis is achieved and maintained throughout the case. In many cases thrombin and Gelfoam are useful adjuncts.
6. Next, dissection is directed through the septum. This allows identification of the preaponeurotic fat pad.
7. With gentle countertraction on the lid directed inferiorly, the preaponeurotic fat pad is retracted superiorly and the fine connective tissue attachments between the posterior-inferior aspect of the fat pad are carefully lysed.

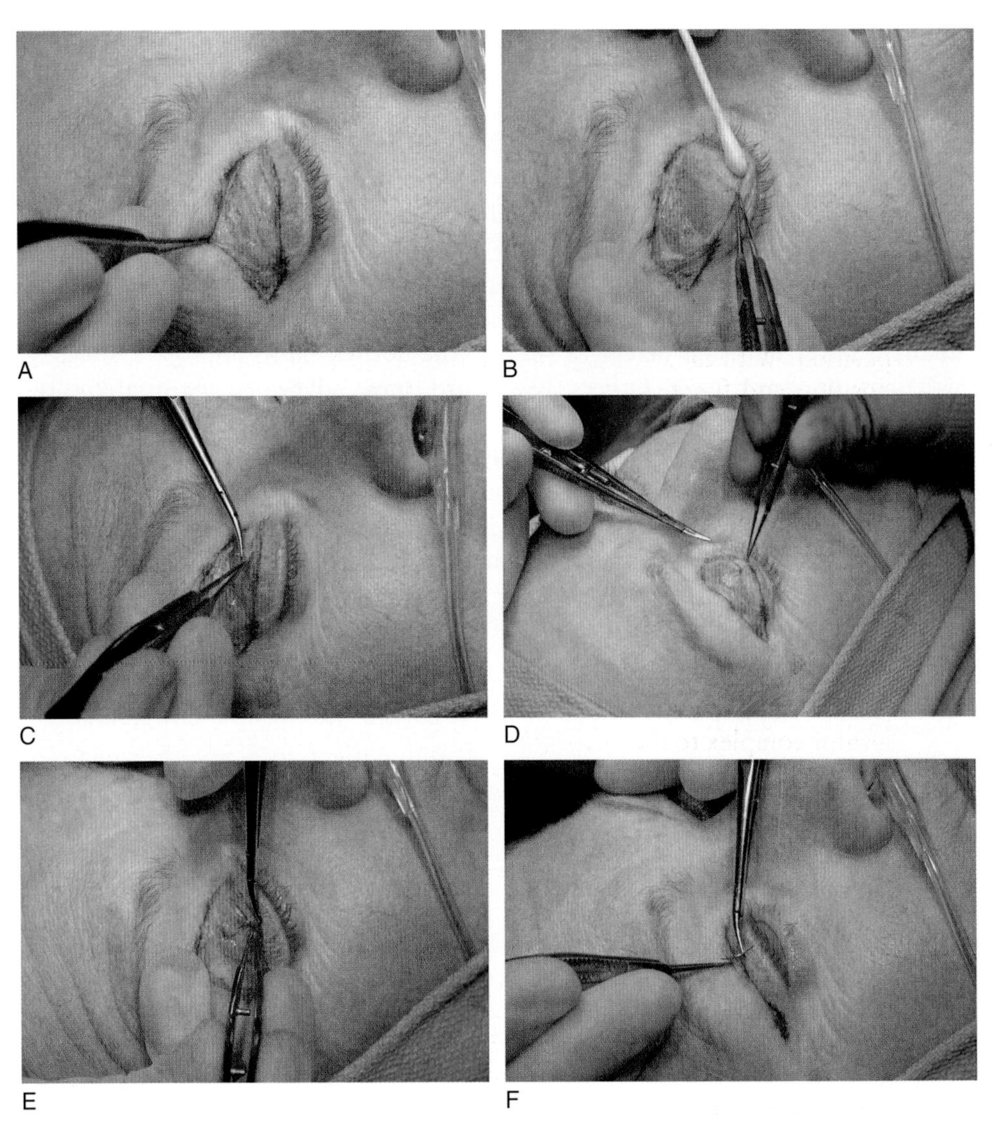

Figure 9-3 External levator aponeurotic approach. (A) The right upper eyelid is opened with preaponeurotic fat and levator complex exposed. (B) Forceps pulling levator aponeurosis inferiorly. Musculoaponeurotic junction is visible. (C) A 6-0 polypropylene suture is used in a horizontal mattress fashion to advance the levator complex onto the anterior surface of the tarsus. (D) The suture is tied. (E) The lid crease is reformed by approximating the pretarsal orbicularis to the levator complex. (F) The orbicularis is closed at three or four points in a buried interrupted fashion with 7-0 polyglactin, followed by closure of the skin edges with 6-0 fast-absorbing gut suture.

8. The musculoaponeurotic junction is identified, as is the levator muscle superiorly and its aponeurosis inferiorly.
9. Next, a suborbicularis/pretarsal dissection is performed with the monopolar unit or Westcott scissors to expose the anterior-superior aspect of the tarsus.
10. In bilateral cases the other lid is dissected to this point, and then the propofol sedation is stopped.
11. A nonabsorbable suture (such as 6-0 polypropylene or 5-0 nylon) is passed in a horizontal mattress fashion through the levator aponeurosis (typically near

the level of the musculoaponeurotic junction) from superiorly to inferiorly. The suture is then passed partial thickness through the anterior-superior aspect of the tarsus at a horizontal position at or just medial to the pupil. The lid is everted to ensure that the suture passage is partial thickness. The suture is then redirected through the levator aponeurosis from inferiorly to superiorly. This cardinal suture is then tied in a temporary slip-knot fashion.

12. In bilateral cases the cardinal suture is placed in the other lid, advancing the levator complex onto the anterior surface as described in Step #11.
13. The corneal protectors are removed and the patient is placed in the seated position. With the effects of the sedation largely worn off, the patient's lid position and function are inspected in primary gaze, up gaze, and down gaze. Eyelid closure is also assessed.
14. If the contour is undesirable or the elevation is insufficient, the cardinal sutures are replaced as needed and lid position and contour are reassessed with the patient in the seated position.
15. Supplemental levator-tarsus sutures are placed as needed (medial and/or lateral to the cardinal suture), and lid height and contour are again inspected.
16. The sutures can be adjusted as needed and are then tied in a permanent fashion.
17. Redundant levator aponeurosis is trimmed as needed.
18. Lid crease reformation is performed by suturing the terminal aspect of the levator complex to the pretarsal orbicularis at the desired lid crease position as needed along the incision line.
19. The orbicularis is closed with 7-0 polyglactin suture at three or four sites along the incision line, and the skin is closed with 6-0 fast-absorbing gut suture or other suture.

9-5-2 *Small-Incision External Levator Repair.* The progressive movement toward more minimally invasive surgical techniques has led to the development of small-incision or minimally invasive external levator repair. The goals of such modifications include more accurate positioning of the eyelid; reduction of bleeding, bruising, and scarring; and decreased operative time.

The small-incision external levator repair is generally reserved for patients with minimal (0 or 1+ on scale of 4) dermatochalasis and levator excursion of 8 mm or more. If significant lash ptosis is present, a standard ptosis repair that allows correction of the lash ptosis across the entire eyelid is preferred. Some of the surgical principles and attendant benefit of this technique may also be applied during ptosis surgery when it is combined with upper blepharoplasty.

9-5-2-1 *Technique*

1. Local infiltrative anesthesia is achieved using approximately 0.6 mL of 2% lidocaine with 1:100,000 units of epinephrine.
2. The skin of the intended incision site is marked. The position of this marking should be at the horizontal position of the eyelid that will achieve the best contour when elevated. In the original description of the technique, an 8-mm incision length was used. The author currently prefers an incision length of 12 mm that extends from the horizontal position of the medial corneoscleral limbus to the lateral limbus with the eye in primary gaze. This slight lengthening of the incision facilitates the dissection and advancement

of the levator while preserving the minimally invasive advantages of the technique.

3. The skin is incised.
4. With an assistant providing traction in an inferior and anterior direction, the surgeon grasps the superior edge of the incision and retracts superiorly. Dissection through the orbicularis just superior to the top of the tarsus is performed with a microdissection needle on the monopolar electrosurgical unit.
5. At this point, a small amount of blunt dissection through the orbital septum with a cotton-tipped applicator is often helpful, along with additional sharp dissection with the microdissection needle.
6. The preaponeurotic fat pad and the musculoaponeurotic junction of the levator complex should be identified. No dissection is necessary on the posterior surface of the levator aponeurosis.
7. The anterior superior surface of the tarsus is exposed in a standard fashion, but the dissection is limited to the portion of the tarsus overlying the cornea.
8. A 6-0 Prolene suture (or other similar nonabsorbable suture) is passed in a horizontal mattress fashion, first through the levator complex at the level of the musculoaponeurotic junction and then partial thickness through the superior third of the tarsus, and finally back through the levator complex at the level of the musculoaponeurotic junction. Restricting the tarsal bites to the superior third of the tarsus minimizes the likelihood of contour abnormalities from the cardinal suture or other supporting sutures. The suture is tied in temporary fashion.
9. The patient is placed in the seated position, and eyelid height and contour are carefully inspected in primary gaze, up gaze, and down gaze. The cardinal suture is adjusted as needed. If needed for contour or if desired, a supporting suture of 6-0 polypropylene is placed medial and/or lateral to the cardinal suture.
10. The polypropylene sutures are tied in a permanent fashion.
11. Eyelid crease reformation is not recommended with this technique.
12. The orbicularis is reapproximated with one or two buried interrupted sutures of 7-0 polyglactin.
13. The skin is closed with 6-0 fast-absorbing plain gut suture.

9-4-3 *Conjunctival Müllerectomy (Putterman Technique)*. The conjunctival müllerectomy (Putterman) procedure can be viewed as a significant modification of the Fasanella-Servat procedure with several advantages. Conjunctival müllerectomy is an excellent choice for limited degrees of ptosis, typically approximately 2 mm. Preoperative testing with phenylephrine drops is useful in predicting the results of conjunctival müllerectomy. This technique's advantages include lack of a skin incision, predictability of results, and ease and speed of performance. The technique can also be graded in a quantitative fashion to address mild to moderate ptosis of varied severity (8 mm resection → 2 mm elevation, 6 mm resection → 1.5 mm elevation, and 4 mm resection → 1 mm elevation). The above advantages make the technique particularly valuable in the armamentarium of cosmetic oculofacial surgery. Conjunctival müllerectomy has been performed safely in patients with dry eye and also in patients with glaucoma filtering blebs. The author's slight modification of the conjunctival müllerectomy is described below.

9-4-3-1 *Technique*

1. The procedure may be performed under local anesthesia, sedation, or general anesthesia.
2. The center of the upper lid margin is marked with a surgical marking pen.
3. Local anesthesia (such as 0.5 mL of 2% lidocaine with 1:100,000 units of epinephrine) is injected into the anterior lamella at the marked position of the eyelid margin. Topical anesthetic is administered to the ocular surface.
4. A 4-0 silk suture is passed partial thickness through the margin near the centering mark. This suture is used as a traction suture to evert the upper lid.
5. The upper lid is everted over a Desmarres retractor.
6. Calipers are used to measure the distance of the desired resection from the superior aspect of the tarsus toward the superior fornix, and a 6-0 silk suture is passed horizontally in several passes across the superior fornix as a marking suture at the desired measured level.
7. Additional local anesthetic is now injected into the conjunctiva and Müeller's muscle.
8. Toothed forceps are used to mobilize the conjunctiva and Müeller's muscle from the levator complex.
9. The Putterman clamp is used to incorporate the desired conjunctiva and Müeller's layers. The silk marking suture should just be engaged in the edge of the clamp, and the preseptal skin should be easily drawn away from the clamp.
10. A double-armed 5-0 plain gut suture is passed from lateral to medial in a serpentine fashion approximately 1.5 mm below the clamp.
11. The conjunctiva and Müeller's muscle engaged in the clamp is now excised with a scalpel. Care is taken to avoid cutting the previously passed suture.
12. Next the suture is used to approximate the conjunctiva and Müeller's muscle on one side of the incision with the conjunctiva and tarsus on the other side of the incision. A simple running technique is used from a medial to lateral direction.
13. Both ends of the suture are now passed through the conjunctival wound, passed transcutaneously, and tied externally at the level of the lid crease. This is done to reduce the possibility of corneal irritation from the knot.

9-4-4 *Frontalis Suspension Procedures.* When levator function is poor (4 mm or less), most surgeons prefer frontalis suspension over levator resection surgery. Patients and relevant family members need to understand from preoperative counseling that frontalis suspension is a very imperfect solution. Possible problems such as overcorrection, undercorrection, asymmetry, eyelid contour abnormalities, lagophthalmos, ocular surface exposure, and need for additional surgery should be discussed thoroughly preoperatively. Continued ptosis in up gaze and retraction in down gaze are predictable and should be discussed preoperatively so that expectations are appropriate.

The material used for suspension should be discussed and decided on preoperatively. Some of the more commonly used materials are autologous fascia lata, banked homologous fascia lata, and commercially available silicone rod. Other options for frontalis suspension include temporalis fascia or frontalis muscle advancement. Many surgeons consider autologous fascia lata to be the gold standard, but not all studies have demonstrated superior results over homologous fascia lata or other autologous materials. There are many published techniques of fascial lata suspension; references are provided at the end of the chapter. Several references regarding frontalis suspension materials are also provided at the end of this chapter.

9-5 POSTOPERATIVE COMPLICATIONS

Owing to the many variables encountered during repair of ptosis, ideal results can sometimes be difficult to achieve. In patients with normal levator function, excellent results are often achievable. When levator function is poor, results are necessarily limited with current approaches and available techniques.

The incidence of complications can be reduced by a thorough knowledge of eyelid anatomy and a careful preoperative workup. Proper surgical planning is especially important in ptosis repair, as there are numerous surgical options. In the operating room, efforts should be made to minimize variables in order to achieve consistent results. Anesthetic considerations, including the volume and concentration of local anesthetic as well as the depth of sedation, are important. Minimizing intraoperative bleeding is also important to optimize ptosis surgery results. Eliminating antiplatelet and anticoagulant drugs preoperatively, as possible, is rewarded with a drier, more precise surgical field. Multiple observations of the patient in primary gaze, up gaze, and down gaze while the patient is in the seated position with minimal sedation can improve the accuracy of ptosis surgery performed under sedation or local anesthetic.

Undercorrection appears to be the most prevalent complication of ptosis surgery. It has two principal causes: inadequate resection or advancement of the levator muscle or improper choice of operation. Overcorrection is a less frequent complication of ptosis surgery, particularly if levator excursion is subnormal, as in levator maldevelopment ptosis. Lagophthalmos may accompany ptosis overcorrection or may occur in rare cases in which the orbital septum is inadvertently incorporated in the closure. When substantial undercorrection, overcorrection, or contour abnormality occurs, early surgical revision can often be performed in the office 2 to 3 weeks postoperatively.

Worsening of dry eye symptoms or mild superficial punctuate keratopathy is not a rare development after ptosis surgery. Lubrication with artificial tears and ointments is usually sufficient, as mild exposure keratopathy typically improves over time. Severe exposure or cases unresponsive to conservative therapy must be managed with surgical revision. On rare occasion, a satisfactory result in terms of lid height and palpebral fissure can produce intolerable exposure keratitis. Such postoperative exposure can be anticipated in chronic progressive external ophthalmoplegia with progressive loss of ocular motility and loss of Bell's phenomenon. The desired result in such cases is a functional undercorrection (i.e., elevation of the eyelids only minimally above the visual axis).

Issues of eyelid symmetry and topography are sometimes bothersome postoperatively to both patient and surgeon. Although these are not typically vision-threatening, care in avoiding them is certainly warranted. Attention to symmetry of the surgical markings, especially placement of the intended lid crease, will help increase the chance of symmetry after surgery. Careful preoperative measurements and good surgical technique are the means of preventing a misplaced lid crease. Substantial variations in lid crease configuration are seen in patients of different ethnicity. When the lid crease is not distinct preoperatively, appropriate presurgical discussion of this issue is important. Such a discussion is almost always necessary with patients of Asian ethnicity undergoing upper eyelid surgery. Failure to remove skin from the upper eyelid after levator resection may result in dermatochalasis obscuring the lid crease. Reformation of a lid crease is performed by closing the skin or orbicularis at the incision with sutures into the underlying levator complex.

Abnormal eyelid contour can usually be avoided. Care in placing the cardinal sutures into the appropriate horizontal position along the tarsus during external levator repair will help avoid an aesthetically displeasing eyelid contour. Placing additional supporting sutures medial and/or lateral to the central cardinal suture is often necessary to avoid contour abnormalities, particularly peaking centrally or flatness medially or laterally. Similarly, attention is required when suturing fascia lata to tarsus in order to achieve a pleasing upper eyelid contour.

Conjunctival prolapse occurs occasionally, especially in severe cases of ptosis where the dissection has to be carried far above the superior upper fornix, causing the suspensory ligaments of the conjunctival fornix to be separated. Prolapse or ectropion is also a result of edema, and spontaneous resorption usually occurs. Topical antibiotic–steroid eye drops can be used four times a day for 2 to 3 weeks. If drops fail, gentle repositioning with a muscle hook after topical anesthesia may be attempted. If this fails to reduce persistent prolapse, the surgeon may try either hyaluronidase (150 USP/1 cc normal saline solution) directly into the prolapse or excision and replacement with three double-armed sutures (5-0 chromic gut) through the full thickness of the eyelid. These sutures exit through the previous skin crease and are tied externally. No stents are used.

Infection may occur postoperatively as with surgery anywhere else in the body. Fortunately, infection after ptosis surgery is rare because of the excellent blood supply to the lids. Postoperative hemorrhage can destroy an excellent result and can even result in loss of vision. This complication is rather unusual. Hemostasis should be meticulously performed before closure. Aspirin products should be avoided for 1 week before and immediately post-operatively as possible. Any trauma to the lids should be guarded against for 3 weeks postoperatively.

SUGGESTED READINGS

GENERAL

Callahan MA, Beard C. *Beard's Ptosis*. 4th ed. Birmingham, AL: Aesculapius Publishing Co., 1990.

Dortzbach RK, Gausas RA, Sherman DD. Blepharoptosis. In: Dortzbach RK, ed. *Ophthalmic Plastic Surgery: Prevention and Management of Complications*. New York: Raven Press, 1994.

LEVATOR SURGERY

Anderson RL, Beard C. The levator aponeurosis. *Arch Ophthalmol.* 1977;95:1437–1441.

Anderson RL, Dixon RS. Aponeurotic ptosis surgery. *Arch Ophthalmol.* 1979;97:1123–1128.

Anderson RL, Dixon RS. The role of Whitnall's ligament in ptosis surgery. *Arch Ophthalmol.* 1979;97:705–707.

Beard C. A new treatment for severe unilateral congenital ptosis and for ptosis with jaw winking. *Am J Ophthalmol.* 1965;59:252–258.

Beard C. The surgical treatment of blepharoptosis: a quantitative approach. *Trans Am Ophthalmol Soc.* 1966;64:401–487.

Berke RN. Results of resection of the levator muscle through a skin incision in congenital ptosis. *Arch Ophthalmol.* 1959;61:177–201.

Dortzbach RK, Kronish JW. Early revision in the office for adults after unsatisfactory blepharoptosis correction. *Am J Ophthalmol.* 1993;115:68–75.

Dortzbach RK, Sutula FC. Involutional blepharoptosis: a histopathologic study. *Arch Ophthalmol.* 1980;98:2045–2049.

Frueh BR, Musch DC, McDonald HM. Efficacy and efficiency of a small-incision, minimal dissection procedure versus a traditional approach for correcting aponeurotic ptosis. *Ophthalmology.* 2004;111:2158–2163.

Jones LT. The anatomy of the upper eyelid and its relation to ptosis surgery. *Am J Ophthalmol.* 1964;57:943–959.

Jones LT, Quickert MH, Wobig JL. The cure of ptosis by aponeurotic repair. *Arch Ophthalmol.* 1975;93:629–634.

Lucarelli MJ, Lemke BN. Small incision external levator repair: technique and early results. *Am J Ophthalmol.* 1999;127(6):637–644.

Paris GL, Quickert MH. Disinsertion of the aponeurosis of the levator palpebrae superioris muscle after cataract extraction. *Am J Ophthalmol.* 1976;81:337–340.

POSTERIOR APPROACH PTOSIS SURGERY

Agatston SA. Resection of the levator palpebrae muscle by the conjunctival route for ptosis. 1942;27:994–996.

Ben Simon GJ, Lee S, Schwarcz RM, McCann JD, Goldberg RA. Müller's muscle-conjunctival resection for correction of upper eyelid ptosis: relationship between phenylephrine testing and the amount of tissue resected with final eyelid position. *Arch Facial Plast Surg.* 2007;9:413–417.

Dresner SC. Further modifications of the Müller's muscle-conjunctival resection procedure for blepharoptosis. *Ophthal Plast Reconstr Surg.* 1991;7:114–122.

Fasanella RM, Servat J. Levator resection for minimal ptosis: another simplified option. *Arch Ophthalmol.* 1961;65:493–496.

Putterman AM, Fett DR. Müller's muscle in the treatment of upper eyelid ptosis: a ten-year study. *Ophthalmic Surg.* 1986;17:354–360.

Putterman AM, Urist MJ. Müller muscle-conjunctiva resection. Technique for treatment of blepharoptosis. *Arch Ophthalmol.* 1975;93:619–623.

Rose JG, Lemke BN, Dresner SC, Lucarelli MJ. Blepharoptosis treatment options during upper eyelid cosmetic blepharoplasty. *Am J Cosm Surg.* 2003;20:73–82.

FRONTALIS SUSPENSION

Ben Simon GJ, Macedo AA, Schwarcz RM, Wang DY, McCann JF, Goldberg RA. Frontalis suspension for upper eyelid ptosis: evaluation of different surgical designs and suture material. *Am J Ophthalmol.* 2005;140:877–885.

Callahan A. Correction of unilateral blepharoptosis with bilateral eyelid suspension. *Am J Ophthalmol.* 1972;74:321–326.

Carter SR, Meecham WJ, Seiff SR. Silicone frontalis slings for the correction of blepharoptosis: indications and efficacy. *Ophthalmology.* 1996; 103:623–630.

Crawford JS. Repair of ptosis using frontalis muscle and fascia lata. *Trans Am Acad Ophthalmol Otolaryngol.* 1956;60:672–678.

Dailey RA, Wilson DJ, Wobig JL. Trans-conjunctival frontalis suspension. *Ophthalmic Plast Reconstr Surg.* 1991;7:284–297.

DeMartelaere SL, Blaydon SM, Cruz AA, Amato MM, Shore JW. Broad fascia fixation enhances frontalis suspension. *Ophthal Plast Reconstr Surg.* 2007;23:279–284.

Esmaili B, Chung H, Pashby RC. Long-term results of frontalis suspension using irradiated, banked fascia lata. *Ophthal Plast Reconstr Surg.* 1998;14:159–163.

Fox SA. Congenital ptosis frontalis sling. *J Pediatr Ophthalmol.* 1966;3:28.

Hersh D, Martin FJ, Rowe N. Comparison of Silastic and banked fascia lata in pediatric frontalis suspension. *J Pediatr Ophthalmol Strabismus.* 2006;43:212–218.

Kersten RC, Bernardini FP, Khouri L, Moin M, Roumeliotis AA, Kulwin DR. Unilateral frontalis sling for the surgical correction of unilateral poor-function ptosis. *Ophthal Plast Reconstr Surg.* 2005; 6:412–417.

Leone CR Jr, Shore JW, Van Gemert JV. Silicone rod frontalis sling for the correction of blepharoptosis. *Ophthalmic Surg.* 1981;12:881–887.

Mauriello JA Jr, Abdelsalam A. Effectiveness of homologous cadaveric fascia lata and role of suture fixation to tarsus in frontalis suspension. *Ophthal Plast Reconstr Surg.* 1998;14:99–104.

Naugle TC Jr, Fry CL, Sabatier RE, Elliott LF. High leg incision fascia lata harvesting. *Ophthalmology.* 1997;104:1480–1488.

O'Reilly J, Lanigan B, Bowell R, O'Keefe M. Congenital ptosis: long-term results using stored fascia lata. *Acta Ophthalmol Scand.* 1998;76:346–348.

Wasserman BN, Sprunger DT, Helveston EM. Comparison of materials used in frontalis suspension. *Arch Ophthalmol.* 2001;119:687–691.

10

Management of Eyelid Retraction

ALEXANDER TAICH, MD, AND
ADAM S. HASSAN, MD

Eyelid retraction has numerous causes (Table 10-1).[1] Most notably eyelid retraction is caused by thyroid eye disease (TED), trauma, and postsurgical changes. The upper eyelid margin is typically measured at 3.5 to 4.5 mm above the center of the cornea. The lower eyelid margin is typically situated at the inferior border of the limbus. Eyelid retraction is a condition in which the upper eyelid margin is displaced superiorly or the lower eyelid margin is displaced inferiorly. Eyelid retraction may result in exposure keratopathy and disturbing ocular symptoms, including blurred vision, photophobia, foreign body sensation, burning, and reactive tearing.

Table 10-1 Causes of Eyelid Retraction

Inflammatory
Thyroid eye disease
Orbital pseudotumor
Cicatricial conjunctival disease
Chronic dermatitis
Scleroderma
Traumatic
Eyelid laceration
Orbital floor fracture
Inferior rectus disinsertion

continued

Table 10-1 (Continued)

Postoperative
Blepharoplasty
Blepharoptosis repair
Eyelid tumor resection and reconstruction
Orbital floor fracture repair
Inferior rectus recession
Superior rectus recession
Retinal detachment surgery (scleral buckle)
Glaucoma filtering surgery with prominent bleb
Involutional, Congenital, Neurogenic
Facial nerve palsy
Aberrant regeneration of oculomotor nerve
Marcus Gunn jaw-winking
Sympathetic overactivity (Claude Bernard syndrome)
Midbrain lesion (Collier's sign)
Pseudoretraction from contralateral ptosis (Hering's law)
Metabolic
Cirrhosis
Hypokalemic periodic paralysis
Uremia
Cushing syndrome
Pharmacologic
Sympathomimetic agents (phenylephrine, apraclonidine)
Botulinum toxin injection
Corticosteroids
Proptotic, Myopic
Contact Lens Wear

10-1 MECHANISMS OF LID RETRACTION IN TED

Eyelid retraction in TED is thought to be due to a combination of inflammation, fibrosis, and adrenergic stimulation of the eyelid retractors.[2] Proptosis can also contribute to eyelid retraction. In the upper eyelid, factors responsible for eyelid retraction include (1) inflammation and fibrosis of the levator and Müller's muscles,[3,4] (2) adrenergic stimulation of Müller's muscle, and (3) inflammation and fibrosis of the inferior rectus muscle, causing hypodeviation of the globe and compensatory overaction of the superior rectus–levator complex. In the lower eyelid, factors responsible for eyelid retraction include (1) inflammation and fibrosis of the inferior rectus muscle with consequent traction on its anterior extension, the capsulopalpebral fascia, which is the main lower lid retractor, and (2) adrenergic stimulation of the smooth muscle fibers within the lower lid retractor complex.

10-2 EXPOSURE KERATOPATHY IN TED

A combination of eyelid retraction and proptosis in TED may result in ocular exposure with symptoms of ocular irritation, an undesirable cosmetic appearance, corneal erosion and infection, or (rarely) globe luxation. Mild exposure problems can be managed with topical lubricants. Guanethidine, a topical sympatholytic agent, is of limited usefulness in the management of eyelid retraction due to its variable efficacy and frequent ocular side effects, including irritation, hyperemia, photophobia, pain, edema, burning sensation, and punctate keratitis.[5] It may be more tolerable if used in lower concentrations.[6]

Exposure problems in the inflammatory phase of the condition present a special challenge as surgical correction of eyelid retraction is best performed in the post-inflammatory, stable phase. Several reports[7–12] have described using Botulinum toxin injections, 2.5 to 15 U, either subconjunctivally or percutaneously, just above the superior border of the tarsus. The lowering of the eyelid can be variable, sometimes requiring titration of the administered dose. The duration of the effect is likewise variable, but may last up to 6 months or longer.[7] The predictable complications of ptosis and diplopia are transient. Overall, chemodenervation with Botulinum toxin can be recommended as a temporary adjunctive treatment of upper eyelid retraction in the inflammatory phase.

Exposure problems in the stable phase that are not adequately relieved by topical lubricants require surgical intervention.

10-3 ORBITAL DECOMPRESSION AND EYELID SURGERY IN TED

Some cases of TED are best managed with only eyelid retraction surgery, others with surgical orbital decompression alone, and still others with a combination of the two treatments, usually separated by an interval of time. Preoperative diplopia and anatomic relationships require rehabilitative surgery to be staged in a specific sequence, starting with orbital decompression, followed by eye muscle surgery, followed by eyelid repositioning. The two surgical procedures are not mutually exclusive. The choice between the two surgical approaches must be made in light of multiple variables, and individualized for each patient. If orbital decompression surgery is being contemplated, eyelid surgery must be delayed until following the decompression surgery. In cases of mild proptosis and retraction, combined as opposed to staged decompression and retraction surgery has been reported.[13]

Although a complete discussion is beyond the scope of this chapter, orbital decompression is indicated for some cases of TED-associated optic neuropathy. In the presence of marked proptosis, orbital decompression may also be necessary to provide optimal relief of exposure symptoms and acceptable cosmesis. Likewise, in cases of unilateral or highly asymmetric proptosis, an optimal cosmetic result may be achieved only with orbital decompression.

10-4 TIMING OF EYELID SURGERY IN TED

It is critical to perform eyelid retraction surgery in TED when the disease is in a quiescent state. Failure to do so may compromise surgical results. The systemic thyroid status and eyelid position on serial examinations should be stable for 6 to 12 months before surgery. Severe exposure keratitis unresponsive to medical management may necessitate earlier intervention in rare instances; an easily reversible tarsorrhaphy or Botulinum toxin injection may also be considered in this setting.

As the therapies for other manifestations of Graves disease can affect eyelid position, eyelid retraction surgery should be delayed until after these treatments have been completed and their effects have stabilized. The therapeutic modalities that, if indicated, should precede eyelid retraction surgery include radioactive iodine or other treatments for hyperthyroidism, systemic corticosteroids, orbital irradiation, orbital decompression, and extraocular muscle surgery for diplopia.[14]

10-5 UPPER EYELID SURGERY IN TED

A variety of procedures have been described to surgically treat upper eyelid retraction, and surgeons continue to refine their techniques. In all of these procedures, alterations are made in one or both of the upper eyelid retractors—that is, Müller's muscle and the levator palpebrae superioris. A recently popularized procedure involves full-thickness blepharotomy.[14–17] In other approaches, Müller's muscle is sometimes excised[18–21] or recessed.[22–26] The levator aponeurosis is sometimes recessed,[22–24,26–29] stretched,[18–20] disinserted,[25,30] myotomized,[31] and transposed.[21,29] Adjustable sutures have been used.[27,28] In the past, materials were sometimes implanted between the recessed upper lid retractors and the tarsus. Although such "spacers" remain useful in the treatment of lower eyelid retraction, their use in the upper eyelid has largely been abandoned because of complications. The upper lid retractors may be weakened either with a posterior approach through a conjunctival incision or with an anterior approach through a cutaneous incision.

10-5-1 *Full-Thickness Blepharotomy in* TED. Leo Koornneef developed a rapid, trancutaneous, graded full-thickness blepharotomy technique in the 1990s. It has since been adopted and described[15–17] by several surgeons. It has been found to achieve consistent eyelid height and contour while relieving the symptoms of exposure keratopathy.

After symmetric upper eyelid crease incisions are marked, anesthesia is accomplished with local infiltration with 0.5% bupivacaine mixed in equal parts with 1% to 2% lidocaine with epinephrine 1:100,000 (Fig. 10-1A). The skin is incised in the relevant portion (central, medial, or lateral) of the marked crease. Subsequent dissection through the orbicularis oculi muscle for the length of the incision exposes the levator aponeurosis inferior to its confluence with the orbital septum near the superior border of the tarsal plate (Fig. 10-1B). The levator aponeurosis, Müller's muscle, and conjunctiva are then incised at the superior border of the tarsal plate in the area of greatest retraction, creating a full-thickness blepharotomy (Fig. 10-1C). The dissection is usually initiated at the junction of the lateral and central thirds of

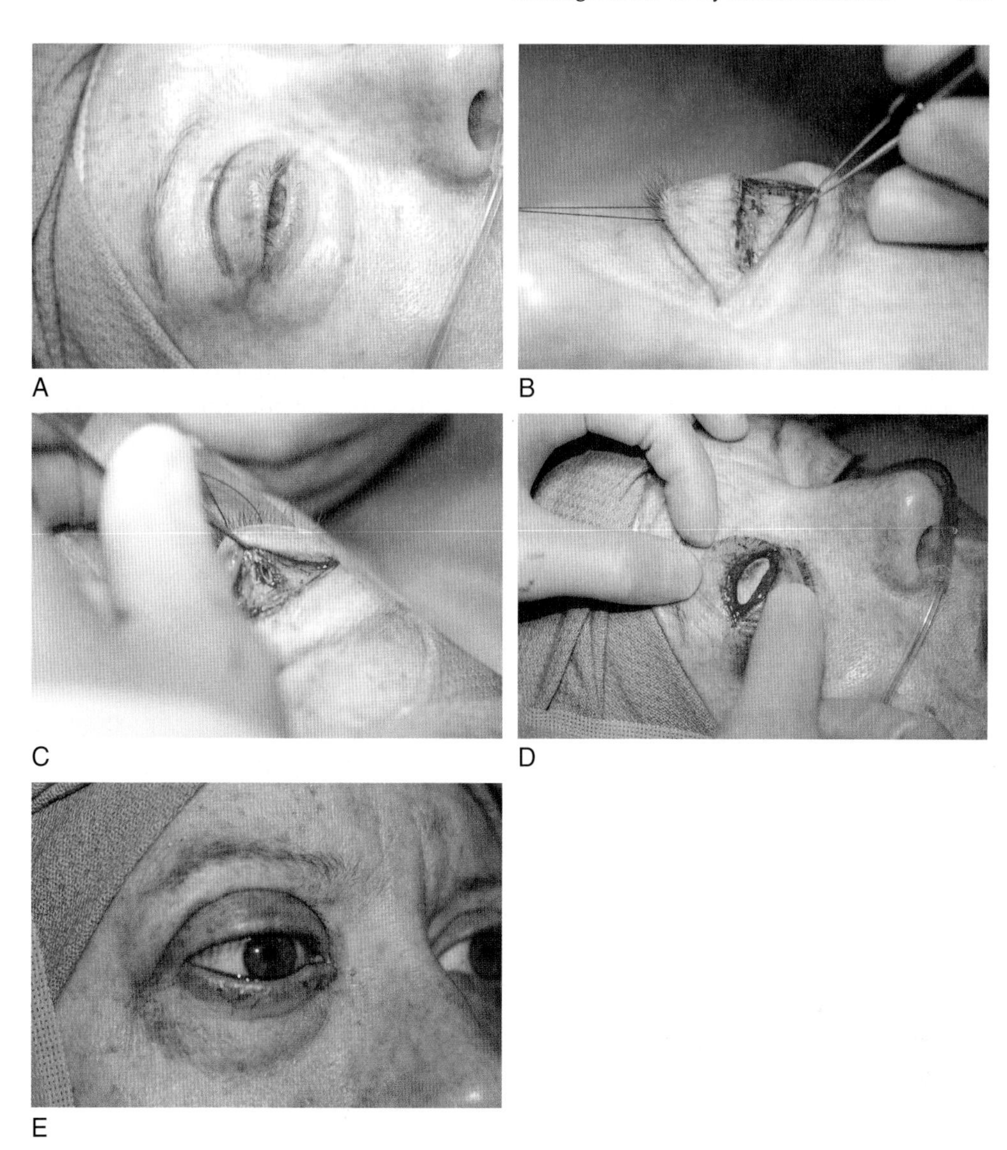

Figure 10-1 Full-thickness blepharotomy in TED. (A) The upper eyelid crease is marked and anesthetized with local infiltration. (B) Dissection through the orbital septum exposes the pre-aponeurotic fat pads and the levator aponeurosis. (C) The levator aponeurosis, Müller's muscle, and conjunctiva are incised to create a buttonhole through the eyelid. (D,E) The full-thickness blepharotomy is then continued medially and laterally in a graded fashion until the desired eyelid height and contour is achieved. (Photos courtesy of Michael T. Yen, MD)

the upper eyelid. The full-thickness blepharotomy is then extended medially and laterally along the superior tarsal border in a graded fashion based on the unsedated patient's eyelid height and contour while seated and in primary gaze (Fig. 10-1D,E). The upper eyelid is recessed to obtain a final postoperative margin to reflex distance between 2 and 4 mm, depending on the severity of exposure symptoms or the height of the other eyelid in unilateral cases. In cases with temporal flare, full-thickness dissection is performed laterally to the superior crus of the lateral canthal ligament, cutting the lateral horn of the levator aponeurosis inferior to the lacrimal gland ducts. The incisions are extended horizontally as needed—in some cases across the entire eyelid.

When extensive medial dissection results in flattening of the upper eyelid contour, a single 6-0 polyglactin mattress suture is placed between the levator aponeurosis and tarsal plate in the flattened area to restore a desirable upper eyelid contour. In select cases, a central bridge of conjunctiva 3 to 4 mm wide can be left intact in the pupillary axis, preventing central ptosis.[17] In severe cases of retraction, this central bridge of conjunctiva must be incised to fully address the eyelid retraction. Limited bipolar cautery can be used for hemostasis.

The procedure is completed by a simple skin closure with a continuous 6-0 nylon or 6-0 polypropylene. No temporary tarsorrhaphy or traction sutures are placed. An example of a patient who underwent unilateral full-thickness blepharotomy for TED-related upper eyelid retraction is illustrated in Figure 10-2.

Alternative anterior approaches[22–24,27–31] utilize transcutaneous levator aponeurotomy or myotomy with or without Müller's muscle myotomy or excision with additional modifications, including adjustable sutures and levator transpositions. None of these techniques addresses the diffuse nature of Graves eye disease, including conjunctival fibrosis,[16] and they suffer from highly variable results in our experience.

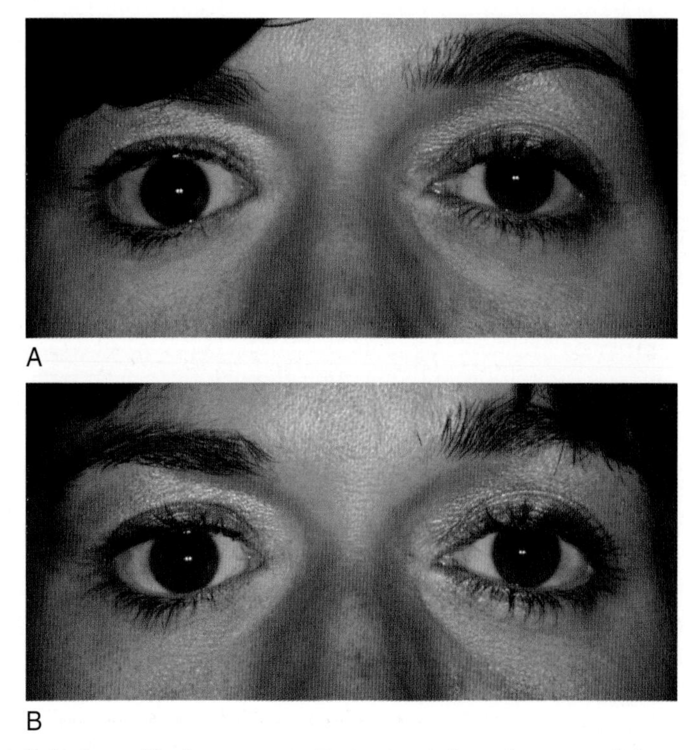

Figure 10-2 Full-thickness blepharotomy in TED. (A) Unilateral upper eyelid retraction in TED. (B) Postoperative result after unilateral full-thickness blepharotomy.

10-6 LOWER EYELID SURGERY IN TED

Various surgical procedures have been described for lower eyelid retraction, all of which involve recession of the lower eyelid retractors. The lower eyelid retractors may be approached through a conjunctival incision, an infraciliary incision, and/or a lateral canthotomy and inferior cantholysis. Unlike the treatment of upper eyelid retraction, most surgeons think that recession of the lower eyelid retractors alone is insufficient to fully correct all but the mildest cases of lower lid retraction, in part because of the effects of gravity. Hence, most surgeons augment lower eyelid retractor recession with one or more additional surgical maneuvers, which fall into two broad categories: (1) alteration of the lateral canthus and (2) implantation of material between the recessed lower eyelid retractors and the tarsus (i.e., spacers). When midfacial descent contributes to the loss of lower eyelid support, some surgeons[32,33] employ pre- or subperiosteal midface lifts in addition to the above techniques.

Alterations in the lateral canthus that have proved useful in the treatment of lower eyelid retraction include the tarsal strip procedure[34–37] and tarsorrhaphy.[36] In the tarsal strip procedure[37] the lower eyelid is disinserted near the lateral orbital rim and reattached to the lateral canthal area in a location different from its original site of insertion, generally more superior and more anterior. The purpose of the tarsal strip procedure in the treatment of ectropion or entropion differs from its purpose in Graves disease. In ectropion or entropion repair, the main purpose is to tighten a lax lower lid, whereas in Graves disease, the purpose is to position the temporal lower lid more superiorly to counteract lid retraction and more anteriorly to counteract proptosis. Excessive tightening of the lower eyelid in the presence of a proptotic eye can worsen lower eyelid retraction by pulling the lower eyelid under the globe. Tarsorrhaphy can also be used to diminish the amount of ocular exposure and to make the eye appear less proptotic, both by narrowing the palpebral fissure and by reducing temporal eyelid retraction.

A variety of spacer materials have been implanted between the recessed lower lid retractors and the tarsus. Cadaveric sclera preserved in ethanol has been the material most commonly used in the past. Other materials that have been successfully used as spacers include upper eyelid tarsus,[38,39] hard palate mucosa,[32,33,40–46] and auricular cartilage.[47–51] Porous polyethylene (MedPore) has been tried, but its use results in a high number of complications requiring further surgery, including exposure.[52,53] Acellular human dermis (AlloDerm) has been tried[54] with good early results. One of the authors (A.S.H.) has been using porcine dermal collagen (ENDURAGen[55]) with early success. The following section presents a technique that combines lower eyelid retractor recession, a tarsal strip procedure, lateral tarsorrhaphy, and placement of a spacer.[56] Different spacer materials can be used.

10-6-1 *Surgical Procedure.* Local anesthesia is preferred so that the eyelid level can be more accurately assessed intraoperatively. A 2% solution of lidocaine with 1:100,000 epinephrine is used to infiltrate the lower lid and lateral canthal area as well as the central upper lid adjacent to the margin. A 4-0 silk suture is placed through skin, orbicularis, and superficial tarsus of the upper eyelid and is used to provide traction upward.

A tarsal strip procedure is initiated.[57] A lateral canthotomy is performed, and the inferior crus of the lateral canthal tendon is isolated from overlying orbicularis and underlying conjunctiva. The inferior crus of the tendon is then lysed adjacent to the lateral orbital wall.

At this point, the lower lid retractors are released. A 4-0 silk suture is placed nasally, centrally, and temporally on the internal surface of the lower eyelid through the conjunctiva and tarsus at the superior aspect of the tarsus. This suture is placed to provide traction outward. The lower eyelid is everted over a Desmarres retractor to expose the surface of the internal lid.

Westcott scissors are used to enter the space temporally between the capsulopalpebral fascia and the orbicularis muscle. The blades are then withdrawn from the wound; one blade is reinserted into the separated plane between the capsulopalpebral fascia and the orbicularis muscle and then moved to the level beneath the inferior tarsal border. The tissues below the inferior tarsus (i.e., conjunctiva and capsulopalpebral fascia) are severed (Fig. 10-3A). The capsulopalpebral fascia is then dissected from the orbicularis muscle to the level of the inferior orbital rim (Fig. 10-3B). Excessive orbital fat, if present, is excised at this time.

The formation of the tarsal strip is then completed. The amount of excess lower lid is determined by overlapping the temporal cut edge of the upper lid with the lower lid at the lateral canthus. A mark is then made with a sterile marker on the lower eyelid margin at the point of overlap; this mark delineates the extent of the future tarsal strip. Westcott scissors are used to make a cut along the gray line corresponding to the tarsal strip. Skin and orbicularis and eyelid margin epithelium are then removed from the strip. The conjunctival epithelium is scraped off the posterior aspect of the strip with a #15 Bard-Parker blade. A 4-0 double-armed polypropylene suture is placed in a double-locking manner through the medial aspect of this strip. The suture arms are then passed either through the periosteum of the lateral orbital

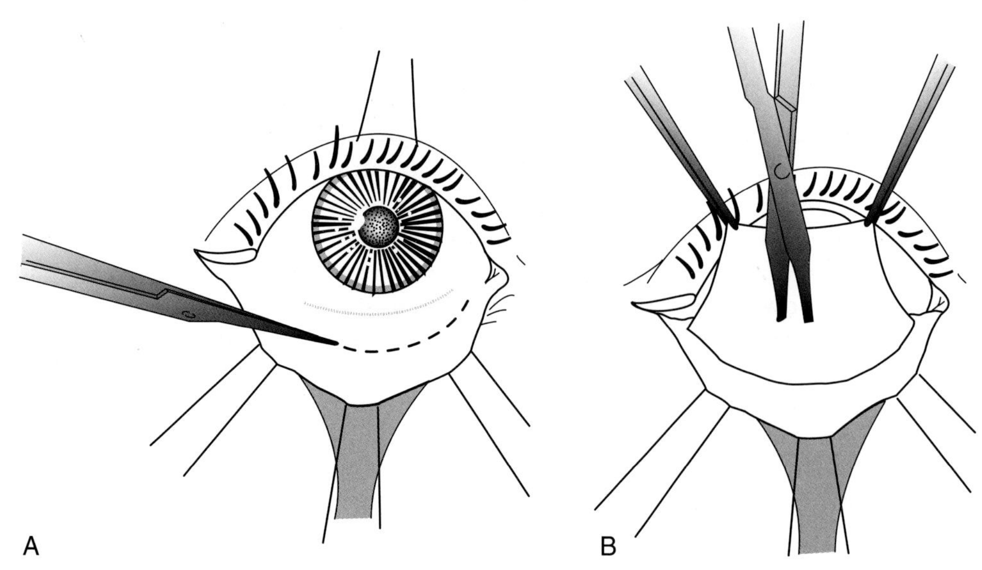

Figure 10-3 (A) Conjunctiva and lower lid retractors are released at the level of the inferior tarsal border. (B) Capsulopalpebral fascia is separated from orbicularis to level of inferior orbital rim.

rim or through the superior crus of the lateral canthal tendon at the desired level. Normally, the lateral canthal angle is reformed 2 mm higher than the medial canthal angle; however, this amount varies from patient to patient as individual needs are assessed. In patients with more pronounced exophthalmos, the suture is often placed more anteriorly than normally done, to prevent the lower lid from being pulled under the globe. The polypropylene suture arms are left untied at this stage of the procedure.

A desired spacer material is brought in or harvested at this point. An implant is then fashioned. As a general rule, in patients with thyroid disease, the width of the implant strip is four times the amount of retraction as measured from the lower lid to the inferior limbus nasally, centrally, and temporally. (In retraction not related to thyroid disease, the scleral strip need be only three times as wide as the amount of lower eyelid retraction. Many configurations and materials for interposition have been described, but they may be less important than the vertical dimension and the relationship to the retraction.)

The implant is sutured to the edge of the capsulopalpebral fascia inferiorly by a running 5-0 chromic suture, with the knot buried nasally and temporally. This step is done with the lower lid everted over a Desmarres retractor to facilitate exposure. The implant is then sutured superiorly to the inferior tarsal border with a running 5-0 chromic suture. If excessive implant material is evident, it is trimmed before suturing. The polypropylene suture from the tarsal strip is tied temporally with the first tie of a surgeon's knot over a piece of 4-0 silk suture to be used as a releasing suture, and the patient is brought to a sitting position. The placement of the suture is adjusted until an optimal lid level is reached, and then the suture arms are tied permanently.

At this point, the patient is again brought to a sitting position and the lid level is evaluated. Once the surgeon is satisfied with the amount of tarsorrhaphy, the anterior lamella from the lower lid is dissected free as a skin–orbicularis flap and is draped superiorly over the corresponding upper lid skin. Skin and orbicularis are then removed from the upper lid in the area of the overlap. The flap from the lower lid is sutured into the newly created defect with interrupted 6-0 silk sutures.

The final step in the procedure involves elevation of the lower lid to prevent wrinkling of the graft. Two 4-0 silk double-armed sutures are passed through the lower eyelid and above the eyebrow. The sutures enter the skin several millimeters beneath the lower lid cilia, pass beneath the orbicularis, and exit through the gray line. Each arm then passes through skin–orbicularis and above the brow. One set of sutures is placed at the junction of the nasal and central third of the lid, and the other at the junction of the central and temporal third of the lid. Ophthalmic antibiotic ointment is applied to the eye and to all skin sutures. According to the surgeon's preference, either a mild pressure patch or ice packs are applied to the eye over the closed lids for 2 days (the day of the surgery and the day after). The sutures are removed 5 to 7 days after the surgery.

10-7 EYELID RETRACTION IN SETTINGS OTHER THAN TED

10-7-1 *After Trauma.* Previously lacerated eyelids may become retracted from loss of tissue and/or cicatrization involving multiple layers of the eyelid. Surgical correction of posttraumatic eyelid retraction may therefore require some combination of lengthening of the anterior lamella with a skin graft, lengthening of the posterior lamella by recession of the eyelid retractors with or without a spacer, and/or excision of foci of scar tissue. Traumatic loss of the tarsus may require posterior lamellar flaps or grafts similar to those used in eyelid reconstruction after tumor resection. All of these surgical maneuvers may not be necessary in every patient; selection of these surgical options must be individualized to the patient's anatomic needs.

In contrast to posttraumatic eyelid retraction, the cicatricial process that results in eyelid retraction in quiescent TED does not involve the skin. Lengthening of the eyelid in thyroid disease almost never requires skin grafting.

Surgical correction of posttraumatic eyelid retraction is usually deferred until at least 6 months after the injury to allow the cicatricial process to stabilize. Some cases of retraction resolve spontaneously during this period. Most patients can be kept comfortable with ophthalmic lubricants during this time, but intractable corneal exposure occasionally necessitates earlier surgical intervention.

Upper eyelid retraction after trauma is often most noticeable in down gaze and may be associated with lagophthalmos. A patient requiring a full-thickness skin graft and excision of deep scar bands is illustrated in Figure 10-4.

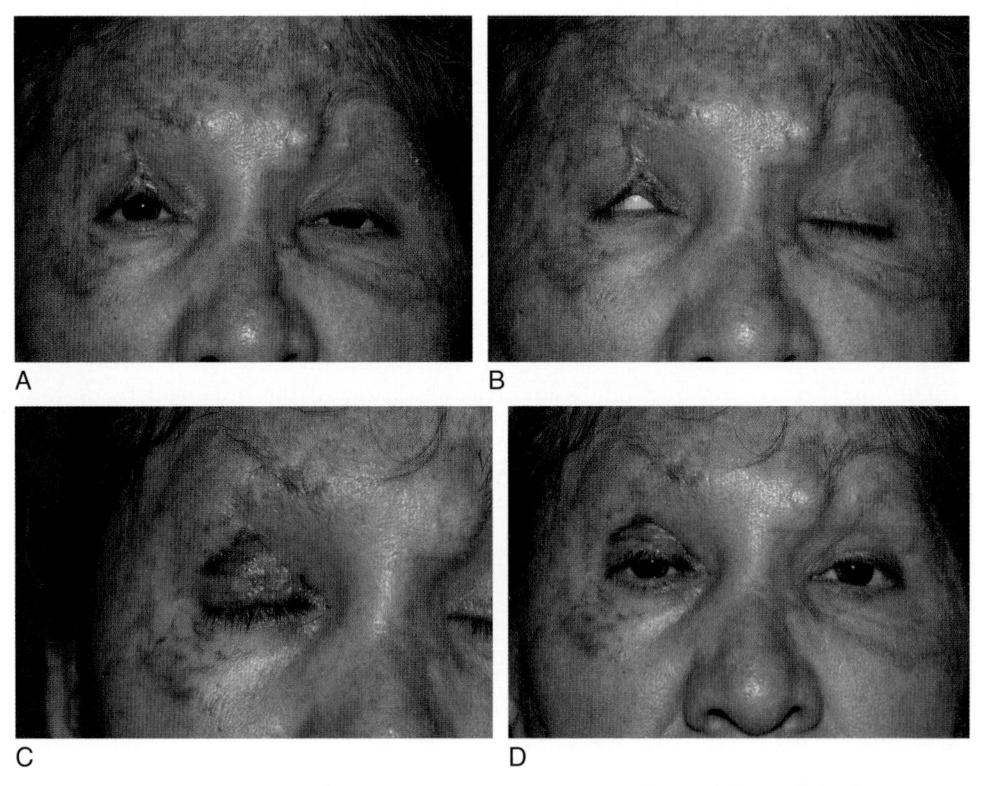

Figure 10-4 (A) A patient with cicatricial ectropion and peaking of the eyelid after a motor vehicle accident. (B) With attempted eyelid closure, the scarred eyelid is peaked and a lagophthalmos is present. (C) A full-thickness postauricular skin graft was placed into the eyelid after releasing the cicatrix. (D) Postoperatively, there is good correction of the deformity and lagophthalmos. (Photos courtesy of Michael T. Yen, MD)

In lower eyelid retraction after trauma, a tarsal strip procedure is employed in the vast majority of cases. In patients without prominent eyes, a tarsal strip is used to tighten the lower eyelid, the lower eyelid retractors are recessed, and a posterior lamellar spacer may not be necessary. In patients with prominent eyes, repair becomes more analogous to that performed in thyroid disease; the tarsal strip is used to reposition the lower lid, but not tighten it, and placement of a posterior lamellar spacer between the inferior tarsal border and the recessed lower lid retractors may be necessary.

10-7-2 *After Blepharoplasty.* Lower eyelid retraction after transcutaneous lower lid blepharoplasty can be a consequence of excessive skin resection, scarring at the level of the orbital septum, and/or lower eyelid laxity.[58] Excessive skin resection may require full-thickness skin grafting, but the cosmetic results of skin grafting in this setting may be variable. Lower eyelid retraction following blepharoplasty can be avoided by a conservative approach to skin excision in lower eyelid blepharoplasty and avoidance of suturing the orbital septum. For mild cases of retraction upward massage can be employed with some success.

A variety of approaches are considered for the late correction of lower eyelid retraction after transcutaneous lower lid blepharoplasty due to orbital septal scarring.[32–35] In patients without prominent eyes, a tarsal strip is used to tighten the lower lid, the lid retractors are recessed, and a posterior lamellar spacer may not be necessary. In patients with prominent eyes, a tarsal strip is used to reposition (but not tighten) the lower lid, and a posterior lamellar spacer is interposed between the inferior tarsal border and the recessed lid retractors. Frequently, to further recruit anterior lamella, elevation of the midface may be required.[32,33]

10-7-3 *After Ptosis Surgery.* Unexpected overcorrection after blepharoptosis surgery may result in upper lid retraction. Overcorrection after levator aponeurosis advancement can be treated the first week after surgery by pulling apart the lid-crease wound and adjusting the amount of advancement.[59,60] Later correction after levator advancement or resection can be accomplished by full-thickness blepharotomy as described above.[61]

10-7-4 *Facial Nerve Palsy.* Facial nerve palsy affects the function of both lower and upper eyelids. Unopposed by the protractor tone of the paralyzed orbicularis oculi, the retractors of the lower and upper lids reset the lids lower and higher than normal, respectively. In addition, lower lid ectropion often accompanies lower lid retraction in this setting. Lagophthalmos often exacerbates corneal exposure problems.

Lower lid retraction and ectropion can be treated by canthal ligament tightening,[62] spacer implantation,[48] midface elevation,[32,33,63] and tarsorrhaphy. In the upper lid, tarsorrhaphy can also be used, but is usually disliked by the patient. Other methods include reanimation with nerve grafts, gold weight implantation,[64] and placement of palpebral springs.

REFERENCES

1. Bartley GB. The differential diagnosis and classification of eyelid retraction. *Trans Am Ophthalmol Soc.* 1995;93:371–389.

2. Char DH. *Thyroid eye disease*, 3rd ed. Boston: Butterworth-Heinemann, 1997.
3. Cockerham KP, Hidayat AA, Brown HG, et al. Clinicopathologic evaluation of the Mueller muscle in thyroid-associated orbitopathy. *Ophthalmic Plastic Reconstructive Surg.* 2002;18(1):11–17.
4. Shih MJ, Liao SL, Kuo KT, et al. Molecular pathology of Müller's muscle in Graves' ophthalmopathy. *J Clin Endocrinol Metab.* 2006;91(3):1159–1167.
5. Fraunfelder FT, Fraunfelder FW, Randall JA. *Drug-induced ocular side effects*, 5th ed. Boston: Butterworth-Heinemann, 2001.
6. Haddad HM. Müller's muscle: to relax or to incise. *Metabolic, Pediatric, and Systemic Ophthalmology.* 1995;18(1-4):15–18.
7. Chuenkongkaew W. Botulinum toxin treatment for upper lid retraction of dysthyroidism. *J Med Assoc Thailand.* 2003;86(11):1051–1054.
8. Ebner R. Botulinum toxin type A in upper lid retraction of Graves' ophthalmopathy. *J Clin Neuro-ophthalmol.* 1993;13(4):258–261.
9. Morgenstern KE, Evanchan J, Foster JA, et al. Botulinum toxin type a for dysthyroid upper eyelid retraction. *Ophthalmic Plastic Reconstructive Surg.* 2004;20(3):181–185.
10. Shih MJ, Liao SL, Lu HY. A single transcutaneous injection with Botox for dysthyroid lid retraction. *Eye.* 2004;18(5):466–469.
11. Traisk F, Tallstedt L. Thyroid associated ophthalmopathy: botulinum toxin A in the treatment of upper eyelid retraction—a pilot study. *Acta Ophthalmol Scand.* 2001;79(6):585–588.
12. Uddin JM, Davies PD. Treatment of upper eyelid retraction associated with thyroid eye disease with subconjunctival botulinum toxin injection. *Ophthalmology.* 2002;109(6):1183–1187.
13. Ben Simon GJ, Mansury AM, Schwarcz RM, et al. Simultaneous orbital decompression and correction of upper eyelid retraction versus staged procedures in thyroid-related orbitopathy. *Ophthalmology.* 2005;112(5):923–932.
14. Shorr N, Seiff SR. The four stages of surgical rehabilitation of the patient with dysthyroid ophthalmopathy. *Ophthalmology.* 1986;93(4):476–483.
15. Elner VM, Hassan AS, Frueh BR. Graded full-thickness anterior blepharotomy for upper eyelid retraction. *Trans Am Ophthalmol Soc.* 2003;101:67–75.
16. Elner VM, Hassan AS, Frueh BR. Graded full-thickness anterior blepharotomy for upper eyelid retraction. *Arch Ophthalmol.* 2004;122(1):55–60.
17. Hintschich C, Haritoglou C. Full thickness eyelid transsection (blepharotomy) for upper eyelid lengthening in lid retraction associated with Graves' disease. *Br J Ophthalmol.* 2005;89(4):413–416.
18. Chalfin J, Putterman AM. Müller's muscle excision and levator recession in retracted upper lid. Treatment of thyroid-related retraction. *Arch Ophthalmol.* 1979;97(8): 1487–1491.
19. Putterman AM. Surgical treatment of thyroid-related upper eyelid retraction. Graded Müller's muscle excision and levator recession. *Ophthalmology.* 1981;88(6):507–512.
20. Putterman AM, Fett DR. Müller's muscle in the treatment of upper eyelid retraction: a 12-year study. *Ophthalmic Surg.* 1986;17(6):361–367.
21. Khan JA, Garden V, Faghihi M, Parvin M. Surgical method and results of levator aponeurosis transposition for Graves' eyelid retraction. *Ophthalmic Surgery and Lasers.* 2002;33(1):79–82.
22. Levine MR, Chu A. Surgical treatment of thyroid-related lid retraction: a new variation. *Ophthalmic Surg.* 1991;22(2):90–94.
23. Harvey JT, Corin S, Nixon D, Veloudios A. Modified levator aponeurosis recession for upper eyelid retraction in Graves' disease. *Ophthalmic Surg.* 1991;22(6):313–317.

24. Older JJ. Surgical treatment of eyelid retraction associated with thyroid eye disease. *Ophthalmic Surg.* 1991;22(6):318–323.
25. Ben Simon GJ, Mansury AM, Schwarcz RM, et al. Transconjunctival Muller muscle recession with levator disinsertion for correction of eyelid retraction associated with thyroid-related orbitopathy. *Am J Ophthalmol.* 2005;140(1):94–99.
26. Looi AL, Sharma B, Dolman PJ. A modified posterior approach for upper eyelid retraction. *Ophthalmic Plastic Reconstructive Surg.* 2006;22(6):434–437.
27. Collin JR, O'Donnell BA. Adjustable sutures in eyelid surgery for ptosis and lid retraction. *Br J Ophthalmol.* 1994;78(3):167–174.
28. Woog JJ, Hartstein ME, Hoenig J. Adjustable suture technique for levator recession. *Arch Ophthalmol.* 1996;114(5):620–624.
29. Ceisler EJ, Bilyk JR, Rubin PA, et al. Results of Mullerotomy and levator aponeurosis transposition for the correction of upper eyelid retraction in Graves disease. *Ophthalmology.* 1995;102(3):483–492.
30. Mourits MP, Sasim IV. A single technique to correct various degrees of upper lid retraction in patients with Graves' orbitopathy. *Br J Ophthalmol.* 1999;83(1):81–84.
31. Grove AS, Jr. Eyelid retraction treated by levator marginal myotomy. *Ophthalmology.* 1980;87(10):1013–1018.
32. Ben Simon GJ, Lee S, Schwarcz RM, et al. Subperiosteal midface lift with or without a hard palate mucosal graft for correction of lower eyelid retraction. *Ophthalmology.* 2006;113(10):1869–1873.
33. Patel MP, Shapiro MD, Spinelli HM. Combined hard palate spacer graft, midface suspension, and lateral canthoplasty for lower eyelid retraction: a tripartite approach. *Plastic Reconstructive Surg.* 2005;115(7):2105–2117.
34. Holds JB, Anderson RL, Thiese SM. Lower eyelid retraction: a minimal incision surgical approach to retractor lysis. *Ophthalmic Surg.* 1990;21(11):767–771.
35. Small RG, Scott M. The tight retracted lower eyelid. *Arch Ophthalmol.* 1990;108(3):438–444.
36. Feldman KA, Putterman AM, Farber MD. Surgical treatment of thyroid-related lower eyelid retraction: a modified approach. *Ophthalmic Plastic Reconstructive Surg.* 1992;8(4):278–286.
37. Anderson RL, Gordy DD. The tarsal strip procedure. *Arch Ophthalmol.* 1979;97(11): 2192–2196.
38. Gardner TA, Kennerdell JS, Buerger GF. Treatment of dysthyroid lower lid retraction with autogenous tarsus transplants. *Ophthalmic Plastic Reconstructive Surg.* 1992;8(1):26–31.
39. Malhotra R, Selva D. Free tarsus autogenous graft struts for lower eyelid elevation. *Ophthalmic Plastic Reconstructive Surg.* 2005;21(2):117–122.
40. Bartley GB, Kay PP. Posterior lamellar eyelid reconstruction with a hard palate mucosal graft. *Am J Ophthalmol.* 1989;107(6):609–612.
41. Cohen MS, Shorr N. Eyelid reconstruction with hard palate mucosa grafts. *Ophthalmic Plastic Reconstructive Surg.* 1992;8(3):183–195.
42. Kersten RC, Kulwin DR, Levartovsky S, et al. Management of lower-lid retraction with hard-palate mucosa grafting. *Arch Ophthalmol.* 1990;108(9):1339–1343.
43. Patel BC, Patipa M, Anderson RL, McLeish W. Management of postblepharoplasty lower eyelid retraction with hard palate grafts and lateral tarsal strip. *Plastic Reconstructive Surg.* 1997;99(5):1251–1260.
44. Patipa M, Patel BC, McLeish W, Anderson RL. Use of hard palate grafts for treatment of postsurgical lower eyelid retraction: a technical overview. *J Cranio-maxillofacial Trauma.* 1996;2(3):18–28.

45. Siegel RJ. Palatal grafts for eyelid reconstruction. *Plastic Reconstructive Surg.* 1985;76(3): 411–414.
46. Wearne MJ, Sandy C, Rose GE, et al. Autogenous hard palate mucosa: the ideal lower eyelid spacer? *Br J Ophthalmol.* 2001;85(10):1183–1187.
47. Baylis HI, Perman KI, Fett DR, Sutcliffe RT. Autogenous auricular cartilage grafting for lower eyelid retraction. *Ophthalmic Plastic Reconstructive Surg.* 1985;1(1):23–27.
48. Krastinova D, Franchi G, Kelly MB, Chabolle F. Rehabilitation of the paralysed or lax lower eyelid using a graft of conchal cartilage. *Br J Plastic Surg.* 2002;55(1):12–19.
49. Marks MW, Argenta LC, Friedman RJ, Hall JD. Conchal cartilage and composite grafts for correction of lower lid retraction. *Plastic Reconstructive Surg.* 1989;83(4):629–635.
50. Matsuo K, Hirose T, Takahashi N, et al. Lower eyelid reconstruction with a conchal cartilage graft. *Plastic Reconstructive Surg.* 1987;80(4):547–552.
51. Moon JW, Choung HK, Khwarg SI. Correction of lower lid retraction combined with entropion using an ear cartilage graft in the anophthalmic socket. *Korean J Ophthalmol.* 2005;19(3):161–167.
52. Tan J, Olver J, Wright M, et al. The use of porous polyethylene (Medpor) lower eyelid spacers in lid heightening and stabilisation. *Br J Ophthalmol.* 2004;88(9):1197–1200.
53. Wong JF, Soparkar CN, Patrinely JR. Correction of lower eyelid retraction with high density porous polyethylene: The Medpor((R)) Lower Eyelid Spacer. *Orbit,* 2001;20(3): 217–225.
54. Taban M, Douglas R, Li T, et al. Efficacy of "thick" acellular human dermis (AlloDerm) for lower eyelid reconstruction: comparison with hard palate and thin AlloDerm grafts. *Arch Facial Plastic Surg.* 2005;7(1): 38–44.
55. Gurney TA, Kim DW. Applications of porcine dermal collagen (ENDURAGen) in facial plastic surgery. *Facial Plastic Surg Clin North Am.* 2007;15(1):113–121.
56. Beard C. Canthoplasty and brow elevation for facial palsy. *Arch Ophthalmol.* 1964;71:386–388.
57. Tenzel RR, Stewart WB. Eyelid reconstruction by the semicircle flap technique. *Ophthalmology.* 1978;85(11):1164–1169.
58. Baylis HI, Nelson ER, Goldberg RA. Lower eyelid retraction following blepharoplasty. *Ophthalmic Plastic Reconstructive Surg.* 1992;8(3):170–175.
59. Shore JW, Bergin DJ, Garrett SN. Results of blepharoptosis surgery with early postoperative adjustment. *Ophthalmology.* 1990;97(11):1502–1511.
60. Dortzbach RK, Kronish JW. Early revision in the office for adults after unsatisfactory blepharoptosis correction. *Am J Ophthalmol.* 1993;115(1):68–75.
61. Demirci H, Hassan AS, Reck SD, et al. Graded full-thickness anterior blepharotomy for correction of upper eyelid retraction not associated with thyroid eye disease. *Ophthalmic Plastic Reconstructive Surg.* 2007;23(1):39–45.
62. Tenzel RR, Buffam FV, Miller GR. The use of the "lateral canthal sling" in ectropion repair. *Can J Ophthalmol.* 1977;12(3):199–202.
63. Elner VM, Mauffray RO, Fante RG, et al. Comprehensive midfacial elevation for ocular complications of facial nerve palsy. *Arch Facial Plastic Surg.* 2003;5(5):427–433.
64. Gladstone GJ, Nesi FA. Management of paralytic lagophthalmos with a modified gold-weight implantation technique. *Ophthalmic Plastic Reconstructive Surg.* 1996;12(1): 38–44.

11

Management of Blepharospasm and Hemifacial Spasm

HEERAL SHAH, MD, AND MICHAEL T. YEN, MD

Benign essential blepharospasm and hemifacial spasm are chronic and disabling medical conditions. Both disorders can result in uncontrollable blinking or frank spasms of the eyelids and face, which may interfere with the activities of daily living and may even render a patient functionally blind and occupationally handicapped. Often, when untreated, the eyelid and facial spasms are so emotionally unsettling that the patients become withdrawn, frustrated, and desperate.

11-1 BLEPHAROSPASM

Essential blepharospasm is the most common manifestation of orofacial movement disorders. The term is used to describe a movement disorder limited to the eyelid protractors without a secondary inciting cause, and is characterized by spontaneous, repetitive, forceful eyelid closure. Benign essential blepharospasm is caused by forceful contraction of the eyelid protractors, which include the orbicularis oculi, corrugator supercilii, and procerus muscles. The prevalence is 32 in 100,000 and women are more commonly affected than men (3:2). The peak onset is in the fifth to sixth decades, and symptoms peak 3 years after onset. When contractions are limited to the orbital and periorbital muscles, the term "benign essential blepharospasm" is used. Often, subsequent contractions of lower face and neck occur concurrently. This is termed Meige syndrome, orofacial dystonia, or oromandibular dystonia (Brueghel syndrome). Furthermore, dystonia outside of the facial nerve distribution is called segmental cranial dystonia or craniocervical dystonia.

Initially, benign essential blepharospasm can manifest as increased frequency in blinking in response to several stimuli, including wind, air pollution, sunlight, noise, and movements of the head or eyes. It can significantly impair quality of life by causing difficulty in reading, writing, and driving. In severe cases, patients may be functionally blind. Several eyelid changes have been noted with longstanding blepharospasm including dermatochalasis, eyelid and brow ptosis, entropion, and canthal tendon abnormalities.

Common symptoms that precede the official diagnosis of benign essential blepharospasm include eye irritation, photophobia, tearing, and ocular pain. Early symptoms include an increase in blink rate (77%), lid spasms (66%), ocular irritation (55%), midfacial or lower facial spasm (59%), brow spasm (24%), and eyelid tic (22%). Several conditions relieve blepharospasm; these include sleep, relaxation, inferior gaze, artificial tears, traction on eyelids, and humming.

Benign essential blepharospasm is a diagnosis of exclusion. Thorough examination is necessary to diagnose conditions that may cause secondary eyelid spasm. These commonly include eyelid inflammation, ocular irritation, and photophobia. For example, blepharitis, infection of the eyelids, keratoconjunctivitis sicca, trichiasis, and corneal disease can cause eyelid spasms, or coexist and aggravate benign essential blepharospasm.

Eyelid spasms are also often observed in patients with neurodegenerative or postencephalitic diseases—for example, Parkinson disease, Wilson disease, Huntington's chorea, Sydenham's chorea, postencephalitic syndromes, and midbrain cerebrovascular disease. These are characterized by tonic, involuntary movements, initiated by voluntary eyelid closure. Drug-induced tardive dyskinesia may occasionally mimic benign essential blepharospasm. However, the characteristic rapid and continuous licking, lip-puckering movements are not common in patients with benign essential blepharospasm. See Table 11-1 for a list of differential diagnoses.

Although mental stress and other psychological factors seem to exacerbate eyelid spasms, studies have demonstrated that the physical condition persists even when the psychiatric condition is cured. Also, if benign essential blepharospasm were a purely psychiatric disorder, it would appear earlier in life, have an episodic course, and demonstrate a consistent history of a premorbid emotional disorder. Regardless, evidence does suggest there is a psychological component to benign essential blepharospasm, and patients often benefit from a combination of emotional and physical treatment.

11-2 PATHOPHYSIOLOGY OF BENIGN ESSENTIAL BLEPHAROSPASM

It is hypothesized that an increased excitatory drive from the basal ganglia may stimulate or perpetuate blepharospasm. While the neuronal reflex arcs of cranial nerves V and VII are normal, an increased excitability of corneal reflexes and shortened recovery cycles of the blink reflex suggest a miscommunication to and from the basal ganglia. Similar eyelid spasms are noted in patients with basal ganglia disease, implicating a basal ganglia abnormality in benign essential blepharospasm.

Table 11-1 Differential Diagnosis of Benign Essential Blepharospasm

Parkinson disease
Huntington disease
Creutzfeldt-Jakob disease
Postencephalitic syndrome
Reflex blepharospasm
Ocular myokymia
Myotonic dystrophy
Encephalitis
Tardive dyskinesia
Tetany
Facial nerve misdirection
Medications: levodopa, antipsychotics, antiemetics
Conjunctival disease
Corneal disease
Iritis
Functional blepharospasm, spurious blepharospasm, seizure blepharospasm

However, it is unlikely that an abnormality at a specific center leads to blepharospasm; the idea of a defect in circuit activity has been recently adopted. One aspect of this circuit is the sensory limb, which responds to a variety of stimuli, including light, corneal irritation, pain, emotion, stress, and so forth. The responses are relayed to the control center, which may be abnormal and therefore unable to regulate the positive feedback involving primarily the motor pathway. This motor pathway consists of the facial muscles, facial nerve, orbicularis oculi, corrugator, and procerus muscles. However, dopamine depletion and alterations in norepinephrine concentrations have also been implicated in other studies. It is evident that the etiology of benign essential blepharospasm is multifactorial, and a definite cause remains to be known.

11-3 TREATMENT OF BENIGN ESSENTIAL BLEPHAROSPASM

The first line of treatment for benign essential blepharospasm is directed toward the sensory pathway of the blepharospasm cycle. This includes wearing tinted glasses with ultraviolet blocking to decrease photo-oculodynia, lid hygiene to decrease irritation, and use of artificial tears and punctual occlusion for dry eye symptoms.

Primary medical treatment for benign essential blepharospasm is botulinum toxin A. This is a large protein with a molecular weight of 900,000 Da that can be split into two subunits. Each subunit is split into three peptide chains with a molecular weight of 150,000 Da. One of these chains possesses neurotoxic activity. Botulinum toxin binds to cell surface receptors at the neural synapse, enters the axon, and inhibits acetylcholine release by interfering with a membrane-bound calcium-dependent enzyme responsible for acetylcholine release. Seven different exotoxins are produced by *Clostridium botulinum*: A, B, C1, D, E, F, and G. Of these botulinum toxin A is the strongest, followed by B and F. The exotoxin may take effect 2 to 4 days following injection, due to the continued release of acetylcholine from vesicles. After 2 or 3 months, when the neuromuscular junction recovers and produces new nerve terminals, the effects begin to fade. More than 95% of patients with benign essential blepharospasm report improvement after treatment.

It is important to realize every patient is different and will respond differently when treated with varying doses of botulinum toxin A. Clinical judgment must be used when considering the number and location of injection sites as well as the dose to be injected. It is generally recommended that the first treatment be approximately 25 units per eye, divided among four to six periocular sites, subcutaneously over the orbicularis oculi and intramuscularly over the corrugator and procerus muscles (Fig. 11-1). The patient's response to the first dose should help determine subsequent doses. Most require another treatment in 3 to 4 months, but this period can range from 1 to 5 months.

Although antibodies to the toxin develop with chronic use, with the low doses used in benign essential blepharospasm, the antibodies are non-neutralizing. Differences in the bioavailability of active toxin among vials, sensitization, or saturation of binding sites by inactive toxin result in variable responses.

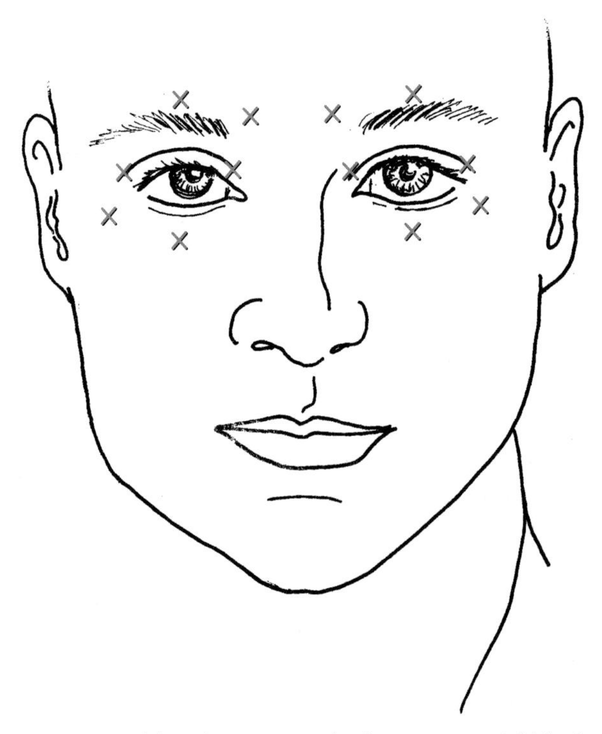

Figure 11-1 Injection pattern of botulinum toxin for benign essential blepharospasm, targeting the pretarsal orbicularis oculi muscle of the upper and lower eyelids as well as the corrugator muscles underneath the eyebrows.

Systemic complications are rare due to the small dose of botulinum toxin injected. However, possible systemic complications are thirst, flulike syndrome, mild rash, and the potentiation of neurologic diseases, including myasthenia gravis. Several local complications have been reported: ptosis (7% to 11%), corneal exposure due to lagophthalmos (5% to 12%), entropion, epiphora, ectropion, photophobia (2.5%), diplopia (<1%), ecchymosis, and lower facial weakness. Ptosis often results when the toxin diffuses from an injection site to the levator muscle. Contraindications to botulinum toxin include pregnancy, lactation, human albumin allergy, neuromuscular diseases, and peripheral neuropathy.

Although numerous systemic medications have been used to treat benign essential blepharospasm, none has completely eradicated the eyelid spasms. They are often used to ameliorate the symptoms, and one or two are tried before forgoing systemic therapy. Options include muscle relaxants, analgesics, antihistamines, antidepressants, anticholinergics, antiepileptics, lithium, antiparkinsonian agents, and serotonin antagonists.

If botulinum toxin becomes ineffective with time, surgical myectomy becomes an alternative. This involves removal of the orbicularis oculi, procerus, and corrugator muscles and allows for correction of concurrent eyelid malposition. A limited myectomy includes the removal of the pretarsal, preseptal, and orbital parts of the upper and lower orbicularis oculi muscle, whereas extended myectomy involves removal of the procerus and corrugator muscles. Although 50% of patients require botulinum toxin after a myectomy, studies have shown an improvement in response to botulinum toxin in these patients

During the limited myectomy, muscle is removed through an eyelid crease incision. The pretarsal muscle is extirpated down to the eyelid margin. The preseptal and orbital orbicularis is excised up to the orbital rim. The corrugator muscle can also be excised through this incision. Care must be taken to avoid the supraorbital neurovascular bundle. Following the myectomy, drains and compressive patches may be used for 24 to 48 hours. Hematomas observed after removal of the patches must be molded flat soon after removing the patches. Complications of this procedure include infection, lagophthalmos, forehead anesthesia, and lymphedema (Fig. 11-2).

In the subgroup of patients who do not get adequate relief from botulinum toxin injections and a myectomy, differential section of the facial nerve is an alternative. This involves facial nerve avulsion, transection, or stretching to isolate and remove the branches of cranial nerve VII that innervate the involved muscles responsible for the eyelid spasms. The main disadvantage is the need for general anesthesia during the procedure in order to use intraoperative nerve stimulation to identify the branches that need to be transected. Furthermore, eyelid deformities are not corrected; paralysis including facial droop can occur, and lid spasms can recur. Although it is known to reduce symptoms in 50% of patients, the complication rate is high.

The sensory component of benign essential blepharospasm is often difficult to quantify. This involves ocular surface irritation and debilitating sensitivity to light or photo-oculodynia. Most patients with photo-oculodynia fail to respond to treatment with botulinum toxin despite weakening of the orbicularis muscle. To diagnose

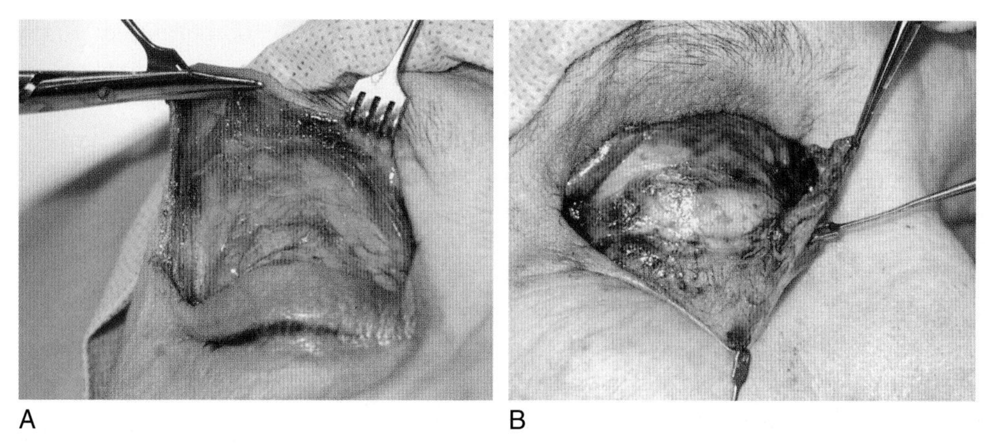

A B

Figure 11-2 The limited myectomy of the upper eyelids is performed through a standard eyelid crease incision. (A) The preseptal and orbital orbicularis is dissected away from the overlying skin and then excised. (B) The pretarsal orbicularis is excised down to the eyelid margin.

photo-oculodynia, a simple test can be performed. The patient is instructed to look into a 25-watt light bulb 3 feet away. Patients who have pain and spasm are diagnosed with photo-oculodynia. Studies have shown a decrease in these symptoms in two thirds of patients following a superior cervical ganglion block. This treatment is reserved for patients with photo-oculodynia, as it is more invasive than botulinum toxin. Patients may also benefit from the use of tinted eyeglass lenses such as the FL-41 lens tint (BPI, Miami, FL).

11-4 HEMIFACIAL SPASM

Hemifacial spasm is characterized by unilateral, clonic or tonic contraction of the muscles innervated by cranial nerve VII with concurrent facial weakness. These muscles include the orbicularis oculi, orbicularis oris, platysma, and other superficial muscles. The contractions begin with forceful closure of the eyelids, and then the lower face is progressively involved. The prevalence is 9 in 100,000, and women are more often affected than women.

Hemifacial spasm is usually due to a vascular stricture that compresses cranial nerve VII at its root of exit. This compression results in nerve demyelination, resulting in poor communication between axons. The blood vessels most commonly at fault include the anterior and posterior inferior cerebellar arteries and vertebral artery. Occasionally, tumors of the cerebellopontine angle or lesions of the temporal bone or parotid gland can cause hemifacial spasms. However, concurrent findings lead to the diagnosis in these mass lesions. For example, symptoms of decreased taste, decreased hearing, or vertigo point may be present with hemifacial spasm if a tumor is the cause. Furthermore, the disease in infants is likely due to serious intracranial disease. Therefore, in typical cases without concurrent neurologic findings, routine MRI or CT scanning of the head is unnecessary. Other factors for which neuroimaging is warranted include young age, parotid mass, bilateral hemifacial spasm, or if surgical decompression is a consideration.

11-4-1 *Anatomy of the Seventh Cranial Nerve.* Cranial nerve VII is a mixed sensory and motor nerve. Its motor nucleus is located in the caudal third of the pons. Four subgroups within the nucleus innervate specific facial muscles; the ventral portion of the intermediate group supplies the axons to the orbicularis oculi. The part of the nucleus supplying the upper half of the face receives corticobulbar input from both cerebral hemispheres. The lower half of the face is influenced by corticobulbar fibers from the opposite cerebral hemispheres.

The sensory nucleus of cranial nerve VII is the rostral portion of the tract. It is lateral to the motor and parasympathetic nuclei in the caudal pons. Sensations of taste from the anterior two thirds of the tongue are carried by special visceral afferent fibers to this nucleus. The impulses travel along the lingual nerve and chorda tympani and reach the brain through the nervus intermedius. Cranial nerve VII, the nervus intermedius, and cranial nerve VIII pass together through the lateral pontine cistern in the cerebellopontine angle and enter the internal auditory meatus. The seventh cranial nerve and intermedius nerve then enter the fallopian canal, which is the longest bony canal traversed by any cranial nerve (30 mm). Through this canal, cranial nerve VII is divided into three segments: labyrinthine segment, tympanic segment, and mastoid segment. The seventh nerve trunk exits the skull at the stylomastoid foramen and separates into a large temporofacial and a small cervicofacial

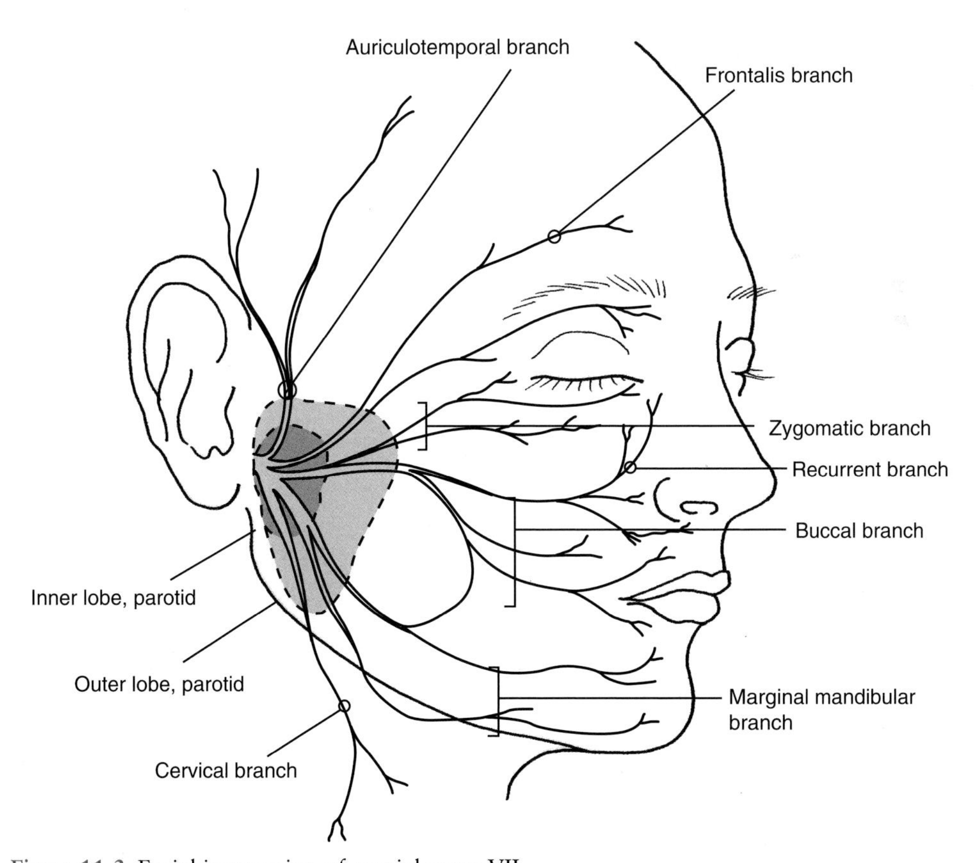

Figure 11-3 Facial innervation of cranial nerve VII.

division between the superficial and deep lobes of the parotid gland. The temporofacial division gives rise to the temporal, zygomatic, and buccal branches. The cervicofacial division is the origin of the marginal mandibular and colli branches. The temporal branch supplies the upper half of the orbicularis oculi, and the zygomatic branch supplies the lower half. The frontalis, corrugator supercilii, and pyramidalis muscles are innervated by the temporal branch (Fig. 11-3).

11-4-2 *Treatment of Hemifacial Spasm.* The primary treatments for hemifacial spasm include neurosurgical decompression of cranial nerve VII and Botulinum toxin. Since the late 1980s, botulinum toxin has become the preferred initial treatment choice. When used in hemifacial spasm, in contrast to blepharospasm, Botulinum toxin provides a longer symptom-free period and is often used only twice a year in these patients. In cases refractory to botulinum toxin type A, a recent study was performed using botulinum toxin type B, resulting in beneficial effects that lasted a shorter time than botulinum toxin type A.

Microvascular decompression is an alternative when obvious compression at the exit zone of the facial nerve root is identified. Vertebral angiograms can localize the site of compression, therefore increasing the safety and efficacy of treatment. Various prostheses are inserted between the artery and site of compression, relieving the pressure. Studies have proven microvascular decompression to be effective and safe in a 3-year follow-up, resulting in an increase in the quality of life. There is a possibility of late effect, resulting in a 1-year lag period before results are observed. In the mid-1990s, a combined endoscopic and microscopic approach was introduced, and it has significantly reduced the morbidity and has increased the success rate of surgery. However, a risk of adverse effects still exists, including a 5.4% chance of delayed facial palsy, 0.6% chance of acute facial palsy, and 0.5% chance of hematomas.

Benign essential blepharospasm and hemifacial spasm are potentially debilitating diseases. The use of botulinum toxin has significantly altered the management of the disease. Furthermore, pharmacotherapy and surgical procedures continue to prove beneficial in patients with resistant pathology.

12

Management of Facial Palsy

RALPH E. WESLEY, MD

Facial palsy can devastate patients. Facial appearance can be grossly distorted by the sagging of half the face, often accompanied by drooling of food and saliva from the paralyzed lip. Blurred vision and ocular pain from exposure and dryness may interfere with the patient's ability to perform an occupation or interact socially. Many patients with facial palsy experience depression or severe discouragement. Effective management of ocular problems by the ophthalmologist can have a profound effect on the patient's rehabilitation.

The ophthalmologist managing facial palsy should be aware of wide-ranging choices in the medical and surgical armamentarium to treat facial palsy. This chapter describes the varying clinical dimensions of facial palsy so that treatment can be individualized for effective management.

12-1 CLINICAL ANATOMY OF FACIAL NERVE

The facial nerve (cranial nerve VII) has four important functions:

1. The facial motor nucleus controls muscles of facial expression, including the orbicularis oculi.
2. The superior salivatory nucleus sends parasympathetic fibers for lacrimal gland secretion and salivary secretion.
3. The nucleus solitarius receives sensory fibers of taste for the anterior two thirds of the tongue.
4. The trigeminal sensory nucleus receives sensory fibers for a small portion of the external ear.

Facial motor fibers constitute about 58% of the 7,000 fibers of the facial nerve, while preganglionic fibers for tearing and salivation represent about 24%.[1,2]

The facial nerve leaves the cerebellopontine angle caudal to the trigeminal nerve adjacent to the nervus intermedius and then enters the internal auditory canal of the temporal bone. Large lesions of cranial nerve VII or VIII may cause loss of corneal sensation from pressure on the trigeminal nerve. The 30-mm course through the temporal bone is the longest interosseous course of any cranial nerve, which makes the facial nerve vulnerable to swelling.

Three branches leave the facial nerve within the temporal bone (Fig. 12-1). The first, and most important, arises at the geniculate ganglion just as the nerve makes a sharp bend, or genu, to head posteriorly. These fibers for lacrimal and palatine gland secretion constitute the greater superficial petrosal nerve carrying lacrimal

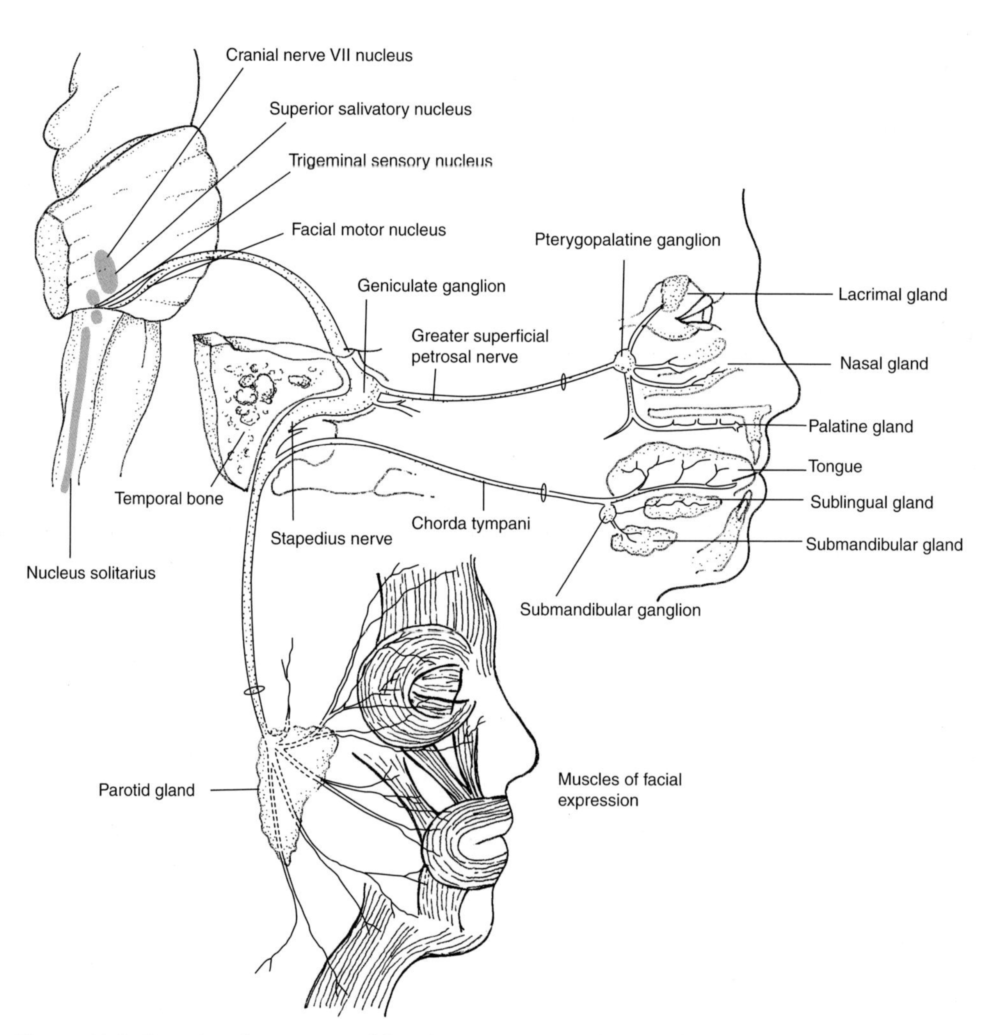

Figure 12-1 Functional anatomy of facial nerve. Lacrimal secretory fibers separate from facial motor fibers deep inside temporal bone at geniculate ganglion. Facial nerve lesions from geniculate ganglion proximally affect tear production as well as lid closure.

secretory fibers to the pterygopalatine ganglion. Postganglionic fibers for tear secretion then follow the infraorbital nerve and branch off with frontozygomatic branches that innervate the lacrimal gland. (The lacrimal branch of the ophthalmic division of the trigeminal nerve provides sensation but no secretory function of the lacrimal gland.)

The other branches of the facial nerve include a small branch to the stapedius muscle within the middle ear and a branch, the chorda tympani, receiving fibers of taste from the tongue and sending fibers to innervate the salivary glands.

The facial motor fibers exit at the stylomastoid foramen between the mastoid and the styloid tip to supply the muscles of facial expression. The facial nerve runs through the parotid gland to innervate the facial musculature through several branches with numerous anastomoses and terminal contacts, usually from the underside of the facial muscles.

Facial nerve lesions above the geniculate ganglion cause more severe symptoms because lacrimal secretion and orbicularis closure are both involved. Central lesions can cause "crocodile tears" when regenerating fibers of the chorda tympani, which normally innervate the salivary glands, grow down the lacrimal secretory neural pathway. When the patient chews, the salivatory nucleus sends nerve innervation that is misdirected to the lacrimal gland, causing the patient's eye to water during mastication.

12-2 DIFFERENTIAL DIAGNOSIS

In many instances, the cause of facial palsy is well established, as in a patient with facial nerve palsy following the removal of an acoustic neuroma. In other cases, the ophthalmologist is usually the first physician to evaluate a patient with a recent-onset presumed Bell's palsy. Acute facial palsy, however, is not always Bell's (idiopathic) palsy.

The most frequent causes of facial palsy are discussed below to give an appreciation for the various clinical settings in which facial palsy occurs. This knowledge allows for therapy to be tailored for each case. A palsy of long duration requires more aggressive treatment than one in which the facial nerve deficit may be mild or of short duration.

12-2-1 *Bell's Palsy.* Bell's palsy is the most likely cause of facial paralysis encountered by the general ophthalmologist, although facial palsy after acoustic neuroma surgery may be more common in referral medical centers. Bell's is the most frequent cause of facial palsy, regardless of the patient's age or sex.[3–5] Bell's palsy is a diagnosis of exclusion because the definition of Bell's palsy is an idiopathic facial paralysis.

Bell's palsy usually occurs on one side of the face, has a sudden onset, and most often improves within 6 months. A simultaneous bilateral facial palsy is said to rule out Bell's palsy, although 6% of patients have developed a palsy on the opposite side.[6,7] Most patients recover from Bell's palsy, but a permanent facial paralysis can occur from idiopathic Bell's palsy. When facial palsy progresses beyond 3 weeks or when function fails to return by 6 months, neoplasm becomes a greater likelihood.

The Schirmer tear test can determine whether lacrimal secretory fibers are affected, in addition to facial motor fibers. A normal Schirmer tear test indicates that the major disease process is peripheral to the geniculate ganglion, where parasympathetic lacrimal secretory fibers travel with the greater superficial petrosal nerve. Patients with Bell's palsy whose lacrimal secretory function is intact usually have a palsy of shorter duration, with greater return of facial function and fewer ocular symptoms. Bell's palsy patients with reduced lacrimal secretion are more likely to have prolonged facial palsy and keratitis even with adequate closure.

12-2-2 *Acoustic Neuroma.* Acoustic neuroma of the adjacent nerve VIII and other cerebellar pontine angle tumors, such as a meningioma or a tumor of the glomus jugulare, are usually often associated with facial nerve weakness after surgery, as opposed to a preoperative tumor compression. Patients with acoustic neuroma are much more likely to complain of a unilateral dry eye or tinnitus than facial weakness. The occurrence of facial palsy prior to acoustic neuroma surgery raises the question of whether a seventh (facial nerve) neuroma rather than true acoustic neuroma (cranial nerve VIII) may exist. Magnetic resonance imaging of the cerebellar pontine angle usually establishes the diagnosis of a tumor.

Management of patients with facial palsy after removal of an acoustic neuroma or a cerebellar pontine angle tumor depends on information provided by the neuro-otologist. In some instances, the nerve has been merely bruised or stretched during removal of the tumor from the adjacent nerve VIII. In other cases with firm attachment of the acoustic eighth nerve tumor to the facial nerve, the deficit is likely to be longer or more severe. If the acoustic tumor cannot be dissected free, the facial nerve must be cut and the gap resutured.

Less likely to demonstrate nerve recovery would be patients in whom such a large segment of the facial nerve had to be removed that the two ends of the nerve cannot be resutured; a nerve graft (e.g., the sural nerve) must be inserted between the two ends. The most severely affected group are those in whom the tumor requires removal of nerve VII with nerve VIII back to the brain stem, in which case no graft can be performed.

Facial palsy after acoustic neuroma surgery means both facial motor function and lacrimal secretory function are involved, because tumors are situated proximal to the geniculate ganglion. Electrical monitoring of facial nerve function during surgical procedures has improved preservation of the facial nerve during surgery.[8,9] Younger patients generally tolerate facial palsy better and have return of facial nerve function more completely and sooner than older patients. Patients with larger tumors may also have loss of corneal sensation, which has important prognostic and management implications.

12-2-3 *Malignant Tumor.* Much less commonly, a malignant tumor of the external auditory canal, such as a squamous cell carcinoma or an adenoid cystic carcinoma, can extend into the temporal bone and cause facial motor palsy. Metastatic lesions from the orbit, lung, breast, or kidney can on rare occasions affect the facial nerve.[10–12] Malignant facial skin lesions and parotid tumors may cause peripheral facial palsy.

12-2-4 HIV *Infection*. Facial palsy can be the first presentation of patients with AIDS (acquired immunodeficiency syndrome), although most cases are reported in patients who are chronically infected with HIV (human immunodeficiency virus).[13] Patients immunocompromised from HIV can present with facial nerve palsy due to a supranuclear, nuclear, or infranuclear lesion.[14,15] In the early stages, this condition may present a diagnostic problem because HIV serologic testing may be negative.[16] Suspected individuals may need follow-up testing. Facial palsy with HIV may occur over a period of hours to days and resolve without treatment in 2 to 10 weeks. These patients may have other neuropathies.

12-2-5 *Lyme Disease*. Lyme disease transferred by the bite of the deer tick (*Ixodes dammini*) by the spirochete *Borrelia burgdorferi* can present with isolated facial palsy. In one study of facial palsy, 19 of 38 patients had neurologic involvement with Lyme disease.[17] One third of these patients had bilateral facial nerve disease.

Lyme disease should be considered in pediatric facial palsy. In one study of 27 children with acute peripheral facial palsy, 16 had Lyme disease.[18] Bilateral facial palsy occurred only in children with Lyme borreliosis. Each child had a history of tick bite and/or erythema migrans in the head and neck region and contracted ipsilateral neurologic deficit, suggesting direct nerve invasion by the *Borrelia burgdorferi* organism. Serologic testing with enzyme-linked immunoabsorbent assay (ELISA) provides the best sensitivity and specificity for detecting Lyme disease. This condition should be treated with antibiotics appropriate for the organism *Borrelia burgdorferi*. The prognosis is good for return of facial function.

12-2-6 *Trauma*. Facial nerve palsy may initially be masked in severely traumatized patients. The mechanism usually occurs by laceration externally or by fracture of the temporal bone internally. With earlier recognition of the trauma to the facial nerve, the otolaryngologist may have a better chance of repairing or decompressing the facial nerve.

12-2-7 *Otitis Media*. Facial palsy from acute otitis media has become a rarity because of the wide availability of effective antibiotics. Facial palsy occurs four to five times more commonly with chronic otitis media. Malignant external otitis is extremely rare, but in patients with metabolic, hematologic, or immunologic-compromising conditions, mortality can reach as high as 50%.[19–23] With antibiotic treatment, facial nerve function returns in 50% of the survivors.

12-2-8 *Ramsay Hunt Syndrome*. Ramsay Hunt syndrome (herpes zoster oticus) deserves emphasis because the findings are diagnostic. Herpes zoster usually incites a painful facial palsy with herpetiform vessels that can be identified at the external ear canal. Recognizing this condition is important because acyclovir can be used for dramatic pain relief. The frequency of severe keratitis requires aggressive ophthalmic care.

12-2-9 *Leprosy*. The lepromatosis type of leprosy (*Mycobacterium leprae*) or the tuberculoid type can cause facial nerve palsy.[24,25] The severity of the corneal complications is greatly increased if the trigeminal nerve is involved, with decreased corneal sensation noted in 60% of patients.[26]

12-2-10 *Sarcoidosis.* Facial palsy can accompany sarcoidosis as the only sign of neurologic involvement, with an acute palsy usually followed by spontaneous recovery.[27] Treatment of sarcoid facial palsy with corticosteroids is controversial because of the high incidence of spontaneous recovery.

12-2-11 *Stroke.* Cerebral vascular accidents can cause facial weakness from either facial nuclear or supranuclear paralysis. Most strokes occur as supranuclear palsy involving the corticobulbar tracts and sparing the facial nucleus. Because the upper face has bilateral innervation, facial weakness may be seen on the opposite side, with sparing of the upper facial movement.

12-2-12 *Pediatric Facial Palsy.* A definitive diagnosis of facial palsy is more likely to be established in the pediatric age group. Lyme disease, as discussed above, is a common cause. Other causes that are easily documented include birth trauma, congenital malformations, hematopoietic derangements, immune disorders, and neoplasms. Traumatic neonatal facial palsy occurs most often in the setting of an uncomplicated forceps delivery. The facial nerve apparently is vulnerable at the lateral stylomastoid foramen when compressed against the maternal sacrum during a prolonged, difficult labor.[28,29] The infant may also have ecchymosis, tics, and synkinesis without craniofacial abnormality. The return of function has been reported to be as good as 41 of 45 in one series.[30] Facial palsy from congenital malformations has a poor prognosis for return of function, but despite reduced closure the pediatric cornea usually tolerates the facial palsy well when accompanied by good Bell's protective ocular movement and good tear production.

12-3 CLINICAL EXAMINATION

Facial palsy is managed primarily based on the patient's facial motor function, lacrimal secretion, and corneal sensation. Several protocols have been published for clinical evaluation and follow-up of facial nerve motor function. Table 12-1 shows a simple system that rates the facial nerve motor function by six degrees to allow consistent clinical evaluation of facial movement. Grade 1 signifies normal facial function. Grade 6 is total loss of facial function (i.e., paralysis). Grade 2 is minimal loss of function, and grade 5 is minimal return of function. Grades 3 and 4 are essentially everything in between, with grade 3 being patients with moderate dysfunction who can force their eyes closed or elevate their brows and grade 4 those with moderate dysfunction who cannot elevate the brows or force the eyelids completely closed. Using a system such as this to follow facial nerve motor function has been shown to be more consistent than either still photographs or videography.[31] The ocular findings help to define not only the state of the eye but also the prognosis. This is valuable in determining both medical and surgical management.

Visual acuity testing can be misleading from two standpoints. Therapeutically applied ointment protects the eye but also blurs vision. In patients with ointment in their eyes, several good blinks should be given actively (or passively by the examiner) to smooth the tear layer and obtain the most accurate visual acuity. On the other

Table 12-1 Rating Facial Nerve Function

Grade	Description	Characteristics
1	Normal	Normal facial function in all areas
2	Mild dysfunction	*Gross*: slight weakness noticeable on close inspection, may have very slight synkineses *At rest*: normal symmetry and tone *Motion*: forehead—moderate to good function; eye—complete closure with minimum effort; mouth—slight asymmetry
3	Moderate dysfunction	*Gross*: obvious but not disfiguring difference between the two sides; contracture and/or hemifacial spasm *At rest*: normal asymmetry and tone *Motion*: forehead—slight to moderate movement; eye—complete closure with effort; mouth—slightly weak with maximum effort
4	Moderately severe dysfunction	*Gross*: obvious weakness and/or disfiguring asymmetry *At rest*: normal asymmetry and tone *Motion*: forehead—none; eye—incomplete closure; mouth—asymmetric with maximum effort
5	Severe dysfunction	*Gross*: only barely perceptible motion *At rest*: asymmetry *Motion*: forehead—none; eye—incomplete closure; mouth—slight movement
6	Total paralysis	No movement

hand, the patient's functional vision is often much less than that determined by high-contrast black letters on a white background when compared with sophisticated contrast-sensitivity tests. The loss of contrast sensitivity is more disabling than is suggested by visual acuity testing.

The degree of facial motor nerve palsy can be graded by simple criteria (see Table 12-1), which allow the examiner to focus on the amount of deficit or the return of facial nerve function. Generally, the temporal branches above the brow are the most severely affected and the last to return.

Some patients can close the eye but have a poor blink. The normal eyelid gives a good, full blink, while the eyelid with facial palsy has only a slight flutter. Such patients have poor wetting of the cornea due to the lack of a "windshield wiper" action of the eyelid sweeping up and down across the cornea. Other patients appear to close the eye satisfactorily while sitting upright, but during sleep, the eye may drift open all night, causing a severe keratitis. In the early postoperative period after acoustic neuroma surgery, swelling of the eyelids and orbicularis muscle can cause a patient with a completely paralyzed face to have what appears to be an almost normal blink with full speed and extent of closure. Lagophthalmos will occur as the swelling decreases and the patient develops a staring eye that fails to close.

The Bell's protective mechanism should be determined because patients who have a good Bell's phenomenon may tolerate poor closure much better than those who have virtually no upward movement of the eye on forced closure. A family member may be able to give valuable information as to whether the cornea is exposed at night during sleep. The eyelids open at night may be protected from exposure when the cornea rolls up underneath the lid with a good Bell's phenomenon.

The lower lid position should be noted. A sagging ectropion from the lack of orbicularis support and the weight of atonic muscle affects whether tears, drops, or ointments will be kept in contact with the cornea. In some cases, frank ectropion results. In other cases, the lid is still apposed to the globe but sags downward, producing scleral show. In either case, the eye tends to have greater drying. The normal position of the lid margin at the lower limbus helps to keep ointment or drops in contact with the cornea for the best possible lubrication. Deviation from this position can increase corneal exposure and irritation. In patients with intact tear production, sagging of the medial eyelid with punctal ectropion may produce epiphora.

Tear production is often the most overlooked factor in facial nerve palsy. Patients with Bell's palsy frequently tolerate poor closure because they have normal lacrimal secretion. On the other hand, patients who have fairly good closure may have severe keratitis and severe ocular pain due to unrecognized reduction in tear production. The Schirmer test will help detect patients with abnormal lacrimal secretory function, although the test can be difficult to perform or interpret in patients who have ointment or artificial tears in their eyes.

Corneal sensation should be carefully tested and compared to the normal side. Acute loss of corneal sensation indicates a severely guarded prognosis for patients with facial palsy and demands aggressive treatment.

12-4 GENERAL TREATMENT CONSIDERATIONS

All therapies either add moisture or provide better closure. The most important principle in the management of facial palsy is to prevent the eye from getting into difficulty rather than to try to get the eye out of difficulty.

The ophthalmologist should make the best determination possible as to the severity and duration of the facial palsy to decide which of the medical and surgical treatments to use. A patient who is improving from a mild Bell's palsy will be treated differently from a patient who has had complete resection of nerve VII and loss of nerve V corneal sensation that is expected to be permanent. A younger person generally tolerates facial nerve injury better and experiences regeneration earlier than an older individual.

Low tear production usually has a much more serious prognosis than poor closure. Acute loss of corneal sensation, combined with decreased tearing and decreased closure, constitutes a triad predictive of severe keratitis and the development of recurrent corneal erosions. The patient's overall health, age, immune status, and accessibility to medical care will also affect whether the treatment is primarily medical or whether more aggressive surgical procedures for eyelid closure should be performed.

12-4-1 *Peripheral Facial Nerve Injuries.* Peripheral facial nerve injuries encompass traumatic laceration and injury from oculofacial plastic procedures such as endoscopic brow lift, midfacial lift, or conventional face lift. Tumor removal from the parotid or external ear can produce a permanent or transient palsy. With bilateral intractable blepharospasm, differential section of the facial nerve was the primary treatment prior to development of Botulinum toxin.

The facial nerve typically has five branches: frontal, zygomatic, buccal, mandibular, and cervical. Distal anastomoses are common, but the frontal and marginal mandibular branches appear to be more vulnerable to injury due to the reduced number of anastomotic fibers. The frontal branch is particularly vulnerable crossing the zygomatic arch. The nerve can be injured during endoscopic forehead-lifting surgery with blunt trauma of an endoscope raising the flap from below even though the frontal branch has not been transected. With endoscopic brow lifting, the patient does not usually notice the facial nerve weakness since the brow has been significantly elevated and improved.

Peripheral facial nerve injuries are usually treated with observation except for traumatic transaction, which should receive urgent repair.

12-5 MEDICAL TREATMENT

The most common treatment for facial palsy is to add lubricants to the eye. Ointment provides longer-lasting protection than drops for an exposed or dry cornea, but with more blurring. In most cases, drops are used frequently during the day, when clear vision is required, and ointments are used to provide longer-term protection from prolonged corneal exposure at night.

As with keratitis sicca, most patients fail to use ointment and drops frequently enough. Patients need to be encouraged to use drops more often than they think is needed and to be told that they will not overdose or harm themselves by putting in drops frequently. Patients who have prolonged facial palsy should be treated with an ointment without preservative to avert any sensitivities to the preservatives. Non-preservative drops are now available in multidose formulations that do not require disposal after a single use.

A humidifier in the bedroom may add enough moisture to cut down on drying symptoms. Patients should avoid irritants such as tobacco smoke, chlorinated swimming pools, air conditioners, aerosol sprays, and eyelid-margin cosmetics. During an airplane flight, the eye often becomes irritated from the dry air and increased ozone content in the pressurized cabin. A plastic bubble can be placed around the patient's glasses to act as a moisture shield that increases humidity around the eye and also decreases the irritation and drying from dust. A moisture-tight occlusive bubble can be placed over the eye at night to cut down on evaporation. Because such bubbles are generally expensive, the traditional method of applying Vaseline around the orbit and then plastic wrap is an inexpensive, effective way to cover an eye that doesn't close at night. Alternatively, tape can be used to pull the upper lid down over the lower lid. Full closure must be ensured to prevent further trauma to the cornea by the tape or dressing. Bandage contact lenses tend to be more helpful in the short run, as opposed to an effective therapeutic alternative. However, some patients have achieved success with bandage lenses. Tinted lenses can help reduce the symptoms of photophobia that may occur in bright sunlight. In severe situations, the eye can be patched for 48 hours to eliminate corneal exposure. In chronic facial palsies, antibiotic drops may be necessary from time to time when mucus turns purulent.

12-6 SURGICAL TREATMENT

Most surgical procedures for facial palsy are designed to increase the closure or coverage of the eye, but procedures that block lacrimal drainage and effectively increase moisture, such as punctoplasty or temporary punctum plugs, should be strongly considered. This section describes three relatively simple procedures to provide relief of facial palsy and then covers more advanced options. The simple procedures that provide relief in most situations include (1) closure of the punctum with cautery or temporary plugs, (2) ectropion repair, and (3) closure of the lid with gold weights or tarsorrhaphy. More advanced procedures to close the lid, including wire-spring insertion, silicone-band placement, and temporalis muscle–fascia transposition, are discussed in a separate section.

12-6-1 *Punctal Closure.* Punctal closure is a simple procedure that can in many instances make a dramatic difference in the patient's management. In patients who cannot be satisfactorily managed with ointment and drops or who have a prognosis for severe dysfunction (for example, after resection of an acoustic neuroma with decreased closure and tear production), closure of the punctum appears to have two important benefits. First, it keeps the patient's own tears in contact with the cornea rather than allowing the tears to drain into the nose. Second, artificial tears will remain in contact with the cornea longer.

Closure of the punctum can be carried out with local anesthesia. Usually, a few drops of topical anesthetic are applied to the conjunctiva with a cotton-tipped applicator. After a few minutes, the injection of local anesthetic through the conjunctiva with a 30-gauge needle near the punctum is better tolerated. A disposable two-battery hand-held cautery is preferred. The tip can be brought to the edge of the punctum to seal and close the epithelium. The cautery should be used in a brief touching action as opposed to a prolonged "cooking" action. With this method, the punctum can later be opened with a simple snip procedure if the patient's normal tear production returns. In some instances, the punctum does not seal down and the treatment needs to be repeated. However, lighter cautery as opposed to going deep into the punctum and canaliculus ensures the ability to snip open the punctum later if need be.

Disposable punctum plugs have the advantage of easy removal if the patient develops tearing instantly or at a later date as lacrimal function returns. Punctum plugs can be difficult to insert in some patients even under local anesthesia. Occasional patients complain of irritation from the caps of the punctum plug, even though the plug appears to be properly fitted. Silicone plugs provide better closure than do the dissolvable collagen plugs.

12-6-2 *Ectropion Repair.* Ectropion that is symptomatic or permanent can be repaired with local anesthesia by a lateral canthoplasty that avoids the notching or trichiasis sometimes associated with central full-thickness eyelid resection. This approach was described and popularized by Bick in the 1950s. With local anesthesia, an incision is performed with a scalpel or with scissors, splitting the upper and lower lids down to the periosteum at the lateral canthus and approximately 1 cm out through the skin. Remnants of the lower lateral canthal tendon should be incised so that the lower lid will be free. Next, the cut edge of the lower lid is grasped and pulled up so that the lid is somewhat overtightened. In many instances, 5 or 6 mm of lower lid margin will be marked and then excised at an angle that meets the most lateral portion of the previous incision.

Once this tissue is excised, hemostasis is obtained and a 4-0 polyglycolic acid mattress suture can be placed from below upward through the cut edge of the tarsus and then into the periosteum at the lateral orbital rim. The suture is cinched up and the knot tied. Also, 6-0 plain gut sutures can be used in a running or an interrupted manner to close the skin–muscle layer of the incision. If ectropion recurs, additional resection can be repeated to tighten the lid. The lid should look somewhat taut for the first week, allowing for some natural tissue relaxation that will occur.

Some surgeons prefer a variation of this technique called the *tarsal strip* or the *lateral canthal sling procedure*, originally described by Tenzel in 1969. After the lower lid is freed, the lateral portion of the lid is de-epithelialized of skin and conjunctiva and then anchored with mattress sutures into the lateral orbital rim.

12-6-3 *Simple Lid-Closure Procedures.* Lateral tarsorrhaphy and placement of a gold weight are procedures that help provide better closure. A lateral tarsorrhaphy is more likely to provide some minor disfigurement but is simpler than the gold-weight procedure. A lateral tarsorrhaphy of 4 or 5 mm produces a minimal blemish and yet may reduce the amount of lagophthalmos by 70% or 80%. A tarsorrhaphy greater than 5 mm will be more cosmetically noticeable but provides better closure.

Placing a gold weight in the upper lid, on the other hand, usually helps the lid to close without producing much cosmetic blemish. When the swelling subsides, patients may be able to feel or see the outline of the gold weight with the lid closed, but rarely when the lid is open. Some patients develop a minimal ptosis with the gold weight, but most have a normal open eyelid position. Gold weights are not totally predictable with respect to lid closure, but most lids close completely, both during the day and at night. The gold weight is based on the dead-weight principle rather than any sort of accelerating spring action. The weight has to pick up speed slowly by gravity rather than by acceleration, as with silicone bands or springs (described later). Thus, when the patient blinks, the normal eye blinks but the gold weight rarely has time to allow the eye to close.

12-6-3-1 *Lateral Tarsorrhaphy.* The development of long-acting absorbable sutures has revolutionized the lateral tarsorrhaphy technique. Previously, most tarsorrhaphies were performed by creating a raw area on the lateral upper and lower lids and then sewing the upper and lower lids together with stitches that were bolstered over rubber pegs. The pegs were left in place for several weeks to give the tarsal plates a chance to fuse.

With the advent of long-acting absorbable sutures, such as polyglycolic acid, a small raw area on the lid margin can be created in the upper and lower lids laterally, and then buried sutures can be used to sew the lids together in a mattress fashion that will hold them long enough to allow the eyelids to fuse. A thin adhesion can be created with enough strength to keep the lids together and yet provide ease of separation at a later date if the patient's facial palsy resolves.

The upper and lower lids should be anesthetized with a local anesthetic containing epinephrine for hemostasis, if not contraindicated by either hypertension or arrhythmia. A #15 Bard-Parker blade can be used to mark approximately 4 mm from the lateral canthus in both the upper and the lower lids. Then a horizontal incision is made at the margin of the lid from this mark over to the lateral canthus. Sharp scissors or a #15 Bard-Parker blade can then be used to remove 0.5 or 1 mm of lid tissue posteriorly that will not create cicatricial entropion or trichiasis (Fig. 12-2).

Next, 5-0 polyglycolic acid sutures are used to bring the upper and lower lids together in a mattress fashion, with the knot tied away from the cornea. Furthermore, 6-0 plain catgut can be used externally for skin closure to reinforce the tarsorrhaphy. The wound essentially requires no care other than gentle washing, although antibiotic ointment is usually applied. The sutures will dissolve and the lids should be fused laterally. Greater amounts of tarsorrhaphy will produce a much more noticeable cosmetic effect, with small amounts of increased closure. The amount of closure with a tarsorrhaphy varies from patient to patient, but even a subtle lateral tarsorrhaphy is frequently enough to provide increased comfort.

12-6-3-2 *Gold-Weight Insertion*. Insertion of a gold weight requires a horizontal incision in the upper lid, dissection down to the tarsal plate, creation of a space between the orbicularis muscle and the tarsal plate, and fixation of the weight to the tarsal plate.[32] The size of gold weight to be inserted can be determined by taping or gluing a weight onto the upper eyelid and noting whether it produces closure of the eyelid without inducing ptosis. Generally, a 1.0- or 1.2-gram weight is used.

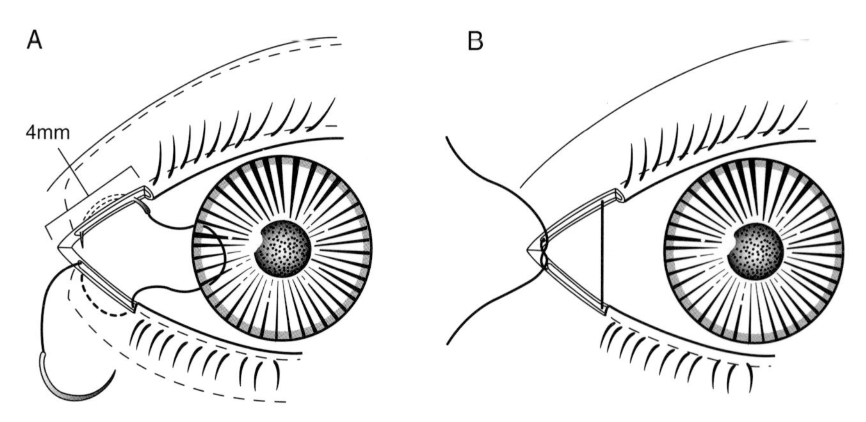

Figure 12-2 Lateral tarsorrhaphy with absorbable sutures. About 4 mm of upper and lower lid margin laterally is carefully excised. (A) Then, 5-0 polyglycolic acid double-armed mattress sutures are passed into upper and lower tarsi. (B) Knot is tied laterally, away from cornea. Skin closure completes repair.

With the patient having local anesthesia and a corneal protector in place, a horizontal incision is made approximately 1 cm in length down a few millimeters from the lid crease (Fig. 12-3). An incision at this level helps avoid injury to the retractors of the upper eyelid that might produce ptosis. Once the incision is made through the skin, vessels should be cauterized. Then the orbicularis muscle is grasped and opened with scissors down to the tarsal plate. After the glistening white tarsal plate is identified, a space should be opened medially and laterally and also inferiorly toward, but short of, the lash roots. The weight is usually fixed with 7-0 silk sutures through the holes with partial-thickness bites in lamellar fashion

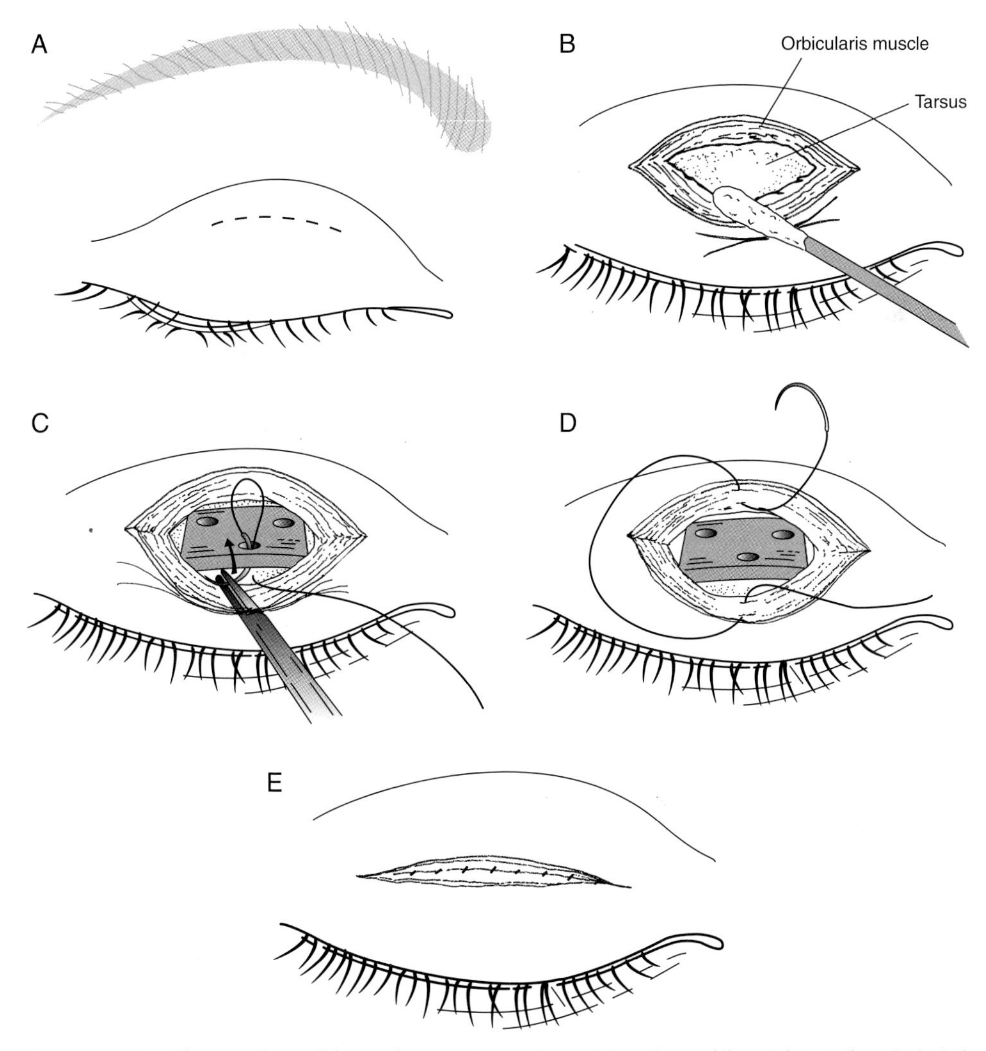

Figure 12-3 Technique for gold-weight insertion. (A) Incision for gold weight is placed slightly below lid crease. Dissection through orbicularis is angled slightly inferiorly to avoid ptosis from injury to levator aponeurosis or Müller's muscle. (B) Tarsal plate is exposed, with pocket for placement of weight shown. Gold weight is inserted to compare size, and 7-0 silk is passed into epitarsal tissue. (C) Needle is passed backward through gold weight. (D,E) After weight is secured to tarsus, orbicularis is closed meticulously with 7-0 polyglactin.

into the tarsal plate. Care should be taken to attach the weight without buckling the tarsal plate. The orbicularis muscle should be closed over the weight with interrupted 7-0 polyglactin (Vicryl) sutures and the skin closed with 6-0 plain gut sutures. Some surgeons prefer to place the weight higher on the tarsal plate or even up on the external surface of the levator aponeurosis. More superior placement requires a heavier weight.

Typically, the patient immediately experiences full closure from the swelling of the orbicularis muscle that takes place after insertion of the weight. Over the course of a few days, as the swelling goes down, the lid may be somewhat stiff. Then, over the next month, most patients experience complete lid closure. Insertion of a gold weight can be combined with procedures to close the punctum and also to correct lower lid ectropion.

Complications are generally minimal or reversible. Bruising and swelling can occur, although they can actually be helpful in the short run by producing some increased tightness of eyelid closure. A patient allergic to gold may develop what appears to be a chronic cellulitis until the weight is removed. Most patients develop a thin capsule around the weight, although in some individuals the capsule attains some thickness and a slight redness that resolves when the gold weight is removed. Swelling and intermittent redness around the weight do not necessitate removal if no other difficulty is encountered. Ptosis of 1 to 2 mm is common and generally resolves after removal of the gold weight.

Gold weights can be left in permanently. However, the question frequently arises as to whether and when a weight may be removed. As patients achieve closure and any keratitis is resolved, measurement of tear production can be helpful in determining whether the weight should be removed.

To determine whether a patient recovering from facial motor palsy can close adequately without the gold weight, the patient should be asked to blink both eyes rapidly. If the affected side has a quick blinking action, the orbicularis muscle is causing the lid to close rather than the gold weight. Another method of evaluation is to place fingers on the upper and lower lids to see if some force is generated by the orbicularis muscle on closure. The Parrish maneuver came from an ingenious patient who hung upside down from the side of her bed to show that the upper lid could be closed against the downward gravitational force of the gold weight.

The gold weight can be removed under local anesthesia by opening the original incision down onto the outer surface of the gold weight. Dissection should be carried on the external surface between the gold weight and the capsule that has formed. The 7-0 silk sutures and fibrous bands through the holes should be cut and then the weight will slip out. The incision can be closed with 6-0 plain gut sutures.

If the patient has more than a minor ptosis, this should be repaired by bringing some of the levator aponeurosis down onto the tarsal plate. A simple way to do this is to grasp the tissue between the tarsal plate and the skin and place a 6-0 polyglycolic acid suture through the tissue. This suture should be stitched to the inferior portion of the wound, which will effectively bring the retractors down and correct the ptosis. Prior to placing this stitch, the surgeon administers local anesthesia, grasps the superior tissue with forceps, and has the patient look up to verify a transmission of the force of the levator aponeurosis.

12-6-4 *Advanced Lid-Closure Procedures.* Although most cases of lid paresis can be managed with the protocols described above, three additional procedures can be used for closure of the eyelid. Two of these procedures, the silicone rod and the orthodontic spring, depend on foreign materials; the third, the temporalis muscle tendon transfer, relies on autogenous tissue. The silicone-rod cerclage consists of placing a rod of silicone around the upper and lower lid. When the eyelid opens on levator function, tension is placed on the cerclage. When the patient relaxes the levator muscle, the stretched cerclage forces closure of the eyelid. With the palpebral spring, a piece of orthodontic wire is fashioned into a spring and placed laterally on the eyelid. As the eyelid is opened, tension is placed on the wire. Once the levator muscle relaxes, the tension of the palpebral spring causes the eyelid to close. With the temporalis muscle tendon transfer, the force of closure is generated by a cerclage around the eyelid of temporalis fascia tendon, which is innervated via the temporalis muscle. When the patient clenches the jaw, using nerve V function of the temporalis muscle, tension is placed on the eyelid to close.

Each of these procedures has advantages and disadvantages. The silicone cerclage can give more effective closure than a gold weight but may result in lagophthalmos. The palpebral spring can provide tight closure, but often the patient has ptosis and an abnormal contour to the upper eyelid. Both the silicone cerclage and the palpebral spring cause the levator muscle to load against an increasing amount of force as the spring or cerclage is pulled open. Consequently, the force of the levator muscle may be overcome prior to reaching full fissure height, which results in ptosis. A gold weight, on the other hand, has a constant loading weight that actually is slightly less as it arcs over the globe. Therefore, the gold weight can be inserted without producing ptosis, but the closure is not as tight as with a spring or cerclage.

Both the silicone-cerclage and the palpebral-spring procedures are technically more difficult than inserting a gold weight. Like all foreign materials under tension, the cerclage and the spring have a tendency in the long run to extrude. Nevertheless, these two procedures can provide tight closure where the slow, gentle closure of a gold weight may not be satisfactory.

The temporalis muscle tendon transfer does not involve a foreign material but requires a conscious effort by the patient to clench the jaw in order to close the lid. Consequently, at night, when the patient relaxes the jaw, the eye may drift open. The fascia, which provides passive lid support, also tends to loosen over the years.

In level of difficulty, the silicone-rod cerclage is perhaps the simplest. The next most complicated is probably the palpebral spring, and the most difficult is the temporalis muscle tendon transfer.

12-6-4-1 *Silicone-Rod Cerclage.* A 1-mm silicone rod should be inserted and adjusted so that the upper eyelid overrides the lower by approximately 1 to 2 mm. Postoperatively, after the swelling and tightness resolve, the patient may actually have a slight amount of lagophthalmos. A tighter cerclage increases the chances of eyelid malposition or cerclage extrusion.

The cerclage can be inserted using local anesthesia with a corneal protector in place. The first incision is made at the medial canthus, exposing the external head of the medial canthal tendon. A second lateral incision should expose the lateral orbital rim. The silicone rod is sewn through the medial canthal tendon with a small-eye needle and is further fixed with a separate nonabsorbable suture. A Wright fascia needle or a hemostat is then used to pass the silicone rod from the medial canthus to the lateral canthus, staying close to the lid margin to avoid rotational ectropion of the upper or lower lid. Placement is easier if silicone is passed to the middle of the upper or lower lid, brought out through a small incision, and then a second pass used to bring it to the lateral canthus.

At the lateral rim, two holes are drilled in the bone to allow for fixation of the rod. One should be placed above the lateral canthal tendon, and one below the lateral canthal tendon. The silicone rod should be crossed so that the lower band goes through the upper hole and vice versa to produce the normal direction of canthal forces. The silicone rod should be handled with toothless forceps to avoid microfractures that may later cause the rod to break.

The rod is then passed through a Watzke sleeve, which allows the rod to be tightened with the 1- to 2-mm override of the upper lid versus the lower lid. A permanent suture is tied around the sleeve to prevent the rod from slipping or loosening in the Watzke sleeve.

This procedure provides immediate improvement in eyelid closure. The Watzke sleeve provides the advantage of permitting adjustment of the tightness on the cerclage later, with local anesthesia, by opening the incision and exposing the Watzke sleeve. A colored permanent suture around the Watzke sleeve makes identification of the sleeve easier because the grayish fibrous tissue around the sleeve may blend with the silicone rod. Inadvertent dissection is avoided by identifying the colored suture and dissecting straight down to the middle of the sleeve, then exposing the silicone rod superiorly and inferiorly. This procedure can be carried out in patients who have had previous lateral tarsorrhaphies, gold-weight insertions, or other closure procedures.

12-6-4-2 *Palpebral Spring.* The palpebral spring provides tighter closure than does the silicone cerclage. To obtain proper results, a springy rather than a malleable orthodontic wire should be selected. Orthodontic wire in the diameter of 0.010 or 0.008 inch with springiness should be used, as opposed to wire with better twisting characteristics, which are preferred for repairing facial fractures. Orthodontic tools are required to achieve uniform, round bending of the loops for proper working of the spring; hemostats and ophthalmic needle holders do not provide satisfactory results. Reviewing the technique with an orthodontist will help the ophthalmologist understand the physics of springs and master the techniques of working with wire materials.

Round-nosed orthodontic pliers can be used to fashion a round spring much like that found in the bend of a safety pin. The diameter of the loop should be approximately 5 mm. The spring should be given a contour in the horizontal direction that will match the arc/contour of the globe, because the eyelid twists open rather than opening in a linear fashion. Making a smaller loop will give a stiffer action to the spring.

At the time of surgery, the upper eyelid and lateral canthus should be infiltrated with a local anesthetic agent that contains epinephrine to provide better hemostasis. A corneal protector is employed. An incision should be made below the brow or through the eyelid crease to expose the orbital rim (Fig. 12-4). A second incision is made in the upper eyelid slightly medial to the midline.

The spring should be adjusted to a position that matches the rim-to-closed position of the eyelid. An 18-gauge needle is passed from the ciliary incision to the lateral aspect of the brow incision, permitting one arm of the spring to be inserted through the needle. Then the needle is withdrawn through the supraciliary incision, leaving the spring in place and making sure that no tarsal penetration has occurred.

The fulcrum of the spring should be anchored laterally over the orbital rim as far as possible without bending toward the temporal muscle fossa. A permanent suture such as 5-0 polypropylene (Prolene) can be used to hold the fulcrum in place at the bony rim.

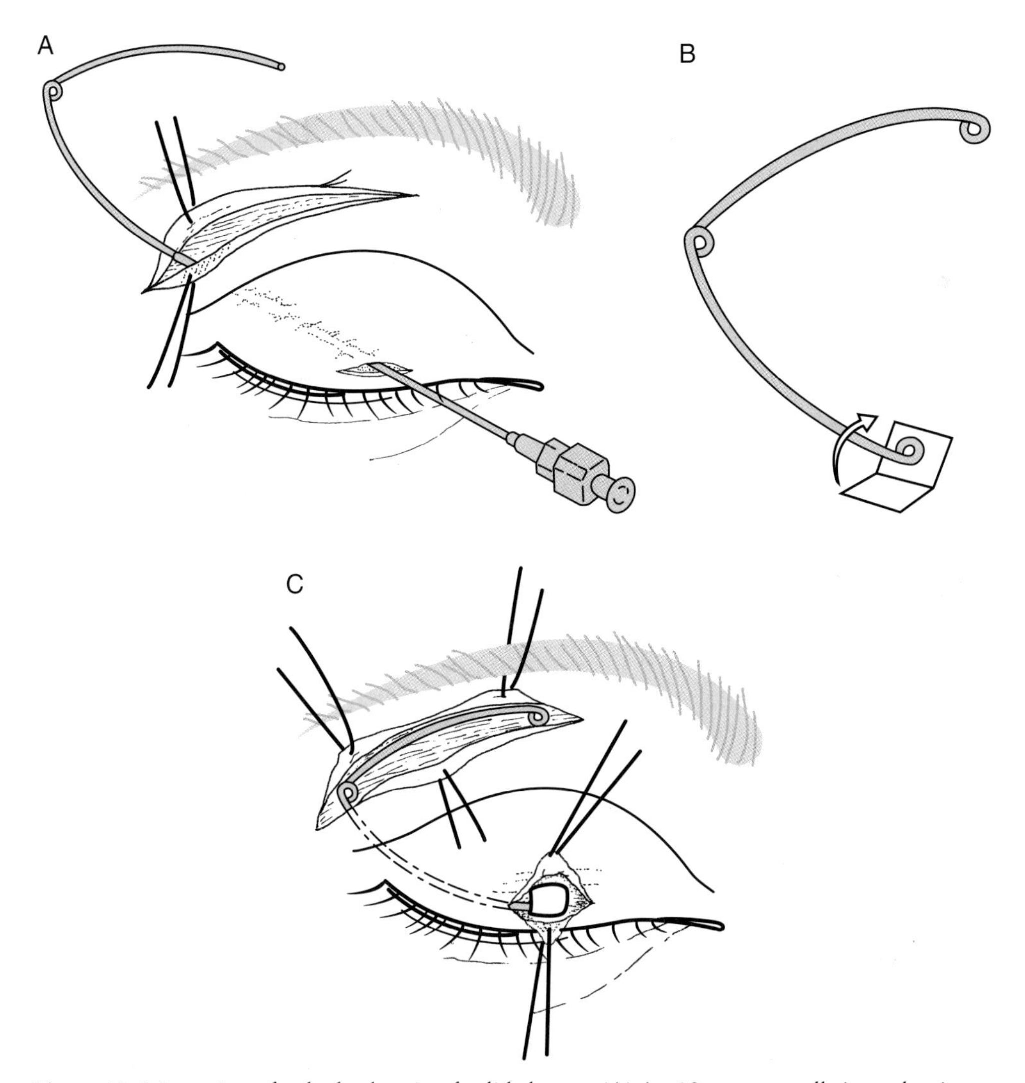

Figure 12-4 Insertion of palpebral spring for lid closure. (A) An 18-gauge needle is used to insert spring into lid incisions. Spring is positioned after each end is twisted. (B) Dacron patch is placed over lid portion of spring. Tightness is adjusted at central twist. (C) Final placement of spring before wound closure.

Orthodontic pliers are then used to blunt each end of the spring and allow for fixation. The upper limb is fixed medially to the periosteum with a second 5-0 polypropylene suture, with another suture halfway between the fulcrum and the end of the upper limb.

The lower limb can be fixed using a 0.2-mm Dacron patch (not mesh) prepared in a Gelfoam press that has been folded over the end of the spring and sutured to the upper tarsal tissue with a permanent (e.g., 7-0 silk) suture. The twist at the end of the lower eyelid arm must be aligned perfectly in a horizontal plane with the rest of the spring, so that the wire will not work through the orbicularis muscle and skin externally or the tarsal plate internally. Orthodontic pliers or a needle holder can be used at the outer canthus to adjust the tightness of the spring.

Separating the arms causes tighter closure. The wound should be closed with good orbicularis closure over the metal spring. A 6-0 polyglycolic acid suture can be used superiorly for muscle closure and 6-0 plain catgut externally. For the lower portion, 6-0 polyglycolic acid skin sutures are used to take deep bites of the orbicularis muscle so that the spring is well covered.

The spring can be adjusted later in the office by exposing the area nearest the fulcrum under sterile conditions. The spring can be set for tight closure as needed, although a tight spring is more likely to produce ptosis or a temporal drooping and abnormal contour of the eyelid. Moderate closure usually provides adequate corneal coverage with fairly reasonable corneal contour.

A spring can extrude, but breakage from material fatigue appears to be extremely rare. Most commonly, the spring extrudes through the supraciliary incision. Frequently, this can be repaired with local anesthesia in the office. A posterior extrusion through the tarsal plate is a serious occurrence that threatens the cornea. Cause for the gravest concern is a posterior extrusion of the spring in an anesthetized cornea so that the patient is not even aware of the problem.

The most cumbersome problem with the palpebral spring is the poor contour that frequently occurs even in the most skilled hands. The palpebral spring dependably provides tight closure, but the side effects are not insignificant. Several authors have commented on the possibility of an eyelid spring moving or vibrating during magnetic resonance imaging.[33–35]

12-6-4-3 *Temporalis Muscle Transfer.* The temporalis muscle tendon fascia transfer can provide permanent closure of the eyelids, using innervation of cranial nerve V rather than the paralytic cranial nerve VII and avoiding the use of foreign materials. The patient must make a chewing action or clench the temporalis muscle to provide the force for blink or closure.

The temporalis fascia can be exposed through a vertical incision at the hairline. The most common technical mistake is to dissect down to the superficial temporalis fascia, which is an extension of the galea rather than the true temporalis fascia that lines the temporalis muscle and goes beneath the zygomatic arch. Strips for the sling can be marked so that the base is attached superiorly to the strip of temporalis muscle mobilized, effectively providing the length necessary for the sling to reach across the eyelids.

An incision should be made at the lateral canthus for passage of the fascia across the eyelids and for receiving the temporalis muscle flap. The subcutaneous tunnel is made from the hairline incision to the lateral canthal incision to pass the flap. A medial canthus incision is made similar to that used for the silicone cerclage. A Wright fascia needle or a hemostat can be used to pass the fascia from the lateral to the medial canthus.

The fascia should be fixed around the external head of the medial canthal tendon and pulled tight to bring the upper lid into apposition with the lower lid under tension. The fascia should then be fixed with a permanent suture. The sling should be fixed tighter than might appear to be optimal, to allow for the relaxation that will occur over subsequent months.

The fascia should be passed fairly close to the lashes to avert a rotational entropion of the upper or lower lid. However, the fascia should be deep to the orbicularis muscle and superficial to the tarsus. Patients can then achieve eyelid closure by a chewing motion on the temporalis muscle. Infection or rejection does not appear to be a problem. Laxity over the long run is the major concern. Contour problems and ptosis are unusual.

This procedure should be used for patients with permanent facial palsy who are not candidates for facial nerve transfer procedures, such as patients who have had facial palsy for years. A facial nerve substitution procedure (also known as a reanimation technique)—for example, the facial hypoglossal transfer described in Section 12-7-1—must be performed within a year for the distal facial nerve to be viable.

12-7 OTHER REHABILITATIVE PROCEDURES

With the loss of facial function, temporal branch paresis and loss of innervation to the frontalis muscle may result in a unilateral brow droop severe enough to cause some impairment of visual field as the brow sags and as the atonic orbital orbicularis muscle pushes the upper lid downward. A direct brow lift provides better correction of this unilateral problem than does a coronal approach. Even with a brow lift, the side with palsy will have a noticeable lack of wrinkles in older individuals. A coronal lift can provide better symmetry by eliminating wrinkles on the normal side, though actual lifting of the brow is best accomplished with the unilateral direct lift.

A simple technique for lifting and stabilizing a brow can be performed by excising a strip of skin approximately 1 cm in height 1 cm above the brow. A sigmoid-shaped spindle with a vertical height of 10 mm is drawn, incised, and removed. The inferior portion of the incision is undermined subcutaneously but not the superior portion. Closure can then be carried out with 5-0 polyglycolic acid subcutaneous sutures and 6-0 nylon mattress stitches.

The more standard technique of making an incision closer to the brow results in the closure trying to match thinner skin near the brow with thicker skin 1 cm higher. With the excision of skin made in the exposed area 1 cm above the brow, the closure is exposed but generally heals well and is less noticeable.

A face lift can be performed on the sagging side to ameliorate the "sad" appearance caused by facial weakness. Occasionally a procedure is required on the other side as well to provide best symmetry.

In patients who have had no return of facial nerve function, a static sling on the involved side of the face may be performed with autogenous fascia to pull the lip and face upward toward the zygomatic arch. This procedure also eliminates the downward pull of the sagging face from the lower lid. The fascial strips must be inserted from the muscles around the mouth and lip subcutaneously, using an instrument such as the Wright fascia needle. The strips are fixed near the zygomatic arch. The strips should be tightened as much as possible, as the sling will eventually sag. This procedure can be used in patients with longstanding facial palsy who are not candidates for facial nerve reinnervation, such as the hypoglossal facial nerve procedure described below.

Blepharoplasty may be of value in patients with persistent sagging skin and muscle in the upper eyelid. This operation should be considered only after the patient has stabilized, as initially the heavy skin may help the patient to close the upper lid. A conservative blepharoplasty should be performed and a high fixation technique of lid crease to upper tarsal or levator aponeurotic tissue employed, to fold the excess tissue up toward the superior sulcus with less risk of corneal exposure.

12-7-1 *Nerve Substitution*. The most effective facial reanimation technique is direct repair of the facial nerve with an end-to-end anastomosis or even with a short interpositional graft. Nerve substitution must be used when the nerve cannot be repaired directly or with a cable graft.

The nerve-substitution procedures graft a normal nerve to the facial nerve. In the case of the spinal accessory/facial anastomosis, the posterior portion of cranial nerve XI is sutured to the distal facial nerve. Movement of the shoulder causes contraction of the facial musculature.

The facial hypoglossal anastomosis appears to be the most reliable form of reinnervation of the facial nerve. The nerves match well in size and can be approximated without tension. The tongue may show varying degrees of atrophy, but the impact on chewing, speaking, and swallowing is frequently minimal. Generally, the return of lower facial function is better than that of the forehead. The face may sag slightly in a resting state, but movement is usually good. The amount of facial expression on the reinnervated side may not match the movement on the opposite side. With fatigue, the face tends to droop.

Eyelid closure seems to return early in the course of reanastomosis, but this procedure does not provide reinnervation of lacrimal gland secretory function. Patients with the facial hypoglossal anastomosis usually develop functional adaptation such that they do not consciously have to think about moving the tongue to innervate the face. Apparently, some substitution of cranial nerve XII for VII occurs through a poorly understood brain stem mechanism that links facial and hypoglossal nuclei.[36]

Newer techniques of cross-facial nerve grafting, dural muscular island pedicles, muscle transfer, free muscle grafting, and free muscle nerve grafts with neurovascular anastomosis can be used alone or in combination with the other substitution procedures, such as the facial hypoglossal anastomosis. These procedures occasionally provide outstanding results but are not generally as dependable as the hypoglossal facial nerve graft for facial reinnervation.

REFERENCES

1. Esselan E. *The Acute Facial Palsies.* Berlin: Springer-Verlag, 1977:7.
2. Van Burskirk C. The seventh nerve complex. *J Comp Neurol.* 1945;82:303–333.
3. Brewis M, Paskanzer DC, Rolland C, et al. Neurological disease in an English city. *Acta Neurol Scand.* 1966;42(suppl 24):1–89.
4. Logan WPD, Cushion AA. *Morbidity Statistics from General Practice.* London: Her Majesty's Stationery Office, Vol. 1, 1958.
5. Mellotte G. Idiopathic paralysis of the facial nerve. *Practitioner.* 1961;187:349–353.
6. May M, Hardin WB. Facial palsy: interpretation of neurologic findings. *Laryngoscope.* 1978;88:1352–1362.
7. Peitersen E. The natural history of Bell's palsy. *Am J Otol.* 1982;4:107–111.
8. Kartush JM. Electroneurography and intraoperative facial monitoring in contemporary neurotology. *Otolaryngol Head Neck Surg.* 1989;101:496–503.
9. Leonetti JP, Matz GJ, Smith PG, Beck DL. Facial nerve monitoring in otologic surgery: clinical indications and intraoperative techniques. *Ann Otol Rhinol Laryngol.* 1990; 99:911–918.
10. Fisch U, Ruttner J. Pathology of intratemporal tumors involving the facial nerve. In: Fisch U, ed. *Facial Nerve Surgery.* Birmingham, AL: Aesculapius Publishing Co., 1977:448.
11. Jackson CG, Glasscock ME, Hughes GB, et al. Facial paralysis of neoplastic origin: diagnosis and management. *Laryngoscope.* 1980;90:1581–1595.
12. Kisimoto S, Saito H. Facial nerve neurolemmoma: a case report and review. *Pract Otolaryngol (Jpn).* 1978;71:817–824.
13. Neeley GJ, Alford BR. The facial nerve in lesions of the temporal bone: clinical considerations. In: Graham J, House WF, eds. *Disorders of the Facial Nerve: Anatomy, Diagnosis and Management.* New York: Raven Press, 1982:191.
14. Belec L, Gherardi R, Georges AJ, et al. Peripheral facial paralysis and HIV infection: report of four African cases and review of the literature. *J Neurol.* 1989;236:411–414.
15. Schielke E, Pfister H, Einhaupl KM. Peripheral facial nerve palsy associated with HIV infection [letter]. *Lancet.* 1989;1:553–554.
16. Sloand EM, Pitt E, Chiarello RJ, Nemo GJ. HIV testing: state of the art. *J Am Med Assoc.* 1991;266:2861–2866.
17. Pachner AR, Steere AC. The triad of neurologic manifestations of Lyme disease: meningitis, cranial neuritis, and radiculoneuritis. *Neurology.* 1985;35:47–53.
18. Christen HJ, Bartlau N, Hanefeld F, et al. Peripheral facial palsy in childhood—Lyme borreliosis to be suspected unless proven otherwise. *Acta Paediatr Scand.* 1990; 79:1219–1224.
19. Chandler JR. Malignant otitis externa. *Laryngoscope.* 1968;78:1257–1294.
20. Kettel K. Facial palsy of otitic origin. *Arch Otolaryngol.* 1938;27:395–401.
21. Pollock RA, Brown LA. Facial paralysis in otitis media. In: Graham J, House WF, eds. *Disorders of the Facial Nerve: Anatomy, Diagnosis and Management.* New York: Raven Press, 1982:221.
22. Hawthorne T, Jonkees LBW. Surgical classification of the paralysis of the facial nerve with guidelines for differential diagnosis and therapy. In: Miehlke A, ed. *Surgery of the Facial Nerve.* 2nd ed. Philadelphia: WB Saunders Co., 1973:52.

23. Shambaugh GE, Glasscock ME. Facial nerve decompression and repair. In: Shambaugh GE, Glasscock ME, eds. *Surgery of the Ear.* Philadelphia: WB Saunders Co., 1980:530.
24. Shields JA, Waring GO III, Monte LG. Ocular findings in leprosy. *Am J Ophthalmol.* 1974;77:880–890.
25. Dethlefs R. Prevalence of ocular manifestations of leprosy in Port Moresby, Papua New Guinea. *Br J Ophthalmol.* 1981;65:223–225.
26. Spaide R, Nattis R, Lipka A, D'Amico R. Ocular findings in leprosy in the United States. *Am J Ophthalmol.* 1985;100:411–416.
27. Silverstein A, Fever MM, Siltzbach LE. Neurological sarcoidosis: study of 18 cases. *Arch Neurol.* 1965;12:1–9.
28. Kaplan JM, Quintana P, Samson J. Facial nerve palsy with anaphylactoid purpura. *Am J Dis Child.* 1970;119:452–453.
29. Linthicum FH. Facial nerve paralysis in children. *Otolaryngol Clin North Am.* 1974;7:433–436.
30. Smith JD, Crumley RL, Harker LA. Facial paralysis in the newborn. *Otolaryngol Head Neck Surg.* 1981;89:1021–1024.
31. Smith IM, Murray JA, Cull RE, Slattery J. Facial weakness: a comparison of clinical and photographic methods of observation. *Arch Otolaryngol Head Neck Surg.* 1991; 117:906–909.
32. Wesley RE, Jackson CG, Tiedeken PT, Glasscock ME. Reconstruction of the eyelid after facial nerve paralysis. *Ophthalmol Clin North Am.* 1991;4:47–71.
33. Seiff SR, Vestel KP, Truwit CL. Eyelid palpebral springs in patients undergoing magnetic resonance imaging: an area of possible concern [letter]. *Arch Ophthalmol.* 1991;109:319.
34. Gardner TA, Rak KM. Magnetic resonance imaging of eyelid springs and gold weights [letter]. *Arch Ophthalmol.* 1991;109:1498.
35. Beyer TL, Sinha S. Eyelid pain after magnetic resonance imaging–induced palpebral spring vibration [letter]. *Arch Ophthalmol.* 1991;109:1503.
36. Glasscock ME, Jackson CG, Hays JW. Facial hypoglossal anastomosis for treatment of facial paralysis. In: Silverstein H, Norrell H, eds. *Neurologic Surgery of the Ear.* Birmingham, AL: Aesculapius Publishing Co., 1979;88:189.

III

Lacrimal System

13

Evaluation of the Lacrimal System

JOHN V. LINBERG, MD

The common complaint of a watering eye may be caused by a variety of problems, including lacrimal hyposecretion, lacrimal hypersecretion, or blockage of the lacrimal drainage system. This system is a complex membranous channel whose function depends on the interaction of anatomy and physiology. Effective tear drainage depends on a variety of factors, including the volume of tear secretion, eyelid position, and anatomy of the lacrimal drainage passages. Epiphora is defined as an abnormal overflow of tears down the cheek. The patient with symptomatic tearing may have a normal lacrimal drainage system overwhelmed by primary or secondary (reflex) hypersecretion or a drainage system that is anatomically compromised and unable to handle normal tear production. On the other hand, a patient with partial drainage obstruction may have a concomitant reduction in tear production and therefore be completely asymptomatic or may even suffer from symptomatic dry eye syndrome. Epiphora is determined by the balance between tear production and tear drainage, not by the absolute function or dysfunction of either one.

The causes of lacrimal drainage problems can be divided into two categories: anatomic and functional. Anatomic obstruction refers to a mechanical or structural abnormality of the drainage system. The obstruction may be complete, such as punctal occlusion, canalicular blockage, or nasolacrimal duct fibrosis, or partial, caused by punctal stenosis, canalicular stenosis, or mechanical obstruction within the lacrimal sac (i.e., dacryolith or tumor). In patients with functional obstruction, epiphora results not from anatomic blockage but from a failure of lacrimal drainage physiology. This failure may be caused by anatomic deformity such as punctal eversion or other eyelid malpositions, but can also result from lacrimal pump inadequacy caused by weak orbicularis muscle action.

13-1 CLINICAL DIAGNOSTIC EVALUATION

It is helpful to determine whether the patient's complaint is true epiphora or a "watery eye." Detailed history-taking and careful examination will help direct the evaluation of a tearing eye. A host of clinical tests have been described, and the selection of appropriate tests will depend on the initial history and ophthalmic examination.

13-1-1 *History-Taking.* Any clinical evaluation should begin with a thorough history. A complaint of watery eye does not necessarily imply a lacrimal drainage problem. Other possibilities, including lacrimal secretory deficiency, ocular irritation, or allergy, need to be considered. Sometimes, when basic lacrimal secretion is reduced moderately, corneal dryness will cause an intermittent increased reflex tear secretion. These patients complain of a foreign-body sensation with episodic tearing when, in fact, the basic problem is dry eye. In addition, some patients may describe a wet eye when, in fact, only a small amount of mucoid secretion is present in the conjunctival sac. Excess mucus may result from any source of irritation, including smoke, smog, wind, dry climate, and pollutants. These sources or irritation also may cause reflex hypersecretion.

Additional history may point to the cause of lacrimal drainage obstruction. Some topical medications, including glaucoma medications such as echothiophate iodide and chemotherapeutic agents (5-fluorouracil and taxotere), are associated with lacrimal obstruction. A history of severe or recurrent allergic or infectious conjunctivitis or ocular pemphigus should lead the physician to suspect canalicular occlusion or acquired punctal stenosis. A history of recurrent dacryocystitis strongly suggests distal nasolacrimal duct obstruction as well as potential stenosis of the proximal system.

A history of facial trauma, previous sinus surgery, or rhinostomy should alert the physician to the possibility of nasolacrimal duct injury. Epiphora associated with bloody tears, nasal obstruction, or epistaxis should raise suspicion of a nasal, sinus, or lacrimal sac tumor. A review of systems may disclose a history of systemic disease that can involve the lacrimal system, such as sarcoidosis or Paget disease, or a history of Bell's palsy as the cause of epiphora.

13-1-2 *External and Slit-Lamp Examination.* Together with a thorough history, a good external examination will guide the physician toward a diagnosis and specific diagnostic tests. As mentioned previously, the complaint of a tearing eye should not divert attention from the possibility of a dry eye. Potential signs of dry eye syndrome include abnormalities in the quality or stability of the tear film, the size of the tear meniscus, and the condition of the corneal epithelium. There may be conjunctival hyperemia, loss of luster of the conjunctiva, limbal congestion, or tenacious conjunctival secretion. The corneal reflex is dull with superficial punctate corneal erosions, epithelial filaments, and sometimes corneal ulceration. Lacrimal hyposecretion may be present in all degrees, from the mildest to the most severe.

Numerous relatively minor abnormalities of the eyelids and conjunctiva may be responsible for reflex hypersecretion of tears. Conjunctival concretions, aberrant cilia, molluscum contagiosum, papillomata, and chalazia involving the eyelid margin may all cause excessive tearing.

Malformations and malpositions of the eyelid margins can be responsible for abnormal tearing. The most common of these are ectropion and entropion. Eversion of the lacrimal puncta may escape casual inspection but can be observed by having the patient rotate the eye maximally upward. If the punctum can be seen without manual eversion of the eyelid, its position is not normal and may be responsible for the epiphora. Redundant and mobile conjunctiva, usually termed conjunctival chalasis, may cause tearing when a fold of redundant conjunctiva hangs over the lid margin covering the puncta. Because the orbicularis oculi muscle is the source of the tear pump mechanism, deficiency in orbicularis function will result in epiphora. A patient with a seventh cranial nerve (facial) paralysis, or lower eyelid laxity, may exhibit epiphora.

A careful biomicroscopic evaluation may disclose punctal stenosis. Mucoid reflux with lacrimal sac massage is pathognomonic for a lower system obstruction. Mass lesions in the medial canthal region, such as a sac mucocele, may cause mechanical obstruction of the tear drainage. Mass lesions extrinsic to the lacrimal drainage system, such as an ethmoid mucocele, may also compress the sac and cause obstruction.

Chronic canaliculitis is characterized by epiphora and fullness in the region of the canaliculus. It can often be due to retained canalicular foreign bodies such as canalicular plugs or punctal plugs that have migrated. Infectious canaliculitis may be caused by bacterial, viral, chlamydial, or mycotic organisms. However, the most common cause is the filamentous gram-positive rod *Actinomyces israelii.* Often yellow particles can be expressed from the punctum when pressure is applied over the canaliculus. Canaliculitis tends to affect only one eyelid and for some reason generally does not involve the adjacent lacrimal sac. The diagnosis can sometimes be confirmed by instilling a drop of topical anesthetic into the conjunctival sac and then gently massaging the canaliculus between two cotton-tipped applicators to express the concretions. The diagnosis can also be made by microscopic examination of the purulent secretion without stain, after adding a drop of potassium hydroxide. Mycelia may be found in such fresh wet preparations.

13-1-3 *Tear Production Measurement.* Approximate measurement of tear production is provided by the Schirmer test without topical anesthetic. The Schirmer I test is used to assess stimulated tear production. The test should be performed in subdued lighting, and both eyes may be tested simultaneously. One end of the filter paper strip is folded and hooked over the lateral third of the inferior eyelid margin. Wetting of the strip is measured at 5 minutes; the average normal measurement is between 10 and 30 mm. Unfortunately, the stimulus to the eye from the filter paper strip is great, and the reflex tearing measured by this test may not reflect normal physiology. The amount of ocular stimulation can be reduced, but not eliminated, by anesthetizing the conjunctiva with topical agents. When the Schirmer test is performed with topical anesthetic, the term *basic secretion* is often used, suggesting that basal secretion is not related to reflex stimuli. A broad range of recent research indicates that all tears are produced in response to neurologic ("reflex") stimuli, so that the simplistic distinction between reflex and basal secretion may be inaccurate. A Schirmer test result of less than 5 mm of wetting, using topical anesthesia, is abnormal. All Schirmer testing is highly variable, and the test should be repeated in an effort to verify the results of an initial test.

Rose bengal is a chloride-substituted iodinated fluorescein dye that stains devitalized epithelial cells. Increased staining of the conjunctival and corneal epithelium is a sensitive indicator of inadequate tear function regardless of the Schirmer test results.

The tear breakup time is a simple test for evaluation of the tear film stability that depends on the basal mucous layer. One drop of fluorescein is placed in the eye, and the patient is asked to blink once. The tear film on the cornea is observed with cobalt-blue light until the film breaks up, exposing dry spots on the cornea. Normal breakup time is 15 to 30 seconds. A tear breakup time of less than 10 seconds is abnormal. The presence or absence of the tear meniscus or its height is a useful finding in ascertaining dry or wet eye. Enhancing the tear meniscus with fluorescein allows better visualization of the strip and its contents.

13-2 LACRIMAL DRAINAGE EVALUATION

After examination of tear secretion and the ocular surface, the lacrimal drainage system may be evaluated with the following tests, in recommended order:

1. Fluorescein dye disappearance test
2. Lacrimal irrigation
3. Probing of canaliculi
4. Dacryocystography
5. Nasal endoscopy

13-2-1 *Fluorescein Dye Disappearance Test.* The fluorescein dye disappearance (FDD) test is a quick, simple, and physiologic method for assessing the lacrimal drainage system.[1] The FDD test is an extremely valuable and practical clinical tool, since it is entirely safe and painless and requires no special instrumentation. The test is most meaningful when both eyes are compared simultaneously. One drop of 2% fluorescein is instilled into the lower fornix of each eye. The patient is instructed not to touch or dab the eye and to blink normally. Both the intensity of the color and the volume of tears are assessed after 5 minutes. As originally described by Zappia and Milder,[1] a residual of 0 or +1 dye is designated as a positive test, indicating probable normal drainage outflow; whereas a residual of +2 to +4 represents a negative test, indicating partial or complete obstruction or pump failure. Other authors have found it more practical to grade the residual dye in only three grades, and to use the more common medical convention that defines an abnormal test result as positive.[2] In this version, trace or no residual dye is considered a negative test (normal); minimal residual dye (+1) is considered a low positive; and marked residual dye (+2) is considered a high positive test suggestive of a delay or impairment in tear drainage.

Although the FDD test is simple to perform and effective as an initial screening test, it is nonspecific and may give false-positive results in the elderly and in dry-eyed patients secondary to excessive conjunctival staining. If the FDD test results are normal, significant lacrimal drainage dysfunction is very unlikely. However, intermittent obstruction from allergy, dacryolith, or nasal polyps may still be a possibility. If the fluorescein dye disappearance is delayed, the test cannot distinguish between physiologic and anatomic causes of drainage dysfunction, nor can it determine whether the abnormality is in the upper or lower outflow system. Thus, a delayed fluorescein dye disappearance is an indication for further testing, and the author's next step is lacrimal irrigation.

13-2-2 *Lacrimal Irrigation*. Gentle irrigation should be performed to evaluate the anatomic patency of the lacrimal drainage system. A drop of topical anesthetic is instilled into the conjunctival sac. Some examiners anesthetize the medial conjunctival cul-de-sac, using 4% lidocaine on a cotton pledget or applicator prior to probing and/or irrigation. The punctum is dilated with a punctal dilator (Fig. 13-1A), and a lacrimal cannula is inserted about 5 to 6 mm into one canaliculus to irrigate with saline. The irrigation is initially performed without occlusion of the opposite punctum. It is important to hold the irrigation cannula gently in the anatomic position of the canaliculus (Fig. 13-1B), because kinking or pressure against the wall of the canaliculus will produce a false sensation of obstruction.

In a normal drainage system, the fluid will easily flow into the nasopharynx, with little or no reflux from the opposite punctum. Reflux in the opposite punctum documents patent canaliculi but suggests distal obstruction. Irrigation with occlusion of the opposite punctum documents mechanical patency at nonphysiologic pressures if fluid passes into the nasopharynx. However, these elevated pressures may force fluid through a partially or physiologically obstructed drainage system.

13-2-3 *Probing of Canaliculi*. When the irrigation test indicates obstruction, gentle probing using a #0000 probe should be performed to palpate the site of the obstruction. If a small probe is used, it is rarely necessary to dilate. The probe is gently advanced through the canaliculus until an obstruction is encountered; force

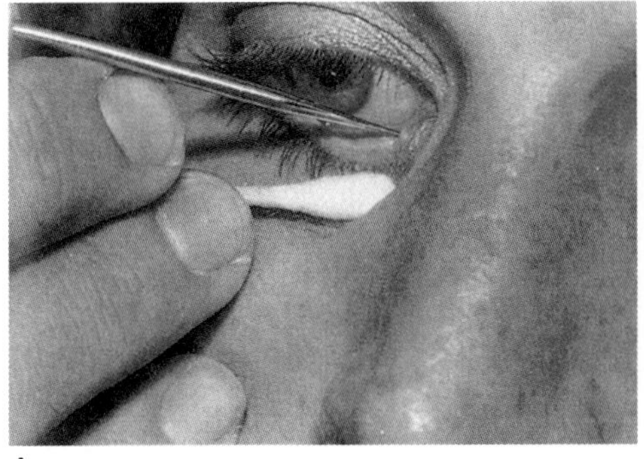
A

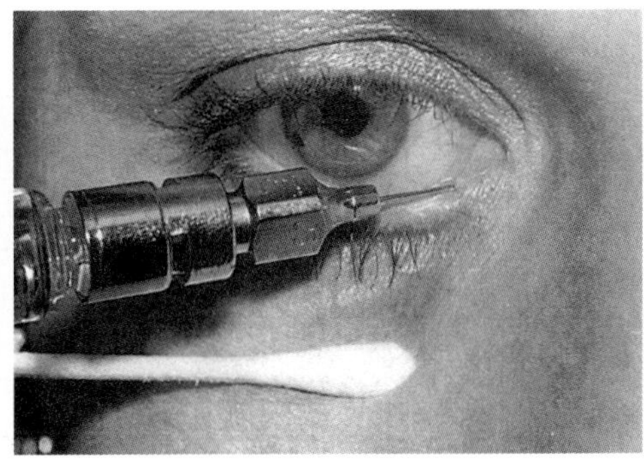
B

Figure 13-1 Lacrimal irrigation. (A) Punctum is dilated with punctal dilator. (B) Cannula is held in anatomic position in canaliculus.

is not appropriate. The probe can be grasped with forceps at the punctum and then withdrawn to measure the distance from the punctum to the obstruction. The nasolacrimal duct in adults should never be probed because the probing is not therapeutic and causes significant pain. Thus, gentle probing is used to localize a site of obstruction within the canaliculi, but not in the lacrimal sac or nasolacrimal duct. The degree of stenosis can sometimes be estimated by using progressively larger probes, but a large probe should never be forced through an obstruction. Probing is diagnostic, not therapeutic, in the evaluation of epiphora. Occasionally, the examiner will detect a gritty sensation during probing, which suggests concretions associated with canaliculitis.

13-2-4 *Jones Dye Test.* In any discussion of the evaluation of the lacrimal drainage system, the Jones dye test should be included. The interpretation of the results of the protocol needs to be understood by ophthalmologists. In 1961, Jones described the use of fluorescein to test lacrimal outflow function.[3] In the primary dye test (Jones I), one drop of 2% fluorescein is instilled into the conjunctival sac. After the nose has been sprayed with 4% tetracaine for comfort, a fine cotton-tipped applicator is inserted beneath the inferior turbinate at 2 minutes and again at 5 minutes. If fluorescein is recovered, the test is positive, indicating a patent system.

If no fluorescein is recovered in the primary test, the secondary dye test (Jones II) is performed. A topical anesthetic is instilled in the conjunctival cul de sac and residual fluorescein is flushed from the conjunctival sac. The patient's head is tilted over an emesis basin, and the canaliculus is irrigated with clear saline. If the irrigant is fluorescein-stained, the test is positive, indicating a patent proximal system. If the irrigant is clear, the test is negative, suggesting stenosis of the punctum or canaliculus. If fluid does not reach the nose at all, then complete obstruction of the system exists.

A positive dye test (Jones I) indicates a normal drainage system. Unfortunately, it is possible for fluorescein dye to pass through a normal drainage system and into the nasal cavity without being detected by the examiner. Even in expert hands, the primary dye test has a high incidence of false-negative results.[4,5] Some authorities have shown that the addition of nasal endoscopy to detect fluorescein in the inferior meatus makes the test more reliable.[6]

In addition, the secondary dye test is not physiologic. It does not establish the functional condition of the lacrimal sac, because the irrigating solution is forced into the nose under nonphysiologic pressures (Table 13-1). Although the Jones fluorescein dye tests have been widely used since they were first described in 1961, the author has not found them to be useful or practical. Since I have found it difficult to obtain consistent results with these tests, I use alternate tests including the FDD test, irrigation, probing, dacryocystography, and nasal endoscopy.

13-2-5 *Dacryocystography.* Dacryocystography (DCG) provides imaging of anatomic details that are not available by any other nonoperative technique. I do not routinely employ special imaging techniques in the everyday evaluation of patients with lacrimal problems. However, DCG is indicated for patients with suspected lacrimal sac tumors or those who may have abnormal anatomy (whether due to

TABLE 13-1 Results of Primary and Secondary Jones Tests

Jones I		
+	Patent system, probable normal physiologic function	
–	False-negative: physiologic dysfunction, anatomic obstruction	
Jones II		
+	Dye in nose	Partial block at lower sac or duct
–	Saline in nose	Punctal or canalicular stenosis
–	Regurgitation at opposite punctum with dye	Complete nasolacrimal duct obstruction
–	Regurgitation at opposite punctum without dye	Complete common canaliculus obstruction
–	Regurgitation at same punctum with dye	Complete common canaliculus obstruction

trauma, reoperations, or congenital anomalies). In addition, DCG may be indicated in selected patients with partial or functional obstruction of the nasolacrimal duct. We recommend the use of computerized digital subtraction DCG over standard DCG to obtain better imaging of the lacrimal system[7,8] (Fig. 13-2).

This study can be performed in the angiography suite of the radiology department. The patient is placed supine on the angiography table. Topical anesthetic drops are placed over the puncta of both eyes. The lower puncta are dilated with a punctal dilator. A sialography catheter is inserted into the lower canaliculus of each

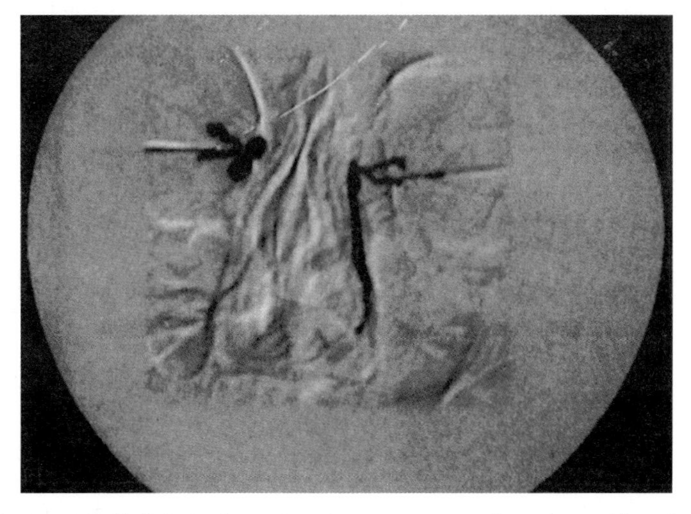

Figure 13-2 Computerized digital subtraction dacryocystogram in patient with unilateral epiphora after facial trauma. Right lacrimal sac is dilated and obstruction is noted at sac–duct junction. Left side shows normal-caliber lacrimal system.

eye and taped in place on the patient's cheek and forehead for later injection of contrast material. Then, the patient is positioned underneath the x-ray beam to allow simultaneous imaging of both lacrimal systems. Each catheter is connected to a 3-cc syringe filled with a warmed contrast agent (iophendylate). The imaging starts as the lacrimal system in both eyes is injected simultaneously with 2 to 3 cc of contrast material. The lacrimal system is visualized on the monitor screen as the contrast agent flows down the pathway. Selected prints can be made to illustrate the flow through the system. Films can be obtained 10 minutes later to evaluate dye retention. Visualization of the site of the obstruction or stenosis by DCG helps determine the surgical plan.

If a functional or partial obstruction of the nasolacrimal duct is suspected with a normal irrigation to the nose, a simplified DCG can be ordered. Only the late film is of interest in these cases, because retention of contrast material in the sac after 10 minutes is clear evidence of distal functional obstruction. The contrast agent can be injected in the clinic and the patient sent to radiology for a single posteroanterior Waters view film. This approach avoids the need for a separate appointment with radiology and the expense of a full DCG.

13-2-6 *Dacryoscintigraphy.* Dacryoscintigraphy uses radionuclei tracer [^{99m} Tc] pertechnetate in saline or technetium sulfur colloid to image the lacrimal system. A drop of the tracer is instilled in the conjunctival cul de sac and the lacrimal system is imaged with a gammagram. The advantages of using the isotope study are its sensitivity, ease of performance, and noninvasiveness. Dacryoscintigraphy and contrast DCG provide different types of information. Scintigraphy is more sensitive for the diagnosis of incomplete blocks, especially in the upper system.[8,9] In addition, the amount of radiation exposure to the lens is less than 2% of that for a complete DCG. However, dacryoscintigraphy does not provide the detailed anatomic visualization available with contrast DCG.

13-2-7 *Computed Tomography.* Computed tomography (CT) of the lacrimal system is generally not used in the evaluation of a tearing patient. However, when epiphora follows trauma and other studies have demonstrated nasolacrimal duct obstruction, CT may reveal orbital rim or maxillary fractures compressing the sac or duct. In the evaluation of an infant with a congenital cystic mass in the medial canthus, a CT scan may be necessary to differentiate an amniocele from a meningocele. In cases of suspected malignancy, a CT scan will demonstrate a soft-tissue mass of the sac or adjacent paranasal sinuses and guide the approach to surgical excision. CT can actually be combined with DCG to provide imaging of the lacrimal drainage system, bone, and soft tissues for the evaluation of complicated cases.

13-2-8 *Nasal Endoscopy.* Nasal endoscopy has revolutionized the visualization of nasal anatomy and has become an important tool for the otolaryngologist in sinus surgery. In the past, the results of lacrimal surgery have generally been evaluated in terms of functional success rather than actual visual inspection of an anatomic result. For the ophthalmologist, the endoscope provides excellent visualization of the intranasal aspect of lacrimal surgery and takes the guesswork out of postoperative evaluations.

Two areas of principal interest in lacrimal surgery are (1) the opening of the nasolacrimal duct under the inferior turbinate and (2) the site of a dacryocystorhinostomy ostium anterior to the middle turbinate. These areas are accessible to rigid endoscopes with conventional solid optical elements. I have experience with the Hopkins telescopic endoscope, which is used in a variety of other fields such as urology, laparoscopy, arthroscopy, and otorhinolaryngoscopy.[10] This instrument is widely available in most general hospitals so that the lacrimal surgeon can use endoscopy without having to purchase one. For the initial attempt with endoscopy, the ophthalmologist may want to ask for assistance from an otolaryngologist.

The technique is simple and easily performed in an outpatient setting using topical anesthesia and no sedation: 4% lidocaine hydrochloride applied with a nasal atomizer works well. Nasal decongestion with 0.25% or 0.5% phenylephrine hydrochloride or Afrin nose spray will shrink the nasal mucosa and facilitate manipulation of the endoscope. A good view of the dacryocystorhinostomy ostium is obtained using the 5.5-mm-diameter Hopkins telescopic endoscope with a 30-degree view angle or the 0-degree wide-angle instrument. The examiner introduces the rod through the nares with its axis parallel to the septum and at an angle of about 45 degrees in relation to the frontal plane of the face. The viewing port is directed laterally away from the midline.

The opening of the nasolacrimal duct under the inferior turbinate is more difficult to visualize because of limited space. A smaller-diameter (2.4-mm) endoscope is introduced through the nares along the floor of the nose, with the viewing port directed upward. Packing the area briefly with a cocaine-moistened pledget of cotton will shrink the mucosa to increase the available space and comfort.

Endoscopy can be very useful in the evaluation of dacryocystorhinostomy failures. The distinction between closure of the nasal ostium and common canalicular stenosis is sometimes difficult to establish by probing or irrigation. Endoscopy is especially helpful in the postoperative care of Jones tubes, because visualization assists in the diagnosis and management of problem cases. In addition, skill in using an endoscope is essential for endonasal dacryocystorhinostomy.

REFERENCES

1. Zappia RJ, Milder B. Lacrimal drainage function, 2: the fluorescein dye disappearance test. *Am J Ophthalmol.* 1972;74:160–162.
2. Meyer DR, Antonello A, Linberg JV. Assessment of tear drainage after canalicular obstruction using fluorescein dye disappearance. *Ophthalmology.* 1990;97:1370–1374.
3. Jones LT. An anatomical approach to problems of the eyelids and lacrimal apparatus. *Arch Ophthalmol.* 1961;66:111–150.
4. Wright MM, Bersani TA, Frueh BR, Musch DC. Efficacy of the primary dye test. *Opthalmology.* 1989;96(4):481–483.
5. Guzek JP, Ching AS, Hoang TA, et al. Clinical and radiologic lacrimal testing in patients with epiphora. *Opthalmology.* 1997;104(11):1875–1881.
6. Becker BB. Flexible endoscopy in primary dye testing of the lacrimal system. *Ophthalmic Surg.* 1990;21(8):577–580.
7. Hurwitz JJ, Victor WH. The role of sophisticated radiologic testing in the assessment and management of epiphora. *Ophthalmology.* 1985;92(3):407–413.

8. Guzek JP, Ching AS, Hoang TA, Dure-Smith P, Llaurado JG, Yau DC, Stephenson CB, Stephenson CM, Elam DA. Clinical and radiologic lacrimal testing in patients with epiphora. *Ophthalmology*. 1997;104(11):1875–1881.
9. Rose JD, Clayton CB. Scintigraphy and contrast radiography for epiphora. *Br J Radiol.* 1985;58:1183–1186.
10. Linberg JV. Endoscopy. In: Linberg JV, ed. *Lacrimal Surgery*. New York: Churchill Livingstone, 1988:297–314.

14

Management of Pediatric Nasolacrimal Duct Obstruction

ASHVINI K. REDDY, MD, AND KIMBERLY G. YEN, MD

Tearing is a common presenting complaint in infants referred to an ophthalmologist and may be the first sign of something as benign as an impermanent anatomic defect or as grave as congenital glaucoma. When tearing is chronic, parents of an affected infant are often frustrated by the persistent accumulation of fluid and mucopurulent material in the eye and on the eyelids and anxious that the condition may be a sign of a more serious problem. The best initial management of tearing in an infant is to take a detailed history, which often provides important clues as to the cause of tearing, and then to perform a thorough, systematic ophthalmic examination.

Tears serve four main functions: (1) they form a tear film to keep the eye moist, (2) they lubricate the eye, (3) they keep the eye clear of particulate matter and debris, and (4) they provide a refractive surface on the corneal epithelium. The tear film comprises three layers: a thin inner layer of proteinaceous mucin coats and protects the eye, an aqueous layer keeps the eye moist and lubricated, and an outer lipid layer slows evaporation of the aqueous layer.

Basal tears are produced by the accessory lacrimal glands located in the conjunctiva and keep the eye moist under steady-state conditions; normal patients have a tear meniscus (or "tear lake") visible along the inner lower eyelid as a result of basal tear production. Irritation or emotional extremes can trigger reflex tear production by the main lacrimal gland in the superotemporal quadrant of the orbit, "flooding" the tear lake. The level of the tear lake is highest when the rate of tear production by the lacrimal glands exceeds the rate of tear drainage into the nasolacrimal system.

Tears normally drain out of the eye through puncta located on the nasal portion of the upper and lower eyelids (Fig. 14-1). They then enter the upper and lower

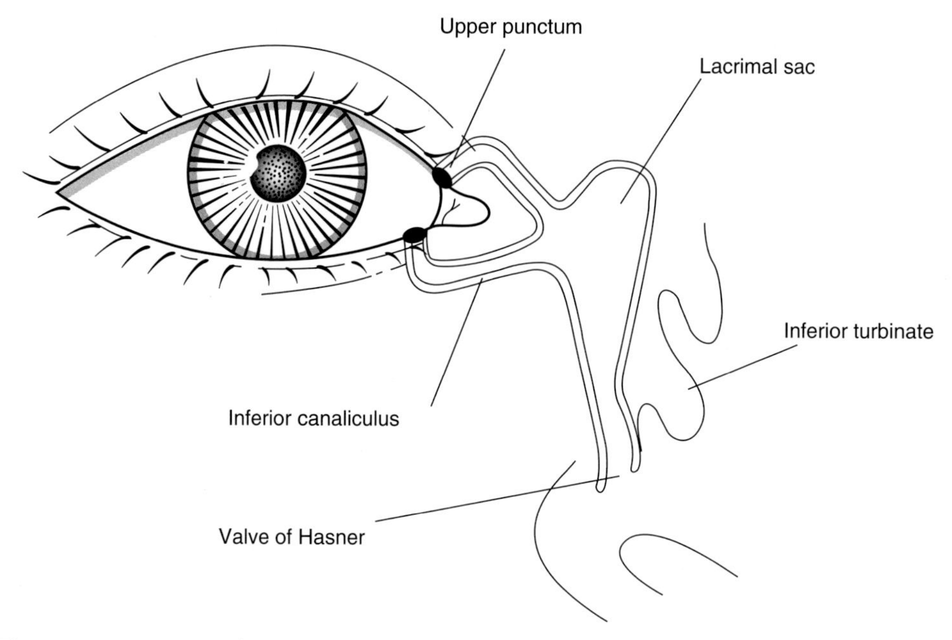

Figure 14-1 Anatomy of nasolacrimal duct system.

canaliculi, which run inferiorly and medially before joining to form the common canaliculus, which conducts tears through the valve of Rosenmuller and into the lacrimal sac. Tears flow out of the lacrimal sac into the nasolacrimal duct and past the valve of Hasner before emptying into the nose just below the inferior turbinates. An obstruction at any point in the drainage system causes tears and mucus to collect proximally, raising the level of the tear meniscus until tears spill over the lower eyelid and onto the cheek (epiphora). Persistent exposure to the mucoid fluid expressed from the duct may also lead to chronic erythema and irritation of the eyelids.

The most common cause of congenital epiphora is nasolacrimal duct obstruction. Approximately 6% of all newborns do not have patent lacrimal drainage systems[1] secondary to the persistence of a residual membrane just before the valve of Hasner, obstructing the distal end of the nasolacrimal duct and impeding the flow of tears into the nose. Less frequently, the obstruction occurs more proximally along the nasolacrimal drainage system. About 80% to 90% of these membranes become patent spontaneously in the first 6 months of life; therefore, tearing from a congenital nasolacrimal duct obstruction is often temporary.[2,3]

Other congenital anomalies of the ductal system include maldevelopment of the tear sac or canalicular system, imperforate puncta or punctal atresia, obstruction from bony abnormalities or a cyst, and congenital lacrimal sac fistulas.[4] Because imperforate puncta prevent tears from entering the lacrimal system, afflicted patients generally present with milder symptoms, and compression of the lacrimal sac will not express the mucoid reflux typical of nasolacrimal duct obstruction. Management may be as simple as perforating the membrane with a pin or punctal dilator.[5] Lacrimal sac fistulas occur when there is a fistula from the lacrimal sac draining directly through to the skin (Fig. 14-2). This fistula may drain tears or

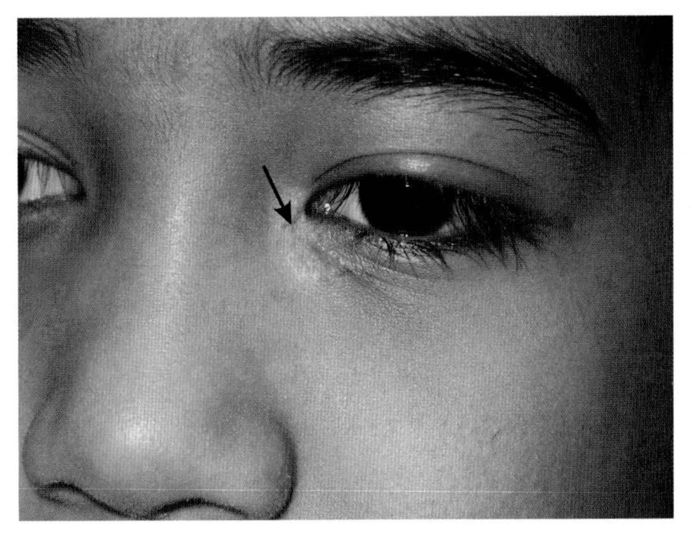

Figure 14-2 Contents of the lacrimal sac may exit below the medial canthus through a congenital lacrimal sac fistula (*arrow*). The chronic tearing may lead to dermatologic lesions of the eyelid.

mucopurulent material and may require excision or marsupialization of the fistula.[5] Occasionally, children may also present with congenital alacrima, an otherwise asymptomatic condition in which reflex tearing is absent.[5]

14-1 DACRYOCELES AND DACRYOCYSTITIS

A congenital dacryocele is a specific type of duct obstruction that presents at birth and occurs due to defects both proximal and distal to the lacrimal sac such that the sac fills with tears and cannot drain. Dacryoceles present in newborns as bluish, cystic masses below the medial canthus in the area of the nasolacrimal sac. The distal obstruction occurs at the valve of Hasner and a functional proximal obstruction occurs at the level of the common canaliculus or the valve of Rosenmuller. As fluid is trapped in the lacrimal system and the sac is distended, the skin overlying the dacryocele below the medial canthus appears characteristically swollen and blue (Fig. 14-3). These patients have an increased risk of infection and associated inflammation (dacryocystitis) that can extend beyond the lacrimal sac, causing cellulitis, orbital infection, and sepsis.

Differential diagnosis of dacryoceles includes capillary hemangiomas and meningoceles. If the mass is pulsatile or not located below the medial canthus, an ultrasound or CT scan examination may be warranted. Patients may also present with intranasal cysts that arise due to prolapse of the lacrimal sac tissue through the inferior meatus. Because infants are obligate nasal breathers, these intranasal cysts may obstruct the nasal passage, causing respiratory distress.[6] Marsupialization of the cyst may be required in such cases,[7] occasionally with nasal endoscopy. In some instances, dacryoceles can be decompressed into the nose with massage.[6] If they cannot be decompressed, probing should be performed to prevent dacryocystitis.

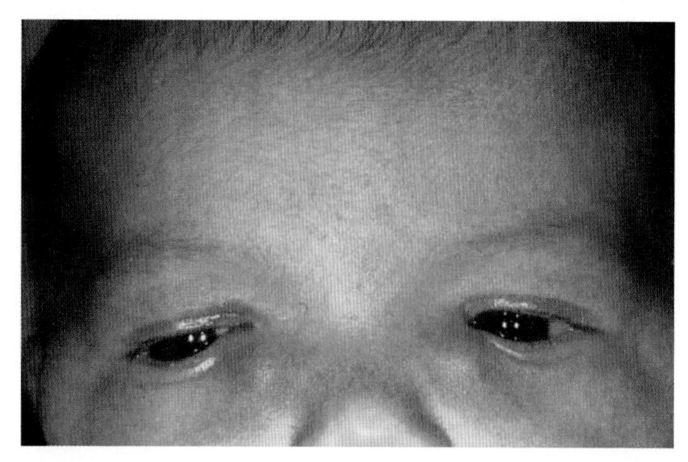

Figure 14-3 Newborns may present with dacryoceles and dacryocystitis, necessitating immediate probing and silicone intubation. This patient presents with bilateral dacryoceles.

Dacryocystitis, or inflammation of a dacryocele, initially presents as erythema over the cystic mass with acute distention and inflammation in the lacrimal sac region. Oral antibiotics should be administered in the presence of mild dacryocystitis. Severe or unresponsive dacryocystitis often requires intravenous antibiotics and more urgent surgical intervention. In these cases, antibiotic treatment and probing are necessary to drain the infected lacrimal sac as soon as possible to prevent the spread of infection. If probing fails to resolve the condition, repeat probing, balloon dilation of the ductal system, dacryocystorhinostomy, or conjunctivodacryocystorhinostomy may be indicated. While still considered controversial by some physicians,[6] broad-spectrum antibiotics are generally given prior to probing to quiet the eye and treat any associated system infection. Surgical intervention should occur after the acute infection has been treated with antibiotics, generally after 24 to 72 hours of antibiotic treatment. Studies have demonstrated a lower success rate of probing procedures in patients with dacryocystitis, possibly because the intranasal component of the cyst wall is thickened, causing the hole made by the probe to close more quickly.[6]

14-2 DIAGNOSING A NASOLACRIMAL DUCT OBSTRUCTION

Tearing in an infant that occurs independent of nasolacrimal duct obstruction may be due to a variety of causes, including external and corneal abnormalities, tear film abnormalities, conjunctivitis, intraocular inflammation, and vision-threatening congenital glaucoma.[8] External eyelid abnormalities, especially misdirection of the eyelashes secondary to epiblepharon and entropion, are seen frequently in young children. Patients with an imbalance of the three main tear film components (particularly the lipid layer) may have a tear breakup time less than 10 seconds secondary to increased evaporation of the aqueous layer. Corneal abnormalities can be detected by slit-lamp examination. Conjunctivitis may be caused by bacterial infection, viral infection, allergy, or irritant exposure. The hallmarks of bacterial and viral

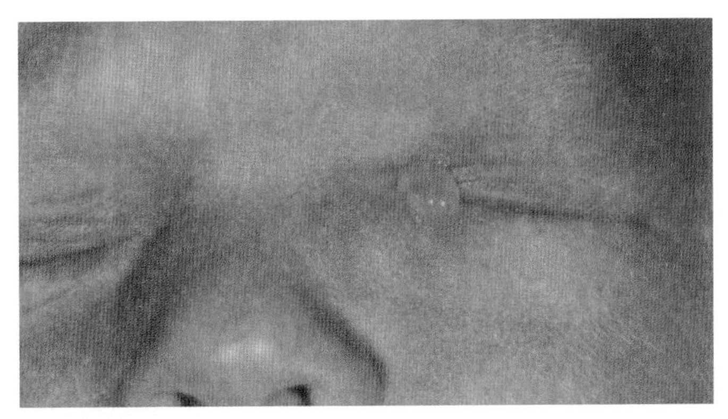

Figure 14-4 Nasolacrimal duct obstruction often manifests with a mucopurulent discharge. This can often be elicited with massage of the lacrimal sac.

conjunctivitis are purulent and watery discharge, respectively, sometimes with evidence of recent or current systemic infection. Allergic conjunctivitis typically involves both eyes and is classically associated with itchiness and, in chronic cases, "allergic shiners." Uveitis presents with redness, tearing, photophobia, and severe pain. The hallmarks of congenital glaucoma are buphthalmos and Haab striae secondary to chronically elevated intraocular pressure. These patients usually also present with photophobia or a history of intermittent clouding of the cornea.

Nasolacrimal duct obstruction typically presents in the pediatric population with chronic epiphora and mattering of the child's eye.[8] Parents may also report periodic redness of the eye without any evidence of pain, irritation, or photophobia and that mucoid material sometimes "glues" the eyelids together overnight while the child is sleeping. Mild cases may simply be associated with an elevated tear meniscus or a glossy, wet look to the affected eye. Symptoms are often exacerbated by an upper respiratory infection or wind exposure (Fig. 14-4). Gentle pressure over the lacrimal sac may produce reflux of mucoid material.

The fluorescein dye disappearance test can be used to confirm nasolacrimal duct obstruction in cooperative patients. This test is discussed fully in Chapter 13: Evaluation of the Lacrimal System.

14-3 CONSERVATIVE MANAGEMENT OF NASOLACRIMAL DUCT OBSTRUCTION

During the initial visit, the physician's role is to examine the patency and position of the puncta as well as to palpate the lacrimal sac to evaluate for inflammation or purulence. In infants without dacryocystitis or children under 6 months of age, conservative management is generally recommended initially. The physician may demonstrate lacrimal sac compression and massage to the parents and recommend that they perform the maneuver four times a day or with each feeding to mechanically force tears that have accumulated in the lacrimal sac through the duct. Compression of the sac is performed by applying downward pressure over the sac with a finger and rocking the finger over the tear sac area. The maneuver should be a rolling, motion that sweeps downward and nasally over the lacrimal sac.[4] This may be combined with the administration of topical antibiotic drops for a short period of time if infection is present.

14-4 SURGICAL INTERVENTION

Although the majority of obstructed nasolacrimal ducts will open during the first 6 months of life, some studies suggest that resolution may occur as late as 12 to 24 months of age.[1] If the obstruction does not resolve spontaneously by 6 to 12 months of age and conservative medical treatment has been unsuccessful, nasolacrimal duct probing is indicated.

Controversy exists over the ideal age for pediatric lacrimal probing. Young infants can be restrained manually for an office procedure, but older, uncooperative children require general anesthesia for sedation. Some physicians advocate early office probing to avoid the risks of general anesthesia, relieve parental anxiety, and decrease the potential long-term risks associated with chronic inflammation.[1,2] Those who prefer to delay probing until the child is older cite the high percentage of cases that resolve spontaneously and/or feel that general anesthesia offers better control during the probing procedure.[2,8] In our practice, we offer probing to children up to 12 months of age who have significant tearing, discharge, or recurrent infection. Children under 7 months of age are generally considered for probing only if recurrent infections or severe symptoms are present.[7]

We perform probing on infants in the office after they have been mummified or papoosed. An able assistant is always present to restrain the child's head. Probing is performed through the lower punctum. A tapered punctal dilator is used to dilate the punctum and a Bowman probe is passed through the nasolacrimal duct to the nose. This is repeated with an irrigating cannula attached to balanced salt solution on a syringe. Patency of the lacrimal system is confirmed by irrigating the balanced salt solution through the punctum, which causes the child to cough when the fluid reaches the nasopharynx.

If the probing is performed under general anesthesia, the nose is first examined for polyps and turbinate hypertrophy. Shrinking the nasal mucosa with cottonoids moistened with oxymetazoline HCl 0.05% can facilitate visualization of the probe as well as minimize nasal bleeding. Dilation of the puncta is then achieved with a tapered punctal dilator. A Bowman probe, generally size 0 or 1, is passed through to the nose. In most children up to 2 years of age, it is important to remember that the floor of the nose is reached when less than half of the length of the probe from the tip to the center part of the handle has been passed, about 20 to 25 mm.

There are three main means of confirming patency of the nasolacrimal duct during probing under general anesthesia. The first (considered the gold standard) is to confirm metal-on-metal contact in the nose by passing a larger probe under the inferior turbinate (Fig. 14-5). Alternatively, one can also directly visualize the probe under the inferior turbinate with the aid of a headlight. In this case, the surgeon may choose to bend the metal probe slightly prior to the procedure so that it may be more easily visualized and located when confirming metal-on-metal sensation (Fig. 14-6).

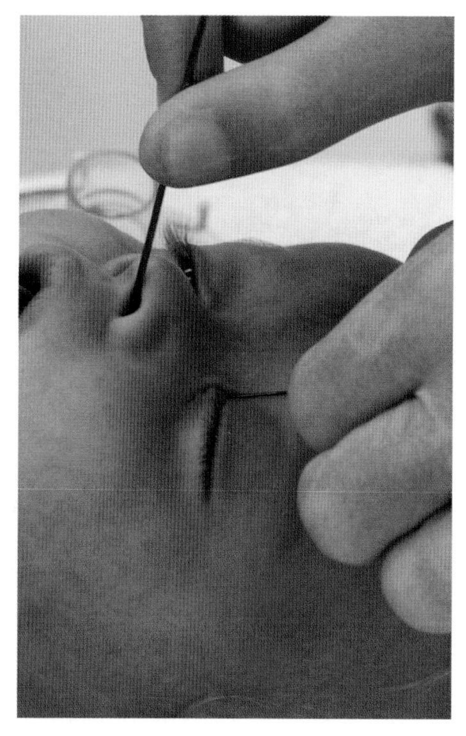

Figure 14-5 Metal-on-metal sensation should be confirmed in the nose to ensure a successful probing.

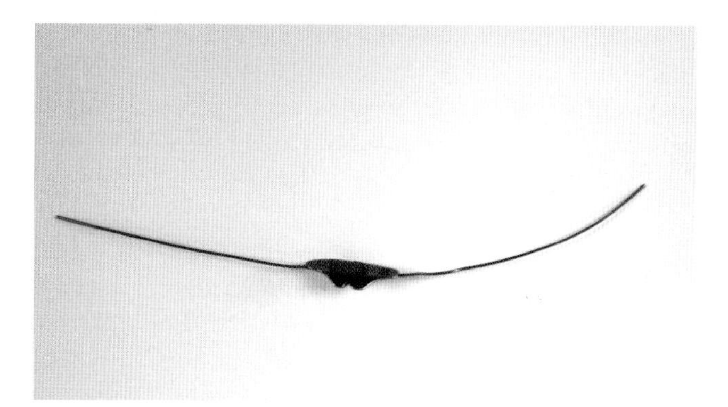

Figure 14-6 Placing a slight anterior curve in the probe or Crawford tubes prevents posterior migration, aids in visualization, and facilitates retrieval.

Third, irrigating fluorescein-stained saline through the lacrimal system and aspirating the fluid out of the nose with a clear suction catheter will confirm patency of the duct. Infracture of the nasal turbinate should be performed if the turbinate appears to be obstructing the exit site of the nasolacrimal duct or is impacted against the lateral nasal wall.

Some studies have demonstrated that initial probing and irrigation resolves 90% to 95% of congenital nasolacrimal obstructions in children up to 36 months of age.[7]

Other studies, however, have shown that the success rate of probing and irrigation decreases significantly after 13 to 18 months of age.[1]

To maintain patency and promote reepithelialization of the duct following probing, silicone lacrimal tubes may be placed temporarily. Absolute indications for such tubes include canalicular or bony abnormalities, technical difficulty during the probing, and dacryocystitis. We prefer silicone lacrimal intubation for any child who undergoes a probing under general anesthesia to avoid a second trip to the operating room. Coating the introducer attached to the silicone tubes with antibiotic ointment or Lacrilube prior to intubation can ease passage of the tubes through the canaliculus.

Retrieval of silicone tubes from the nose may be performed using the traditional Crawford hook or simplified with the use of a groove director (Fig. 14-7A,B). Groove directors have been reported to minimize trauma to the nasal mucosa and can also be used to infracture the inferior turbinate during the procedure.[11] The Ritleng system is an alternative instrument for insertion of the tubes; rather than an olive tip for retrieval with a hook, the system uses a thread-guided system. Although bicanalicular intubation has been traditionally used, studies have demonstrated that monocular intubation is an acceptable alternative and has an equal success rate.[12] With bicanalicular intubation, the tube is secured with a knot between the two tube ends in the nose, tied with a silk suture end to end from the lumens of the tube, or tied side by side with a dissolvable suture to the lateral wall of the nose. Monocanalicular tubes do not need to be secured in the nose, but should be placed so the collarette is positioned properly in the punctum.

Silicone tubing should be left in place in the nasolacrimal duct system for at least 2 to 3 months. During follow-up, the surgeon should observe for punctal erosion, granuloma formation, or corneal or conjunctival irritation, in which case the tubes should be removed immediately.[3] Otherwise, there is no specific contraindication to leaving the tubes in place for an extended period of time. Removal of the tubes

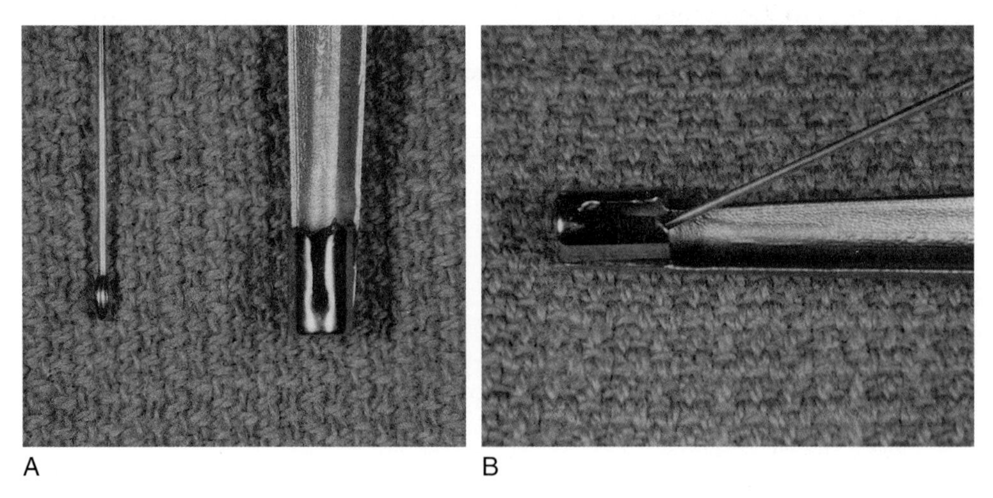

Figure 14-7 (A) A groove director simplifies removal of the silicone lacrimal tubes and minimizes trauma to the nasal mucosa. (B) The olive tip of the metal Crawford probe slides easily into the basket and is engaged by the keyhole of the groove director.

can be performed in the office with an able assistant restraining the child's head. If the ends are knotted together, the knot can be rotated into the palpebral fissure in clinic and the tube cut and pulled from the canalicular system. If dissolvable suture is used to tie the tubes side by side, the tubes can be removed painlessly with a blunt hook or forceps in clinic without rotating the tubes. Monocanalicular stents can be removed by using forceps to securely grasp and pull the collarette out of the punctum.

An alternative method of managing nasolacrimal duct obstruction is balloon catheter dilatation.[13] This method can be used in older patients, those who have failed previous probings, or patients with craniofacial anomalies.[14] It is considered an alternative or adjunct procedure to traditional probing and silicone intubation and is even preferred by some surgeons as a primary intervention. Recent data suggest that balloon dacryocystoplasty does not offer an advantage over simple probing as an initial treatment for congenital nasolacrimal duct obstruction, even up to age 36 months.[15]

Operative fistulization of the lacrimal sac into the nasal cavity, or dacryocystorhinostomy, is typically considered only when all other options have been exhausted, specifically in cases of persistent epiphora that is socially unacceptable or affects vision, chronic or recurrent dacryocystitis, and dacryolith formation. The surgical approach may be external or endoscopic and may include the application of topical mitomycin C, though this remains controversial.[16] Though recent studies have documented the safety and reliability of endoscopic procedures,[17] many practitioners prefer an external approach.

14-5 SUMMARY

The approaches to treating nasolacrimal duct obstruction in an infant are diverse and controversies exist. However, the combination of these various techniques resolves 98% to 99% of nasolacrimal duct obstruction in children. The parents are generally satisfied and appreciative. Only a few children will require a dacryocystorhinostomy, and in these cases referral to an experienced lacrimal surgeon is usually required.

REFERENCES

1. Katowitz JA, Welsh MG. Timing of initial probing and irrigation in congenital nasolacrimal duct obstruction. *Ophthalmology* 1987;94:698–705.
2. Robb RM. Probing and irrigation for congenital nasolacrimal duct obstruction. *Arch Ophthalmol* 1986;104:378–379.
3. Buerger DG, Schaeffer AJ, Campbell CB, Flanagan JC. Congenital lacrimal disorders. In: Nesi FA, Lisman RD, Levine MR. *Smith's Ophthalmic Plastic and Reconstructive Surgery* 2nd ed. St. Louis: Mosby, 1998:649–660.
4. Tan AD, Rubin PAD, Sutula FC, Remulla HD. Congenital nasolacrimal duct obstruction. *Int Ophthalmol Clin* 2001;41(4):457–469.
5. Calhoun. Problems of the lacrimal system in children. *Pediatr Clin North Am* 1987;34(6):1457–1465.

6. Becker BB. The treatment of congenital dacryocystocele. *Am J Ophthalmol.* 2006; 142(5):835–838.
7. Paysse EA, Coats DK, Bernstein JM, Go C, deJong AL. Management and complications of congenital dacryocele with concurrent intranasal mucocele. *J AAPOS* 2000;4(1):46–53.
8. Schwartz BA, Manley DR. Disorders of the lacrimal apparatus in infancy and childhood. In: Nelson LB *Harley's Pediatric Ophthalmology* 4th ed. Philadelphia: W.B. Saunders Company, 1998:345–352.
9. Del Monte M. *Atlas of Pediatric Ophthalmology and Strabismus Surgery.* Churchill Livingstone, 1992:209–221.
10. Robb RM. Success rates of nasolacrimal duct probing at time intervals after 1 year of age. *Ophthalmology* 1998;105:1307–1309.
11. Anderson RL, Yen MT, Hwang IP, Lucci LM. A new groove director for simplified nasolacrimal intubation. *Arch Ophthalol* 2001;119:1368–1370.
12. Engel JM, Hichie-Schmidt C, Khammar A, Ostfeld BM, Vyas A, Ticho BH. Monocanalicular silastic intubation for the initial correction of the congenital nasolacrimal duct obstruction. *J AAPOS.* 2007;11:183–186.
13. Hutcheson KA, Drack AV, Lambert SR. Balloon dilatation for treatment of resistant nasolacrimal duct obstruction. *J AAPOS.* 1997;1(4):241–244.
14. Lueder GT. Balloon catheter dilation for treatment of persistent nasolacrimal duct obstruction. *Am J Ophthalmol* 2002;133:337–340.
15. Gunton KB, Chung CS, Schnall BM, Prieto D, Wexler A, Koller HP. Comparison of balloon dacryocystoplasty to probing as the primary treatment of congenital nasolacrimal duct obstruction. *J AAPOS.* 2001;5(3):139–142.
16. Nemet AY, Wilcsek G, Francis IC. Endoscopic dacryocystorhinostomy with adjunctive mitomycin C for canalicular obstruction. *Orbit.* 2007;26(2):97–100.
17. Yigit O, Samancioglu M, Taskin U, Ceylan S, Eltutar K, Yener M. External and endoscopic dacryocystorhinostomy in chronic dacryocystitis: comparison of results. *Eur Arch Otorhinolaryngol* 2007;264(8):879–885.

15

Surgery of the Lacrimal System

ROGER A. DAILEY, MD, FACS, AND MAURICIO R. CHAVEZ, MD

Obstruction of the tear outflow system can occur anywhere along its course from the tear lake to the inferior meatus of the nose. Surgical techniques designed to relieve this functional or complete obstruction have been available for a long time. Toti of Italy described the dacryocystorhinostomy (DCR) procedure in 1908 as a treatment modality for obstruction of the nasolacrimal duct. His technique did not make use of mucosal flaps. Dupuy-Dutemps of France, on the other hand, encouraged the use of flaps. He recommended suturing together the nasal mucosal and lacrimal sac flaps. The success rate of the operation improved dramatically. Today the external DCR procedure makes use of modifications of both of these historically described procedures.

In recent years, intranasal DCR has enjoyed renewed popularity. This procedure had been performed by Lester Jones and others for years but was dropped because the success rate was 80% at best. Although the use of endoscopic techniques and laser technology has been advocated by some authorities, the success rate (approximately 70%) with relatively short-term follow-up has limited its acceptance. More recently, Javate and associates reported a series of patients undergoing endoscopic DCR with the radiofrequency Ellman unit. Their reported success rate of 90% compared favorably with a 94% success rate in 50 age-matched patients undergoing external DCR with a follow-up of 9 months. This rate also compares favorably to the present authors' success rate of approximately 95% in uncomplicated cases undergoing external DCR and a similar rate with the endoscopic approach without use of a laser. Therefore, the laser does not appear to offer any significant advantage over more traditional intranasal approaches, and the cost may actually be a financial disincentive to its use. The benefit of mitomycin continues to be debated. You and associates performed a prospective study showing favorable long-term success rates with the use of mitomycin. On the other hand, Liu and associates performed a prospective study that demonstrated no benefit.

While the DCR works well for lacrimal sac or nasolacrimal duct obstruction, it does not address obstructions of the puncta and canaliculi. Multiple procedures are available to the lacrimal surgeon for obstructions in the upper system and are discussed in this chapter. The definitive procedure for significant canalicular obstruction is the conjunctivodacryocystorhinostomy (CDCR), which was initially described by Lester Jones. The DCR was performed to the point of mucosal flaps and then a polyethylene tube was placed from the medial canthus into the nasal cavity posterior to the anterior lacrimal sac mucosal flap and the nasal mucosal flap. Because of the improved capillary attraction of glass, these were later changed to Pyrex tubes, which demonstrated improved effectiveness, and they remain the standard today despite efforts to find substitute autogenous and synthetic materials. In 2002 we began using frosted Jones Pyrex tubes and in 2004 we reported their effectiveness in treating patients who had extrusion of their smooth Jones Pyrex tubes. The frosted treatment of the outer surface retains all the benefits of the original tube but appears to decrease tube extrusion. The frosted outer surface seems to allow the contracting scar tissue to fix the tube more securely in place by simple friction while still allowing easy manual removal for fittings and cleanings.

15-1 DACRYOCYSTORHINOSTOMY

DCR, as performed today, has proven to be beneficial for the treatment of acute or chronic nasolacrimal duct obstruction, as well as functional obstruction of the lacrimal outflow system. Functional obstruction is diagnosed using the Jones dye tests. The Jones I in this case would be negative (no dye), and the Jones II would be positive, indicating that the dye was unable to pass from the eye to the nose in approximately 10 minutes without assistance; however, fluid can be forced through the duct by the examiner using a syringe and cannula. This procedure can be performed through an external or endoscopic approach.

15-1-1 *Anesthesia*. Cooperative adult patients are urged to have the procedure performed with local infiltrative anesthetic combined with intravenous sedation or monitored anesthesia care (MAC). Recovery is generally shorter and easier for the patient and there is less intraoperative hemorrhage than with general anesthesia.

The eye is topically anesthetized with proparacaine hydrochloride. Subcutaneous infiltration of 2% lidocaine with epinephrine (1:100,000) in the operative area below the medial canthus and in the region of the infratrochlear nerve above the medial canthal tendon is performed. Half-inch packing gauze or cottonoids saturated with cocaine hydrochloride 4% to 5% and phenylephrine hydrochloride 2% are packed into the nose in the region of the anterior tip of the middle turbinate. When general anesthetic is used, the same infiltration and nasal packing are employed.

15-1-2 *External Approach Technique*. The skin incision is made 11 mm nasal to the medial commissure, starting just superior to the insertion of the medial canthal tendon and extending inferiorly and slightly laterally for about 20 mm (Fig. 15-1).

The knife should not cut deeper than the subcutaneous fascia. After cutting through the remaining subcutaneous tissue with sharp Stevens scissors, the surgeon should insert a self-retaining, spring-type retractor such as the Agrikola. Hemostasis is obtained with a battery cautery unit, which facilitates initial orbicularis fiber separation as well.

With two Freer elevators, the angular artery and vein are located as they cross the medial canthal tendon (Fig. 15-2). The vessels are retracted to the medial or

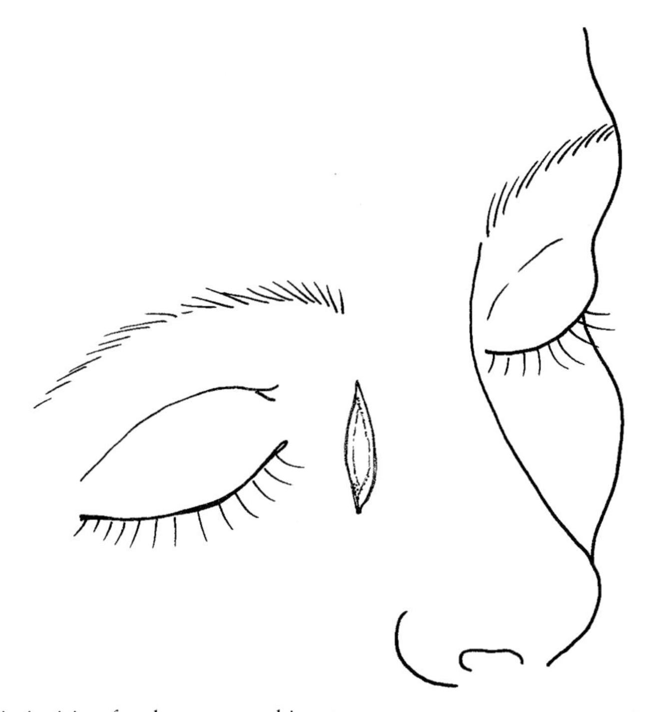

Figure 15-1 Skin incision for dacryocystorhinostomy.

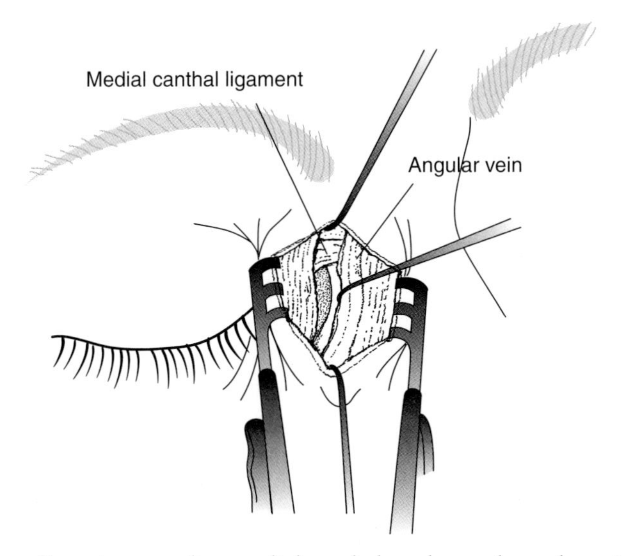

Figure 15-2 Deeper dissection revealing medial canthal tendon and angular vein.

lateral side with one elevator, while the other elevator begins the separation of the muscle and periosteum exactly beneath the point where the medial canthal tendon attaches to the bone. With pressure against the bone, the tip of the elevator is directed inferiorly and outwardly until the region below the spine of the anterior lacrimal crest is reached. The periosteal division will be about 3 to 5 mm medial and will extend inferiorly to the margin of the anterior lacrimal crest. The periosteum is elevated on both sides of this incision and reflected over the anterior lacrimal crest; then the sac is elevated posteriorly beneath the tendon to the posterior lacrimal crest. Next, the nasolacrimal duct is freed from the bone inferiorly as far as possible in the nasolacrimal canal.

The lacrimal sac is infiltrated with local anesthetic, and a 0.5-inch square cottonoid is inserted between the soft tissue of the lacrimal sac and the bony lacrimal fossa. The cottonoid serves three purposes: hemostasis, anesthesia, and protection of the sac during bone removal.

At this time, the spring retractor is exchanged for one with longer teeth, such as a Goldstein, which will reach the periosteum and give better deep exposure. The nasal packing is removed in preparation for bone removal. Using a drill with a 4- to 5-mm dental burr, the surgeon removes an oblong area of bone anterior to the lacrimal crest, taking care not to injure the nasal mucoperiosteum. Irrigation is done to prevent excessive heat buildup and to facilitate visualization. The nasal mucoperiosteum is separated from the underside of the bone with a dental burnisher. The cottonoid is extracted and the nasal mucoperiosteum is injected with the local anesthetic.

A 45-degree Kerrison punch is then used to enlarge the vertical dimensions of the bony opening (Fig. 15-3). The most important area to remove is just in front of the posterior lacrimal crest and under the medial canthal tendon. The tendon can be elevated but typically is not, as it is a most important guide to adequate removal of the bone beneath its insertion.

The bony bridge of anterior lacrimal crest that remains is then removed with a rongeur. This step occasionally leads the surgeon into the anterior ethmoid air cells, typically posing no problem. The authors suggest a conservative "deskeletonization" of these cells. The last portion of bone to be removed is the medial half of the nasolacrimal canal. First the nasal mucoperiosteum is separated from the canal down to the inferior turbinate. A rongeur can then be used to remove this bone, thereby avoiding the postoperative "sump" syndrome described by Richard Welham, MD. The Kerrison rongeur is helpful to smooth the rough edges of the bone where the anterior and posterior lacrimal crests meet inferiorly. A good rule in all tear sac surgery is never to have a bony margin closer than 5 mm to the common canaliculus.

Attention is now focused on the tear sac. The Goldstein retractor is loosened and a #0 probe inserted through either canaliculus "tents" the medial wall toward the nasal mucoperiosteum (Fig. 15-4). A #11 Bard-Parker blade is used to cut through both the periosteal and the mucosal layers of the medial wall of the sac slightly lateral to the tip of the probe. When the wall has been perforated, the scalpel is removed and one blade of a sharp curved Stevens or iris scissors is inserted into the sac. The incision is extended to the top of the fundus and to the bottom of

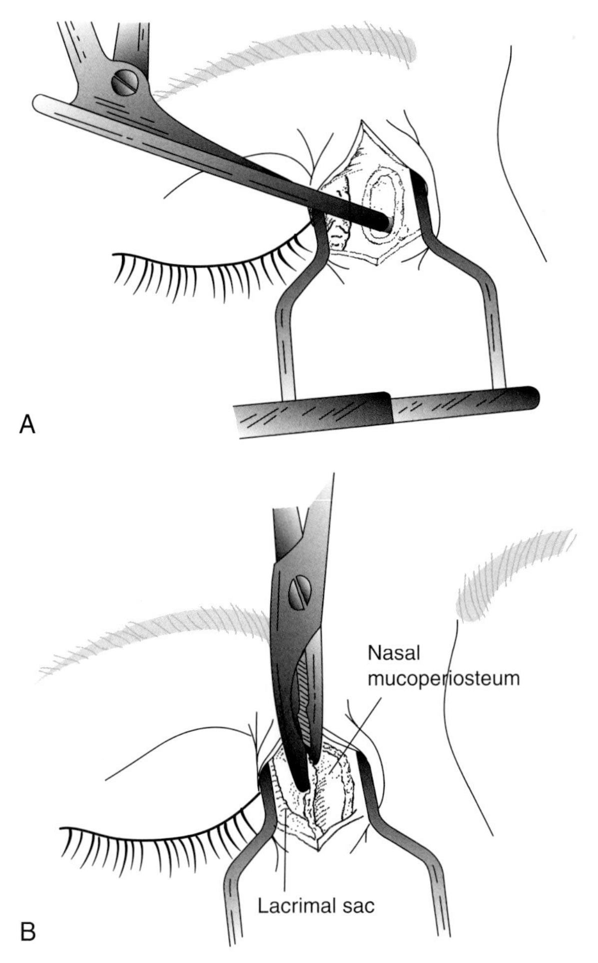

Figure 15-3 Enlarging bony ostium. (A) Using Kerrison punch to enlarge vertical dimensions of bony opening. (B) Further enlargement of bony ostium with removal of medial wall of nasolacrimal duct.

the exposed nasolacrimal duct. A similar incision is made in the nasal mucoperiosteum adjacent to and parallel with the one in the tear sac. The posterior flap of the tear sac and nasal mucoperiosteum are removed with forceps and scissors. There is no need to sew these flaps together.

Both canaliculi are now intubated by Quickert probes with silicone tubing. The silicone is brought out through the nose and at the end of surgery is tied with a square knot, cut, and allowed to retract into the nose. The surgeon should ensure that there is no tension on the puncta, which could lead to punctal erosion. If bleeding is a problem, 0.5-inch gauze with petroleum jelly can be placed up the nose as an anterior pack, or an adequate amount of Instat, a collagen absorbable hemostat, can be placed beneath the flaps anterior to the tip of the middle turbinate.

Silicone tubing is not always necessary; it is suggested for pediatric patients, canalicular stenosis, and reoperations. The alternative is to place an antibiotic

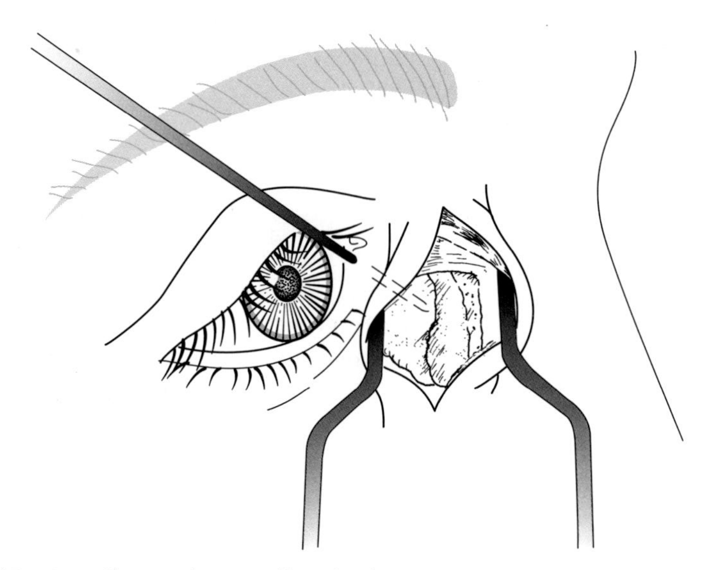

Figure 15-4 Tenting of lacrimal sac to allow for fenestration.

ointment–soaked strip of 0.25-inch packing gauze behind the anterior nasal and sac flaps. The packing is removed through the nose in approximately 2 weeks. This can be impossible to do in infants or children and in adult patients who are uncooperative unless a general anesthetic is used.

The anterior flap of the tear sac is now approximated with the anterior-based flap of the nasal mucosa using two interrupted 5-0 polyglactin 910 sutures on a P-2 needle. The retractor is removed. The periosteum and orbicularis muscle are now closed as a single layer using running or interrupted 6-0 polyglactin 910 sutures. A running 5-0 plain fast-absorbing gut suture is used to close the skin. An antibiotic ointment is then placed on the wound, and covered with a small bandage. If petroleum-jelly gauze was used for hemostasis, it is removed through the nose the following day. If Instat was used, it can remain. The silicone tubing is usually retained for 6 weeks. The tubing can be removed through the nose after being cut in the medial canthus, or it is cut and then pulled through the upper canaliculus.

15-1-3 *Endoscopic Approach Technique.* Adequate preparation of the nose will make the surgery easier. Preoperative vasoconstriction of the nasal cavity is achieved by using a long-acting nasal decongestant 2 hours and 1 hour before the operation. In the operating room, infiltration of the mucosa at the internal ostium site and the middle turbinate with Xylocaine with epinephrine 1 to 100,000 is done. Nasal packing follows it with a strong vascoconstrictor like cocaine 4% to induce long-lasting decongestion of the nasal cavity to aid in exposure of the surgical site and to minimize bleeding.

It is mandatory when performing nasal endoscopic procedures to use proper, high-quality instruments. A 0-degree 4-mm endoscope is used, although a 30-degree angle is nice to have available for special situations where visualization is more difficult. A high-powered xenon light source is essential to keep visualization to an optimal level. A high-resolution monitor at least 19 inches wide placed close to the head of the patient at the level of the eyes of the surgeon will complete the video unit necessary to perform the operation.

The nasal packing is removed and, using the endoscope, the middle turbinate is identified. A Freer elevator can be used to firmly displace the turbinate toward the septum to enhance exposure of the uncinate process when necessary. A small ridge formed by the projection of the frontal process of the maxilla can usually be seen anterior to the uncinate process at approximately the same level as the anterior projection of the middle turbinate. The anterior incision is made with a crescent knife or the sharp edge of the Freer elevator several millimeters anterior to the ridge below the insertion of the turbinate. The posterior incision is made parallel to the first one just anterior to the uncinate process over the lacrimal bone. The incisions are joined superiorly and inferiorly, and the mucosa can be elevated using a Freer periosteal elevator (Fig. 15-5A). The mucosa is then removed using a grasping forceps. Electrocautery should be avoided if possible as it leads to nasal crusting postoperatively. The frontal process of the maxilla and its suture line with the lacrimal bone are easily seen. The osteotomy is started by removing the frontal process of the

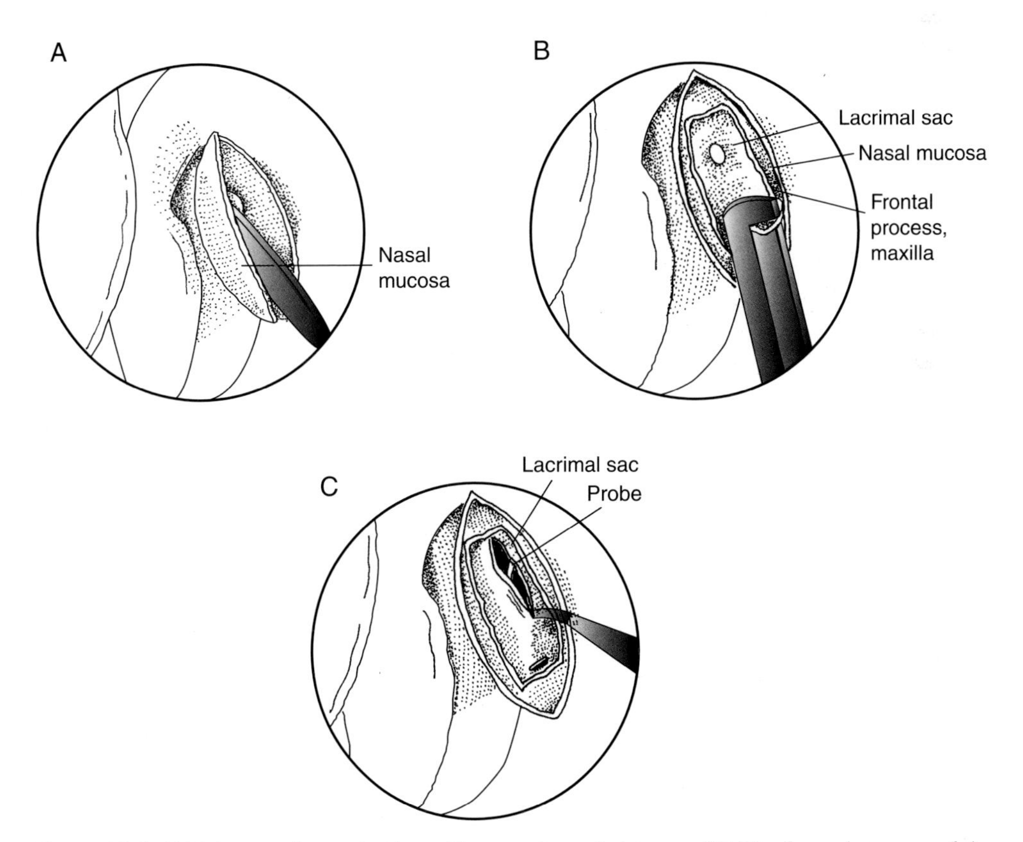

Figure 15-5 (A) Mucosa elevated using a Freer periosteal elevator. (B) The frontal process of the maxilla is removed using a Kerrison rongeur. (C) The lacrimal sac is opened with small horizontal incisions and a third vertical incision close to the maxillary bone edge joins the two previous ones.

maxilla with a Kerrison rongeur. With the tip of the rongeur, the ledge formed by the thick maxillary bone can be felt and the rongeur is inserted just under it. Usually three or four bites are necessary to uncover the anterior part of the lacrimal cylinder (Fig. 15-5B). Care is taken to slip the instrument between the bone and the lacrimal mucosa to avoid undue bleeding and distortion of the anatomy. Using a periosteal elevator, the lacrimal bone is lifted from the lacrimal mucosa. Posteriorly, this dissection often involves the uncinate process, especially if one plans to remove the medial wall of the sac. A Blakely forceps is used to remove the elevated lacrimal bone and the uncinate process. If the uncinate process is to be removed it should be cut at its upper and lower insertion. The lacrimal sac is opened with a vertical incision. Superior and inferior incisions can be made as needed, forming trap door–like flaps (Fig. 15-5C). A zero Bowman probe is then inserted through either canaliculus into the lacrimal sac and is seen behind the flap. The angulated micro-Blakely forceps is used to remove the lacrimal flap. By grabbing the flap anteriorly, a controlled posterior tear can be made so that the whole medial aspect of the lacrimal cylinder is removed, ideally in one piece. Leaving the lateral wall of the lacrimal sac intact preserves the mucosal lining and promotes a quick and controlled reepithelialization of the lateral nasal wall by having the nasal mucosa fusing with the lacrimal mucosa. A gentle massage of the lacrimal sac is done externally with the finger to visualize the inner aspect of the sac and to express any dacryolith hidden in the lacrimal sac wall. At the end of surgery, the lacrimal system is intubated with silicone tubing (as described in the previous section). Instat is then placed into the wound area, and the silicone tubing is tied in a square knot, cut, and allowed to retract into the nose.

15-2 CANALICULAR ABNORMALITIES

The lacrimal drainage system may be divided into the upper system (eyelid margins, punctum, and canaliculi) and the lower system (lacrimal sac and nasolacrimal duct). This section deals primarily with diseases and surgery of the upper system. Disorders of the upper lacrimal system may result from congenital disorders, such as agenesis, atresia, or supernumerary channels or diverticula, or may be acquired after trauma, inflammation, neoplastic disease, or medications (idoxuridine or echothiophate iodide).

15-2-1 *Punctal Disorders.* Stenosis of the punctum is treated conservatively by dilating first with a Jones punctum dilator and then the Ziegler dilator. If inspection reveals a closed punctum, it can frequently be opened using a #75 Beaver blade or a #11 Bard-Parker scalpel blade. Once the punctum has been opened, weekly dilation is advisable until it remains open. Loupes, a biomicroscope, or an operating microscope can be helpful.

Chronic spastic closure of the punctum and conditions leading to phimosis of the punctum are repaired by a one-snip technique. This simple office procedure preserves the pumping action of the ampulla. Proparacaine is instilled in the conjunctival cul de sac, and cocaine solution on a cotton-tipped applicator is applied to the punctum for several minutes. One blade of an iris scissors is inserted vertically into the ampulla, while the other blade remains on the conjunctival side

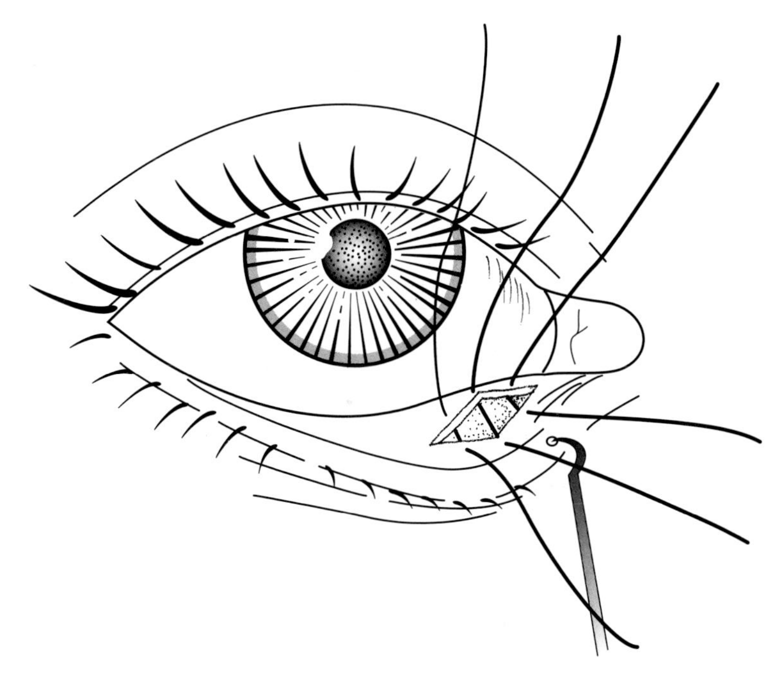

Figure 15-6 Closure of diamond-shaped wedge excision for punctal eversion.

of the eyelid. To avoid pain, the scissors are closed quickly, snipping the canal vertically. If the one-snip procedure fails, then a second snip is made at the inferior margin of the vertical incision, progressing medially for 3 mm.

Eversion of the punctum due to mild medial eyelid ectropion is repaired by a diamond-shaped wedge resection (Fig. 15-6). A diamond-shaped section of the conjunctival and subconjunctival tissue is removed just inferior to the punctum. The conjunctiva and submucosa are grasped with forceps inferior to the punctum. When the forceps are elevated, small curved iris scissors are placed horizontally beneath the forceps, pushed toward the eyelid, and brought together. This procedure removes an ellipse or diamond-shaped piece of tissue. The wound is then closed with an interrupted 7-0 polyglycolic acid suture. An alternative is the "window-shade procedure," in which a rectangular flap of conjunctiva–tarsus is dissected toward the punctum. The flap is resected, and its edges are sutured to the cut in the cul de sac with a 7-0 polyglycolic acid suture.

For patients who suffer secondary reflex hypersecretion in association with keratitis sicca, closing the punctum may provide a great deal of relief. If all tests confirm that the patient's epiphora is the result of reflex tearing due to sicca problems such as foreign-body sensation, contact-lens intolerance, or corneal damage, collagen plugs may be placed in the ampulla to temporarily retard or completely block lacrimal outflow. Gentle thermal cautery or electrocautery directed into the punctum may be performed to produce the same temporary effect. If the patient notes definite improvement in symptoms without troublesome epiphora, more vigorous cautery to the entire ampulla epithelial surface can be used to close the ducts permanently. The canaliculus may also be surgically interrupted by dissecting out the canaliculus, while it is defined by a probe, and excising a portion.

15-2-2 *Canalicular Disease*. Scarring of the canaliculi may follow severe conjunctival infections, inflammations, allergies, burns, and reactions to drugs, such as glaucoma medications. Idiopathic canalicular obliteration is present in a small percentage of patients, who may develop closure at any point in the canalicular system. Sealing frequently commences at the common canaliculus and progresses to complete obliteration over time, without evidence of trauma or infection. Canaliculitis is rarely bacterial. However, cultures should be obtained and any potentially causative organisms treated with appropriate antibiotic therapy. Concretions in the canaliculi are usually caused by infection with *Actinomyces israelii*. Some fungi can also be causative. One or both canaliculi may become so dilated that the concretions may be removed with a small ear curette or "milked out" with a glass rod. When all granules appear to have been removed, the canaliculi should be irrigated with normal saline or antifungal solutions. The treatment may be repeated at weekly intervals. Occasionally, a *Streptothrix* granule forms a plug, which must be dislodged.

If the foreign material is not removed, the canaliculus should be opened by an incision into the horizontal limb along the posterior aspect of the eyelid. The vertical limb of the canaliculus and the punctum must be left undisturbed while the canaliculus and ampulla are curetted. Usually, horizontal incisions do not need to be sutured, but if a vertical tear develops in the eyelid margin, it should be closed to prevent gaping and fistulization.

15-2-3 *Punctal and Canalicular Lacerations*. Atraumatic technique is essential in handling tissues that have been lacerated. No sharp instrument should be used until all parts of the lacerated lacrimal system have been identified. It is important that all skin and muscle tissues be preserved.

Although repair of lacrimal lacerations should be done as early as safety permits, it is usually wise to delay surgery 12 to 24 hours if local swelling or hemorrhage is present. Surgery is best undertaken with an operating microscope and an experienced surgical team. An interim treatment consists of compresses and local antibiotics. Lacerations of the punctum on the conjunctival side may be left alone if they are vertical and minimal or if they create a large punctal opening but do not affect the lacrimal pump mechanism.

For skin lacerations and lacerations extending into one or both canaliculi, the Jones dye test will quickly determine if at least one canaliculus is still functioning. An undamaged canaliculus alone may handle the lacrimal drainage. Surgical intervention may not be needed, other than for anatomic repair of the involved canaliculus in the event of a future injury.

When the lateral 2 to 3 mm of the canaliculus has been destroyed by burns or lacerations and is irreparable but the medial canaliculus can be identified, marsupializing the open end of the medial canaliculus may cure the obstruction. It may be necessary to slit the canaliculus to enlarge the ostium or to perform a canaliculoconjunctival anastomosis. The proximal end of the lacerated canaliculus can often be identified more easily with the operating microscope. Saline may be helpful in identifying the lacerated end of the canaliculus by retrograde flow when instilled through the intact part of the system, or the wound can be filled with saline and then air injected through the intact portion of the system. The air bubbles emanate from the end of the lacerated canaliculus, allowing its identification. A flap of skin and muscle may be turned down for better exposure. The medial palpebral tendon may be elevated so that the area of injury is exposed.

The canaliculus is identified and a fine lacrimal probe is passed through the punctum and the lateral canaliculus, across the laceration, and into the medial end of the canaliculus. The probe is replaced by a stent before repair begins. The most popular stent consists of silicone tubing. As popularized by Quickert and Dryden, silicone tubing is attached to a probe that is passed through the lacrimal system. The probe is guided out the nose with the help of a groove director or under direct visualization. The canaliculus is approximated with 9-0 or 10-0 nylon, after which the pretarsal orbicularis muscle, conjunctiva, and skin are closed to complete the repair.

15-2-4 *Strictures at the Common Canaliculus.* Strictures at the common canaliculus may require slitting or excising, often under direct visualization after the lacrimal sac is opened. The stricture, pushed into view in the open sac with a lacrimal probe, may then be incised or excised around the probe. Various methods have been suggested to stent the stricture and prevent its recurrence. This stenting of the opened stricture or obstruction is as important to the success of the surgical procedure as the actual lysis of the tissues.

A 3-0 nylon suture may be passed into the sac, past the stricture site, and out the canaliculus. To this may be attached several additional sutures, which can then be pulled into the stricture; eventually, material as thick as umbilical tape may be added. The external ends of the suture are fixed to the face with adhesive tape. After several weeks, the tape or suture can be pulled through the nose.

An alternative stent has been suggested by Werb and modified by Quickert and others. This procedure consists of exposing and excising the stricture and passing silicone tubing through both the upper and the lower canalicular systems and out the nose, where the two ends of the silicone are attached to each other by a sleeve or suture, or tied in a square knot. The Quickert probes can be used to guide the silicone tubing. The continuous loop of silicone tubing may be directed from the opened internal punctum through the anastomosis of sac and nasal mucosa membrane in the middle meatus during DCR. In some cases, the Quickert probes may be inserted through the occluded common canaliculus and directed down the nasolacrimal duct under the inferior turbinate without the necessity of the accompanying DCR.

15-3 CANALICULODACRYOCYSTOSTOMY

Canaliculodacryocystostomy is done when both canaliculi are obstructed near their juncture with the sac and at least 8 mm of the lower canaliculus is in good condition. Because of the high failure rate, the authors often place a Pyrex tube at the same time. After the silicone has been removed, the Pyrex tube is temporarily obstructed. If the anastomosis stays open, the Pyrex tube can be removed.

The skin incision, beginning at the level of the medial palpebral tendon 11 mm nasal to the medial commissure of the eye, is carried downward and slightly outward for about 20 mm. The lacrimal sac is exposed and the fundus dissected free. A probe

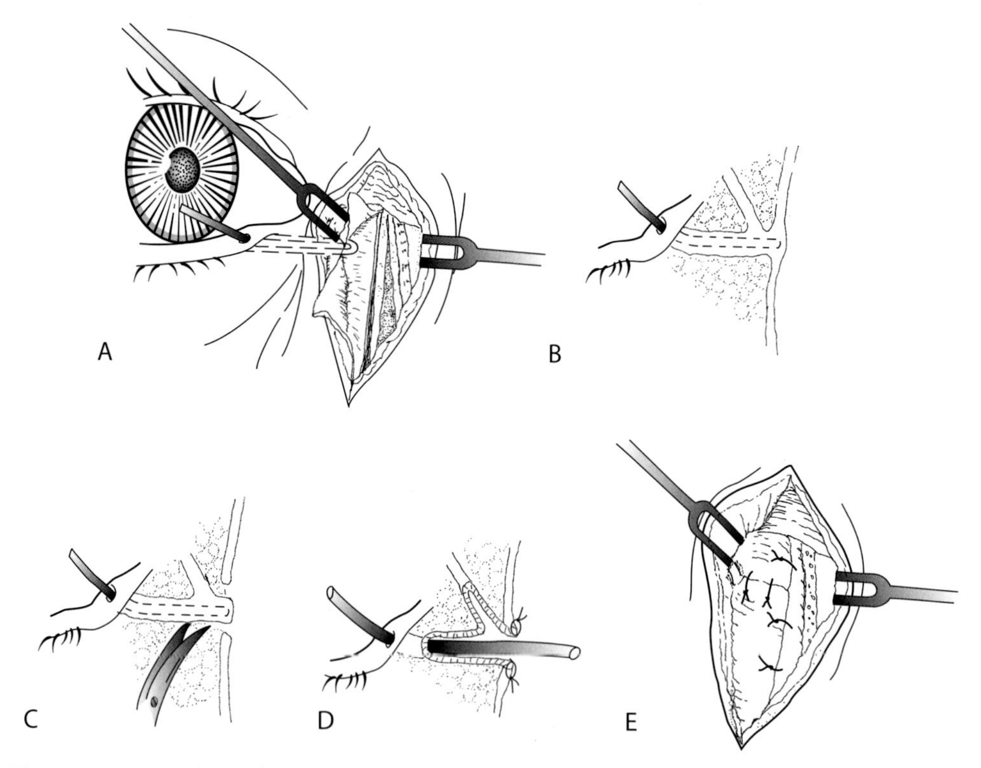

Figure 15-7 Canaliculodacryocystostomy. (A) Dacryocystorhinostomy is finished as far as removal of posterior flaps. (B) Anterior tear sac flap is cut down to probe. (C) Phimosed or obstructed common canaliculus is dissected free and (D) excised. Two sutures are placed from canalicular epithelium to tear sac margin. Silicone tube is inserted and outer end is sutured to lower lid skin. (E) Anterior tear sac flap is repaired and routine closure completed.

is passed into the canaliculus and pressed into the wound beneath and posterior to the orbicularis muscle and tendon. The sac is carefully dissected free at its medial 3 or 4 mm, and a cut is made obliquely into the blind end of the sac so that the resulting beveled opening will be present downward. The dissection is carried around the common canaliculus, and the stricture is resected (Fig. 15-7). Silicone tubing or malleable probes are passed as a stent through the canaliculus and sac and out the nares. The canaliculus is sutured to the sac with 7-0 polyglycolic acid suture so that its mucosa will extend into the sac about 1 to 2 mm. The wound is closed in the usual manner, and the silicone is tied, cut, and allowed to retract into the nose.

15-4 CONJUNCTIVODACRYOCYSTORHINOSTOMY

Conjunctivodacryocystorhinostomy is done when a flaccid canaliculus or complete paralysis of the lacrimal pump is present or when both canaliculi are absent or obliterated. The DCR is performed to the point of anastomosis of the anterior lacrimal flap, without detaching the medial palpebral tendon. If prominent, the caruncle is excised, with care being taken to remove as little conjunctiva as possible. Insert a sharp Stevens scissors into the lacrimal lake 2 mm posterior to the cutaneous margin of the commissure (Fig. 15-8A). Using blunt and sharp dissection, gently manipulate the scissors into the opened tear sac, being sure they are anterior to the body of the middle turbinate. If the anterior tip of the turbinate obstructs the tube's internal aperture, resect it.

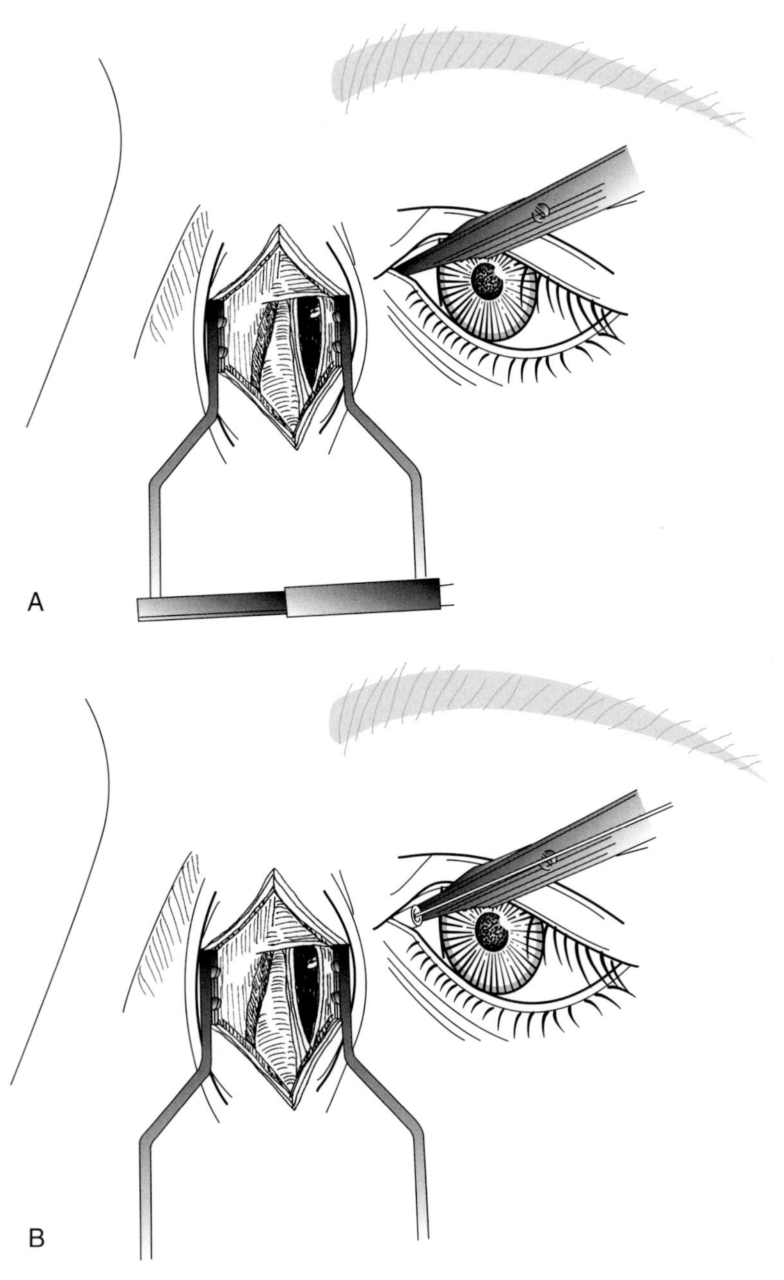

Figure 15-8 (A) Stevens scissors inserted into the lacus lacrimalis 2.5 mm posterior to the cutaneous margin of the commissure. (B) Zero probe with Pyrex tube in place being passed just anterior to the scissors.

With the blades of the scissors in place and held slightly open, pass a zero probe with a 17-mm Pyrex tube (Jones tube) with a 4-mm collar just above or anterior to the scissors, between the opened blades, and into the sac (Fig. 15-8B). Now remove the scissors and simultaneously push the Jones Pyrex tube down the course of the probe into position. Observe the interior of the nose to be certain that the inner end does not touch the septum. If the tube does touch the septum, use a shorter one. Secure the tube in place with a 5-0 polyglycolic acid suture passed around the collar of the tube. Tie the tube in place, and pass the suture through the skin of the canthus and tie it to prevent dislodging of the tube. The remainder of the closure is the same as for DCR.

Postoperatively, patients are seen at 1 day, 1 week, and 6 weeks. At the time of surgery, the authors typically place longer tubes than will ultimately be necessary, to prevent mucosal overgrowth from the nasal sidewall. Because of this length, the tube will occasionally be obstructed by the mucosa of the nasal septum. At the 6-week visit, the tube can be exchanged for a shorter one and the collar size reduced to 3.5 mm to minimize the tube's visibility in the medial canthus.

Patients are warned to hold the tubes or squeeze their eyes closed tightly when blowing the nose, sneezing, or coughing. If the tube becomes dislodged, it must be replaced as soon as possible, because the fistula will close down completely within hours. Patients are instructed to snuff in artificial tears through the tubes, while pinching the nostrils closed, twice a day to help maintain patency. The tubes are removed in the office and cleaned with alcohol every year.

SUGGESTED READINGS

Dailey RA, Tower RN. Frosted Jones Pyrex tubes. *Ophthal Plast Reconstr Surg.* 2005;21:185–187.

Dailey RA, Wobig JL. Use of collagen absorbable hemostat in dacryocystorhinostomy. *Am J Ophthalmol.* 1988;106:109–110.

Javate RM, Campomanes BSA Jr, Co ND, et al. The endoscope and the radiofrequency unit in DCR surgery. *Ophthalmic Plast Reconstr Surg.* 1995;11:54–58.

Jones LT, Linn ML. The diagnosis of the causes of epiphora. *Am J Ophthalmol.* 1969;67:751–754.

Jones LT, Marquis MM, Vincent NJ. Lacrimal function. *Am J Ophthalmol.* 1972;73:658–659.

Liu D, Bosley TM. Silicone nasolacrimal intubation with mitomycin-C: a prospective, randomized, double-masked study. *Ophthalmology.* 2003;110:306–310.

Loff HJ, Wobig JL, Dailey RA. The bubble test: an atraumatic method for canalicular laceration repair. *Ophthalmic Plast Reconstr Surg.* 1996;12:61–64.

Mustarde JC, Jones LT, Callahan A. *Ophthalmic Plastic Surgery: Up-to-Date.* Birmingham, AL: Aesculapius Publishing Co., 1970:100.

Reifler DM. Results of endoscopic KTP laser–assisted dacryocystorhinostomy. *Ophthalmic Plast Reconstr Surg.* 1993;9:231–236.

Wobig JL, Dailey RA. Surgery of the lacrimal apparatus. In: Lindquist TD, Lindstrom RL, eds. *Ophthalmic Surgery: Looseleaf and Update Service.* St. Louis: Year Book Medical Publishers, 1990:VE1–VE17.

You YA, Fang CT. Intraoperative mitomycin C in dacryocystorhinostomy. *Ophthal Plast Reconstr Surg.* 2001;17:115–119.

IV

Orbit

16

Fractures Involving the Orbit

CHRISTINE C. ANNUNZIATA, MD, BOBBY KORN, MD, PHD,
AND DON O. KIKKAWA, MD

Orbital and periorbital injury can occur with localized trauma to the eye or in the setting of multiple trauma associated with injury to other vital organs. A reported 16% of major trauma patients have ocular or orbital injury, and 55% of patients with facial injury have associated ocular or orbital injury. In general, the amount of ocular, soft tissue, and bony damage is related to the amount, duration, and direction of force applied to the orbit and face. Nevertheless, orbital injury is common and can be a subtle finding in the context of other facial or life-threatening injuries.

16-1 ORBITAL ANATOMY

Geometrically, the bony orbit most closely resembles a four-sided pyramid consisting of an apex, a base, and four sides: roof, floor, medial wall, and lateral wall. The absence of the orbital floor posteriorly and the inclination of the lateral wall toward the medial wall changes the geometric shape from a four-sided pyramid to a three-sided pyramid at the orbital apex (Figure 16-1). The bony margin circumscribes the orbital entrance and provides anterior support for the thin bones of the interior walls of the orbit. Rounding of the orbital walls blends demarcation of the superior, medial, inferior, and lateral walls. The entrance measures 40 mm horizontally and 32 mm vertically. The widest portion of the orbital margin lies about 1 cm behind the anterior orbital rim. In adults, the depth from orbital rim to apex varies from 40 to 45 mm. Safe subperiosteal dissection may be accomplished along the lateral wall and orbital floor for 22 mm and along the medial wall and orbital roof for 30 mm. The volume of the orbit is approximately 30 cc.

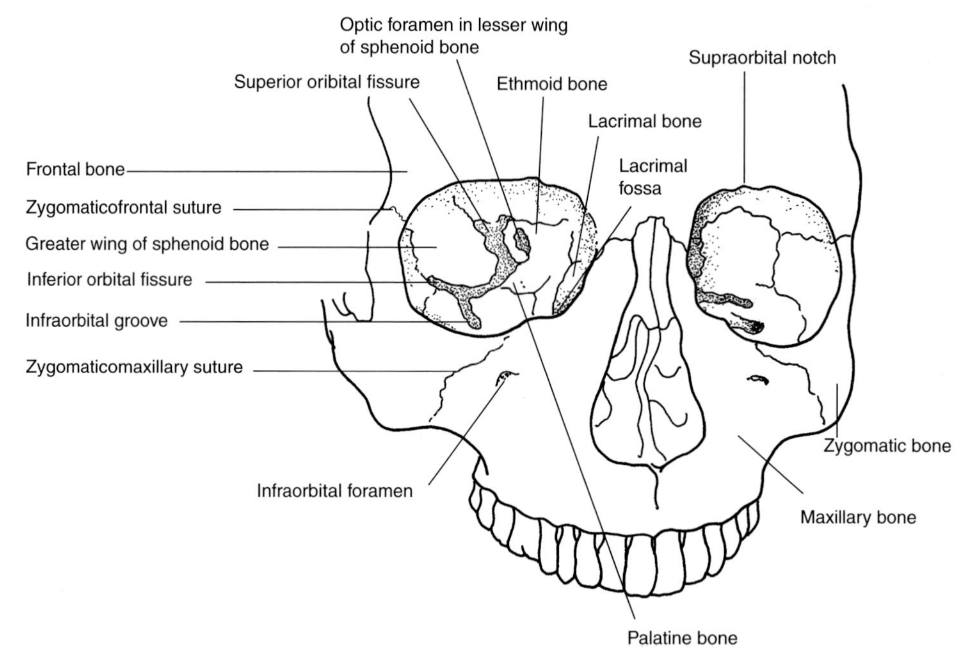

Figure 16-1 Orbital bony anatomy.

The triangular floor of the orbit serves as the roof of the maxillary sinus. Several areas of thin bone create weak points in the orbital floor that are susceptible to fracture. The thinnest portion is medial to the infraorbital groove and canal, particularly posteriorly, where the medial wall has no bony support (Figure 16.2). In the posterior aspect of the floor, the infraorbital fissure extends as the infraorbital canal. This canal travels in a lateral to medial direction across the floor and terminates as the infraorbital foramen 1 cm below the midpoint of the inferior orbital rim. Anteriorly, the fissure is roofed by bone and forms a canal within the orbital floor. Posteriorly, the infraorbital nerve does not have this bony protection and is susceptible to injury with inferior subperiosteal dissection.

The medial wall consists of the sphenoid, maxillary, lacrimal, and ethmoid bones. The medial wall thins as the ethmoid bone is encountered, and pneumatized ethmoidal air cells are visible beneath the lamina papyracea, the thinnest portion of the medial wall. This area is particularly prone to fractures. The anterior and posterior ethmoidal foramina transmit branches of the ophthalmic artery and nasociliary nerve. These are located just superior to the medial canthal ligament approximately 20 mm and 35 mm, respectively, posterior to the anterior lacrimal crest. The optic foramen is located approximately 5 cm posteriorly from the anterior lacrimal crest.

The lateral wall is the thickest of the orbital walls, formed anteriorly by the zygoma and posteriorly by the greater wing of the sphenoid. The superior orbital fissure bounds the lateral wall posteriorly and the inferior orbital fissure bounds the lateral wall inferiorly.

Posteriorly, the lesser wing of the sphenoid bone and superiorly, the frontal bone make up the orbital roof. The roof is comparatively strong relative to the medial wall and floor, and significant frontal trauma is usually required to fracture it.

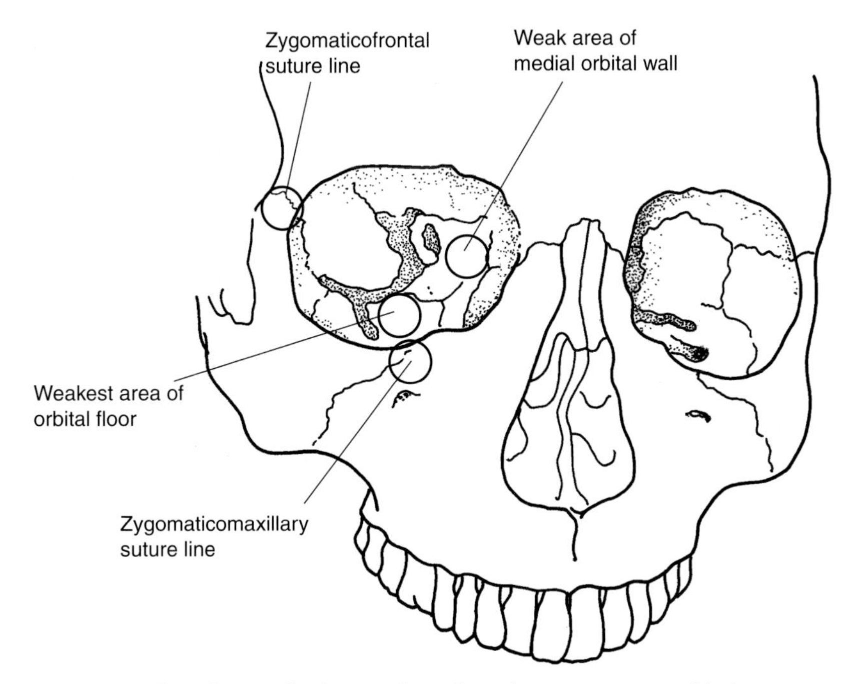

Figure 16-2 Areas of weakness of orbit (*circles*) where fractures are most likely to occur.

The orbital periosteum strongly adheres to the orbit in several places, including suture lines, fissures and canal openings, the trochlear fossa, and the dura mater at the optic canal. In other areas, a subperiosteal dissection plane can be created fairly easily.

16-2 PATIENT EVALUATION

Physical examination should commence after careful history-taking and review of systems is complete. Important historical factors include the exact mechanism of injury and potential comorbidities. The patient's general medical condition should be evaluated and stabilized first, especially when high-velocity injuries have occurred. Potentially life-threatening injuries to the head, chest, or abdomen should be addressed promptly and may take precedence over orbital or ocular examination. In multiple trauma patients, thorough ophthalmologic examination may not be possible because life-threatening injuries are given higher priority in diagnosis and treatment, and because patients are often unable to cooperate fully if at all. This often leads to delay in diagnosis and treatment and has been shown to contribute to late enophthalmos in these patients.

16-3 OCULAR EXAMINATION

One of the main functions of the bony orbit is to protect the eye. The ophthalmologist's primary concern is evaluation of the globe. Assessment of vision and integrity of the globe should be performed as soon and as completely as possible. The severity of an orbital fracture does not necessarily correlate with the degree of injury to the globe. Visual acuity, pupillary reaction and function, intraocular pressure, and confrontational visual field testing can all be tested relatively easily at the bedside with an awake and cooperative patient. Anterior segment examination as well as indirect ophthalmoscopy should also be performed to evaluate for corneal or scleral lacerations, intraocular foreign bodies, lens dislocation or capsular rupture, angle recession or closure, vitreous hemorrhage, choroidal rupture, retinal edema, tears, or detachment.

16-4 MOTILITY EXAMINATION

Examination of the extraocular muscles is critical in assessing patients for potential surgical needs. Ptosis may be caused by roof fractures affecting the levator muscle or oculomotor nerve. If an eyelid laceration involves the levator muscle, an attempt to repair the muscle should be made during the acute phase of injury. However, unless there is permanent nerve injury, ptosis caused by damage to the levator muscle is often temporary. Patients will also often complain of diplopia both in the early and late post-trauma periods. Examination will frequently show limitation of the globe on up gaze and/or down gaze. Limitation of eye movement is seldom found in the horizontal direction unless there is a medial wall fracture or hematoma present. The restriction of vertical movement of the eye commonly is caused by entrapment of the inferior rectus or its associated connective tissues (orbital septa). The inferior oblique muscle is infrequently involved. Pain present on attempted up gaze is often due to increased traction on an entrapped muscle. Entrapment is more likely to occur with small fractures that tightly wedge the muscle or associated connective tissue into the fracture site (Fig. 16-3). In children, orbital fracture of the pliable orbital floor can cause a "trapdoor" effect causing entrapment of the inferior rectus and an associated oculocardiac reflex. However, even in large fractures of longer standing, fibrosis of the prolapsed tissues can significantly limit vertical eye movement.

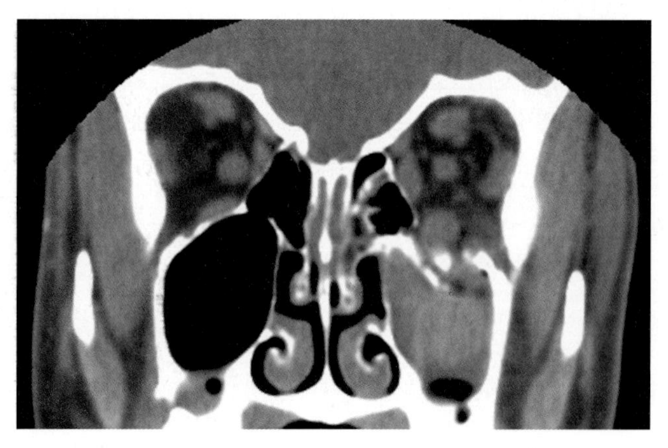

Figure 16-3 Left extraocular muscle and soft tissue entrapment. This may be more likely with smaller fractures and can cause persistent diplopia and motility disturbance.

Forced-duction testing is the most reliable way to evaluate extraocular muscle entrapment at the bedside. It may also release the traction on the involved muscle or connective tissue, and is thus a critical diagnostic and potentially therapeutic test. The examiner first places anesthetic drops in the eye, and then grasps the conjunctiva and Tenon's capsule just inferior to the limbus at the 6 o'clock position. The test is positive if there is resistance as the eye is rotated upward. The test is particularly informative in the presence of radiographic suggestion of entrapment. There are, however, other causes of limited globe movements to keep in mind, such as hematoma or orbital edema, or damage to the extraocular muscles or their innervations.

16-5-1 *Orbitofacial Examination: Inspection.* Orbital fractures are almost always accompanied by other notable periorbital findings, including facial contour abnormalities, hemorrhage and ecchymosis, lacerations, and globe malpositions. Consequently, inspection alone of the associated orbital and facial changes can provide significant diagnostic information to the examiner.

Displaced fractures often create facial contour abnormalities that can be a clue to the location and severity of an underlying fracture. Early assessment of facial contour is critical since these changes can be subtle or absent in the presence of significant edema or hemorrhage. For example, a displaced fracture of the zygoma may cause facial asymmetry secondary to lateral canthal dystopia and depression or flattening of the cheek prominence (Fig. 16-4). Nasoethmoidal orbital fractures typically present with flattening of the bridge of the nose and measurable widening of the intercanthal distance (telecanthus). Soft tissue degloving injuries of the medial canthus usually have a C- or reverse C-shaped skin laceration, ptosis, and lacrimal drainage system injury (Fig. 16-5).

Large or deeper lacerations in the periorbital area often indicate significant force and may be associated with an underlying fracture, particularly if there is associated orbital hemorrhage.

Soft tissue injuries often accompany orbital fractures and often lead to significant periorbital ecchymosis. Preseptal hemorrhage may spread extensively, but postseptal hemorrhages, including subconjunctival hemorrhages, can also occur and are usually self-limited. Subperiosteal hemorrhages occur with orbital floor

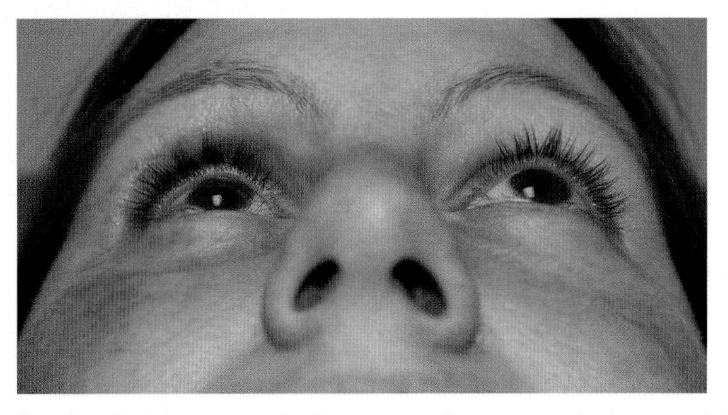

Figure 16-4 Orbitofacial examination. Right zygoma fracture producing enophthalmos and a characteristic flattening of the malar prominence.

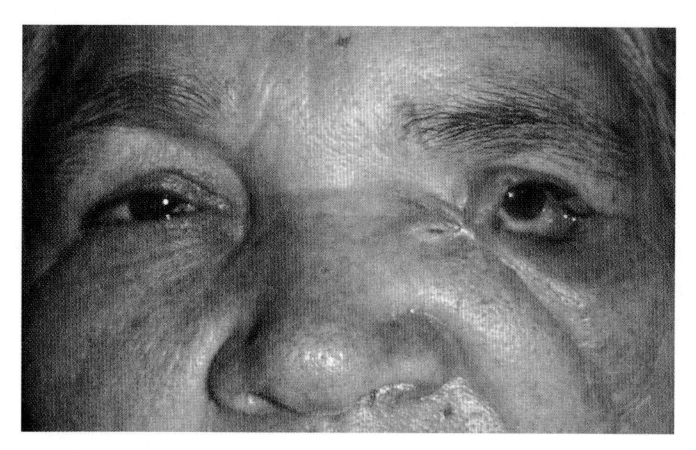

Figure 16-5 Orbitofacial examination. C-shaped laceration, ptosis, and telecanthus in a soft tissue degloving injury of the left medial canthus.

fractures and tend to be of limited size if the periorbita remains intact. These hematomas are also limited by the firm adherence of the periosteum to the bone at suture lines. A subperiosteal hematoma may be visible on computed tomography (CT) as a crescent-shaped area of hyperdensity along the orbital margin. If the periorbita is disrupted, blood can leak anteriorly toward the orbital septum and conjunctiva.

Intraconal hemorrhage can occur if orbital vessels are damaged, and this can result in significant exophthalmos or motility disturbances (Fig. 16-6). These hemorrhages should raise suspicion for the possible presence of an optic canal fracture. Extensive hemorrhage can increase orbital pressure and compromise the retinal vascular circulation, necessitating urgent lateral canthotomy and inferior cantholysis. If vascular compromise persists or vision worsens, surgical bony decompression may be necessary.

Eyelid and globe malpositions may give important clues to underlying problems. Horizontal, vertical, and axial globe positions should be measured. Of note, the Naugle exophthalmometer is usually preferred, but measurement errors can occur when there is significant rim deformity in the presence of maxillary or inferior rim fractures. Alternatively, Hertel exophthalmometers may be inaccurate in the presence of zygomaticomaxillary fractures. If exophthalmos is present, orbital emphysema

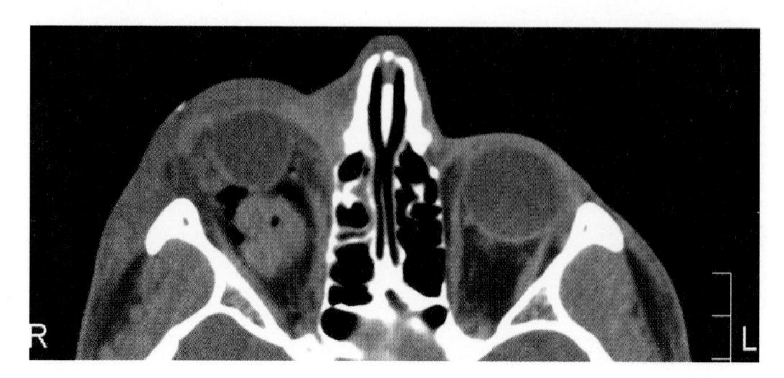

Figure 16-6 CT scan showing right retrobulbar hematoma. This can result in significant exophthalmos requiring urgent lateral canthotomy and inferior cantholysis.

from an underlying fracture involving either the ethmoid or maxillary sinuses, or orbital hemorrhage should be suspected. Enophthalmos may occur secondary to a large fracture of the orbital floor with prolapsed orbital fat and other posterior, medial, and inferior orbital tissues into the maxillary antrum or ethmoid sinuses. Extraocular muscle entrapment can also contribute to enophthalmos, as muscle fibers tether the globe posteriorly. In delayed presentations, atrophy of the orbital fat can further contribute to poor support behind the globe, allowing the eye to recede farther back into the orbit.

In addition to being cosmetically unacceptable, enophthalmos greater than approximately 2 mm decreases support of the upper eyelid, resulting in ptosis and a deepening of the superior sulcus (Fig. 16-7). In large orbital floor fractures with associated damage to Lockwood's ligament and other suspensory structures, ptosis of the globe results from migration of the eye, not only posteriorly in the orbit, but also inferiorly into the maxillary sinus.

16-5-2 *Orbitofacial Examination*: *Palpation*. Gentle palpation of the orbital margin can help define the point of maximal tenderness, which is often coincidental with the fracture site, as well as bone movement or discontinuity. Care should be taken not to displace dislocated fragments along the rim.

Fractures involving the paranasal sinuses and in particular medial wall fractures often cause orbital emphysema and can be palpated as crepitus. When a periosteal defect is present, Valsalva maneuvers or nose blowing can force air through the fracture site and into the orbit, where it can accumulate. Rarely, extensive proptosis with elevated orbital and intraocular pressure can result. Thus, patients should be urged not to blow the nose after orbital fracture for at least 2 weeks.

16-5-3 *Orbitofacial Examination*: *Neurologic Evaluation*. Clinical examination in facial trauma patients should always include an assessment of facial sensation. Since the peripheral branches of the trigeminal nerve lie in close contact with the orbital bones, orbital fractures often lead to sensory nerve damage. Identifying these areas of dysfunction can help identify the location of a fracture site. Contusion injuries to sensory nerves can result in areas of facial anesthesia or hypoesthesia that is typically temporary.

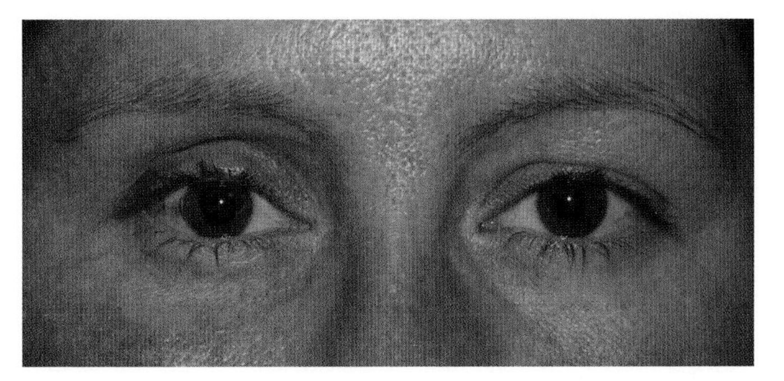

Figure 16-7 Enophthalmos, ptosis, and deepening of the superior sulcus in a patient with a right orbitofacial fracture.

The infraorbital nerve passes along the floor of the orbit and its branches carry sensation from the lower eyelid margin to the ipsilateral upper lip and upper teeth. This nerve and its branches are often involved in orbital floor or inferior rim fractures. Generally, the more posterior the orbital floor injury, the more extensive and inferior the sensory loss.

Orbital roof fractures can damage the supraorbital nerve, producing an area of numbness around the medial upper eyelid and eyebrow.

Lateral wall and zygoma fractures can damage the zygomaticotemporal and zygomaticofacial nerves. Nevertheless, resultant numbness is rare because of considerable redundancy of nerve distribution in this area.

Motor function of the facial nerve should also be evaluated during initial assessment of orbital fractures. Damage along the nerve's course can be extensive and may result in dysfunction of the frontalis, orbicularis, and other facial muscles.

16-5-4 *Orbitofacial Examination: Nasal Evaluation.* The nasal bones are often fractured in facial trauma. Following external inspection and palpation of the nose, internal examination of the septum, mucosa, and turbinates should be performed. A fracture of the cribriform plate or inner table of the frontal sinus can lead to cerebrospinal rhinorrhea and should prompt an evaluation by the neurosurgical team.

Medial orbital fractures may involve the lacrimal drainage system. For example, extensive injury is frequently seen in a naso-orbital-ethmoidal (NOE) fracture when it involves the intraosseous portion of the nasolacrimal duct. Also, the canalicular system can be damaged by medial canthal degloving injuries, which are often associated with NOE fractures. Thus, the patency of the lacrimal drainage system should be determined before and after surgical intervention.

16-6 ORBITAL IMAGING

Orbital CT with coronal and axial views is invaluable in the diagnosis and management of orbital fractures (Fig. 16-8). Non-contrast, thin (1- to 3-mm) cuts, and direct coronal rather than reconstructed views provide the most information but may not be practical to obtain in instances of severe bodily, head, or cervical trauma. The size of the fracture, the extent of soft tissue incarceration, the presence of subperiosteal hematoma, and the location of displaced fragments can all be directly estimated by this technique. In the presence of cervical immobilization, such as by a C-collar, direct coronal images are often not possible. In this instance, coronal views can be reconstructed from axial views. Sagittal views can also be helpful.

If CT is not available, a Waters view of the skull is the best radiologic means for screening patients with potential orbital fractures. This view may show fragmentation of the bone of the floor, prolapsed orbital soft tissues, or a fluid level in the maxillary antrum, and sometimes orbital or eyelid emphysema. A Caldwell view is helpful in screening the ethmoid sinuses for medial orbital wall fractures. Of note, plain radiographs have been reported to have a false-negative rate as high as 50% and are nondiagnostic 30% of the time in some studies.

Magnetic resonance imaging (MRI) shows soft tissue details particularly well. However, because MRI does not image cortical bone, it is not very useful in evaluating

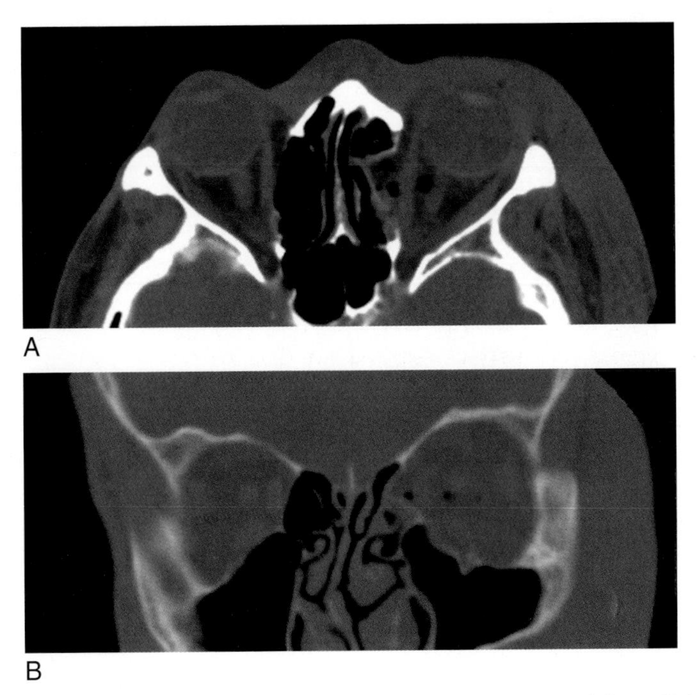

Figure 16-8 Orbital imaging. (A) CT scan, axial view, demonstrating a left medial wall fracture. (B) CT scan, coronal view, demonstrating an additional orbital floor fracture in the same patient.

orbital fractures. Furthermore, MRI is contraindicated in the presence of a metallic orbital foreign body. In cases of possible traumatic optic neuropathy or optic canal fractures, MRI may be particularly helpful in visualizing the course of the optic nerve and evaluating the extent of canal congestion or the presence of displaced fracture fragments. This information can be critical during surgical planning for possible optic canal decompression in the presence of traumatic optic neuropathy.

16-7 FRACTURES INVOLVING THE ORBIT

16-7-1 *Midfacial Fractures.* The midface consists of nine bones that lie between the frontal bone and the mandible. The Le Fort classification of facial fractures helps describe the three most common patterns for facial fractures (Fig. 16-9). They are bilateral by definition and rarely occur in their pure form clinically. The orbit is involved in Le Fort types II and III.

A Le Fort I fracture is a horizontal fracture of the maxilla running from the inferior lateral piriform rim to the pterygomaxillary fissure. The tooth-bearing maxillary fragment is dislocated from the remainder of the facial bones. A Le Fort I fracture is almost always present in a type II or type III fracture.

A Le Fort II or pyramidal fracture is a midface fracture beginning at various levels from the nose bilaterally. The fracture then extends through the inferior orbital rim, the lacrimal bones, and the orbital floor, extending finally to the zygomaticomaxillary buttresses. This configuration of the fracture gives it a pyramidal shape. Damage to the ethmoids always occurs in a pyramidal fracture, and the lacrimal drainage

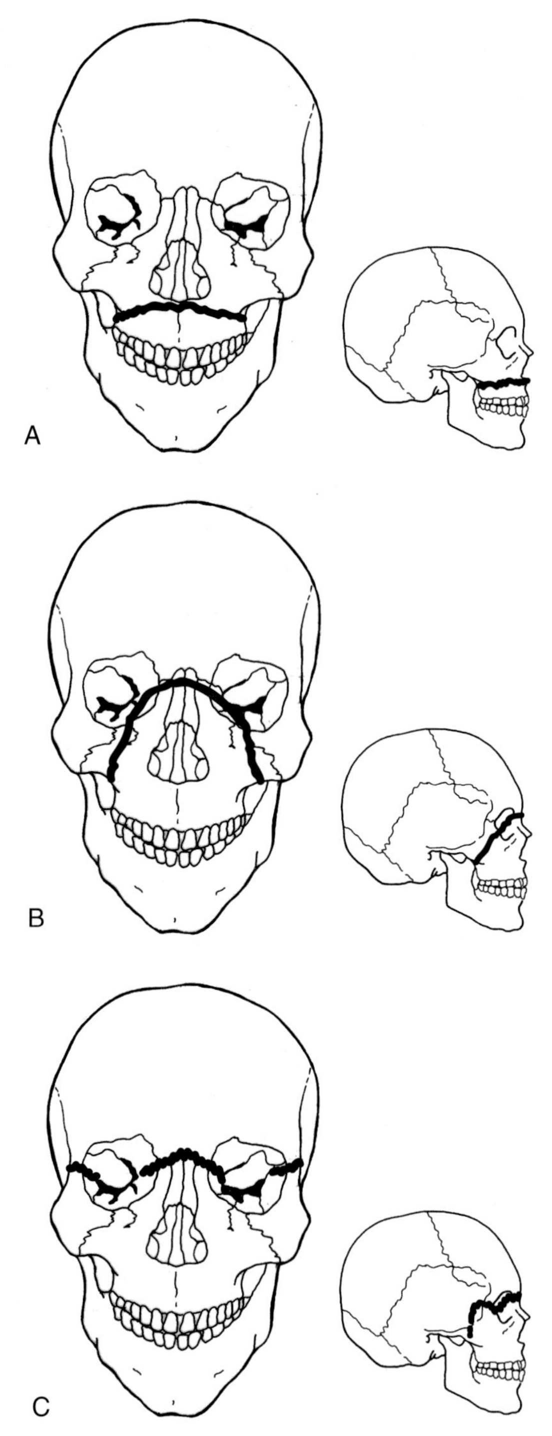

Figure 16-9 Le Fort classification. (A) Le Fort I or transverse fracture: fracture line does not involve orbits. (B) Le Fort II or pyramidal fracture: orbital floors and nasal bones are involved. (C) Le Fort III fracture, or craniofacial dysjunction: both orbits are involved.

system may also be involved. Diplopia is also a common finding following Le Fort II fractures.

A Le Fort III fracture involves a complete craniofacial dysjunction, or complete separation of the face from the cranium. The facial bones are often displaced posteriorly and inferiorly. The fracture line crosses the upper nasal bones and involves the frontomaxillary suture, the ethmoids, the infraorbital fissure, and the optic canal. Laterally, the fracture line crosses the orbital margin near the frontozygomatic sutures and the zygomatic arch.

Surgically, the midface is conveniently accessed through an inferior transconjunctival incision combined with a transoral gingivobuccal incision. If necessary, an upper lid incision may be used to approach the zygoma or arch. Other useful approaches include a transcaruncular incision for medial wall access or a bicoronal flap for wide exposure. Microplating or wiring systems with at least two fixation points are necessary for internal fixation and realignment of the midface bones.

16-7-2 *Orbitozygomatic Fractures.* The zygoma is particularly prone to injury secondary to its anatomic prominence in the anterior lateral orbit. If the fracture is nondisplaced and there is no associated orbital floor fracture or muscle entrapment, no surgical treatment may be necessary. Furthermore, low-velocity, non-comminuted fractures may be externally reduced if they remain stable after reduction.

Dislocation of the zygomatic bone often occurs in high-velocity injuries. Fractures involving the junction of zygomatic process of the frontal bone, the zygomaticomaxillary suture line or infraorbital foramen, and the zygomatic arch are known as tripod fractures. These injuries require open reduction with rigid internal fixation. Furthermore, the orbital floor is usually involved and may require additional treatment.

On clinical examination, patients often have flattening of the cheek, lateral canthal dystopia, and inferior globe displacement. Palpation along the lateral orbital rim and arch can identify gaps, step deformities, and points of tenderness at the fracture site. Subconjunctival, palpebral, and retroseptal or subperiosteal hemorrhage may be present.

The presence of pain with jaw movement or malocclusion of the bite indicates impingement of depressed arch fragments on the coronoid process or associated mandibular or maxillary fractures.

Neurosensory dysfunction is common with lateral wall fractures. Despite frequent disruption of the zygomaticofacial and zygomaticotemporal nerves, redundant nerve distribution often prevents clinical manifestations of injury. However, the infraorbital nerve is frequently involved since the orbital rim is inherently weak at the infraorbital foramen. Hypoesthesia or anesthesia of the lower eyelid and cheek may be present.

Displaced fractures require open reduction and internal fixation. Surgical access to the fracture sites can be obtained through incisions in the gingivobuccal sulcus, transconjunctivally, or through an upper eyelid crease incision. Eyelid crease or lateral brow incisions may help expose the zygomaticofrontal suture and are helpful for plating or wiring free-floating or severely displaced fragments of the lateral orbital rim (Fig. 16-10). Coronal incisions or a temporal approach (Gilles procedure) can be used in cases of severe comminuted fractures of the rim and zygoma that

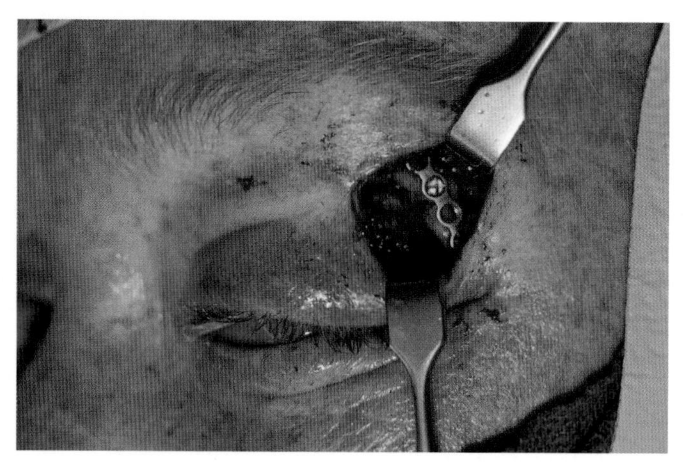

Figure 16-10 Repair of a displaced left zygoma fracture with plating through an eyelid crease incision.

require arch visualization. Usually, the fragments of the zygomatic arch do not need to be fixated with plates or wires if the other two fracture sites are reduced and fixated.

16-7-3 *Orbital Roof and Supraorbital Rim Fractures.* Orbital roof and supraorbital rim fractures often require a multidisciplinary treatment approach. Patients with these fractures often have accompanying intracranial injury and should be evaluated by the neurosurgical service. Also, the increased intracranial pressure associated with high-velocity head injury can herniate intracranial contents downward into the orbit in the presence of a roof fracture (Fig. 16-11). In severe cases, the communication between the intracranial cavity and orbit can lead to symptomatic pulsatile exophthalmos.

Clinical examination often reveals a forehead, brow, or lid laceration overlying the fracture or depression of the supraorbital ridge. A long and sharp object passing through the upper eyelid may perforate the orbital roof without any injury

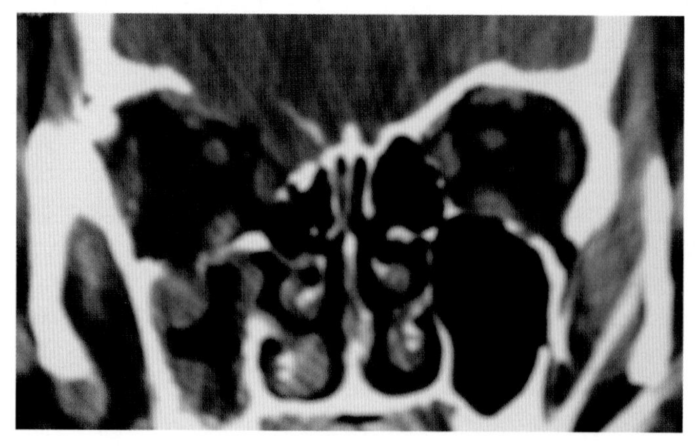

Figure 16-11 Orbital roof fracture. This injury led to severe intracranial injury and herniation of the frontal lobe into the right orbit.

to the globe. This injury can be especially subtle on clinical examination, especially in a child with a small laceration wound of the upper eyelid.

Palpation may reveal a step deformity and a point of tenderness at the site of the fracture. Periorbital edema and ecchymosis is the most common clinical finding. Lid ptosis and motility disturbance may result from a third nerve injury or mechanical damage to the levator muscle or trochlea. Traumatic ptosis following a roof fracture should not be repaired for at least 6 months after the injury because recovery of function may spontaneously occur. The supraorbital nerve is also vulnerable to injury as it exits the supraorbital notch along the superior orbital rim margin.

Orbital emphysema and epistaxis or cerebrospinal rhinorrhea may be present because of involvement of the frontal sinus, the cribriform plate, and the nose. The fracture may also extend posteriorly to the superior orbital fissure or the optic canal, resulting in traumatic optic neuropathy or other cranial nerve injury.

Minimally displaced fractures of the supraorbital rim do not require operative treatment. In some cases of mild fragment displacement, closed reduction may be definitive. If an overlying laceration is present, reduction can be performed through the wound prior to closure.

Occasionally, open reduction of a roof or supraorbital fracture is required, such as in cases involving the superior oblique trochlea or fractures that communicate with the cranial cavity. This repair may be performed with a neurosurgeon, and the surgical approach is through an existing laceration or a coronal incision.

In cases of bony compression of the optic nerve, surgical decompression may be indicated. Recent studies have indicated that approximately 20% to 30% of patients improve spontaneously and that initial visual acuity is the most significant predictive factor affecting the outcome of traumatic optic neuropathy. In particular, patients with no light perception may benefit the most from surgical decompression versus medical management. The surgical approach can be intracranial, transethmoidal, or transorbital.

Traditionally, in the acute phase of an optic canal injury and in the presence of traumatic optic neuropathy, high-dose systemic corticosteroids have been administered as a neuroprotective agent and to minimize inflammation and swelling. Hemorrhage, shearing of optic nerve fibers, or optic nerve edema leads to traumatic optic neuropathy in the absence of radiographic evidence of a canal fracture. Of note, no randomized controlled trials of steroids in traumatic optic neuropathy have been done, and recent studies have identified possible detrimental effects of steroids when used in brain and spinal cord injuries.

If a CT or MRI scan demonstrates an intrasheath hemorrhage compressing the optic nerve, optic nerve sheath fenestration and evacuation of the hematoma should be performed. The best approach for optic nerve fenestration is medially through an upper eyelid crease incision without medial rectus disinsertion. It can also be approached laterally, with or without bone removal if necessary.

16-7-4 *Orbital Floor Fractures.* Fractures of the orbital floor often occur with fractures of the orbital rim and adjacent facial bones. The most common site for a blowout fracture of the orbital floor is the thin portion of the maxillary bone in the posterior medial aspect of the floor. Because the ethmoid bones along the medial orbital wall are also quite thin, there may be significant associated fracture into the ethmoid sinuses. The inferior rectus muscle, with its long course along the floor, is the extraocular muscle most likely to be involved in a floor fracture. The muscle or its connective tissue may be involved through entrapment or by damage to its innervation. The branch of the oculomotor nerve to the inferior oblique passes along the lateral border of the inferior rectus, and trauma to the nerve along this route will cause paresis of the inferior oblique. If a medial orbital wall fracture is associated with a fracture of the floor, the medial rectus muscle or its connective tissue system may be involved and tether the globe, limiting horizontal movement.

The inferior orbital fissure lies between the sphenoid and maxillary bones in the posterior part of the orbit. The infraorbital groove and canal extend anteriorly along the middle of the orbital floor, ending at the infraorbital foramen. The infraorbital groove and canal contain the infraorbital neurovascular bundle, which may be compromised in an orbital floor fracture. Damage to the infraorbital artery leads to hemorrhage, and trauma to the infraorbital nerve causes sensory dysfunction within its distribution on the face.

Historically, the indications for orbital floor fracture repair have been controversial. Initially, surgery was recommended for virtually all patients with the clinical and radiographic features of a fracture. Subsequent studies recommended the nonsurgical management of orbital fractures because relatively few patients who were managed without surgery developed significant enophthalmos and/or diplopia. Current recommendations support surgical repair for selected patients with orbital floor fractures.

Certain guidelines are helpful in determining whether surgery is advisable:

1. Limitation of up gaze and/or down gaze within 30 degrees of the primary position with a positive traction test and with radiologic confirmation of a blowout fracture of the orbital floor is an indication for surgery (Fig. 16-12). These findings indicate extraocular muscle entrapment. Diplopia may improve significantly over the course of the first 2 weeks as edema or hemorrhage in the orbit resolves and as some of the entrapped tissues stretch. However, if there is no significant improvement over the course of 2 weeks after the initial injury

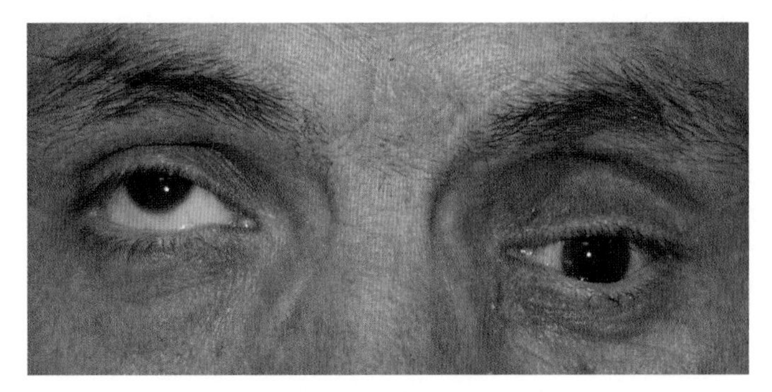

Figure 16-12 Indications for surgery. This longstanding left orbitofacial fracture led to significant limitation of up gaze requiring surgical intervention.

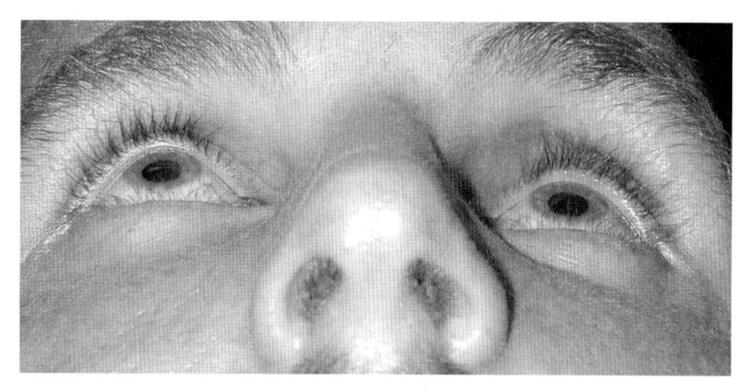

Figure 16-13 Left enophthalmos. This can be cosmetically unacceptable or may cause clinically significant limitation of inferior visual field in down gaze.

and if the above findings are present, surgery is advisable to prevent sequelae. If the entrapped tissues are not freed, vertical diplopia is likely to persist. Furthermore, globe limitation may become worse if significant fibrosis and contracture of the entrapped tissues occurs.

2. Enophthalmos greater than 2 mm that is cosmetically unacceptable to the patient is a reasonable indication for surgery (Fig. 16-13). Enophthalmos commonly is masked by orbital edema immediately after the trauma, and several weeks or months may pass before the extent of this problem is fully appreciated. If significant enophthalmos is present within the first 2 weeks and is associated with a large orbital fracture, greater enophthalmos can be anticipated in the future, and in most cases surgical repair is advisable.
3. A large fracture involving half the orbital floor or more, as determined by CT, particularly when associated with a large medial wall fracture, is an indication for surgery. These extensive floor fractures have a high incidence of subsequent significant enophthalmos and limitation of globe movement. Restriction of the globe may result from progressive fibrosis and contracture of the prolapsed tissues. Cosmetically unacceptable enophthalmos is even more likely to occur when such large orbital floor fractures are associated with a large fracture into the ethmoid sinuses.
4. A patient with an entrapped inferior rectus muscle shown on CT should undergo surgical repair early on. Such a patient will most likely have clinically significant diplopia if untreated.
5. The white-eyed blowout fracture in children from the trapdoor effect should be repaired promptly. The oculocardiac reflex can be activated in cases such as this and constitutes an indication for emergent repair.

The transconjunctival approach to the orbital floor provides good exposure and has the advantages of a largely hidden incision and of minimizing the possibility of postoperative lower eyelid retraction (Fig. 16-14). Care should be taken to keep the orbital septum intact to avoid lower lid retraction during wound closure. An alternative approach involves an infraciliary transcutaneous approach through the lower eyelid. Safe subperiosteal dissection can be accomplished approximately 25 mm posterior to the inferior orbital rim before risking injury to the orbital apex structures. The prolapsing orbital contents are gently lifted out of the fracture,

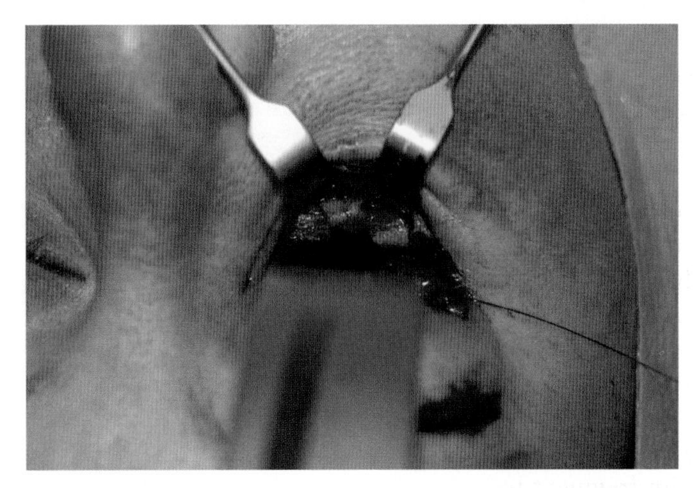

Figure 16-14 Transconjunctival approach to the right orbital floor and inferior orbital rim.

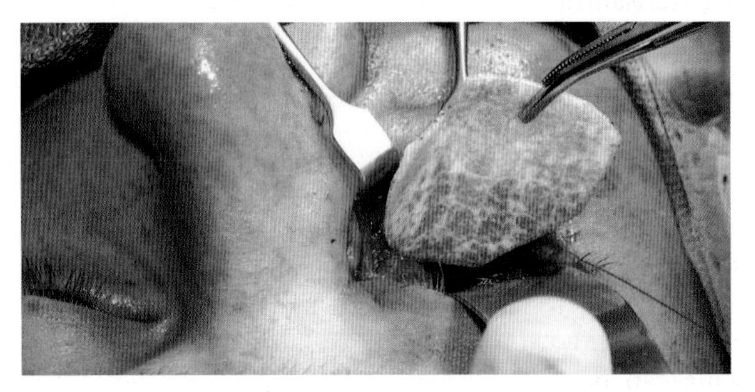

Figure 16-15 Placement of a porous, flexible, orbital implant over a large right orbital floor defect.

and an implant is placed over the fracture to maintain the orbital structures in proper position (Fig. 16-15).

Many different materials have been used as implants to cover the defect in the orbital floor, including autogenous bone or cartilage or allografts such as Supramid or silicone sheets, Vicryl or metallic mesh, porous hydroxyapatite, or porous polyethylene. Autogenous bone grafts have the advantage of being more physiologic and easily penetrated by systemic antibiotics after vascularization has taken place. These bone grafts are more difficult to obtain, however, and sometimes resorb over time. Nonporous allograft materials are easy to mold and handle, but sometimes form capsules and can be complicated by intracapsular hemorrhage requiring removal. Porous implants are being used with increasing frequency because of their ease of use (moldable and easily shaped), as well as their ability to be incorporated into the soft tissue and remain fixated.

16-7-5 *Inferior Orbital Rim Fractures.* The inferior orbital rim lies between the orbital floor and the anterior wall of the maxillary sinus. All three structures are usually involved in high-velocity injury to the inferior rim. Zygomatic fractures are also often coexistent.

Clinical examination can reveal step deformities and a point of maximal tenderness to palpation along the rim. If the maxillary sinus is violated, fragments of bone may be displaced into the sinus cavity, and orbital emphysema may be present. Diplopia may be caused by damage to the inferior oblique muscle at its origin along the rim. Nasolacrimal sac injury or duct obstruction occurs when the intraosseous portion of the lacrimal duct is damaged along the medial inferior orbital rim.

The infraorbital foramen and/or canal are natural weak points and are almost always involved in inferior orbital rim fractures. Sensory deficits along the course of the infraorbital nerve should be assessed before and after surgical repair of the orbital floor or inferior orbital rim. Nerve function may return, but this often takes several months.

Conservative management of these fractures can suffice if there is no or minimal displacement of the anterior orbital rim. In cases requiring surgery, the reduction of a depressed rim fragment is approached through a transconjunctival incision with lateral cantholysis, a transcutaneous approach through an infraciliary incision, or a combined transantral approach with a gingivobuccal sulcus incision and a Caldwell-Luc antrostomy. A periosteal incision is made over the fracture site and a subperiosteal dissection plane is created. The displaced rim fragments are elevated and wired or plated into position.

16-7-6 *Medial Wall Fractures.* Medial wall fractures can occur in isolation but are often associated with other orbital and facial fractures. Frequently, there are few associated clinical signs and symptoms, and these fractures may be easily overlooked. Furthermore, medial wall fractures may not always be demonstrable on imaging because of the thinness of the lamina papyracea. Orbital hemorrhage and emphysema can be present and enophthalmos occurs with large fractures. Hemorrhage can be severe if the ethmoidal arteries are disrupted. Valsalva maneuvers and nose blowing should be avoided. Diplopia occurs when the medial rectus muscle, orbital fat, or fascial connective tissue entrapment limits abduction. Epistaxis is also common but usually self-limited. An intranasal examination can reveal cerebrospinal fluid rhinorrhea or nasoethmoidal instability.

Indications for surgery include a positive forced-duction test of the medial rectus muscle or enophthalmos secondary to significant herniation of orbital contents into the ethmoidal sinus. In many cases, conservative management is adequate. Access to the medial wall is best achieved through a post-caruncular incision at the junction of the caruncle with the plica semilunaris. The periosteum is incised at the level of the posterior lacrimal crest, and the medial canthal tendon is not disrupted. The transcaruncular approach may be combined with a transconjunctival incision with lateral canthotomy and inferior cantholysis if a floor fracture is also present. When necessary, the inferior oblique muscle may be disinserted at its origin to improve exposure. Implants can be applied similarly to floor implants and rarely require fixation. In the presence of a floor fracture, a single implant can often be molded to adequately cover both defects.

16-7-7 *Naso-orbito-ethmoidal Fractures.* NOE fractures result from a high-velocity injury to the central midface and are frequently associated with other orbital and facial fractures. The fracture lines extend through the maxilla and the inferior orbital rim, as well as the medial orbital wall and lateral nasal bones. Flattening of the bridge of the nose is usually accompanied by measurable widening of the intercanthal distance (telecanthus). If soft tissue degloving is also involved, skin lacerations, ptosis, and lacrimal drainage system injury are also commonly present. Depending on the level of damage, a subsequent dacryocystorhinostomy may become necessary.

It is important to reduce unstable nasoethmoidal fractures as early as possible, while the fragments are still mobile. Surgical access is obtained through a combination of external nasal, bicoronal, lower eyelid or transconjunctival, and gingivobuccal sulcus incisions. Internal plates, wires, and transnasal wiring can be used to secure the unstable fragments until healing has occurred. The medial canthal tendon insertion should be preserved or repaired. Probing and silicone intubation of the nasolacrimal system should be performed if the patency of the system is interrupted.

16-8 GENERAL MANAGEMENT OF ORBITAL FRACTURES

Besides those indications listed for orbital floor fractures, common indications for surgical intervention include displacement of bone fragments disfiguring the normal facial contours, interference with mastication in the presence of a zygomatic fracture, or nasolacrimal duct obstruction such as is seen in NOE fractures.

General anesthesia is preferred; however, fracture surgery may be satisfactorily performed with monitored local anesthesia if necessary. A headlight is essential for optimal visualization within the orbit.

The timing of surgical repair depends on the patient's general medical condition, associated ocular injuries, and the type of fracture involved. When the fracture involves the inferior orbital rim, the naso-orbital structures, or the orbital floor, the bones usually can be easily moved into correct position for as long as 7 to 10 days after injury. This allows ample time for the medical stabilization of the patient. During this time, the surgeon can also assess and address any associated intraocular injuries, and fully evaluate the extraocular muscles and nasolacrimal system as the initial swelling and hemorrhage abates. Beyond 2 to 3 weeks, firm adhesions form between the fractured bone fragments. These adhesions may require an osteotomy to disrupt, and this may induce severe orbital trauma or hemorrhage. Thus, most orbital fractures should ideally be repaired within 10 to 14 days of injury.

Zygoma fractures are preferably repaired within the first week, when the displaced fragment is still easily moved. After the first week, the thick zygoma bone becomes adherent with reactive tissue and callus formation, which makes fracture reduction more difficult.

Unlike orbital floor and medial wall fractures, facial and zygoma fractures often require some type of internal stabilization with either wires or plates. The general principle of immobilizing a fracture must be adhered to whether wires or plates are used. Fixation should progress from superior to inferior and from lateral to medial. In most instances, a displaced fracture must be secured in at least two positions to stable bone to prevent rotation. This is especially true of a zygomatic fracture because of significant pull of muscle groups on the fracture fragments.

16-9 POSTOPERATIVE COMPLICATIONS

Numerous complications can occur following orbital blowout fracture repair. For the most part, many of them are correctable.

1. Blindness. Blindness following surgery for orbital fractures is fortunately rare. Such loss of vision is usually caused by either orbital hemorrhage compromising the blood supply to the optic nerve or trauma to the optic nerve by the orbital implant or orbital dissection. The risk of visual loss or injury to a seeing eye must be carefully weighed against the potential benefits of surgery when planning early or late surgical correction of an orbital fracture. The surgeon must be particularly judicious with the use of orbital implants.
2. Residual diplopia. An injured extraocular muscle that has been trapped in the fracture may have impaired function for several weeks or months after it has been freed. This impairment and paresis may result in diplopia postoperatively. Often, the muscle function returns and the diplopia resolves. If muscle imbalance remains after 6 months, the diplopia may be treated by the use of prisms or strabismus surgery.
3. Undercorrection of enophthalmos. Undercorrection of enophthalmos is much more common than overcorrection, and treatment is difficult because of contracture of orbital tissues and atrophy of orbital fat. Attempts to correct this problem usually are made by placing thicker or more posterior implants on the orbital floor. Care should be taken not to create globe elevation or hyperglobus with these thicker implants.
4. Overcorrection of enophthalmos. Overcorrection of enophthalmos is more likely to occur with thicker implants and may be present in the immediate postoperative period, gradually improving over the course of weeks or months as edema resolves and contracture occurs. Reoperation is rarely necessary.
5. Lower eyelid retraction. Apparent lower eyelid retraction may be caused by mechanical elevation of the globe because an implant is too thick. In such cases, the implant should be reduced in thickness or removed completely. True lower eyelid retraction also may occur due to adhesions of the orbital septum to the orbital rims (Fig. 16-16). Such adhesions are particularly likely to occur if the septum is vertically shortened during wound closure. This problem may be corrected by making a horizontal incision along the inferior border of the tarsus and recessing the orbital septum, lower eyelid retractors, and conjunctiva. The development of lower eyelid retraction is less common with the transconjunctival approach than with the infraciliary transcutaneous approach, because the dissection avoids the orbital septum.
6. Infection. Infection is treated with systemic antibiotics, but treatment usually necessitates removal of the orbital floor implant as well.
7. Extrusion of the implant. Extrusion of the implant can result from infection, trauma, an oversized implant, hemorrhage, or poor fixation with implant mobility. Adequate fixation of the orbital implants can be performed with screw fixation. Frequently, an extruded implant does not need to be replaced,

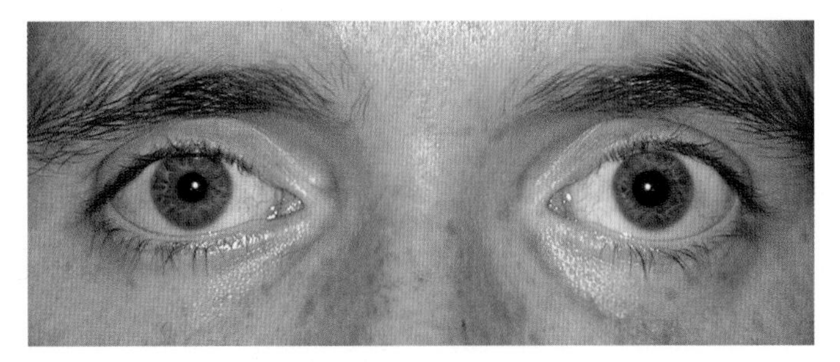

Figure 16-16 Left lower eyelid retraction following orbital fracture repair.

depending on the time of extrusion and the size of the fracture, because scar tissue heals beneath the implant.

8. Lymphedema. Lymphedema is more likely to occur with a lower eyelid crease incision that is curved upward in the lateral canthal area, severing the lymphatic vessel drainage, particularly from the upper eyelid. To avoid this complication, the incision should not be extended into the lateral canthal area. The lymphedema may clear slowly over the course of several months.
9. Infraorbital nerve dysfunction. The infraorbital nerve may be damaged in the initial injury or by the surgeon during exploration of the orbital floor. This damage results in numbness, hypesthesia, or anesthesia in the area of sensory distribution of the nerve. If bone fragments impinge on the nerve, they should be removed. Usually, sensory function of the infraorbital nerve gradually returns over a period of several months to 1 year.

16-10 FRACTURES IN THE PEDIATRIC AGE GROUP

Orbital fractures in children are most commonly due to sports-related injuries. Floor fractures occur most often. Orbital roof fractures also occur more frequently since pneumatization of the frontal sinus absorbs energy from supraorbital rim trauma and the sinuses are not well developed in children. Indications for surgical repair are similar to those in adults, including large fractures, enophthalmos greater than 2 mm, and clinically significant diplopia.

The management of facial and orbital fractures in infants and children is significantly different from the management of adult orbital fractures. Surgical repair of pediatric orbital fractures requires particular attention to potential damage to bony growth plates. For example, injury to permanent tooth buds can occur following maxillary or mandibular fractures and repair. Also, bony overgrowth of internal microplates may require later removal of the hardware in children.

Diplopia, extraocular muscle limitation, and trapdoor or incomplete fractures are more common in children than in adults secondary to increased bone pliability. Consequently, early surgical intervention may be required in the amblyogenic population since extraocular muscle involvement can lead to restrictive strabismus and diplopia. Also, earlier surgical intervention appears to shorten the postoperative recovery time in children, and may be advantageous in this patient population.

SUGGESTED READINGS

Baumann A, Ewers R. Midfacial degloving: An alternative approach for traumatic corrections in the midface. *Int J Oral Maxillofac Surg.* 2001;30(4):272–277.

Brady SM, McMann MA, Mazzoli RA, Bushley DM, Ainbinder DJ, Carroll RB. The diagnosis and management of orbital blowout fractures. *Am J Emerg Med.* 2001; 19:147–154.

Converse JM. On the treatment of blow-out fractures of the orbit. *Plast Reconst Surg.* 1978;62:100–104.

Cruz AA, Eichenberger GCD. Epidemiology and management of orbital fractures. *Current Opinion in Ophthalmology.* 2004;15:416–421.

Eski M, Sahin I, Deveci M, Turegun M, Isik S, Sengezer M. A retrospective analysis of 101 zygomatico-orbital fractures. *Craniofacial Surg.* 2006:17(6):1059–1064.

Garibaldi DC, Iliff NT, Grant MP, Merbs SL. Use of porous polyethylene with embedded titanium in orbital reconstruction: A review of 106 patients. *Ophthalmic Plast Reconstr Surg.* 2007:23(6):439–444.

Gilbard SM, Mafee MF, Lagouros PA, Langer BG. Orbital blowout fractures: The prognostic significance of computed tomography. *Ophthalmology.* 1985;92:1523–1528.

Goldberg RA, Lessner AM, Shorr N, Baylis HI. The transconjunctival approach to the orbital floor and orbital fat: A prospective study. *Ophthalmic Plast Reconstr Surg.* 1990;6:241–246.

Harris GJ. Orbital blow-out fractures: Surgical timing and technique. *Eye.* 2006; 20:1207–1212.

Harris GJ, Garcia GH, Logani SC, Murphy ML. Correlation of preoperative computed tomography and postoperative ocular motility in orbital blow-out fractures. *Ophthalmic Plast Reconstr Surg.* 1998;14:379–390.

Hatton MP, Watkins LM, Rubin PAD. Orbital fractures in children. *Ophthalmic Plast Reconst Surg.* 2001;17:173–179.

Hawes MJ, Dortzbach RK. Surgery on orbital floor fractures: Influence of time of repair and fracture size. *Ophthalmology.* 1983;90:1066–1070.

Hawes MJ, Dortzbach RK. Blow-out fractures of the orbital floor. In: Dortzbach RK, ed. *Ophthalmic Plastic Surgery: Prevention and Management of Complications.* New York: Raven Press, 1994:195–210.

Holk DE, Ng JD, eds. *Evaluation and Treatment of Orbital Fractures.* Philadelphia: Elsevier, 2006.

Hosal BM, Beatty RL. Diplopia and enophthalmos after surgical repair of blowout fracture. *Orbit.* 2002;21:27–33.

Jin HR, Yeon JY, Shin SS, Choi YC, Lee D. Endoscopic versus external repair of orbital blowout fractures. *Otolaryngol Head Neck Surg.* 2007;136(1):38–44.

Kikkawa DO, Lemke BN. Orbital and eyelid anatomy. In: Dortzbach RK, ed. *Ophthalmic Plastic Surgery: Prevention and Management of Complications.* New York: Raven Press, 1994:1–29.

Kim SJ, Lew H, Chun SH, Kook KH, Juan Y, Lee SY. Repair of medial orbital wall fracture: transcaruncular approach. *Orbit.* 2005;24:1–9.

Koorneef L. Orbital septa: anatomy and function. *Ophthalmology.* 1979;86:876–880.

Kwon JH, Moon JH, Kwon MS, Cho JH. The differences of blowout fracture of the inferior orbital wall between children and adults. *Arch Otolaryngol Head Neck Surg.* 2005;131:723–727.

Lemke BN. Anatomy of ocular adnexa and orbit. In: Smith BC, ed. *Ophthalmic Plastic and Reconstructive Surgery,* vol. 1. St. Louis, MO: CV Mosby, 1987:3–74.

Levin LA, Beck RW, Joseph MP, Seiff S, Kraker R. The treatment of traumatic optic neuropathy: the International Optic Nerve Trauma Study. *Ophthalmology*. 1999; 106(7):1268–1277.

Liu D. Blindness after orbital blowout fracture repair. *Ophthalmic Plast Reconst Surg*. 1994;10(3): 206–210.

Poon A, McCluskey PJ, Hill DA. Eye injuries in patients with major trauma. *J Trauma*. 1999;46:494–499.

Putterman AM, Stevens T, Urist MJ. Nonsurgical management of blow-out fractures of the orbital floor. *Am J Ophthalmol*. 1974;77:232–239.

Seider N, Gilboa M, Miller B, Hadar RS, Beiran I. Orbital fractures complicated by late enophthalmos: Higher prevalence in patients with multiple trauma. *Ophthalmic Plast Reconstr Surg*. 2007;23(2):115–118.

Sires BS, Stanley RB Jr, Levine LM. Oculocardiac reflex caused by orbital floor trapdoor fracture: an indication for urgent repair. *Arch Ophthalmol* 1998;116(7): 955–956.

Su GW, Harris GJ. Combined inferior and medial surgical approaches and overlapping thin implants for orbital floor and medial wall fractures. *Ophthalmic Plast Reconstr Surg*. 2006;22(6):420–423.

Yang WG, Chen CT, Tsay PK, deVilla GH, Tsai YJ, Chen YR. Outcome for traumatic optic neuropathy- Surgical versus nonsurgical treatment. *Ann Plast Surg*. 2004;52(1):36–42.

Yu-Wai-Man P, Griffiths PG. Steroids for traumatic optic neuropathy. *Cochrane Database of Systematic Reviews* 2007, Issue 4. Art. No.: CD006032.

Zide BM, Jelks GW. *Surgical Anatomy of the Orbit*. New York: Raven Press, 1985.

17

Evaluation and Spectrum of Orbital Diseases

RAYMOND S. DOUGLAS, MD, ROBERT A. GOLDBERG, MD, AND CATHERINE J. HWANG, MD

Although orbital disorders are not frequently encountered in the comprehensive ophthalmologist's practice, it is essential to be able to diagnose patients with orbital disease and manage them accordingly. Various disease processes can affect the orbit. This chapter endeavors to provide a thoughtful, stepwise, and logical approach to the evaluation of orbital disease. The discussion begins with differential diagnosis, adds an intelligent history-taking and physical examination, and then focuses on efficient use of diagnostic tests to finally arrive at the correct diagnosis. The staging and management of two common orbital disorders, orbital inflammation and thyroid-associated ophthalmopathy, will also be discussed.

17-1 DIFFERENTIAL DIAGNOSIS

The differential diagnosis of orbital disease is extensive, and most listings of orbital disease divide the causes between histopathologic and mechanistic categories.[1–3] This type of grouping is intellectually sound and scientifically useful but does not provide a framework that the clinical practitioner can easily grasp and directly use in sorting through the differential diagnosis of any given patient. In broad terms, orbital disease can be considered in terms of location, extent, and biologic activity.[4] The classification used in this chapter is broken down along clinical lines and takes advantage of the fact that the orbit has a somewhat limited repertoire of ways that it can respond to pathologic conditions.

Orbital disease can be categorized into five basic clinical patterns: inflammatory, mass effect, structural, vascular, and functional. Although many cases cross over into several categories, the vast majority of clinical presentations fit predominantly into one of these patterns. As the clinician walks through each step of the evaluation process—history, physical examination, laboratory testing, orbital imaging—a conscious effort should be made to categorize the presentation within this framework.

If the practitioner approaches orbital disease with this framework of discrete patterns of clinical presentation, then at every step of the diagnostic pathway (history, physical examination, orbital imaging studies, and special tests), he or she can draw from a defined set of differential diagnoses that characterize each pattern of orbital disease and use that information to efficiently and confidently orchestrate diagnosis and management. Often, as the practitioner moves along this diagnostic pathway, a difficult decision encountered is whether to perform an orbital biopsy. This framework can help guide the clinician in distinguishing cases requiring tissue for histopathologic evaluation from cases that can be safely managed, at least initially, without the security of a tissue diagnosis.

17-1-1 *Inflammatory Clinical Pattern.* A large percentage of orbital diseases have orbital inflammation as their primary pattern of clinical presentation (Table 17-1). These cases can be further broken down into acute inflammation (onset over hours to days), subacute inflammation (onset over days to weeks), and chronic inflammation (onset over weeks to months). The classical signs of inflammation are present: pain, redness, edema and chemosis, heat, and eventually dysfunction.

TABLE 17-1 Inflammatory Pattern of Presentation

Acute (Days)
Infection: preseptal cellulitis, orbital cellulitis, abscess
Acute idiopathic inflammation: scleritis, myositis, diffuse anterior, apical
Fulminant thyroid-related orbitopathy
Fulminant neoplasia
Hemorrhage into existing lesion: lymphangioma, hematic cyst, bone cyst
Subacute (Days to Weeks)
Infection: fungal, opportunistic
Specific: thyroid-related orbitopathy, Wegener syndrome, sarcoidosis, vasculitis, etc.
Nonspecific idiopathic ("pseudotumor")
Diffuse
Localized: scleritis, myositis, dacryoadenitis, perioptic neuritis
Chronic (Weeks to Months)
Idiopathic sclerosing inflammation of orbit
Specific: thyroid-related orbitopathy, Wegener syndrome, sarcoidosis, vasculitis, etc.
Masquerade: neoplasm (primary or metastatic)
Retained foreign body

17-1-2 *Mass Effect Clinical Pattern*. Tumors presenting primarily with mass effect are characterized by displacement of the globe (axial or nonaxial proptosis) and in some cases a palpable eyelid mass (Table 17-2).

17-1-3 *Structural Clinical Pattern*. Orbital diseases that present a structural orbital pattern are characterized by enophthalmos, bony asymmetry produced by major

TABLE 17-2 Mass Effect Pattern of Presentation

Soft Tissue
Localized
Cavernous hemangioma
Peripheral nerve tumor (schwannoma, meningioma)
Lymphoma
Lacrimal gland neoplasms
Optic nerve meningioma
Optic nerve glioma
Other soft tissue neoplasms
Idiopathic sclerosing inflammation of orbit ("pseudotumor")
Metastatic neoplasm
Secondary tumor from paranasal sinuses
In infants and children: rhabdomyosarcoma, metastatic neuroblastoma, capillary hemangioma, lymphangioma
Cystic
Dermoid cyst
Epithelial and lacrimal duct cyst
Mucocele
Lacrimal sac mucocele (dacryocele)
Parasitic cyst (echinococcal, cysticercosis)
Hematocele
Lymphangioma or other hemorrhagic tumor
Bone
Sphenoid wing meningioma
Metastatic neoplasm
Osteoma, osteosarcoma, ossifying fibroma
Xanthomatous bone lesion
Plasmacytoma, myeloma, and other marrow neoplasms
Histiocytosis-X, eosinophilic granuloma
Fibrous dysplasia and other idiopathic ossifying syndromes

TABLE 17-3 Structural Pattern of Presentation

Acquired Structural Alterations
Trauma (including postoperative)
Destructive lesions of bone (dermoid cyst, bone cyst, neoplasm)
Congenital Structural Alterations
Encephalocele, meningocele
Sphenoid wing hypoplasia (neurofibromatosis 1)

TABLE 17-4 Vascular Pattern of Presentation

Dynamic* Lesions
Orbital arteriovenous malformation
Cavernous sinus fistula
Dural arteriovenous malformation (fistula)
Varix

*That is, pulsating or responding to changing venous pressure.

structural shifts in the bony orbital framework, or pulsatile proptosis when the bony barrier between the orbit and the intracranial cavity is missing (Table 17-3). The presence of a structural lesion can often be strongly suspected on these clinical grounds, but orbital imaging studies confirm the diagnosis and characterize the precise anatomic nature of the structural defect.

17-1-4 *Vascular Clinical Pattern*. The grouping of vascular orbital lesions is somewhat problematic in that vascular lesions span the spectrum from true active vascular lesions, such as arteriovenous malformation and orbital varix, to neoplasms of cells of vascular origin, such as hemangiopericytomas. Even though their biologic origin is from vascular tissue, vascular neoplasms behave clinically like soft tissue tumors, do not have the characteristics of active vascular lesions, and, for the purposes of this clinically based classification, are not included in the vascular pattern of presentation. The true active vascular lesions in the orbit are characterized by a clinical pattern of dynamic change, either slow dynamic change related to postural changes in venous pressure in the case of varices and related lesions connected to the venous system, or pulsation, thrill, bruit, and generalized vascular congestion seen in arterial lesions such as arteriovenous malformation or cavernous sinus fistulas (Table 17-4).

17-1-5 *Functional Clinical Pattern*. The functional pattern of presentation is characterized by functional deficit out of proportion to mass or inflammation (Table 17-5). Although primarily optic nerve dysfunction is encountered, occasionally involvement of other neurovascular structures at the orbital apex, with ophthalmoplegia or sensory deficit, is seen. The clinical presentation is characterized by decreased vision with an afferent pupillary defect, or ophthalmoplegia.

TABLE 17-5 Functional Pattern of Presentation

Optic Nerve Tumors
Glioma
Meningioma
Orbital Apical Neoplasms
Lymphoma
Idiopathic sclerosing inflammation of orbit
Tolosa-Hunt syndrome
Compression
Fibrous dysplasia or other bony overgrowths
Sphenoid wing meningioma
Indirect optic nerve trauma

17-2 HISTORY-TAKING

In both the history-taking and the physical examination, the clinician (armed with the differential diagnosis discussed above) needs to "think biologically." What is the pattern of disease in the framework above, and is there evidence for destruction of tissue? Destructive biology, which characterizes neoplasia and sometimes severe inflammation, manifests clinically as loss of function: sensorimotor deficits such as optic neuropathy, limitation of movement, or decreased sensation.

Historical information that should be obtained includes the time course of onset, associated symptoms, and modifying factors; old photographs can be very useful to verify the presence or absence of orbital changes. Historical evidence of infiltration or compression (pain, decreased vision, double vision, numbness) should be carefully sought. Systemic disease affects the orbit, and symptoms of thyroid dysfunction, systemic vasculitis, inflammation, or neoplasia may help refine the differential diagnosis as well as detect generalized disease requiring therapy. Previous trauma or surgery, including nasal, sinus, intracranial, or facial, must not be overlooked.

17-3 PHYSICAL EXAMINATION

A careful examination of the globe and ocular adnexa may offer important clues to the underlying diagnosis. A complete, dilated eye examination should be performed in conjunction with a comprehensive orbital examination, which includes assessment for proptosis, resistance to retropulsion of the globe, palpable orbital masses, associated eyelid abnormalities, ocular pulsations, and orbital bruits. Proptosis is quantified by exophthalmometry. A difference of greater than 2 mm between the two eyes on exophthalmometry is likely pathologic. It should be noted whether the proptosis is axial (indicative of a mass behind the globe, usually intraconal) or if the globe is displaced horizontally or vertically (with the direction of proptosis generally opposite the location of the orbital mass lesion). The location of orbital lesions is often helpful in guiding the differential diagnosis. For example, mucoceles are usually superonasal, while lacrimal gland lesions tend to be centered superotemporally.

General physical examination may include inspection of skin, oropharynx, and nasopharynx; palpation of the lymph nodes; auscultation of the lungs; and neurologic testing when indicated. A more thorough systemic examination could reveal evidence of an occult malignancy (breast or prostate mass) or a systemic inflammatory disorder (rheumatoid arthritis, Wegener's granulomatosis, sarcoidosis).

Evaluation of afferent (visual physiology and sensation) and efferent (extraocular motility) function of the eye is an essential part of the examination. This will assist in localization of the lesion, assessment of disease progression on serial examinations, and decision-making regarding the need for prompt intervention, such as surgery or systemic corticosteroids. Eye examination must include testing of visual acuity, pupillary function and assessment for a relative afferent pupillary defect (Marcus Gunn pupil), confrontation visual fields (with formal perimetry when indicated), extraocular motility, and ocular alignment (alternate cover test), in addition to slit-lamp examination, tonometry, and dilated fundus examination. Refraction is important to confirm that decreased vision is truly refractive in nature. If the vision is not correctable to 20/20, then an explanation must be found (corneal epitheliopathy, cataract, maculopathy, choroidal striae, or optic neuropathy). Dyschromatopsia in the affected eye lends further support for optic nerve involvement in a patient with decreased vision and a relative afferent pupillary defect. Corneal sensation should be evaluated and any evidence of dysfunction of cranial nerve II, III, IV, V, VI, or VII noted. A lesion between the orbital apex and the cavernous sinus may affect multiple cranial nerves with minimal or no proptosis. Forced-duction testing may differentiate restrictive from paretic muscle dysfunction and may be useful in some cases.

Table 17-6 summarizes ocular, periocular, and systemic signs that are clinically significant to orbital disease.

17-4 LABORATORY EVALUATION

Particularly in the case of inflammatory disease, orbital disorders are often manifestations of systemic abnormalities. Laboratory testing not only helps to narrow the differential diagnosis by pinpointing systemic disease that may account for orbital findings, but also may be important in identifying systemic disorders that require treatment independent of the orbital pathology. Systemic disorders that commonly affect the orbit and can be evaluated with laboratory testing include Graves thyroid disease (T_3, T_4, sensitive TSH, anti-TSHR), sarcoidosis (angiotensin-converting enzyme, chest x-ray), Wegener's granulomatosis (antinuclear cytoplasmic antibody), myasthenia gravis (acetylcholine receptor antibodies), and specific autoimmune disorders such as lupus or Sjögren's syndrome.

17-5 ORBITAL IMAGING

Orbital imaging is the cornerstone of diagnosis. Imaging technology is continually improving, allowing the practitioner to increasingly refine the differential diagnosis and make an accurate presumed diagnosis based on the imaging findings.[5]

TABLE 17-6 Clinical Significance of Ocular, Periocular, and Systemic Signs

Signs	Diagnoses to Consider
Ocular	
Subconjunctival salmon-colored lesion	Lymphoma
Granulomatous uveitis/retinal periphlebitis	Sarcoidosis
Dilated and tortuous episcleral vessels/ elevated intraocular pressure/dilated retinal veins	Carotid–cavernous sinus fistula, dural or orbital arteriovenous malformation
Increased intraocular pressure on up gaze	Thyroid-related orbitopathy
Optociliary shunt vessels	Optic nerve meningioma
Orbital/Periocular	
S-shaped lid deformity	Plexiform neurofibroma/lacrimal gland fossa mass
Lid retraction/lid lag	Thyroid-related orbitopathy
Prominent lid veins/proptosis worse on bending over or Valsalva maneuver	Orbital varix
Ocular pulsations	Neurofibromatosis, meningoencephalocele
Orbital bruit	Carotid–cavernous sinus fistula, dural or orbital arteriovenous malformation
Lid ecchymosis	Neuroblastoma, leukemia, lymphangioma; trauma
Unilateral vesicular skin lesions	Herpes zoster ophthalmicus
Enophthalmos	Trauma, chronic sinusitis, metastatic breast cancer (scirrhous carcinoma)
Systemic	
Scalp tenderness	Giant cell arteritis
Prominent temple	Sphenoid wing meningioma
Black eschar in nose or mouth	Mucormycosis, phycomycosis
Café-au-lait spots	Neurofibromatosis
Generalized lymphadenopathy	Lymphoma
Weight loss	Malignant neoplasm
Multiple system infection	Immune system compromise

The comprehensive ophthalmologist should have a basic understanding of the relative advantages and disadvantages of each imaging modality, should know which study should be ordered in different clinical situations, and should be able to order the test (e.g., orientation of view, slice thickness, intravenous contrast) to obtain the most information in an efficient and cost-effective manner. Guidelines for ordering orbital imaging studies are summarized in Table 17-7.

TABLE 17-7 Guidelines for Ordering Orbital Imaging Studies

Study	Most Useful	Less Useful	Contraindications	How to Order
Ultrasonography	Vascular tumors (color-flow Doppler)	Deep orbital tumors		Clarify differential diagnosis
	Anterior inflammations	Bony tumors		Skilled operator required
	Dynamic imaging			
Computed tomography (CT)	Trauma	Orbital apex and cavernous sinus	Pregnancy (relative)	Fine orbital cuts 1.5-mm width at 1.0-mm intervals
	Orbital mass	Intravenous dye with renal dysfunction	Direct coronal scans	
	Bone tumors		Dye allergy	
Magnetic resonance imaging (MRI)	Orbital apex, optic nerve, cavernous sinus, skull base tumors	Bony trauma	Claustrophobia	Clarify differential diagnosis
	Vascular lesions		Metal in patient: pacemaker, ocular foreign body	Orbital surface coil
	Inflammatory lesions			
	Staging Graves disease			
Magnetic resonance angiography (MRA)	High-flow vascular lesions: arteriovenous fistula, cavernous dural fistula	Smaller or low-flow lesions	Claustrophobia	Clarify differential diagnosis
			Metal in patient: pacemaker, ocular foreign body	
			Paramagnetic dye allergy (rare)	
Arteriography	High-flow vascular lesions: arteriovenous fistula, cavernous dural fistula		Dye allergy	Clarify differential diagnosis
	Small lesions			
	Neuro-interventional therapy			

17-5-1 *Ultrasonography*. Orbital ultrasonography has generally been replaced by computed tomography (CT) and magnetic resonance imaging (MRI) in orbital diagnosis, but it still plays an important role in selected instances. In thyroid-associated ophthalmopathy, ultrasound often demonstrates enlarged extraocular muscles,[6] but this finding is nonspecific and does not typically refine the differential diagnosis. Ultrasonography has high resolution in the area of the sclera and optic nerve insertion and is particularly useful for evaluating scleritis and other anterior inflammations that produce sub-Tenon's fluid. Ultrasonography lacks the resolution of CT and MRI in the deep orbit but has one very significant advantage: it is performed in real time so that dynamic changes can be readily observed. For example, with eye movements, the optic nerve can be observed to move around a tumor that is separate from the nerve, differentiating it from a tumor attached to the nerve. Also, vascular tumors can be identified by active pulsation or, in the case of venous lesions, by compressibility and demonstrable change in size with the Valsalva maneuver. Color-flow Doppler ultrasonography is particularly sensitive for demonstrating vascular flow and can demonstrate arterialized, retrograde flow in the orbital veins in cases of cavernous dural fistula or arteriovenous malformation.[7]

17-5-2 *Computed Tomography*. Especially at centers where it is less expensive and more easily obtained, CT is the single most useful orbital imaging modality. Compared to MRI, CT scanning is faster, less expensive, and less sensitive to movement artifact. The resolution and soft tissue contrast are adequate to visualize almost any pathologic orbital process, and the bony resolution is superior to all other modalities, making CT ideal for evaluating orbital trauma or bony tumors. To obtain optimal images, the entire orbit should be scanned in fine resolution; fine 1.5-mm cuts at 1.0-mm intervals provide the best possible detail, although thicker slices suffice for many types of disease conditions. Direct coronal scans are obtained by tilting the patient's neck back, and although coronal scans are sometimes limited by neck mobility or by artifacts from dental fillings, they allow excellent views of the extraocular muscles and optic nerve and provide the best view of the orbit to evaluate the roof or floor (for example, blowout fractures) or the extraocular muscles. Multiplanar reformatting allows coronal and sagittal reconstructions when patient positioning is an issue. Technological advances have also made three-dimensional surface shaded CT reconstructions possible, permitting better spatial resolution. Contrast CT studies provide further information; however, the iodinated intravenous dye may be contraindicated in patients with renal dysfunction (e.g., diabetic patients).

17-5-3 *Magnetic Resonance Imaging*. MRI has become an essential tool in the diagnosis of orbital processes.[8] Technological advances are gradually making MRI cost-competitive to CT, and "open" scanners are reducing the claustrophobia induced by confinement in a tight closed gantry. Nevertheless, at present in most centers, MRI is still more expensive and more difficult for the patient. MRI provides soft tissue and bone marrow resolution superior to CT and is particularly useful to evaluate tumors of the cavernous sinus and skull base, including optic nerve tumors that enter the cranial cavity. The radiologist has a number of tools to improve orbital images, including surface coils for increased spatial resolution, various fat-suppression protocols, and intravenous contrast agents (gadolinium). T2-weighted images may be useful for staging Graves orbitopathy by assessing muscle edema, an indicator of active inflammation. Thus, acute and chronic stages of Graves disease can be discriminated. Because bone is not differentiated from air, MRI is not useful for evaluating orbital fractures or differentiating bone and calcium.

MRI and CT can be synergistic in their contribution to diagnosis and, particularly in difficult cases, both studies may be better than either alone. The best results are obtained when the radiologist knows the differential diagnosis so that the appropriate studies can be obtained. Therefore, it is essential to provide the radiologist with as much clinical information as possible and to review the films with the radiologist.

17-5-4 *Angiography and Arteriography.* In the case of orbital vascular lesions characterized by flowing blood and vascular lesions of the cavernous sinus, standard orbital imaging studies often need to be supplemented by specific techniques to evaluate vascular flow patterns. Noninvasive modalities such as magnetic resonance angiography (MRA) and computed tomographic angiography (CTA) have for the most part replaced conventional catheter angiography in the initial evaluation of patients.[9] Standard arteriography, however, is still the gold standard for detecting and characterizing the most subtle lesions, and in patients where a lesion is highly suspected and MRA and CTA findings are equivocal, catheter arteriography should be performed. In addition, catheter angiography allows direct treatment by a transarterial or transvenous route. Arteriography carries a small but real risk of serious complications such as stroke. Working closely with the radiologist is imperative to achieve good diagnostic results with minimal risk when dealing with suspected orbital vascular tumors.

17-6 ORBITAL BIOPSY

Orbital biopsy must be approached with respect. To maximally benefit a patient whose tissue is required for diagnosis, a number of factors must be taken into account. The decision to perform biopsy should be weighed against the relative risks and benefits. In general, the threshold for biopsy should be low, although in the setting of lesions that are benign clinically and radiographically, observation may be appropriate. Also, certain inflammations may be appropriately treated medically, under close observation. Fine-needle aspiration biopsy, in a center with a skilled cytopathologist, is a very useful tool that can obviate the need for a trip to the operating room in cases such as lymphoma or metastatic carcinoma that would not otherwise need surgery.[10] Open biopsy must be performed with care and skill to produce a diagnostic tissue sample with as little damage as possible to normal structures.[11] The removed tissue must be handled gently and fixed immediately; preoperative consultation with a pathologist will identify any special handling of the tissue or special fixatives that might be necessary.

17-7 MANAGEMENT OF ORBITAL DISORDERS

17-7-1 *Orbital Inflammation.* An inflamed orbit with redness and compromised ophthalmic function is a dramatic presentation that, particularly in the fulminant form, can be frightening for both patient and diagnostician. As with all orbital disease, a careful, methodical, and studied approach to formulating and working through a differential diagnosis is required. The history helps to sort through possible antecedent factors such as trauma, foreign body, sinus disease, and pre-existing (local or systemic) disease, including thyroid dysfunction. The history also allows the clinician to characterize the inflammatory disease with regard to timing of onset: Is the presentation acute (evolving over days), subacute (days to weeks), or chronic (weeks to months)? These major categories of onset have significance with regard to constructing a differential diagnosis (see Table 17-1).

It is particularly important to identify treatable inflammations. Obvious in this group is infection, which requires specific and sometimes emergent treatment with antibiotics or surgery. Other inflammations that might respond to treatment include surgical diseases, such as retained foreign body, abscess, or neoplasia, or systemic diseases, such as Wegener's granulomatosis or sarcoidosis, which require systemic treatment that may be life-saving as well as vision-saving.

Because of its overwhelming statistical prominence in orbital disease, thyroid-related orbitopathy should be in the differential diagnosis of virtually every case of orbital inflammation. Atypical presentations of Graves orbitopathy, such as strikingly asymmetric or acute onsets, occur and must be considered.

Unfortunately, the current state of medical knowledge does not allow for a specific diagnosis in many cases of orbital inflammation—hence the "generic" diagnosis idiopathic orbital inflammatory disease. This condition can take an acute, subacute, or chronic form and can involve a specific orbital structure (scleritis, myositis, dacryoadenitis, or perioptic neuritis, for example) or multiple orbital structures. The outdated term *pseudotumor* lumps together a rich variety of specific and nonspecific, diffuse and localized inflammatory syndromes. It should be abandoned for terminology that is as precise as possible with regard to both the localization and the cause of the inflammation.

A prime example of a specific type of inflammation that should not be called a pseudotumor is idiopathic sclerosing orbital inflammatory tumor.[12] This is a type of nonspecific inflammation that has a characteristic pathologic picture with desmoplasia and considerable fibrosis. These tumors form a slow-growing orbital mass that can be associated with significant infiltration and loss of function (Fig. 17-1). Rather than being a "burned-out" acute nonspecific inflammation, these tumors probably represent an entirely different disease and should be treated early and aggressively. The optimal treatment has not been identified, but corticosteroids, surgical debulking, radiotherapy, and immunosuppression with cytotoxic drugs may play a role in selected cases.

17-7-2 *Thyroid-Associated Ophthalmopathy.* Thyroid-associated ophthalmopathy (TAO) is by far the most common disease entity producing orbital signs and symptoms and should always be considered in the differential diagnosis of a patient with

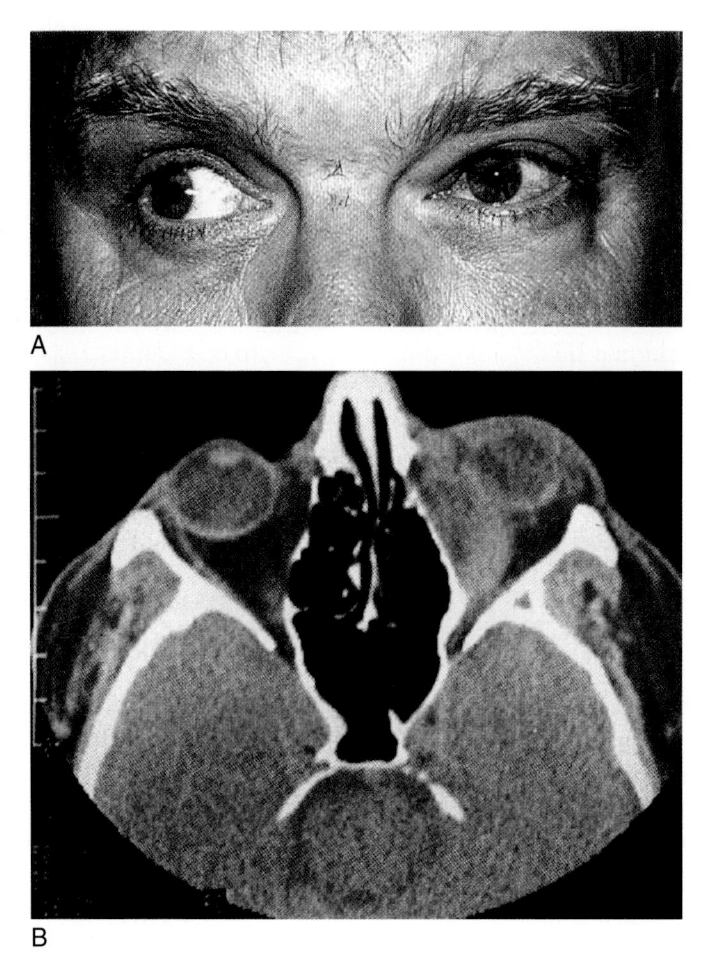

Figure 17-1 Idiopathic sclerosing orbital inflammatory tumor. (A) 40-year-old man with slowly progressive painful proptosis and extraocular motility limitation. (B) Axial CT demonstrates homogeneous medial orbital mass involving medial rectus muscle and apex. Biopsy demonstrated mixed inflammatory response with marked fibrosis, consistent with idiopathic sclerosing inflammatory tumor of orbit. Tumor failed to respond to corticosteroids, radiation, and cytotoxic drugs, and patient eventually required exenteration for pain control.

proptosis or orbital inflammation. Although the classic presentation—with bilateral proptosis, inflammation, extraocular motility restriction, and eyelid retraction—is easily recognized, atypical presentations such as asymmetric or purely unilateral disease, acute severe inflammation, myositis, or subtle noninflamed disease are not infrequent and may be difficult to diagnose, particularly if the diagnostician fails to consider the diagnosis of Graves disease.

TAO is primarily a clinical diagnosis. No laboratory test definitively establishes the diagnosis of thyroid-associated orbitopathy. Patients may be hyperthyroid, euthyroid, or hypothyroid at presentation, and an occasional patient with non-Graves proptosis has thyroid dysfunction coincidentally. Nevertheless, the demonstration of autonomous thyroid functioning with an abnormally low TSH test makes the diagnosis of Graves thyroid disease and therefore Graves orbitopathy extremely likely. Perhaps the most important aspect of assessing thyroid function is to identify patients with hypothyroidism or hyperthyroidism, who should be evaluated by an internist or endocrinologist for long-term management of the thyroid component of the disease.

The pathogenesis of TAO is complex, and it seems that autoimmunity plays a large role. Early in the disease, orbital pathology shows infiltration by immunocompetent cells, predominantly T lymphocytes, mast cells, and mononuclear cells, and an accumulation of glycosaminoglycans with subsequent volume expansion. Cytokines, including IFN-γ, TNF-α, and IL-1, have been found associated with the T-cell infiltrate in the connective tissues. Later in the disease fibrotic changes occur. The structures mainly affected in the disease process are the extraocular muscles and the orbital fatty connective tissue. Some patients have primarily an enlargement of the extraocular muscles, while others have increased orbital fat volume with normal muscles. The reasons for the differing presentations is still being investigated but may be related to the phenotype of the orbital fibroblasts and the various cytokines produced locally.[13]

Clinically significant TAO occurs in approximately 10% to 45% of patients with Graves disease. Patients with TAO typically have a self-limited course, becoming quiescent within 3 to 5 years of onset, although chronic courses can occur.[14] When a patient with TAO is evaluated, it is critical to stage the disease: active, inflammatory phase or congestive, postinflammatory phase. TAO in most patients follows a fairly predictable course with an early inflammatory stage lasting 6 months to 2 years. This phase is characterized clinically by inflammatory signs including eyelid erythema and edema, caruncular and conjunctival injection and edema, and also by fluctuations that can occur daily or weekly. Other manifestations of TAO include upper lid retraction with lateral flare, lower lid retraction, exposure keratitis, diplopia, and exophthalmos. A clinical assessment scale is often used to follow patients and assess disease activity, but a universal classification system is needed in order to better understand the disease course. Imaging studies typically show fusiform expansion of one or more of the extraocular muscles, most often with tendon sparing. The finding of large muscles (greater then 9 mm in width) or a "crowded" orbital apex indicates patients at risk for compressive optic neuropathy,[15] as does restrictive myopathy.[16]

CT without contrast is the most widely used imaging tool in the diagnosis of TAO. Direct axial and coronal fine cuts (2 to 3 mm) are used for assessing the relationship between the extraocular muscles and the optic nerve and are useful for surgical planning. MRI has also been used more in recent years for the evaluation of TAO, as it may be helpful in assessing disease activity. Multiple techniques have been used, including surface coils and various fat-suppression protocols to enhance its sensitivity and specificity. Ultrasonography has limited utility and often shows enlarged extraocular muscles with tendon sparing but does not rule out other disorders; it is therefore not very useful in making treatment or diagnostic decisions, although some evidence suggests that it may be useful in staging the disease.[17] A reasonable guideline is to use orbital imaging as an aid with the differential diagnosis in atypical cases, to evaluate the optic nerve in cases of compressive optic neuropathy,

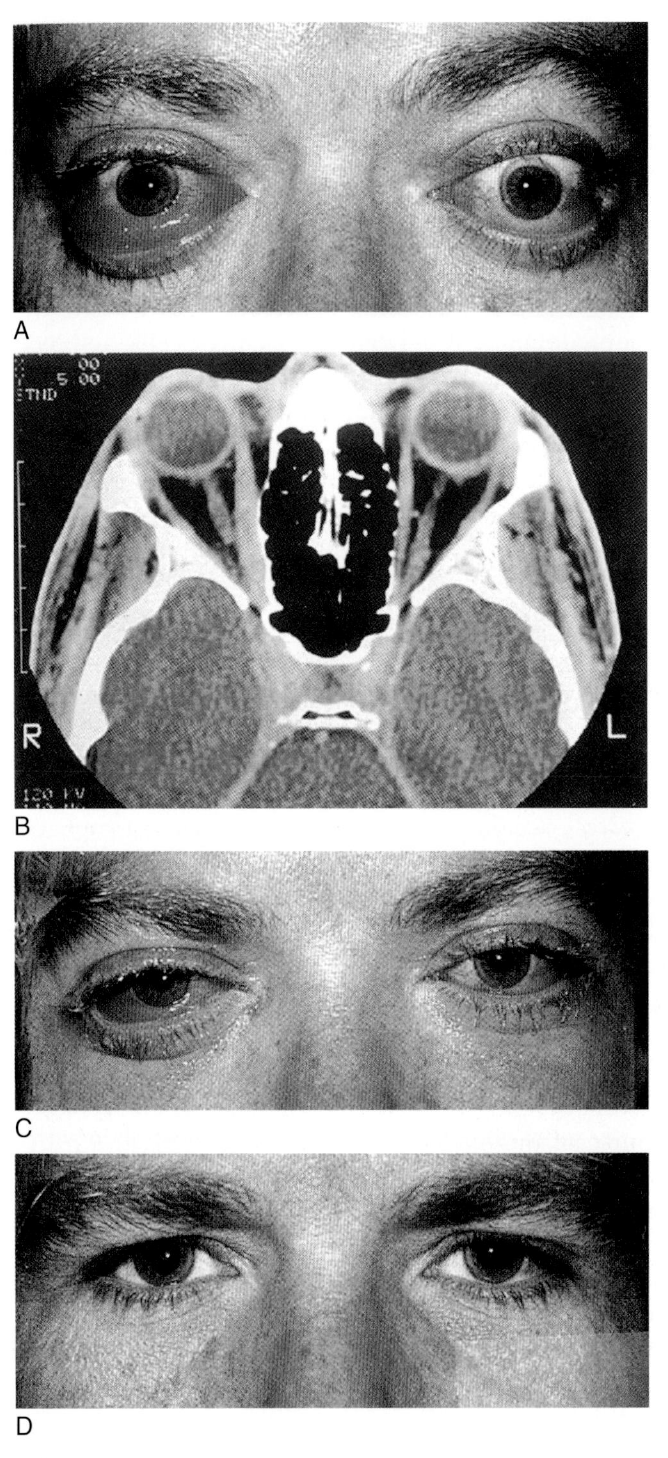

Figure 17-2 Thyroid-associated ophthalmopathy. (A) 35-year-old man developed bilateral acute orbital cellulitis as initial onset of thyroid-associated ophthalmopathy. Lateral cantholysis and pulsed intravenous corticosteroids were initial therapy. (B) Axial CT demonstrates proptosis and moderate enlargement of medial rectus muscle belly. (C) After 1 week of corticosteroid therapy, inflammation decreased significantly. Corticosteroids were tapered over a 3-month period. (D) 1 year later, well after corticosteroids were discontinued, patient demonstrates minimal inflammation; no surgery was required.

as a method to document progression in association with clinical signs and symptoms, or as a planning tool for possible orbital decompression surgery.

TAO treatment has been evolving throughout the years. As a paradigm, thyroid function is optimized and medical therapy is directed to decrease the immune response. Corticosteroids remain the mainstay of treatment, but specific therapies directed at the immune system are being investigated. In addition, smoking cessation is critical in the management of patients with TAO since smokers tend to have more severe ophthalmopathy than nonsmokers.

During the inflammatory phase, treatment may include anti-inflammatory medication such as corticosteroids or radiotherapy (Fig. 17-2).[18] One strategy is to offer a 2-month tapering course of corticosteroids, and if there is a rebound when the corticosteroids are tapered, then radiotherapy (20 Gy given in 10 fractions) is offered along with another course of corticosteroids. Surgery is less predictable and less successful when performed during the inflammatory phase and, except for unusual or emergent circumstances (such as marked exposure keratopathy or severe compressive optic neuropathy unresponsive to anti-inflammatory therapy), is better deferred until the disease stabilizes into the postinflammatory or chronic phase.

Although there can still be waxing and waning smoldering inflammation, the postinflammatory phase is generally characterized by stability and lack of active inflammation, and staged reconstructive surgery is often performed at this time (Fig. 17-3).[19] The order of reconstruction is orbital decompression, strabismus surgery, and last eyelid surgery. The postinflammatory phase is often characterized by considerable orbital congestion related to venous stasis in a compressed orbit and is manifested clinically by edema, chemosis, and commonly a painful pressure sensation. These congestive symptoms must be differentiated from frank inflammation, because congestive disease in the postinflammatory stage responds poorly to anti-inflammatory medications but often responds well to orbital apical decompression surgery, which restores venous outflow.

Compressive optic neuropathy is a vision-threatening complication of Graves ophthalmopathy that requires careful management.[20] It can occur in inflamed orbits early in the course of the disease or late, in the postinflammatory stage, and in proptotic or nonproptotic orbits. It is often but not always associated with orbital apical crowding on imaging studies and with increased intraocular pressure on up gaze. In the inflammatory stage, anti-inflammatory therapy is often effective. Because radiotherapy takes one or more months for maximal effect, corticosteroid therapy is generally preferred for all but the mildest cases, and pulsed corticosteroids can be used in more severe cases. Surgical decompression of the orbital apex is an effective immediate treatment of compressive neuropathy and is used for patients who do not respond quickly (days to weeks) to medical treatment. For the most severe cases—for example, with counting-fingers vision or dense afferent pupillary defect—surgery and anti-inflammatory therapy are provided simultaneously. In the postinflammatory stage, medical therapy is less effective and surgery is the first line of treatment. The optic nerve has considerable reserve when it is compressed slowly, and even cases with severe loss of vision can respond to therapy.

17-7-3 *Benign Tumors.* Benign tumors are characterized biologically by lack of infiltration into surrounding tissues. Therefore, they are often easily dissected from the

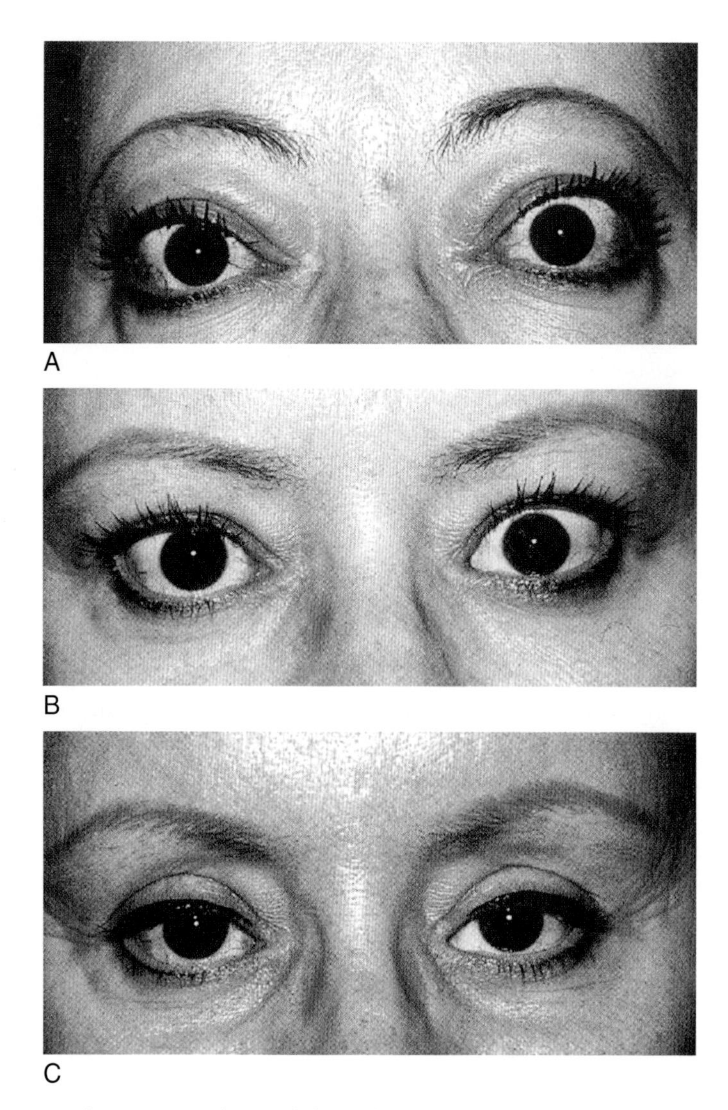

Figure 17-3 Postinflammatory phase of thyroid-associated ophthalmopathy. (A) Patient with stable congestive thyroid-associated ophthalmopathy, 2 years into course. No compressive optic neuropathy is present, but patient has swelling and periocular pressure sensation related to orbital congestion, as well as exposure keratopathy from proptosis. (B) Same patient after orbital decompression: edema and chemosis, as well as orbital pressure sensation, improved following release of orbital apical crowding and venous congestion. When proptosis was reduced, exposure keratopathy was slightly improved. (C) Same patient following eyelid repositioning surgery; exposure keratopathy substantially improved.

orbit, and surgery is indicated when the mass produces symptoms or signs. Orbital imaging studies occasionally pick up small benign orbital tumors. If these are asymptomatic, the best management is generally observation; many benign tumors such as schwannoma and cavernous hemangioma grow very slowly if at all. Benign masses should be excised completely if possible to prevent recurrence. Benign mixed tumor of the lacrimal gland is an example of a tumor that can recur in malignant fashion if not completely excised; lacrimal gland tumors should be approached with care.[21] Recurrences can be much more difficult to manage than the initial tumor because of scar tissue formation.

Some tumors—for example, dermoid cysts—are somewhat difficult to dissect because of chronic low-grade inflammation and possible erosion into surrounding bone; careful dissection and sometimes removal of significant amounts of bone are required. Other benign tumors—for example, lymphangioma and neurofibroma—tend to grow diffusely and intertwine extensively with normal structures, making complete removal difficult or impossible without endangering function. In these cases, subtotal resection is preferable. Optic nerve meningiomas cannot be surgically removed without causing functional damage to the nerve, so surgery is reserved for nonfunctioning nerves or for tumors that have been documented by gadolinium MRI to be growing into the cavernous sinus.

17-7-4 *Vascular Tumors.* From a treatment standpoint, orbital vascular tumors can be categorized by the degree of flow through the lesion.[22] Low-flow vascular lesions such as orbital varices do not always require treatment. If treatment becomes necessary because of growth, compression of vital structures, or disfigurement, these lesions can be removed surgically with wide exposure and careful identification of the feeding veins. The lesions are fragile and surgery is difficult.

High-flow lesions represent abnormal connections between the arterial and venous circulations. These lesions often cause significant functional problems because of the profound alterations in blood flow. High-flow lesions are best treated with a multidisciplinary approach that includes neurovascular embolization combined with surgery.[23]

Capillary hemangiomas and lymphangiomas are examples of tumors that originate from vascular tissue but do not have abnormal connections to the vascular system. They can be removed surgically.[24–26] Capillary hemangiomas, particularly in the growing phase over the first year or two of life, often respond to oral or injected corticosteroids.[27]

17-7-5 *Malignant Tumors.* Malignant neoplasms have the biologic potential to spread aggressively in a localized area and to metastasize to distant sites. Decision-making must take this tendency into account. In general, if careful evaluation suggests that the tumor has not metastasized, cure is possible with complete local resection. In the orbit, resection often but not always involves removal of the globe. If a previous biopsy has been performed, the tract of the biopsy is included in the resection. Incisions for biopsies should be planned with this eventuality in mind. If the tumor has metastasized, there is usually not much role for surgery beyond obtaining an accurate biopsy or palliation. Tumors metastatic to the orbit from elsewhere in the body often respond to radiotherapy.[28,29]

Management decisions are made from permanent histopathologic material and in association with oncologists, radiotherapists, and related surgical specialists. Appropriate surgical treatment of malignant lesions can be effected only when coordinated with chemotherapy, immunotherapy, and radiation therapy. The needs and desires of the patient and family are of paramount importance in the application of all treatment protocols.

REFERENCES

1. Rootman J. Frequency and differential diagnosis of orbital disease. In: Rootman J, ed. *Diseases of the Orbit: A Multidisciplinary Approach*. Philadelphia: JB Lippincott, 1988:119–139.
2. Henderson J. *Orbital Tumors*. New York: Raven Press, 1994.
3. Kennedy RE. An evaluation of 820 orbital cases. *Trans Am Ophthalmol Soc*. 1984;82:134–157.
4. Krohel GB, Stewart WB, Chavis RM. *Orbital Disease: A Practical Approach*. New York: Grune & Stratton, 1981.
5. Lee AG, Brazis PW, Garrity JA, White M. Imaging for neuro-ophthalmic and orbital disease. *Am J Ophthalmol*. 2004;138:852–862.
6. Demer JL, Kerman BM. Comparison of standardized echography with magnetic resonance imaging to measure extraocular muscle size. *Am J Ophthalmol*. 1994;118:351–361.
7. Lieb WE. Color Doppler imaging of the eye and orbit. *Radiol Clin North Am*. 1998;36:1059–1071.
8. Lemke AJ, Kazi I, Felix R. Magnetic resonance imaging of orbital tumors. *Eur Radiol*. 2006;16:2207–2219.
9. Green D, Parker D. CTA and MRA: visualization without catheterization. *Semin Ultrasound CT MR*. 2003;24:185–191.
10. Glasgow BJ, Layfield LJ. Fine-needle aspiration biopsy of orbital and periorbital masses. *Diagn Cytopathol*. 1991;7:132–141.
11. Rootman J, Stewart B, Goldberg RA. *Atlas of Orbital Surgery*. New York: Raven Press, 1995.
12. Gordon LK. Orbital inflammatory disease: a diagnostic and therapeutic challenge. *Eye*. 2006;20:1196–1206.
13. Smith TJ. The putative role of fibroblasts in the pathogenesis of Graves' disease: evidence for the involvement of the insulin-like growth factor-1 receptor in fibroblast activation. *Autoimmunity*. 2003;36:409–415.
14. Rundle F, Wilson C. Ophthalmoplegia in Graves disease. *Clin Sci*. 1944;5:17–29.
15. Feldon SE, Muramatsu S, Weiner JM. Clinical classification of Graves' ophthalmopathy. Identification of risk factors for optic neuropathy. *Arch Ophthalmol*. 1984;102: 1469–1472.
16. Tanenbaum M, McCord CD Jr., Nunery WR. Graves' ophthalmopathy. In: McCord CD Jr., Tanenbaum M, eds. *Oculoplastic Surgery*. New York: Raven Press, 1995: 379–416.
17. Prummel MF, Suttorp-Schulten MS, Wiersinga WM, Verbeek AM, Mourits MP, Koornneef L. A new ultrasonographic method to detect disease activity and predict response to immunosuppressive treatment in Graves ophthalmopathy. *Ophthalmology*. 1993;100:556–561.
18. Marcocci C, Marino M, Rocchi R, Menconi F, Morabito E, Pinchera A. Novel aspects of immunosuppressive and radiotherapy management of Graves' ophthalmopathy. *J Endocrinol Invest*. 2004;27:272–280.
19. Shorr N, Seiff SR. The four stages of surgical rehabilitation of the patient with dysthyroid ophthalmopathy. *Ophthalmology*. 1986;93:476–483.
20. Neigel JM, Rootman J, Belkin RI, Nugent RA, Drance SM, Beattie CW, Spinelli JA. Dysthyroid optic neuropathy. The crowded orbital apex syndrome. *Ophthalmology*. 1988;95:1515–1521.
21. Stewart WB, Krohel GB, Wright JE. Lacrimal gland and fossa lesions: an approach to diagnosis and management. *Ophthalmology*. 1979;86:886–895.

22. Harris GJ. Orbital vascular malformations: a consensus statement on terminology and its clinical implications. *Am J Ophthalmol.* 1999;127:453–455.
23. Rootman J, Kao SC, Graeb DA. Multidisciplinary approaches to complicated vascular lesions of the orbit. *Ophthalmology.* 1992;99:1440–1446.
24. Deans RM, Harris GJ, Kivlin JD. Surgical dissection of capillary hemangiomas. An alternative to intralesional corticosteroids. *Arch Ophthalmol.* 1992;110:1743–1747.
25. Harris GJ, Sakol PJ, Bonavolonta G, De Conciliis C. An analysis of thirty cases of orbital lymphangioma. Pathophysiologic considerations and management recommendations. *Ophthalmology.* 1990;97:1583–1592.
26. Walker RS, Custer PL, Nerad JA. Surgical excision of periorbital capillary hemangiomas. *Ophthalmology.* 1994;101:1333–1340.
27. Haik BG, Karcioglu ZA, Gordon RA, Pechous BP. Capillary hemangioma (infantile periocular hemangioma). *Surv Ophthalmol.* 1994;38:399–426.
28. Goldberg RA, Rootman J, Cline RA. Tumors metastatic to the orbit: a changing picture. *Surv Ophthalmol.* 1990;35:1–24.
29. Ahmad SM, Esmaeli B. Metastatic tumors of the orbit and ocular adnexa. *Curr Opin Ophthalmol.* 2007;18:405–413.

18

Surgical Exploration of the Orbit

PETER J. DOLMAN, MD, FRCSC

The orbit comprises the globe and optic nerve surrounded by a complex tangle of muscles, nerves, and vessels, all cushioned in pockets of fat. While surgery in the anterior orbit is readily performed, the challenge increases significantly for deeper orbital pathology because the bony walls on four sides and the eyeball and lid structures anteriorly limit both access and visibility. The apex is a particularly difficult area because so many vital structures converge in its narrow confines.

18-1 PREOPERATIVE PLANNING

The history and physical examination help narrow the differential diagnosis so that appropriate imaging and special investigations may be arranged. The urgency of these diagnostic tests to allow appropriate medical or surgical intervention is partly determined by the speed of symptom onset and by the presence of significant pain or progressive functional impairment such as vision loss or diplopia.

Computed tomography (CT) scans are usually readily available and help define the tissue characteristics and location of an orbital lesion. Reformatting allows coronal, sagittal, and 3-D views without repositioning the patient, although a true coronal CT scan may be requested if a distensible varix is suspected. Contrast CT scans may be useful for assessing the vascularity of the lesion but require an evaluation of renal function.

Magnetic resonance (MR) scans may characterize certain soft tissue features better, identifying fluid levels and determining whether a lesion involves normal anatomic structures such as the optic nerve, muscle, or lacrimal gland. They are particularly useful in evaluating lesions of the optic nerve and chiasm.

Ultrasounds may help to define certain superficial orbital lesions (distinguishing a lymphoma from a pleomorphic adenoma in the lacrimal gland, for example) and are very useful in assessing intraocular pathology.

Positron emission tomography (PET) scans may help determine the presence of recurrent malignancy or lymphoma in a previously operated or treated site and whole body evaluation may be helpful for staging lymphomas . A trained neuroradiologist can help interpret a complex image.

In general, well-circumscribed, accessible lesions are excised in toto. Poorly defined, infiltrative lesions and those causing tissue destruction (suggestive of malignancy or aggressive inflammation) usually are biopsied, either by needle or with surgery. Most lacrimal gland lesions are biopsied, although a suspected pleomorphic adenoma should be completely excised, avoiding violating the capsule. Abscesses and hematomas causing a compartment syndrome usually require prompt surgical drainage. Small discrete lesions in an area that is difficult to reach surgically and that appear slowly progressive with no visual consequences may be observed with serial clinical examinations and imaging.

Lesions involving the intracranial space, sinuses, or skull base may require the assistance of the neurosurgery, otorhinolaryngology, or craniofacial team. Certain vascular lesions, such as arteriovenous fistulas and venous malformations, are best treated with the assistance of an interventional neuroradiologist or neurosurgeon. A plastic or craniofacial surgeon may help reconstruct large defects resulting from resection of large malignancies or aggressive infections.

The patient should be evaluated preoperatively by all potential surgical team members, as well as by the anesthesiologist if there are medical concerns, and by an oncologist if there is a known malignancy elsewhere and metastasis is suspected. In most cases, a biopsy is performed first to confirm a malignancy, and then further treatment is determined based on the pathology results and subsequent staging by the oncology team.

Patients must be fully informed about their condition and shown their imaging studies. The practitioner must explain the planned surgery, including its purpose, usual recovery period, and potential complications. Often it is helpful to have other family members present during this discussion.

18-2 INTRAOPERATIVE CONSIDERATIONS

Sufficient time should be booked to allow the surgery to proceed in a non-rushed manner. Imaging studies should be visible in the operating suite for intraoperative consultation. Local anesthesia with sedation may be adequate for superficial lesions, including lacrimal gland biopsies. General anesthesia is usually required for deeper lesions or more complex procedures. The anesthesiologist may keep the patient hypotensive to reduce intraoperative bleeding.

The pathologist should be notified if a rush specimen is planned and should advise how tissue should be sent to the laboratory. Many pathologists prefer that specimens are sent fresh to allow gene sequencing, immunostaining, or fixing in media like glutaraldehyde for electron microscopy. If a specimen will be left for several hours before processing, it is often wise to submit a portion in formaldehyde.

During biopsy, the surgeon should obtain a sufficiently large piece to allow interpretation, avoid using cautery on the biopsied tissue, and ensure that the tissue is delicately handled by both the surgeons and the assisting nurses when it is placed in the vial for transfer. The surgeon should describe the location of the lesion and provide some history and a suspected diagnosis to help the pathologist plan appropriate stains and to assist interpretation.

In cases of possible infection, pus or inflamed tissue should be submitted in culture media, and the surgeon should request fungal and tuberculosis cultures if hard tissue suspicious for granulomas is biopsied.

Viewing of the surgical site may be helped with surgical loupes, often combined with a headlight. The operating microscope provides greater magnification for microdissection in sensitive areas, such as optic nerve sheath decompressions. The endoscope is increasingly being employed to view posterior orbital fracture sites or to inspect deep pathology.

18-3 SURGICAL APPROACHES

The surgical approach is chosen preoperatively to provide the most direct access with best visualization and least risk of injury to critical orbital structures. There are five orbitotomy approaches: anterior, lateral, trans-sinus, transcranial, and combined.

18-3-1 *Anterior Orbitotomy.* Anterior access to the orbit is possible through the periorbital skin or through the conjunctiva. Most lesions in the anterior half of the orbit and certain decompressible lesions (like a cavernous hemangioma) from the posterior half of the orbit may be removed from this route, without requiring bone removal.

18-3-1-1 *Transcutaneous.* Skin incisions are chosen in relaxed skin tension lines to reduce postoperative scarring (Fig. 18-1).

A *sub-brow incision* (Fig. 18-1A) affords direct access for lesions involving the superior orbital rim, orbital roof, or frontal sinus (such as a fronto-ethmoidal mucocele). Care must be taken to slant the incision inferiorly to avoid cutting the brow hair roots, and the surgeon must be conscious of the supraorbital nerve coursing superiorly from the notch. A segment of the rim may be excised to improve exposure.

The *Lynch incision* (Fig. 18-1B) curves perpendicular to the medial canthus immediately lateral to the angular vein. A variation on this approach is to create a smaller parallel incision immediately medial to this vessel. The periosteum is opened with a monopolar electrocautery and stripped over the anterior lacrimal crest to expose the lacrimal sac for biopsy or excision of neoplasms. Lateral displacement of the sac provides access to the medial subperiosteal space to reduce a medial wall fracture, to decompress a tight orbit, to drain subperiosteal fluid collections, or to biopsy a lesion in the medial orbit or ethmoid sinus (Fig. 18-2). Caution must be taken to identify and cauterize the anterior and posterior ethmoidal vessels, which are located 24 mm and 36 mm, respectively, posterior to the anterior lacrimal crest. A coronal CT scan should be reviewed to assess for an inferiorly displaced

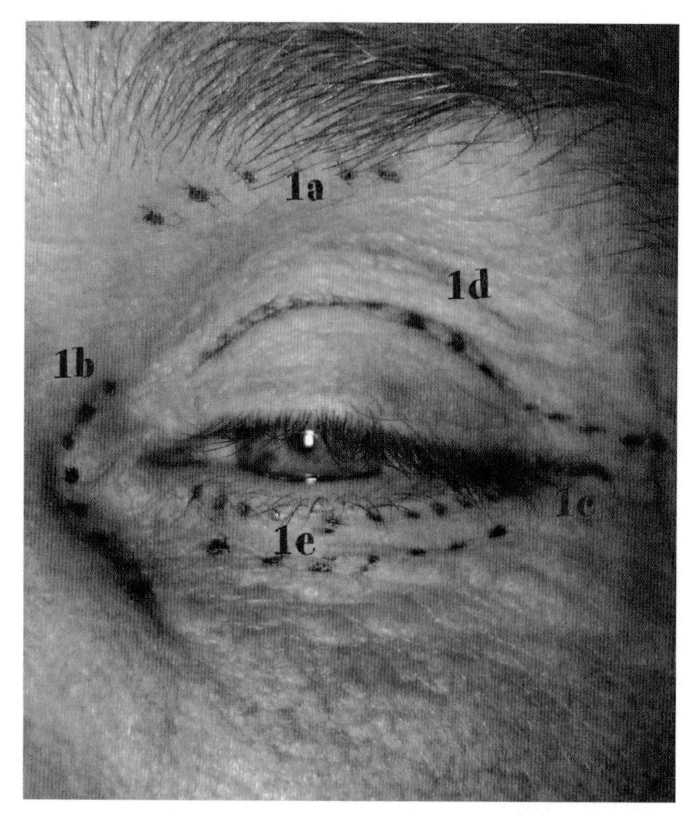

Figure 18-1 Skin incisions for anterior orbitotomies: (A) sub-brow; (B) Lynch; (C) lateral canthotomy; (D) upper lid crease; (E) infraciliary or lower lid crease.

cribriform plate or fovea ethmoidalis, as inadvertent cracks in these structures from ethmoidal bone decompression could lead to cerebrospinal fluid leakage or intracranial hemorrhage.

A *lateral canthotomy* (Fig. 18-1C) provides access to the lateral subperiosteal space and to the lateral bony rim for repair of tripod fractures. An inferior or superior cantholysis permits emergent decompression of an acute compartment syndrome (Fig. 18-3).

The upper lid is usually entered through the *upper lid crease* (Fig. 18-1D). A traction suture through the center of the lid margin facilitates separation of the anatomic planes. The skin is incised with a scalpel, laser, or fine-tipped electrocautery, and dissection is carried through the orbicularis muscle to the level of the conjoint septal-retractor ligaments, with care taken to avoid traumatizing the levator complex. The dissection is carried toward the orbital rim along the avascular suborbicularis fascial plane.

Opening the upper lid septum allows surgical access to lesions involving the orbital lobe of the lacrimal gland, the levator muscle, and the superior peripheral orbital space. A medial upper lid crease approach permits a narrow passage between the medial palpebral horn of the levator and the superior oblique tendon into the medial intraconal space and access to the anteromedial optic nerve (Fig. 18-4).

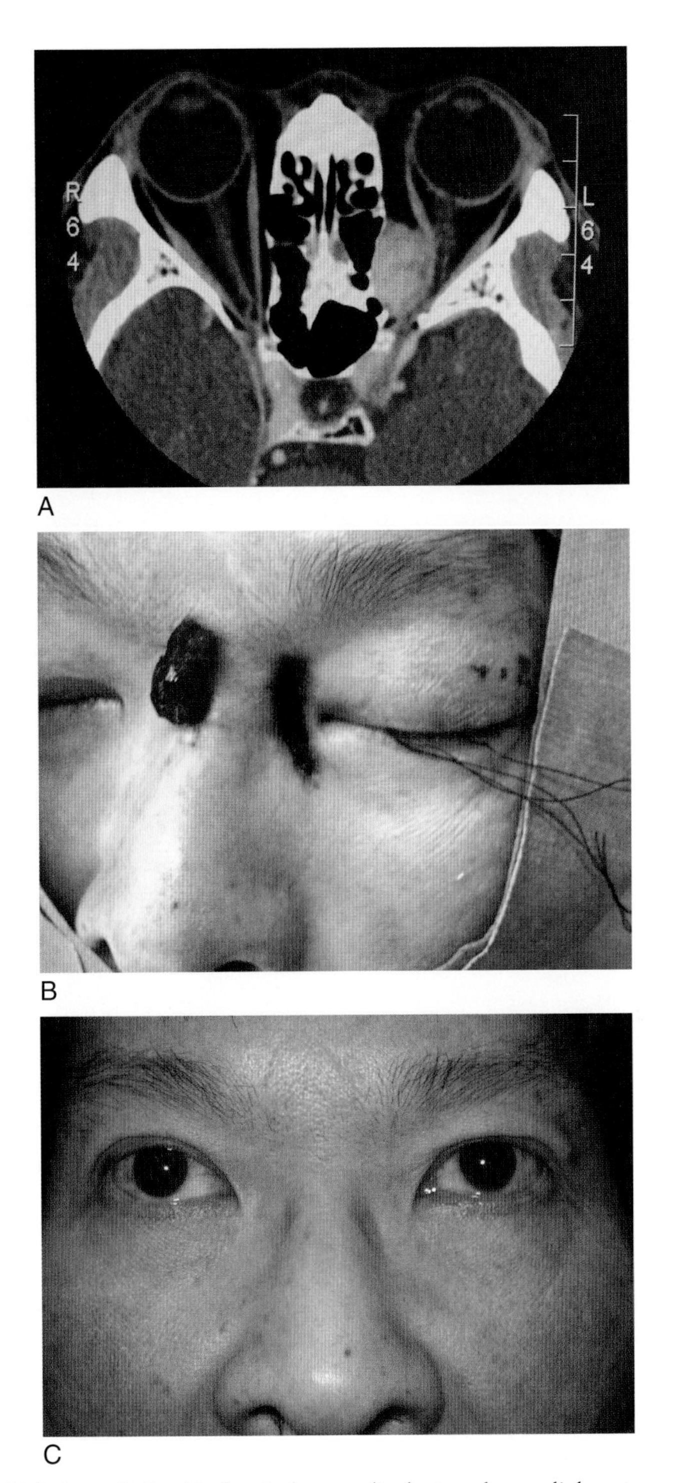

Figure 18-2 (A) Left medial orbital apical mass displacing the medial rectus and optic nerve temporally. (B) Delivery of decompressed hemangioma through a Lynch incision. (C) 2 months postoperative view of same patient showing well-healed left Lynch incision.

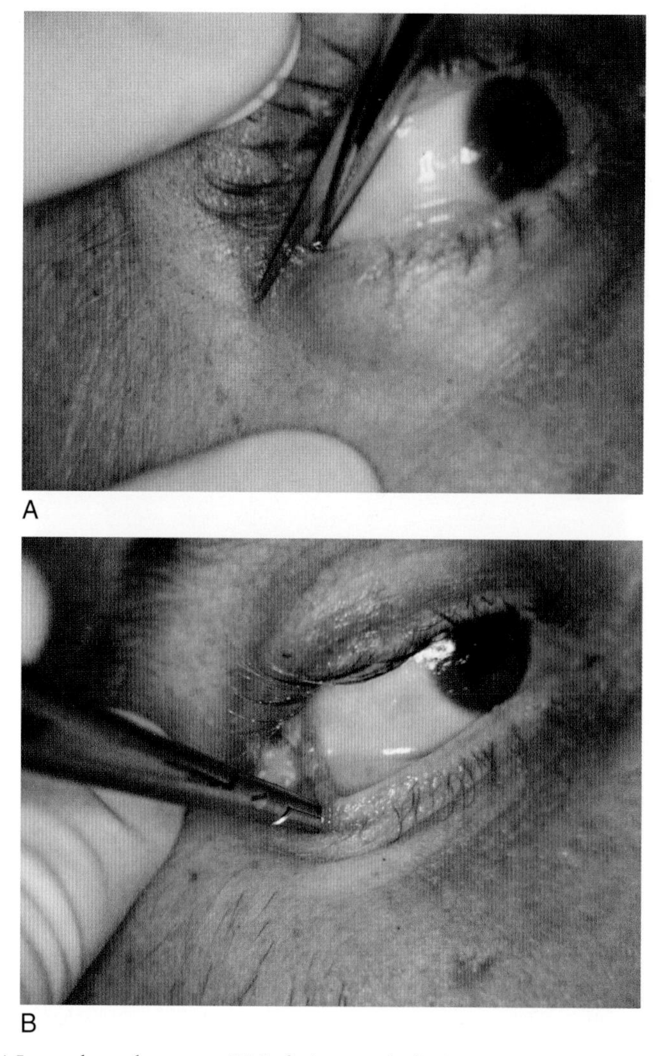

Figure 18-3 (A) Lateral canthotomy. (B) Inferior cantholysis.

Pathology in the subperiosteal space may be reached through the same approach, by dissecting along the septum to the arcus marginalis. The periosteum is opened and peeled posteriorly into the orbit. Bone pathology, including roof fractures, abscesses extending from the frontal sinus, and mucoceles, may be treated by this route (Fig. 18-5). Note should be made of the supraorbital nerve and the trochlea medially to avoid damaging these structures.

The lower lid is often opened through an *infraciliary or lower lid crease* (Fig. 18-1E), and dissection is carried inferiorly in the suborbicularis fascial plane toward the inferior rim. Opening the inferior lid septum allows surgical access to lesions involving the inferior rectus and inferior oblique muscles and the inferior peripheral orbital space. Opening the periosteum at the rim and elevating it posteriorly permits orbital floor fracture repairs, release of subperiosteal pus or hematoma, and bony decompression of a tight orbit.

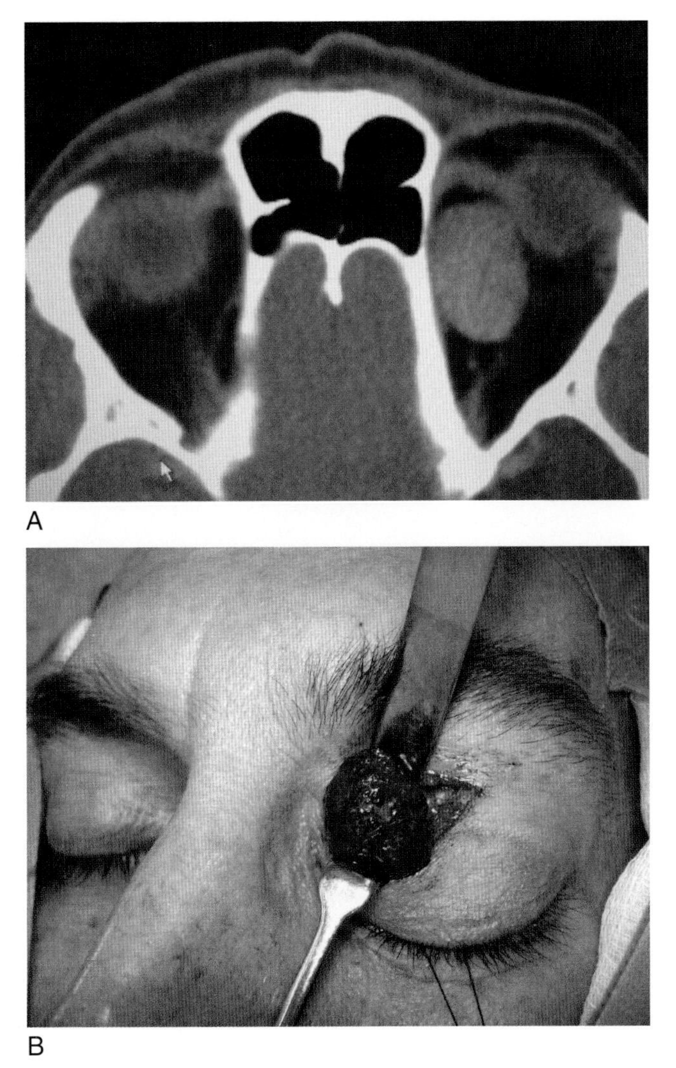

Figure 18-4 (A) Coronal CT showing anterior superomedial intraconal and peripheral orbital mass causing proptosis and visual distortion. (B) Delivery of mass through superomedial upper lid crease incision.

A *bicoronal flap* may be considered for bilateral superior orbital processes such as mucoceles or malignancies.

18-3-1-2 *Transconjunctival.* The conjunctiva provides an alternative route to most areas of the anterior orbit with the exception of the superior orbit, where the lacrimal ductules and intricate anatomy of the superior rectus and levator complex favor the transcutaneous approach.

The *swinging lower lid transconjunctival route* (Fig. 18-6) provides excellent exposure to the inferior peripheral orbit space and the subperiosteal space, with only a tiny canthotomy scar. Lidocaine with epinephrine is injected in the conjunctival fornix and lateral canthus. A retraction suture is placed in the inferior lid margin, and following a lateral canthotomy and inferior cantholysis, the lid is everted over

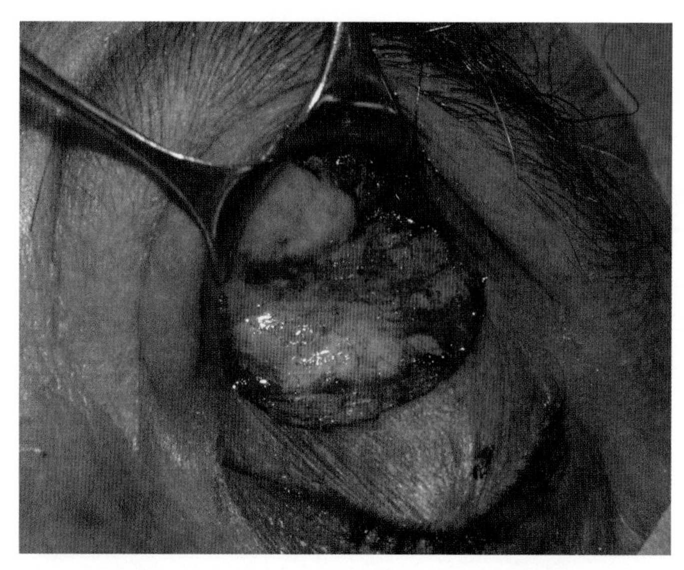

Figure 18-5 Drainage of superior subperiosteal abscess contiguous with frontal sinusitis through a superior lid crease approach.

a Desmarres retractor (Fig. 18-6A). The conjunctiva and lower lid retractors are opened between the inferior tarsal border and the fornix along their length to the inferior punctum (Fig. 18-6B). The conjunctiva and retractors are then dissected towards the rim, and the Desmarres retractor is reversed and used to pull the tarsal edge inferiorly (Fig. 18-6C).

The cut end of the conjunctiva and retractor can then be placed on a superior traction suture and an opening made through the septum to enter the inferior orbital space to access similar lesions described above (lower lid trans-septal) (Fig. 18-7). Alternatively, a ribbon malleable retractor can be used to pull the cut end of the retractors and orbital septum and fat posteriorly against the orbital floor, stretching the tissues over the periosteum anterior to the inferior rim. A monopolar electrocautery is then used to open the periorbita to the bone, and the orbital portion is stripped posteriorly with a Cottle and Freer elevator to expose the orbital floor. During this maneuver, the surgeon must ensure that the assistant is holding the lower lid tissues firmly against the cheek bone, avoiding a fold of lower lid skin being trapped below the Desmarres retractor, which might lead to button-holing with the electrocautery. This approach is very useful for accessing the orbital floor for fracture repair, floor decompressions, and drainage of subperiosteal blood or pus (Fig. 18-8).

The same approach can be used to access the lateral wall of the orbit (for lateral wall decompression), the anterior maxilla for fracture repair or for augmenting the malar prominence, or the medial wall (by extending the conjunctival incision superomedially onto the plica semilunaris). In the latter approach, care should be taken to identify the inferior oblique muscle and lacrimal sac to avoid inadvertent trauma.

The inferior fornix conjunctiva and retractors can be closed with a running absorbable suture (such as Vicryl 6-0), and the lateral canthus closed with a running absorbable suture (such as Vicryl 5-0) from the upper and lower lid margin along the skin incision.

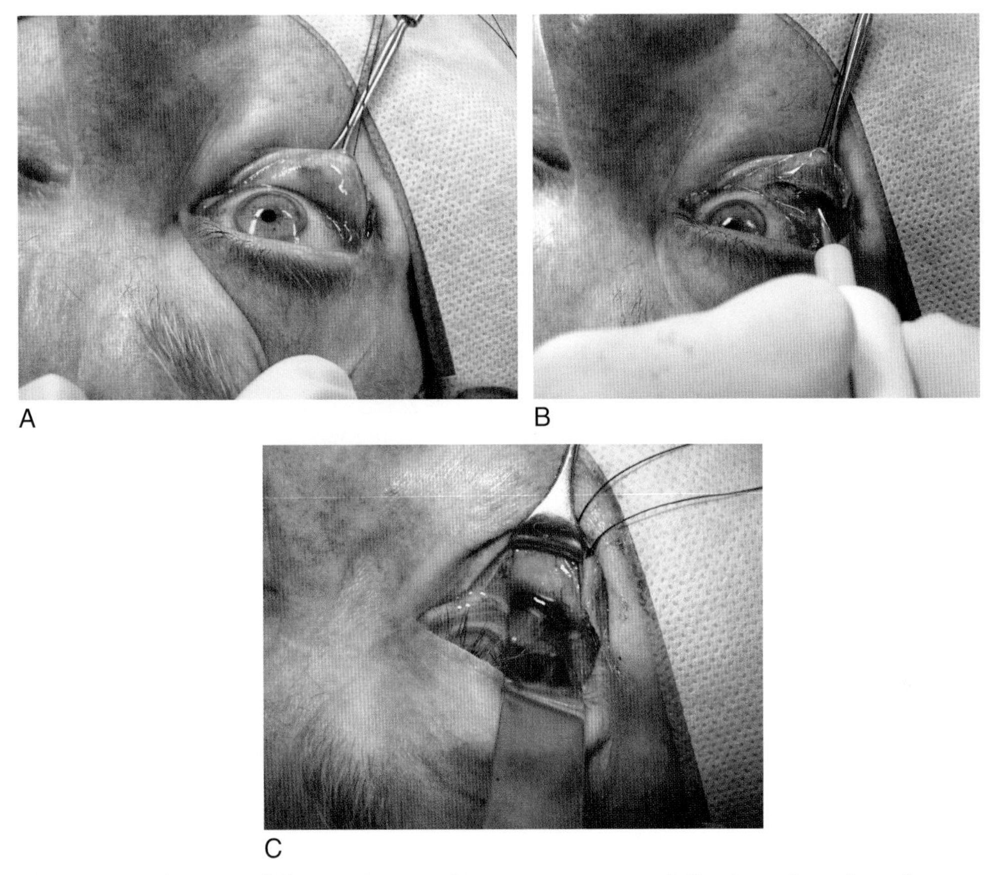

Figure 18-6 (A) Lower lid everted over a Desmarres retractor following a lateral canthotomy and inferior cantholysis. (B) The conjunctiva and lower lid retractors are opened with a hot-wire cautery. (C) The Desmarres retractor is reversed and traction applied inferiorly while dissection is carried inferiorly in the suborbicularis plane to the inferior arcus marginalis.

A deep suture may be placed to reappose the inferior canthal ligament to the periosteum on the inside of the lateral rim, but this step can often be omitted.

The *lateral bulbar conjunctival incision* is made at the limbus or parallel to the limbus midway to the fornix. It provides access to the lateral or superior rectus muscles or the palpebral lacrimal gland, or can be used to reposition or resect prolapsed temporal fat. The lacrimal gland ductules can be identified with a fluorescein strip and avoided.

The *medial bulbar conjunctival incision* (Fig. 18-9) provides access to the medial rectus muscle for biopsy or strabismus repair, and to the posterior intraconal space for incisional or needle biopsies or removal of small lesions. Access to the medial anterior intraconal space is possible by separating the medial rectus muscle at its insertion and distracting it medially while a traction suture in its insertion site is used to fully abduct the globe. Thin tissue malleable retractors can be used to separate the orbital fat vertically as dissection is followed posteriorly along the surface of the globe, identifying the long ciliary nerve behind the equator, until the optic nerve becomes visible (Fig. 18-10A). This approach is particularly useful for biopsies of

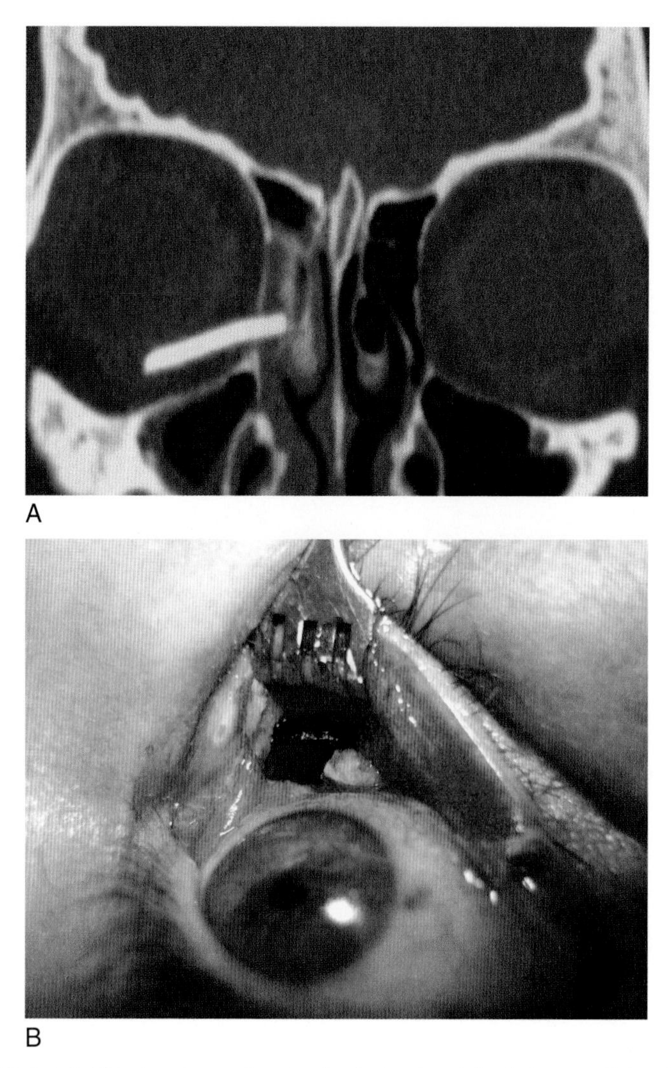

Figure 18-7 (A) Axial CT showing a foreign body in the right inferomedial orbit following a barroom fight. (B) Inferior fornix approach to deliver a large glass fragment.

perineural inflammatory or neoplastic masses, or for optic nerve sheath fenestration (Fig. 18-10B). Also, a medial intraconal hemangioma could be exsanguinated and delivered through this route.

The *caruncular (semilunar fold) incision* provides a similar exposure as the Lynch incision but avoids a potentially unsightly scar. It is most useful for accessing the medial subperiosteal space for reduction of medial wall fractures or for bony decompression. An incision is made along the semilunar fold and dissection is followed posteriorly and medially along the posterior limb of the medial canthal ligament to the posterior lacrimal crest. A thin retractor aids in displacing orbital fat laterally. Once the medial bone is reached, the periorbita can be excised parallel to the crest and elevated posteriorly to expose the surgical space (Fig. 18-11).

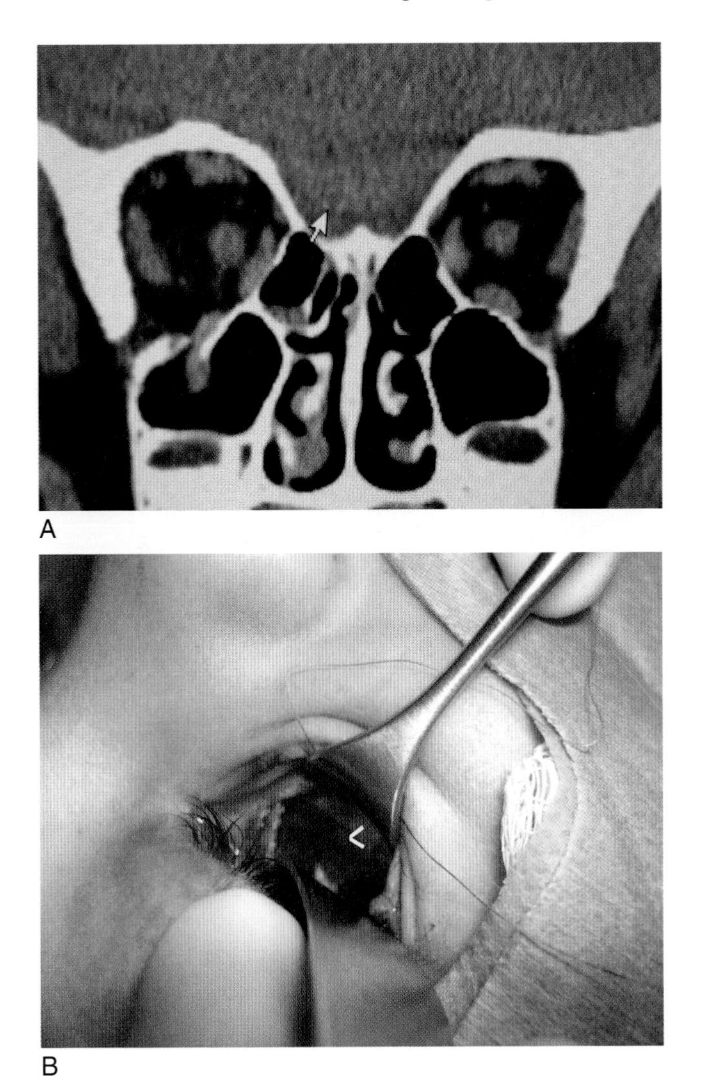

Figure 18-8 (A) Coronal CT shows tethering of the right inferior rectus muscle within a trapdoor floor fracture. (B) Intraoperative view of the right orbital floor with the tethered tissues in the fracture site (*arrow*).

18-3-2 *Lateral Orbitotomy.* Removal of various sections of the lateral orbital rim or wall (lateral orbitotomy) allows for resection of retrobulbar lesions lateral or superior to the optic nerve. It is also the surgery of choice for complete excision of the lacrimal gland for pleomorphic adenomas.

The skin incision for this approach has evolved over the years. Berke modified the standard vertical Kronlein incision to a horizontal incision extending laterally 5 cm. Wright proposed an S-shaped incision from the lateral sub-brow along the lateral rim and then horizontally in a smile-crease. This approach has been recommended by many for lacrimal gland excision. More recently, many surgeons have employed an extended upper lid crease for lateral orbitotomies (Fig. 18-12). A bicoronal flap may also be employed for a lateral orbitotomy, especially when combined with a craniotomy for removal of the orbital roof.

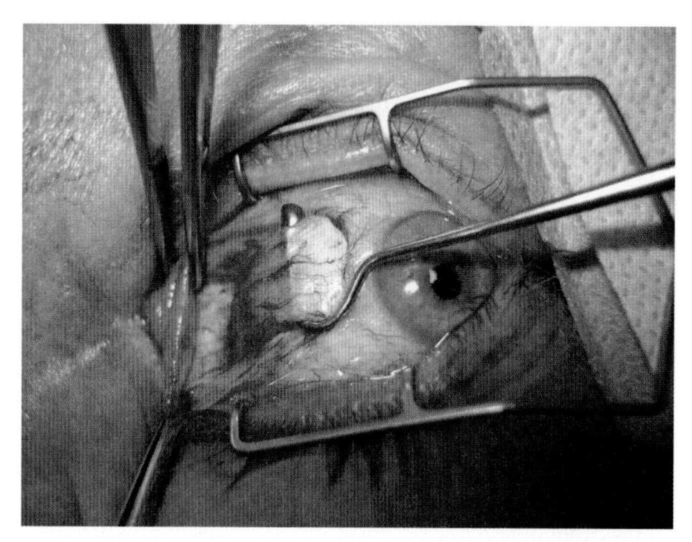

Figure 18-9 Medial bulbar conjunctival incision showing a muscle biopsy for an atypical medial rectus myositis.

In brief, an upper lid crease is marked and infiltrated with lidocaine with epinephrine. A 4-0 silk suture can be placed around the insertion of the superior rectus and lateral rectus muscle to mobilize the globe and to identify these structures during the orbitotomy. A traction suture can also be placed in the upper lid margin for downward traction.

Dissection is carried up to the superior orbital rim in the avascular suborbicularis fascial plane, as described previously (upper lid crease anterior orbitotomy). A Desmarres retractor or Raleigh rakes are used to retract the flap superiorly while a malleable retractor is used to protect the orbital soft tissue structures around the inside of the rim. The bone flap incisions can be outlined with a surgical marker: the standard bone flap to access the lateral peripheral or intraconal orbital space extends from the frontozygomatic suture to the body of the zygoma. The flap may be extended superiorly to include the anterior lip of the superior orbital rim for lesions involving the lacrimal gland or the superior orbit. It may be extended inferiorly to the lateral margin of the inferior orbital fissure for extensive lesions involving the inferior orbit. The periosteum is incised vertically along the rim and relaxing incisions are placed both superiorly and inferiorly. The periosteum is stripped nasally into the orbit beyond the arcus marginalis, with care taken to hug the bone as it reflects sharply backward at the lacrimal gland fossa. The periosteum is reflected laterally over the temporalis muscle, which is separated from the lateral wall with a monopolar electrocautery. With the malleable retractor placed between the exposed bone and the soft tissue of the orbit, a Stryker oscillating blade is used to make the bone cuts. A sturdy end-biting bone rongeur is used to outfracture the segment of lateral bone, which is stored in a saline cloth for later replacement (see Fig. 18-12B). Additional bone can be removed piecemeal with the rongeur toward the posterior orbit. The marrow space in the sphenoid bone lateral to the superior orbital fissure can be drilled with a diamond burr to improve access for apical lateral lesions.

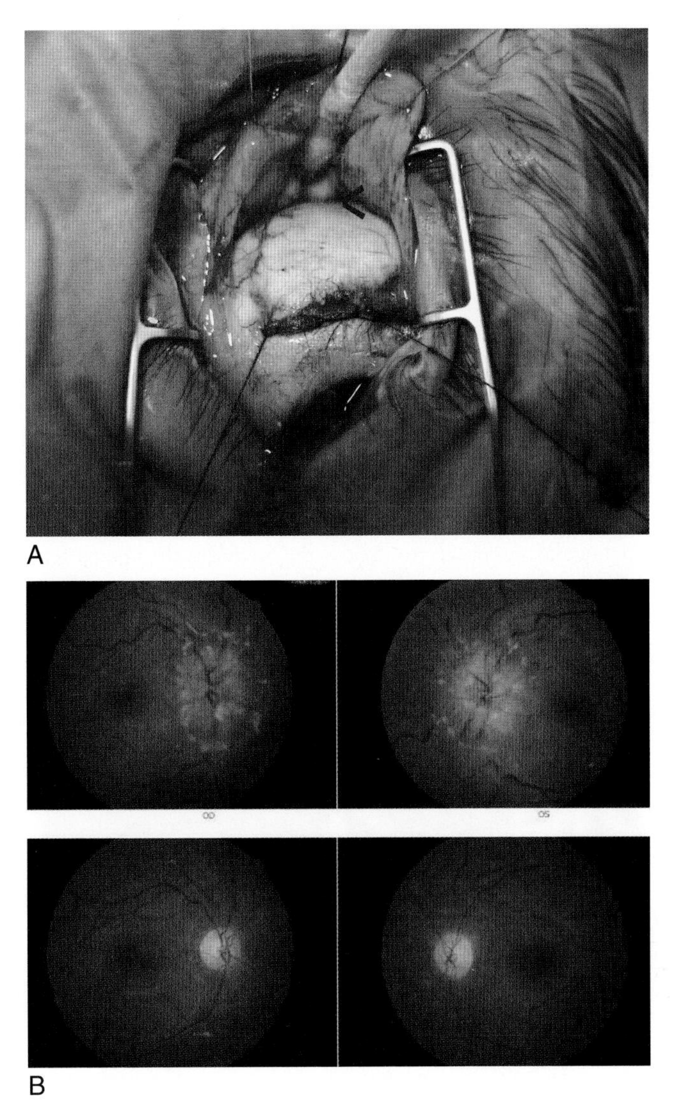

Figure 18-10 (A) Reflected medial rectus muscle with the left eye rotated laterally. The long ciliary nerve is visible as a post-equatorial horizontal line leading to the optic nerve (*arrow*) in a patient with severe benign intracranial hypertension (BIH) with severe vision loss. (B) Preoperative and postoperative (2 months) disc photographs of the same patient who underwent a left optic nerve sheath fenestration for severe BIH. Vision returned from hand motions to 20/25 bilaterally.

The margins of the lesion may be felt through the periorbita, guiding where the periorbita should be opened. The lateral rectus muscle can be tagged with a suture and displaced to facilitate access to the lesion (see Fig. 18-12B). The orbital fat is separated down to the lesion, which is then carefully dissected from surrounding normal tissue. Encapsulated tumors are removed intact; infiltrative lesions may be biopsied for a rush diagnosis to permit further management decisions (see Fig. 18-12C). Bipolar cautery, cottonoid Neuro Patties, and gentle retraction help maintain a bloodless field. Lymphangiomas may require debulking, and a CO_2 laser may help maintain hemostasis.

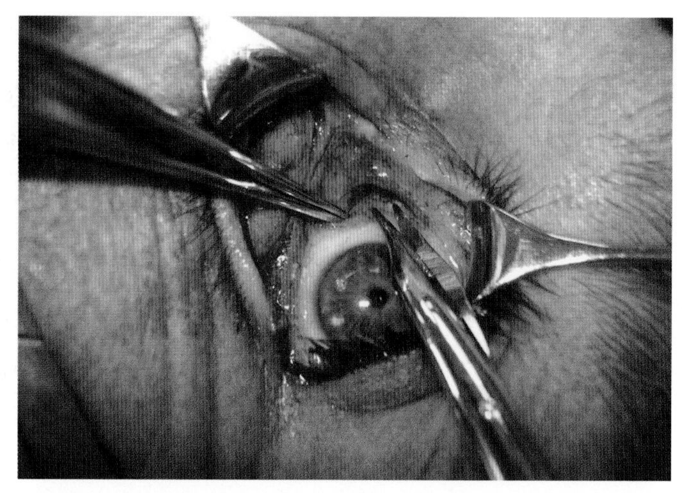

Figure 18-11 A combination of a swinging eyelid fornix approach (to expose the orbital floor) combined with a caruncular approach (to expose the medial wall) in a patient with a combined left orbital floor and medial wall fracture.

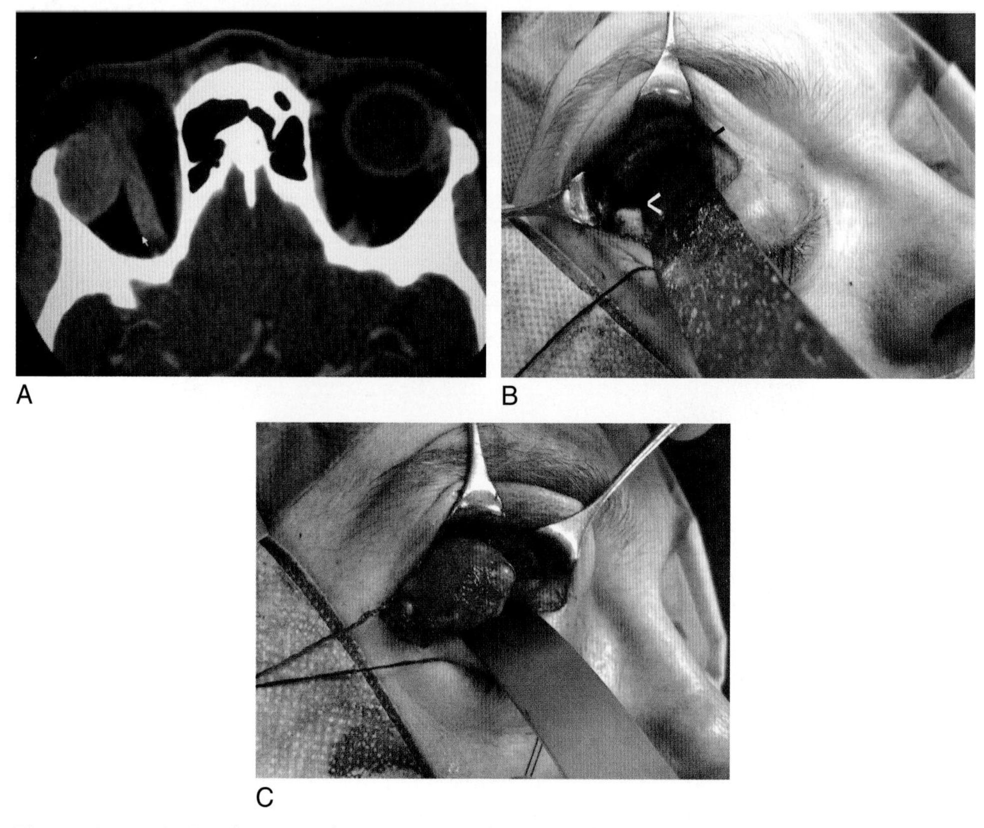

Figure 18-12 (A) Axial CT scan demonstrating a large right lacrimal gland mass. (B) Intraoperative view of a right lateral orbitotomy through an upper lid crease approach following removal of a segment of the superolateral rim (cut edges marked with *arrows*). Notice the sutures in the lateral rectus and upper lid margin and the lacrimal gland mass defined by the malleable retractor. (C) The pleomorphic adenoma is delivered in toto with the periorbita intact over the mass.

Once the lesion has been removed or biopsied, the periorbita is closed with dissolving sutures, and the bone flap is sutured back using predrilled holes at either end of the bone rim and the adjoining rim. The periorbita is then sutured back to the lateral periosteum and the skin of the crease is closed with a running suture. A drain is usually not necessary. Intraoperative intravenous steroids help reduce postoperative edema.

The patient should be monitored for postoperative edema or hemorrhage leading to a compartment syndrome by checking vision and pupil response. The head of the bed is kept elevated and cool compresses are applied.

18-3-3 *Trans-sinus Orbitotomy.* The sinuses are often related to orbital disease: mucoceles, malignancies, and infection may spread from contiguous sinuses into the orbit. Soft tissues may be trapped by bone fractures extending into the sinuses. Certain inflammatory disorders (such as midline granulomatoses) involve both the orbit and sinus cavities.

Surgery for lesions involving both the orbit and adjacent sinuses are often best performed by a combined orbit/ENT team approach (Fig. 18-13).

The sinus cavities may be also used for access into the orbit, sometimes with the assistance of a trained endoscopist: a transantral approach may be helpful in reducing posterior orbital blowout fractures. A posterior medial apical lesion may be accessed through the ethmoid sinuses. Decompression of the optic canal has been described

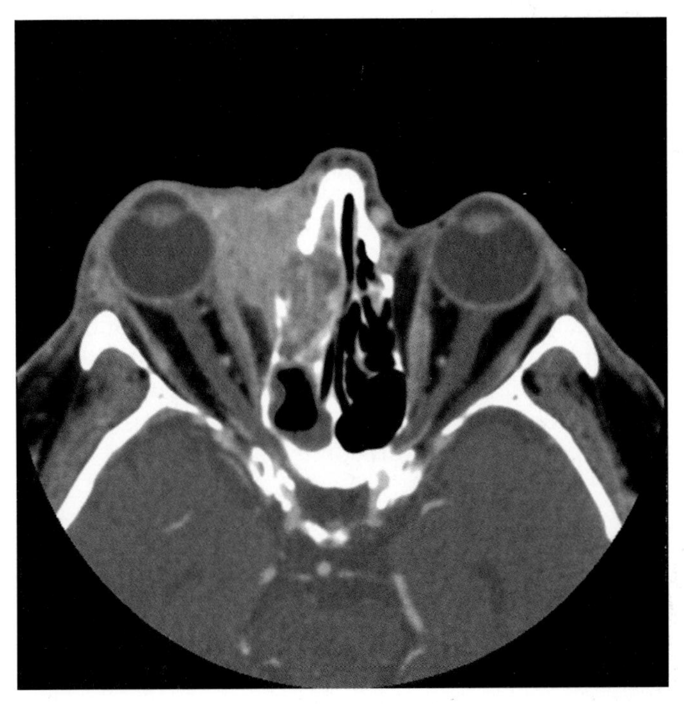

Figure 18-13 A large invasive mass involving the left nasal cavity, ethmoid sinus, and medial orbit. Biopsy identified a squamous cell carcinoma, and exenteration of the orbit and sinuses was performed with a combined otolaryngology and orbital approach.

through a sphenoid approach. The rigid endoscope and the advent of 3-D CT scan localizing software improves the accuracy of these approaches.

18-3-4 *Transcranial Orbitotomy*. A bicoronal flap permits dissection inferiorly to the superior orbital rims and is the standard incision for a frontal or parietal craniotomy. A neurosurgical approach with gentle retraction of the frontal lobe may provide access to the prechiasmal optic nerve for optic canal decompressions or to the orbital roof for superior apical lesions or for lesions involving both the orbit and intracranial cavity.

18-3-5 *Combined Orbitotomy*. Specific lesions may not be accessible for removal through one approach alone. In these cases, a combination of the previous four approaches may be helpful.

1. Combined anterior medial and lateral orbitotomy: A medial apical intraconal lesion may be difficult to reach through a medial limbal conjunctival approach alone, even with disinsertion of the medial rectus muscle. In these cases, a lateral orbitotomy may be helpful to displace the globe laterally so that better visualization of the apex is possible.
2. Combined anterior inferior and lateral orbitotomy: Large lesions of the inferolateral orbit may be more easily reached and removed via a combination of a lateral orbitotomy combined with a swinging lid approach to the inferior orbit. In these cases, a canthotomy may provide sufficient access to the lateral rim with stripping of the periosteum, as well as allowing access to the inferior fornix to create the swinging lid.
3. Combined trans-sinus and anterior orbitotomy: Mucoceles may be exposed from the orbital side but drained from a sinus approach. Lesions involving both the sinus and the orbit may require exposure of the orbital side through a caruncular or Lynch approach as well as removal of the sinus portion using an endoscopic sinus approach. Orbital abscesses are typically drained anteriorly but may benefit from lavage of the contiguous sinus.
4. Combined lateral and transcranial orbitotomy: A panoramic orbitotomy removes en bloc the orbital roof and superior rim, and the lateral wall and rim, using a bicoronal flap approach. This is particularly useful for resection of large malignancies involving the orbit but extending intracranially, or sufficiently large in the posterior orbit that a lateral or anterior orbitotomy alone would not provide adequate exposure. A large optic nerve glioma, particularly if it were extending into the intracanalicular portion of the nerve, is usually more safely resected through this combined route.

18-4 COMPLICATIONS

Preoperative planning reduces the risk of certain complications. Advising the patient to stop all anticoagulants at appropriate intervals (2 weeks for aspirin and nonsteroidal anti-inflammatories, and 2 days for warfarin) helps reduce the risk of excessive bleeding.

Postoperative edema is more likely with extensive or prolonged surgery, particularly if the tissues were already inflamed because of infection or an inflammatory condition.

The use of intraoperative and postoperative corticosteroids may reduce its severity, as will elevating the head of the bed and applying regular cold compresses. Lubricant ointment or drops may help with corneal and conjunctival exposure in the immediate postoperative period; in severe cases with proptosis and poor lid protection, moist chambers or a temporary tarsorrhaphy may be required.

Severe postoperative bleeding or edema might lead to a compartment syndrome. Most orbitotomies do not require placement of a drain, but this may be helpful in extensive or prolonged dissections, or following evacuation of abscesses. The patient should be monitored for a drop in vision or development of an afferent pupil defect in the first 24 hours postoperatively so that appropriate cantholysis or opening of the wounds to relieve orbital pressure can be performed as necessary.

Most orbitotomies do not require perioperative antibiotics. However, systemic antibiotics are typically employed in cases involving transgression of the sinuses, drainage of abscesses, or placement of alloplastic implants.

Functional loss following orbitotomies is usually transient. Ptosis may develop following lacrimal gland excisions or from tumor resections around the superior orbit. Diplopia may occur from apraxia from prolonged compression while operating near the apex, from inadvertent nerve trauma, or from disruption to the trochlea in the superomedial orbit. Forehead numbness or paresthesia may result from injury to the supraorbital nerve near the superior rim, while cheek, nose, and upper jaw dysesthesia may result from orbital floor fracture repair or decompression of the medial wall or floor. Vision loss is fortunately rare and typically arises from an acute untreated compartment syndrome, or from dissection of optic nerve pathology or large lesions in the orbital apex.

Cerebrospinal fluid leaks may arise from damage to the dura directly from roof dissections or indirectly from a fracture in the fovea ethmoidalis during a medial wall orbital decompression.

SUGGESTED READINGS

Harris GJ, Logani SC. Eyelid crease incision for lateral orbitotomy. *Ophthal Plast Reconstr Surg*. 1999;15(1):9–16.

Harris GJ, Perez N. Surgical sectors of the orbit: using the lower fornix approach for large, medial intraconal tumors. *Ophthal Plast Reconstr Surg*. 2002;18(5):349–354.

McCord CD, Tanenbaum M. *Oculoplastic Surgery*. New York: Raven Press, 1987.

Pelton RW, Patel BC. Superomedial lid crease approach to the medial intraconal space: a new technique for access to the optic nerve and central space. *Ophthal Plast Reconstr Surg*. 2001;17(4):241–253.

Rootman J, Stewart B, Goldberg RA. *Orbital Surgery. A Conceptual Approach*. Philadelphia: Lipincott-Raven, 1995.

Tsirbas A, Kazim M, Close L. Endoscopic approach to orbital apex lesions. *Ophthal Plast Reconstr Surg*. 2005;21(4):271–275.

Vijayalakshmi P. The precaruncular approach to the medial orbit. *J AAPOS*. 2007; 11(2):208.

Zide BM, Jelks GW. *Surgical Anatomy of the Orbit*. New York: Raven Press, 1985.

19

Surgical Decompression of the Orbit

J.D. PERRY, MD, AND CRAIG LEWIS, MD

19-1 INTRODUCTION

In 1835 Graves first described the characteristic exophthalmos of thyroid eye disease,[1] and his name has since become synonymous with thyrotoxic ophthalmopathy. Graves disease is relatively common, with a prevalence and incidence of 1% and 0.1%, respectively.[2] Although subtle signs of ophthalmopathy are present in most patients with Graves disease, only 30% have obvious eye findings, and only 5% develop ophthalmopathy severe enough to warrant specific treatment with radiotherapy, immunosuppression, or orbital decompression surgery. Graves disease and Graves ophthalmopathy are more common in females than in males, though males tend to have more severe eye disease. Cigarette smokers have an increased risk of developing Graves disease, an increased risk of developing associated ophthalmopathy, and a progressively increased risk of severe ocular manifestations.[3]

19-2 OVERVIEW OF GRAVES OPHTHALMOPATHY

While the onset of Graves disease usually occurs when people are in their forties, thyroid optic neuropathy tends to occur in the fifties and sixties, underscoring the importance of careful long-term follow-up of these patients.[4,5] The ophthalmopathy of Graves disease is usually associated with hyperthyroidism, but it occurs in euthyroid and hypothyroid patients as well. The clinical course of the ophthalmopathy does not directly correlate with the thyroid status, although more than 80% of thyroid patients who develop severe ophthalmopathy do so within 18 months of the detection of the thyroid disease.[6] The early findings of thyroid ophthalmopathy include conjunctival injection, lacrimation, ocular surface irritation, orbital and periorbital swelling, and mild eyelid retraction. Progression of the disease can result in severe orbital congestion, massive enlargement of the extraocular muscles with secondary diplopia, proptosis, compressive optic neuropathy, prominent eyelid retraction, spontaneous subluxation of the globe anterior to the eyelids, and exposure keratopathy. Treatment options for these serious complications of Graves disease include systemic corticosteroids, radiation therapy, and orbital decompression surgery.

The role of radiation therapy in the management of Graves ophthalmopathy remains controversial. In 1973, Donaldson et al. first reported results of radiotherapy for Graves ophthalmopathy using a megavoltage linear accelerator.[7] This series and multiple subsequent series have reported favorable results in approximately 60% of patients.[8] A more recent prospective study by Gorman et al., however, found that orbital radiotherapy had no beneficial therapeutic effect for moderate Graves ophthalmopathy.[9] Proponents of orbital radiation contend that radiotherapy is most effective for the acute congestive phase of the disease, while proptosis and longstanding eye muscle restriction generally respond poorly. Some orbital specialists have found radiation therapy useful in the management of compressive optic neuropathy and reserve orbital decompression surgery for patients who fail to respond to radiation therapy. Others feel that compressive optic neuropathy from Graves disease is best managed with orbital decompression surgery and reserve orbital radiation for patients who fail to respond favorably to decompression surgery. These surgeons contend that orbital radiation causes a short-term increase in orbital congestion and may not have its maximal effect for several months after treatment, while orbital decompression surgery gives immediate relief of the optic nerve compression.[5] Orbital radiotherapy is contraindicated in patients with preexisting retinopathy, such as diabetic retinopathy, due to the risk of worsening retinal microvasculature disease. The most common complication of orbital radiotherapy is cataract formation.[10] Orbital radiotherapy does not appear to increase the risk of subsequent cancers.[10,11] The American Academy of Ophthalmology recently reviewed the medical literature to evaluate the efficacy and safety of orbital radiation for Graves ophthalmopathy.[12] Regarding efficacy, they concluded that extraocular motility defects may improve with radiotherapy, but that proptosis, eyelid retraction, and soft tissue changes do not improve. Regarding safety, the most significant complication is radiation retinopathy, which occurs between 1% (definite retinopathy) and 21% (possible retinopathy) in the first 10 years after treatment. There was not significant evidence to evaluate the safety and efficacy of radiation therapy for compressive optic neuropathy.[12]

Systemic corticosteroids represent an effective temporizing measure in the acute management of thyroid optic neuropathy, but side effects make this an unattractive alternative for long-term management.[5] Corticosteroids effectively relieve orbital congestion and are often used perioperatively with orbital decompression surgery and in conjunction with orbital radiation. Some recommend prophylactic corticosteroids for high-risk patients to decrease the risk of worsening eye disease after radioactive iodine treatment.[13]

Orbital decompression surgery involves the surgical expansion of the bony orbital cavity and removal of orbital fat to reduce orbital pressure and proptosis.

Decompression surgery effectively relieves dysthyroid compressive optic neuropathy refractory to oral corticosteroids.[14]

19-3 OVERVIEW OF ORBITAL DECOMPRESSION

Orbital decompression techniques involving one, two, three, and four walls have been described for management of Graves ophthalmopathy (Table 19-1). Early orbital decompression surgery involved the removal of a single orbital wall, usually the medial orbital wall (Fig. 19-1). In 1911, Dollinger described the Kronlein lateral orbitotomy approach for removal of the lateral orbital wall and is credited with the

Table 19-1 Anatomic Targets for Orbital Decompression

Decompression targets	Underlying structures	Amount of retrodisplace ment	Approaches	Notes
Medial wall	Ethmoid sinuses	2–5 mm when combined with medial floor	Transcutaneous, transconjunctival, transcaruncular, transantral, endoscopic transnasal	Decompression of posterior medial wall is important for treatment of compressive optic neuropathy; visualize location of cribiform plate to avoid CSF leak
Orbital floor	Maxillary sinus		Same as medial above	Potential for hypoglobus and diplopia, especially if maxillary ethmoid strut removed; risks damage to infraorbital nerve
Anterior lateral wall	Temporalis muscle and buccal fat	1–2 mm	Lateral canthal, upper eyelid crease	
Deep lateral wall	Temporalis muscle fascia and dura of anterior and middle cranial fossa	3–6 mm when combined with anterior lateral wall	Same as anterior lateral plus transcoronal	Potential for CSF leak
Orbital roof	Dura of frontal cranial fossa	Minimal unless combined with deep lateral	Transcoronal, neurosurgical	Potential for CSF leak
Intraconal fat		1–3 mm	Any	Risks bleeding, Adie's tonic pupil

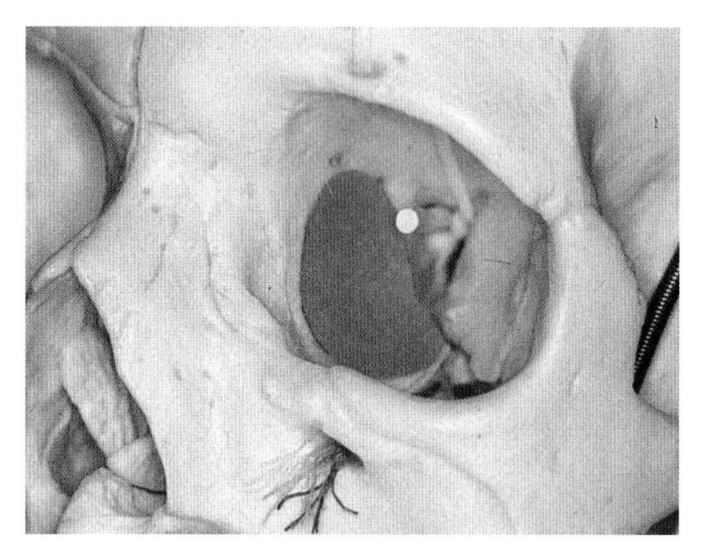

Figure 19-1 Outline of bone removal in a medial orbital wall decompression.

first description of orbital decompression surgery.[15] In the 1930s, Naffziger described the removal of the orbital roof; Sewall, the medial orbital wall; and Hirsch and Urbanek, the orbital floor in an attempt to correct thyroid-related proptosis.[16–18] In 1957, Walsh and Ogura described the simultaneous removal of the medial wall and orbital floor in what amounted to a combination of the Sewall and Hirsch techniques.[19] This two-walled orbital decompression effectively releases pressure on the optic nerve and reduces mild to moderate degrees of proptosis (4 mm).[20]

Many approaches to the bony orbit are described in the literature, including transcutaneous, transconjunctival, transcaruncular, transantral, transcranial, and transnasal approaches (Table 19-2). Newer approaches stress cosmetically hidden or less visible incisions. The advent of miniplate fixation has led to the development of more extensive orbital expansion procedures.[21,22] These include advancement and outward rotation of the lateral orbital wall in an attempt to achieve a greater degree of lateral orbital expansion. In combination with traditional techniques, these procedures may allow for a greater reduction in proptosis (>6 mm).

Advances in endoscopic sinus surgery have led to the development of a "closed" decompression of the medial orbital wall and orbital floor. The endonasal approach has also been used in combination with the open decompression techniques. The endonasal approach may make preservation of the medial orbital strut more challenging, which could lead to higher rates of diplopia.[23]

Recent techniques in orbital decompression surgery attempt to decrease the risk of postoperative diplopia. One such technique, described by Goldberg et al. in 1992, is the preservation of the medial orbital strut at the junction of the maxillary and ethmoid sinuses during medial wall and orbital floor decompressions to decrease postoperative globe displacement and misalignment.[24] Another idea is the "balanced" orbital decompression, which involves decompression of both the medial and the lateral orbital walls and preservation of the orbital floor. This approach has a lower incidence of postoperative muscle imbalance compared to

Table 19-2 Surgical Approaches to Orbital Decompression

Approaches	Accessed areas	Pros	Cons
Medial cutaneous (Lynch)	Medial wall	Good visualization	Visible scar
Inferior eyelid crease	Floor	Good visualization	Visible scar; risks eyelid retraction
Endoscopic transnasal	Medial wall and medial orbital floor	Hidden incision; excellent visualization of deep apex	Requires endoscopic equipment; must remove maxillary ethmoid strut for full decompression
Transantral	Floor and medial wall	Hidden	Must remove maxillary ethmoid strut for full decompression
Transcaruncular (medial transconjunctival)	Medial and inferomedial wall	Hidden	
Inferior transconjunctival	Inferior wall	Hidden	
Superior eyelid crease	Superficial and deep lateral orbit	Incision follows eyelid crease relaxed skin tension line	
Transcoronal	All four surfaces, including deep lateral orbit	Hidden	
Lateral canthal	Lateral wall	Incision follows relaxed skin tension line; combined with inferior transconjunctival incision, provides good lateral wall access	

traditional methods.[25] A lateral wall-only orbital decompression may decrease the risk of postoperative diplopia compared with balanced decompression for patients who require smaller amounts of decompression.[26]

To broaden the scope of the surgical options, Olivari has reported good results with meticulous extirpation of intraconal and extraconal orbital fat without bone removal.[27,28] This fat-removal technique can be used in conjunction with traditional techniques to achieve greater degrees of decompression.

19-4 INDICATIONS FOR ORBITAL DECOMPRESSION

Indications for orbital decompression surgery include visual loss from compressive optic neuropathy, severe proptosis with exposure keratopathy, recurrent globe prolapse anterior to the eyelids, and cosmetically objectionable exophthalmos. Although mild exophthalmos can be masked with eyelid surgery, patients with greater than

24 to 25 mm of proptosis usually require (or desire) orbital decompression surgery prior to eyelid surgery to achieve acceptable cosmetic results. Improved orbital decompression techniques have led to an increase in the number of elective cases for the cosmetic correction of exophthalmos. When possible, orbital decompression surgery should be delayed until the thyroid function has been regulated and the orbitopathy stabilized, with no evidence of progression for several months. In cases of severe visual loss or exposure keratopathy, such postponement may not be possible.

19-5 EVALUATION OF THE THYROID PATIENT

Thyroid patients require a multidisciplinary approach, and their care often involves an endocrinologist, a neuro-ophthalmologist, a strabismus specialist, and an orbital surgeon. Preoperative evaluation and treatment of the thyroid status helps to avoid the risk of thyroid storm. A careful evaluation of visual function, including visual acuity, pupillary examination, color vision evaluation, and formal visual field testing, establishes a baseline level of visual function for future comparison. Slit-lamp biomicroscopy with fluorescein helps identify any corneal surface irregularities, which can contribute to visual impairment and ocular discomfort. A detailed evaluation of extraocular muscle motility is essential and aids in predicting the extent of post-decompression motility disturbance. Preoperative computed tomography (CT) scans should include coronal sections through the orbits to identify the position of the cribriform plate, to visualize ethmoid air-cell anatomy, and to rule out preexisting sinus disease. Although orbital magnetic resonance imaging (MRI) provides excellent soft tissue detail, it does not display the bone detail necessary for preoperative planning.

As orbital decompression often represents the first step in a series of rehabilitative procedures, the surgeon should discuss the treatment plan thoroughly with the patient prior to surgery. Subsequent stages may include extraocular muscle surgery to reduce diplopia and eyelid surgery to correct significant eyelid retraction. A discussion of the surgical risks of orbital decompression surgery should include diplopia, abnormal globe displacement, sinusitis, infraorbital hypesthesia, nasolacrimal duct obstruction, significant blood loss requiring transfusion, cerebrospinal fluid leaks, meningitis, and visual loss.

19-6 TECHNIQUES FOR ORBITAL DECOMPRESSION

The most commonly employed orbital decompression procedures represent modifications of the medial wall and orbital floor technique first described by Walsh and Ogura.[19] Various approaches to these areas have been used, including transantral, transcutaneous via subciliary or external ethmoidectomy incision, transconjunctival, transcaruncular, and transnasal.[14,29,30] Ophthalmologists most commonly use either the transconjunctival, transantral, or the transcaruncular approach. Some advocate a combination of approaches to maximize the amount of decompression and limit the risk of postoperative diplopia.[31]

McCord and Moses first described a lateral canthotomy, transconjunctival approach to avoid cutaneous scar formation and ectropion.[32] Advocates of this anterior orbital approach state that better visualization of the anterior orbital structures, including the infraorbital neurovascular bundle, lacrimal sac, and inferior oblique muscle, reduces morbidity. Some reports suggest that the transantral approach has a greater complication rate, including a higher incidence of strabismus, oroantral fistula, infraorbital hypesthesia, and sinusitis.[33–35] Advocates of the transantral approach, however, believe that this approach provides better exposure of the posterior orbital floor. This may aid in a more complete posterior decompression, a critical factor when dealing with compressive optic neuropathy. More recently, Shorr et al. described a transcaruncular approach to the medial orbit and orbital apex.[36] This approach provides excellent visualization of the medial and inferomedial orbit through a hidden incision, and it allows for preservation of the anterior maxillo-ethmoidal strut to decrease the risk of postoperative strabismus.[14] Good results have been achieved with each of these approaches.

19-6-1 *Inferomedial Orbital Decompression Using a Lateral Canthotomy and Transconjunctival Approach.* This technique is performed under general anesthesia. Once the patient is prepared and draped in the usual sterile fashion, a small amount of 0.5% lidocaine with 1:200,000 epinephrine is infiltrated transconjunctivally into the lateral canthus and lower eyelid. The vasoconstricting effect of the epinephrine reduces intraoperative bleeding. A surgical headlight with or without operative loupes is essential for good visualization of the anatomic landmarks during the procedure.

A lateral canthotomy with an inferior cantholysis is completed to free the lower eyelid, exposing the inferior fornix. Monopolar electrocautery divides the conjunctiva and lower eyelid retractors between the inferior tarsal border and the inferior conjunctival fornix. The fat pockets of the lower eyelid are sequentially exposed and liberally debulked; this step is similar to transconjunctival lower blepharoplasty (Fig. 19-2). Once fat has been removed back to the level of the intraorbital rim, the periosteum is incised along the inner aspect of the orbital rim. A Freer periosteal

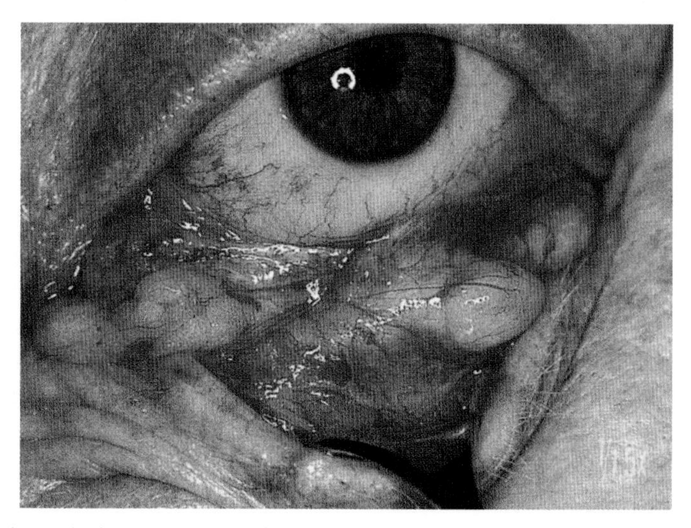

Figure 19-2 Through the lower eyelid fornix incision, the orbital fat is prolapsed forward and excised.

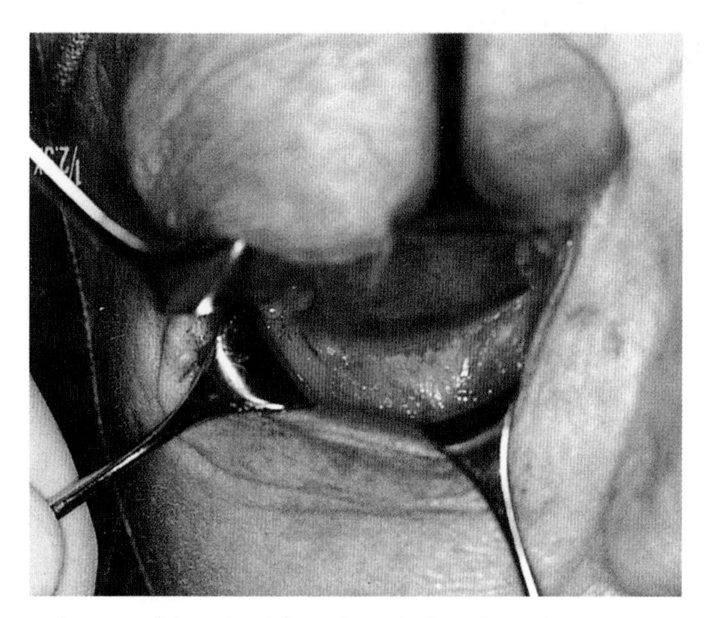

Figure 19-3 Visualization of the orbital floor through the inferior fornix incision.

elevator is then used to elevate the periorbita from the orbital floor. The periosteum is thick and strongly adherent at the orbital rim but dissects off the orbital floor with minimal resistance. A blunt-tipped Freer periosteal elevator reflects the periorbita off the orbital floor more posteriorly (Fig. 19-3).

Inspection of the orbital floor reveals a small elevation over the infraorbital neurovascular bundle. A curved hemostat is used to puncture the anterior orbital floor medial to the neurovascular bundle. Rongeurs are then used to remove the anteromedial orbital floor. The posteromedial orbital floor is removed using a front-biting rongeur. The orbital floor should be removed to the posterior wall of the maxillary sinus. The posterior wall is identified by a thick, three-pronged strut of bone formed by fusion of the orbital floor, superomedial wall of the maxillary sinus, and infralateral wall of the ethmoid sinus. Although removal of this strut may be necessary to treat compressive optic neuropathy, removal can result in a greater degree of postoperative muscle imbalance and diplopia. For this reason, the strut can be spared in cosmetic orbital decompression surgery without optic neuropathy.

The dissection proceeds into the ethmoid sinus posterior to the posterior lacrimal crest. The ethmoid bone, air cells, and mucosa are removed to include posterior ethmoid air cells. Brisk bleeding can occur during ethmoid sinusotomy and is best controlled by the complete extirpation of the ethmoid mucosa. Complete removal of the posterior ethmoid air cells is more important for treatment of compressive optic neuropathy. The dissection is kept below the fronto-ethmoidal suture to avoid inadvertent damage to the cribriform plate. Careful preoperative evaluation of coronal CT images identifies the location of the cribriform plate relative to the ethmoid sinus. The most inferior extension of the cribriform plate is usually into the anterior ethmoid air cells, where great care should be taken to avoid a cerebrospinal fluid leak.

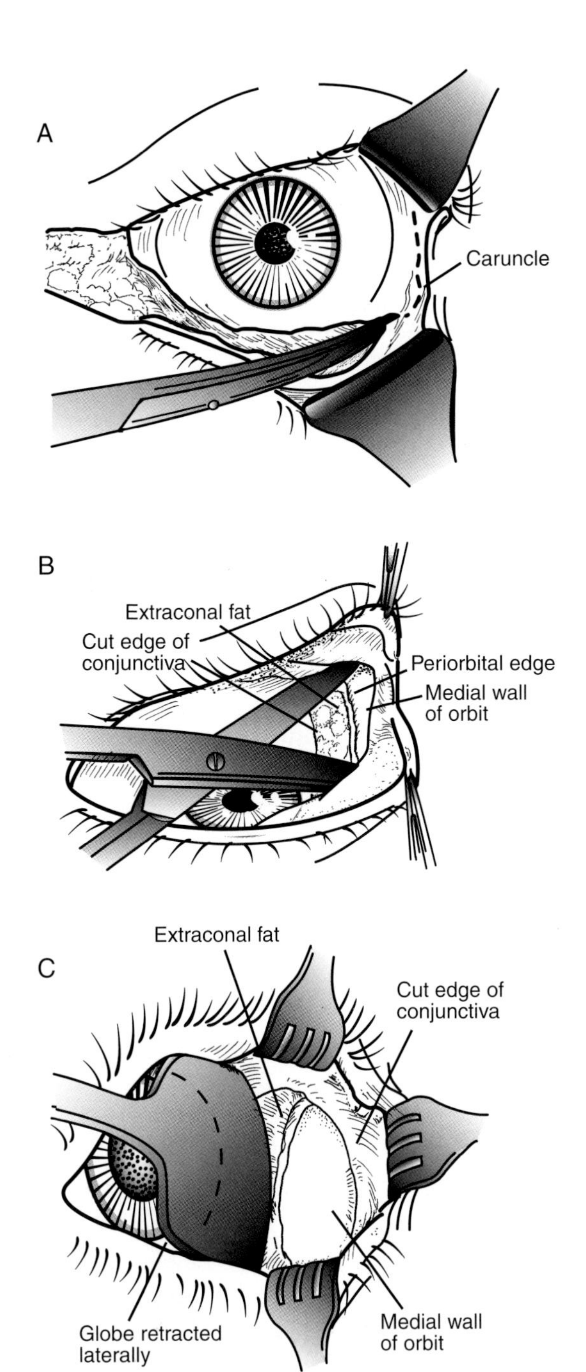

Figure 19-4 (A) Transcaruncular incision extending from the inferior fornix through the caruncle. (B) Dissection is directed posterior to the posterior lacrimal crest. (C) Wide exposure of the medial orbital wall is achieved after placement of an orbital retractor.

Removal of the posterior orbital floor and posterior ethmoid air cells back to the optic canal is essential to reduce pressure on the optic nerve. Visualization of these structures, however, can be difficult with a transconjunctival approach. Digital palpation of the orbital floor and medial orbital wall assists in identifying residual bone struts, which may hinder a complete decompression of the orbital apex. Some surgeons employ the transconjunctival approach inferiorly, combined with either an external ethmoidectomy (Lynch) approach or a transnasal endoscopic approach to the medial orbital wall. These latter approaches may provide better visualization of the posteromedial orbital wall. Alternatively, the transcaruncular approach, described below, provides improved access to the orbital apex.

19-6-2 *Inferomedial Orbital Decompression Using a Transcaruncular Approach.* For the transcaruncular approach, 1 to 3 mL of 1% lidocaine with 1:100,000 epinephrine is infiltrated into the anterior medial canthus under general anesthesia. The posterior lacrimal crest is located by palpation with a malleable retractor. Using Westcott scissors, a 12-mm vertical incision is created through the lateral third of the caruncle, taking care to avoid the semilunar fold (Fig. 19-4). The fibrous layer deep to the caruncle is incised with Stevens scissors in the direction of the posterior lacrimal crest, and the scissors are gently spread to establish the dissection plane. This dissection plane between the orbital septum and Horner's muscle is continued to the periorbita just posterior to the posterior lacrimal crest. The periorbita is exposed with a malleable retractor and incised with a monopolar cautery instrument. A periosteal elevator creates a wide aperture by reflecting the periorbita superiorly and inferiorly. The anterior and posterior ethmoidal arteries are identified and cauterized with bipolar cautery. Next, the periorbita is widely elevated to provide

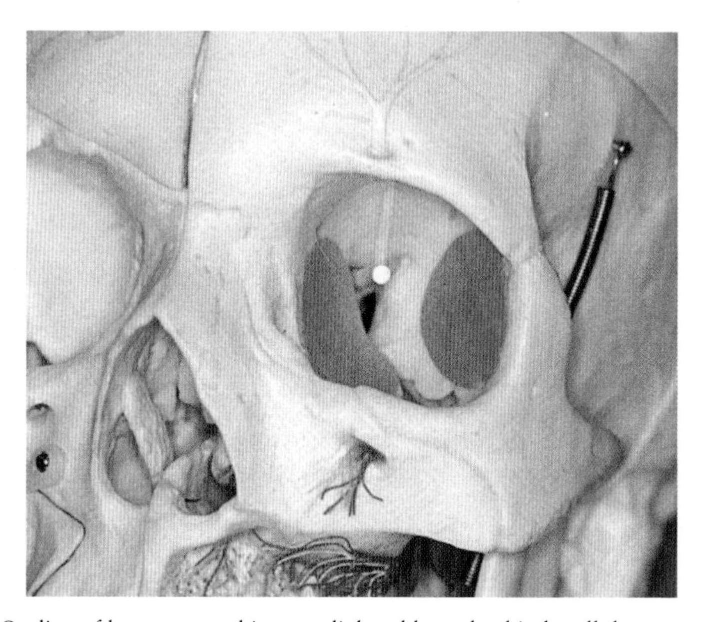

Figure 19-5 Outline of bone removal in a medial and lateral orbital wall decompression.

wide exposure of the entire medial wall, the medial extent of the superior and inferior walls, and the orbital apex. Removal of the medial and inferiomedial walls then proceeds as described previously.

After bony removal, the periosteum is incised, taking care to avoid injury to the medial and inferior rectus muscles. The orbital contents are gently prolapsed through the periosteotomy. Intraconal fat can be excised using a bipolar cautery and scissors. The caruncular incision is closed with interrupted 6-0 plain gut sutures.

19-6-3 *Lateral Orbital Floor and Lateral Wall Decompression Techniques.* For patients with mild proptosis (<24 mm), the inferomedial orbital decompression is generally satisfactory. Patients with moderate proptosis (24 to 28 mm) usually require removal of the lateral orbital floor and lateral wall (Fig. 19-5) in addition to the medial wall. Some surgeons advocate lateral wall-only decompression, combined with fat removal when possible, as a first choice for surgical orbital decompression, adding inferomedial decompression for greater amounts of proptosis reduction.[26]

The lateral orbital floor is most commonly approached through a lateral canthotomy and inferior conjunctival approach, as described previously. After the periosteum is elevated from the lateral floor of the orbit, a curved hemostat or small osteotome can be used to puncture the orbital floor lateral to the infraorbital nerve. The orbital floor is thicker in this area and slightly more difficult to puncture. Front- and back-biting rongeurs are then used to remove the lateral orbital floor back to the infraorbital fissure. Care is taken not to dissect into the infraorbital fissure, where damage to the infraorbital nerve and excessive bleeding can occur. The anterior portion of the infraorbital fissure extends into the mid-orbit and is quickly encountered when dissecting posteriorly along the lateral orbital floor. Even with maximal orbital decompression, a strut of bone should be preserved over the infraorbital nerve to prevent the globe from dropping too far inferiorly (i.e., hypoglobus).

The lateral wall may also be approached through an extended upper eyelid crease incision or through a coronal incision. For lateral wall decompression, the lateral canthal tendon can be disinserted and the inner aspect of the lateral orbital wall either burred away with a power drill or excised with a large rongeur, leaving the orbital rim intact. Moderate lateral expansion of the orbit can be achieved by aggressive bone removal along the posterior lateral orbital wall. Other techniques of lateral orbital decompression include complete removal of the lateral orbital wall through an extended lateral canthotomy incision,[37] advancing or rotating the lateral orbital wall with miniplate fixation,[21,22] and a coronal trans-temporalis approach for removal of the lateral wall while leaving the orbital rim intact.[38]

19-6-4 *Balanced Orbital Decompression.* As mentioned earlier, some orbital surgeons advocate a "balanced" orbital decompression in an attempt to reduce the incidence of postoperative diplopia and globe displacement. The procedure involves decompression of the medial and lateral orbital walls while leaving the lateral orbital floor intact and preserving the maxillo-ethmoidal strut. This technique may be best suited for patients with no preoperative diplopia, moderate to severe proptosis, and no evidence of optic neuropathy.

19-7 ORBITAL FAT DECOMPRESSION

Removal of additional orbital fat can assist in a more complete orbital decompression.[27] Fat from within and around the muscle cone can be removed from the medial, inferior, and lateral orbit through the lateral canthotomy and transconjunctival approach. A second incision in the upper eyelid crease can access the superior orbit for additional fat removal. Great care must be taken when removing intraconal and posterior orbital fat to avoid excessive bleeding and injury to vital structures.

19-8 ADDITIONAL TECHNIQUES FOR SEVERE EXOPHTHALMOS

The advent of miniplate and microplate fixation has ushered in a new era in craniofacial surgery. These techniques have been used to develop more aggressive orbital expansion procedures.[21,22] Advancement and rotation of the lateral orbital wall expands the orbit both internally and externally and can aid in a greater reduction in proptosis. For severe exophthalmos, some authors advocate a neurosurgical approach to a four-walled decompression.[39,40] These four-wall decompressions allow maximal expansion of the orbital volume, resulting in a greater reduction in exophthalmos. Four-wall decompression may involve greater morbidity and is often reserved for patients with severe proptosis (>30 mm).

19-9 COMPLICATIONS OF ORBITAL DECOMPRESSION

Orbital decompression surgery by any approach carries a significant risk of serious complications. Complications include diplopia, obstruction of the maxillary sinus ostium with secondary sinusitis, preseptal and orbital cellulitis, nasolacrimal duct obstruction, lateral canthal deformity, scarring, globe malposition (i.e., hypoglobus), extensive blood loss, cerebrospinal fluid leaks and secondary meningitis, infraorbital hypesthesia, and visual loss.

Maxillary sinusitis may require placement of a nasoantral window to facilitate adequate sinus drainage. Persistent diplopia may require corrective strabismus surgery. Eyelid retraction is not specifically addressed with orbital decompression surgery, and corrective eyelid surgery may be required despite a reduction in proptosis. Temporary numbness of the ipsilateral cheek and gums is common, lasting from 3 to 6 months. Permanent hypesthesia is uncommon. Damage to the lacrimal sac or nasolacrimal duct may lead to permanent nasolacrimal obstruction, requiring secondary dacryocystorhinostomy. Persistent or recurrent optic neuropathy can occur even after maximal orbital decompression surgery. In this event, an orbital CT scan should be obtained to rule out residual bone that may be impinging on the optic nerve. Reoperation may be necessary to remove residual bone struts near the orbital apex. In the face of failed orbital decompression surgery with no evidence of residual bony compression of the optic nerve, systemic corticosteroids and orbital radiation therapy can be considered.

REFERENCES

1. Graves RJ. Clinical lectures delivered at the Meath Hospital during the session 1834-1835. Lecture XII. Newly observed affection of the thyroid. *London Med Surg.* 1835;7:515–523.
2. Jacobson DL, et al. Epidemiology and estimated population burden of selected autoimmune diseases in the United States. *Clin Immunol Immunopathol.* 1997;84(3):223–243.
3. Wiersinga WM, Bartalena L. Epidemiology and prevention of Graves' ophthalmopathy. *Thyroid.* 2002;12(10):855–860.
4. Trobe JD, et al. Dysthyroid optic neuropathy. Clinical profile and rationale for management. *Arch Ophthalmol.* 1978;96(7):1199–1209.
5. Kazim M, et al. Treatment of acute Graves orbitopathy. *Ophthalmology.* 1991;98(9):1443–1448.
6. Gorman CA. Temporal relationship between onset of Graves' ophthalmopathy and diagnosis of thyrotoxicosis. *Mayo Clin Proc.* 1983;58(8):515–519.
7. Donaldson SS, et al. Supervoltage orbital radiotherapy for Graves' ophthalmopathy. *J Clin Endocrinol Metab.* 1973;37(2):276–285.
8. Bartalena L, et al. Orbital radiotherapy for Graves' ophthalmopathy. *Thyroid.* 2002;12(3):245–250.
9. Gorman CA, et al. A prospective, randomized, double-blind, placebo-controlled study of orbital radiotherapy for Graves' ophthalmopathy. *Ophthalmology.* 2001;108(9): 1523–1534.
10. Wakelkamp IM, et al. Orbital irradiation for Graves' ophthalmopathy: Is it safe? A long-term follow-up study. *Ophthalmology.* 2004;111(8):1557–1562.
11. Schaefer U, et al. A long-term follow-up study after retro-orbital irradiation for Graves' ophthalmopathy. *Int J Radiat Oncol Biol Phys.* 2002;52(1):192–197.
12. Bradley EA, et al. Orbital radiation for graves ophthalmopathy: a report by the American Academy of Ophthalmology. *Ophthalmology.* 2008;115(2):398–409.
13. Bartalena L, et al. Relation between therapy for hyperthyroidism and the course of Graves' ophthalmopathy. *N Engl J Med.* 1998;338(2):73–78.
14. Perry JD, et al. Transcaruncular orbital decompression for dysthyroid optic neuropathy. *Ophthal Plast Reconstr Surg.* 2003;19(5):353–358.
15. Dollinger J. Die Drukentlastung der Augenhohl durch Entfernung der auBeren Orbitalwand bei hochgradigen exophthalmos (Morbus Basedow) und konsekutiver Hornhuaterkrangkung. *Dtsch Med Wochenschr.* 1911;37:1888–1890.
16. Hirsch VO, Urbanek GR. Behandlung eines excessiven exophthalmos (Basedow) durch Entfernung von orbital fett von der Kieferhohle aus. *Monatsschr F Ohrenh.* 1930;64: 212–213.
17. Naffziger HC. Progressive exophthalmos following thyroidectomy; its pathology and treatment. *Ann Surg.* 1931;94(4):582–586.
18. Sewell EC. Operative control of progressive exophthalmos. *Arch Otolaryngol Head Neck Surg.* 1936;24:621–624.
19. Walsh TE, Ogura JH. Transantral orbital decompression for malignant exophthalmos. *Laryngoscope.* 1957;67(6):544–568.
20. Soares-Welch CV, et al. Optic neuropathy of Graves disease: results of transantral orbital decompression and long-term follow-up in 215 patients. *Am J Ophthalmol.* 2003;136(3):433–441.
21. Wolfe SA. Modified three-wall orbital expansion to correct persistent exophthalmos or exorbitism. *Plast Reconstr Surg.* 1979;64(4):448–455.
22. Wulc AE, et al. Lateral wall advancement in orbital decompression. *Ophthalmology.* 1990;97(10):1358–1369.

23. Michel O, et al. Follow-up of transnasal orbital decompression in severe Graves' ophthalmopathy. *Ophthalmology.* 2001;108(2):400–404.
24. Goldberg RA, et al. The medical orbital strut in the prevention of postdecompression dystopia in dysthyroid ophthalmopathy. *Ophthal Plast Reconstr Surg.* 1992; 8(1):32–34.
25. Graham SM, et al. Medial and lateral orbital wall surgery for balanced decompression in thyroid eye disease. *Laryngoscope.* 2003;113(7):1206–1209.
26. Goldberg RA, et al. Strabismus after balanced medial plus lateral wall versus lateral wall only orbital decompression for dysthyroid orbitopathy. *Ophthal Plast Reconstr Surg.* 2000;16(4):271–277.
27. Olivari N. Transpalpebral decompression of endocrine ophthalmopathy (Graves' disease) by removal of intraorbital fat: experience with 147 operations over 5 years. *Plast Reconstr Surg.* 1991;87(4):627–643.
28. Richter DF, et al. Transpalpebral decompression of endocrine ophthalmopathy by intraorbital fat removal (Olivari technique): experience and progression after more than 3000 operations over 20 years. *Plast Reconstr Surg.* 2007;120(1):109–123.
29. Anderson RL, Linberg JV. Transorbital approach to decompression in Graves' disease. *Arch Ophthalmol.* 1981;99(1):120–124.
30. Kennedy DW, et al. Endoscopic transnasal orbital decompression. *Arch Otolaryngol Head Neck Surg.* 1990;116(3):275–282.
31. Kulwin DR, et al. Combined approach to orbital decompression. *Otolaryngol Clin North Am.* 1990;23(3):381–390.
32. McCord CD Jr., Moses JL. Exposure of the inferior orbit with fornix incision and lateral canthotomy. *Ophthalmic Surg.* 1979;10(6):53–63.
33. DeSanto LW. Transantral orbital decompression. In: CA Gorman, RR Waller, JA Dyer, eds. *The Eye and Orbit in Thyroid Disease.* New York: Raven Press, 1984:231–251.
34. Warren JD, et al. Long-term follow-up and recent observations on 305 cases of orbital decompression for dysthyroid orbitopathy. *Laryngoscope.* 1989;99(1):35–40.
35. Garrity JA, et al. Results of transantral orbital decompression in 428 patients with severe Graves' ophthalmopathy. *Am J Ophthalmol.* 1993;116(5):533–547.
36. Shorr N, et al. Transcaruncular approach to the medial orbit and orbital apex. *Ophthalmology.* 2000;107(8):1459–1463.
37. McCord C D Jr. Orbital decompression for Graves' disease. Exposure through lateral canthal and inferior fornix incision. *Ophthalmology.* 1981;88(6):533–541.
38. Leatherbarrow B, et al. Three wall orbital decompression for Graves' ophthalmopathy via a coronal approach. *Eye.* 1991;5(Pt 4):456–465.
39. Maroon JC, Kennerdell JS. Radical orbital decompression for severe dysthyroid exophthalmos. *J Neurosurg.* 1982;56(2):260–266.
40. Stranc M, West M. A four-wall orbital decompression for dysthyroid orbitopathy. *J Neurosurg.* 1988;68(5):671–677.

20

Optic Nerve Sheath Decompression

THOMAS N. HWANG, MD, PHD, AND TIMOTHY J. McCULLEY, MD

Optic nerve sheath decompression (ONSD) or fenestration refers to a surgical technique that creates a window through the dural and arachnoid meningeal layers of the retrobulbar optic nerve sheath to release pressure on the optic nerve. ONSD for treatment of visual loss secondary to refractory papilledema was first described by DeWecker in 1872.[1] Later that century, Carter and Müller published the second case series of optic nerve sheath fenestrations.[2] However, despite these and several additional reports, the clinical benefit of performing this procedure was still questioned.[1–4] In addition, alternative cerebrospinal shunting procedures were developed for patients with increased intracranial pressure.[5,6] Renewed interest arose in 1964 when Hayreh demonstrated the effectiveness of ONSD in relieving experimental papilledema in rhesus monkeys.[7] Various supporting clinical publications have since followed, starting with Smith, Hoyt, and Newton's description in 1969 of relief of chronic papilledema by ONSD.[8–14]

20-1 INDICATIONS FOR OPTIC NERVE SHEATH DECOMPRESSION

Surgical intervention is considered for patients with progressive visual loss secondary to elevated intracranial pressure (ICP) in whom conservative management, such as medications (acetazolamide and furosemide) and weight control, has failed.[8–14] Occasionally surgery is used primarily in patients whose visual function has already reached a critical level. Examples include patients in whom vision has declined to a disabling level in hopes that rapid papilledema resolution will result in some visual return. Surgery is also considered primarily in those with little remaining vision, in whom any further visual loss would carry substantial functional impact should conservative management fail.

Once surgical intervention is deemed necessary, ONSD is one of several options. Cerebrospinal fluid (CSF) shunting in the form of ventricular–peritoneal (VP) or lumbar–peritoneal (LP) shunting can be considered. A deciding factor for some is the presence of headache, which is more effectively managed with VP or LP shunting. Comparative trials of ONSD and other CSF shunting procedures are lacking. Consequently, some medical centers opt for ONSD as the first-line surgical option, while others recommend alternative shunting procedures.

At present, the only uniformly accepted therapeutic indication for ONSD is management of visual loss related to elevated ICP. The most common setting for ONSD is idiopathic intracranial hypertension. However, ONSD may restore or stabilize visual loss from elevated ICP secondary to other causes such as sinus thrombosis and cryptococcal meningitis.[15–18] As always, surgical risk must be weighed against the degree of visual loss and progression, and when appropriate, life expectancy is considered.

Some controversy surrounds whether bilateral fenestration should be a consideration. The argument for it is decreasing the number of times a patient must be subjected to general anesthesia. Also, simultaneous bilateral surgery limits the risk for progressive visual loss while waiting for second eye surgery. The argument against simultaneous bilateral surgery is based largely on the fact that in a substantial proportion of patients, bilateral improvement may be seen with unilateral surgery. Sergott et al. reported fellow eye improvement in 12 of 21 patients.[10] Staged surgeries also avoid the possibility of bilateral visual loss should complications occur. If visual loss was encountered with the first ONSD, if needed the second eye could be managed with alternative CSF shunting procedures. Most clinicians recommend against bilateral simultaneous ONSD.

Numerous reports describe ONSD being performed in settings not associated with elevated ICP: arteritic and non-arteritic ischemic optic neuropathy, optic pits with serous retinal detachments, optic neuropathy accompanying acute retinal necrosis, central retinal vein occlusions, optic nerve drusen with progressive visual loss, and traumatic optic neuropathy.[19–24] One series described treatment of 17 patients with retrobulbar optic nerve sheath enlargement from any cause with progressive visual loss, including intracranial hemorrhage and optic nerve meningioma.[25] However, only the treatment of non-arteritic anterior ischemic optic neuropathy (NAION) with ONSD has undergone the scrutiny of a randomized controlled clinical study in the Ischemic Optic Neuropathy Treatment Trial (IONDT). In this cohort, surgery proved to be of no benefit and was possibly detrimental to patients with NAION.[26] Until appropriately established effective outside of the setting of elevated ICP, ONSD should be considered investigational and no more than a last resort in such cases.

The following case is illustrative. A 35-year-old woman presented with severe chronic papilledema. Neuroimaging studies revealed no evidence of a compressive mass lesion. Intracranial pressure was markedly elevated by lumbar puncture. Visual acuity was 20/200 OD, 20/25 OS, and visual fields were markedly constricted in both eyes. Due to the severity of visual loss on presentation, surgery was pursued primarily. ONSD was performed first on the right eye and then on the left eye 1 week later. By 6 weeks after surgery, optic disc swelling had resolved (Fig. 20-1) and visual function had normalized.

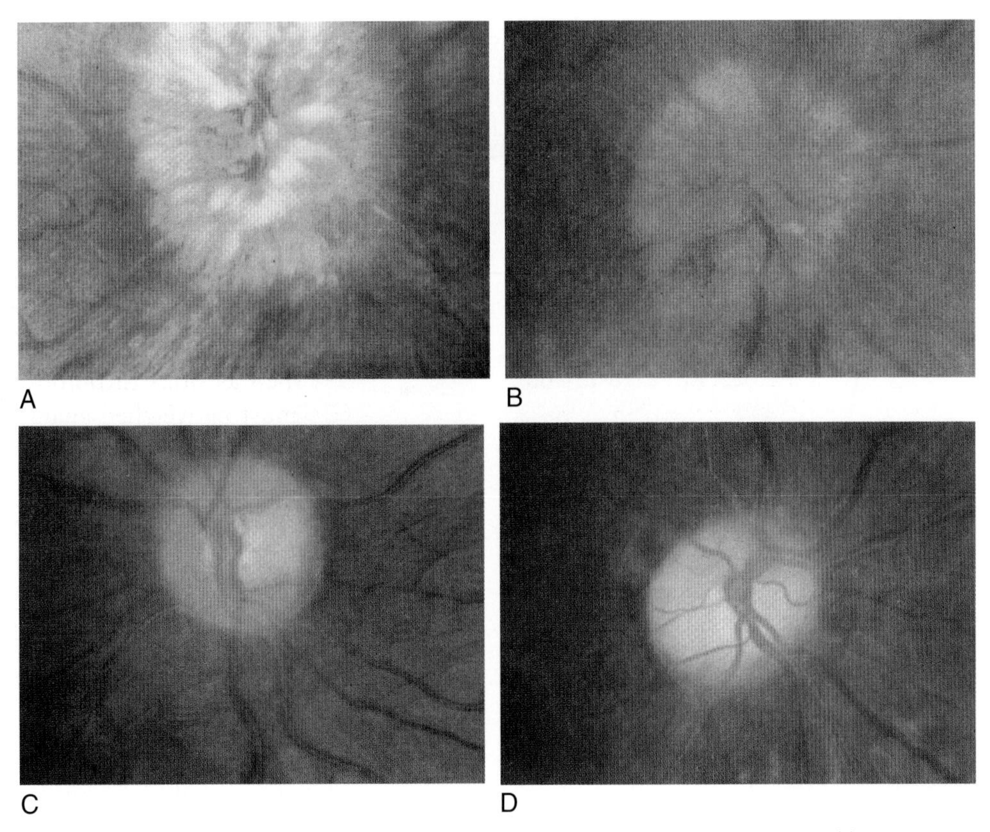

Figure 20-1 Chronic asymmetric papilledema in a patient with idiopathic intracranial hypertension. (A) Right eye. (B) Left eye. Resolution of papilledema after successful ONSD. (C) Right eye. (D) Left eye.

20-2 TECHNIQUES OF OPTIC NERVE SHEATH DECOMPRESSION

ONSD can be performed using a variety of approaches, generally divided into lateral, medial, and superomedial. Almost exclusively done under general anesthesia, ONSD can be theoretically performed with a retrobulbar or peribulbar infiltrative anesthetic if general anesthesia is contraindicated. Positioning of the patient in slightly reverse Trendelenburg can reduce orbital venous pressure during the surgery. The following briefly describes the finer nuances of the various approaches to the optic nerve sheath. Actual fenestration, common to all approaches, is described next.

20-2-1 *Medial Approach.* In 1973, Galbraith and Sullivan published the original description of a medial approach to the optic nerve that involved a transconjunctival medial orbitotomy and disinsertion of the medial rectus muscle.[27] The medial approach provides a direct route to the optic nerve. Because there are fewer short ciliary vessels, the medial approach allows access to the nerve sheath with less disruption of the vessels and nerves (Fig. 20-2). In addition, if the nasal short ciliary vessels are violated or the nasal optic nerve is directly damaged, the resulting injury would

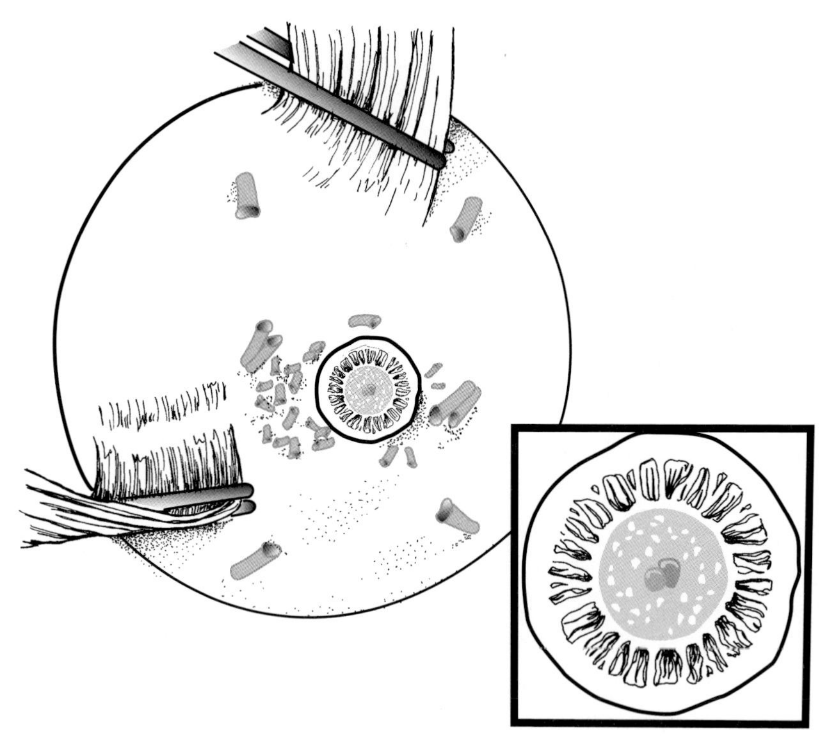

Figure 20-2 View of posterior pole from orbit, showing increased number of short ciliary vessels temporal to optic nerve.

theoretically create visual field deficits farther in the periphery than damage to the lateral optic nerve, which contains the papillomacular bundle.

The medial approach begins with either a 360-degree or a nasal 180-degree peritomy. Tenon's capsule is dissected away from the medial rectus, which is then disinserted from the globe. Traction sutures are either looped beneath the vertical recti muscles or placed through the medial rectus insertion so that the globe can be abducted, swinging the optic nerve closer to the medial incision. The medial rectus is retracted to expose the vortex veins and the long ciliary arteries in the orbital fat (Fig. 20-3). The fat is retracted with cotton-tipped applicators and half-inch neurosurgical cottonoids to reveal short ciliary vessels and nerves identifying the retrobulbar optic nerve sheath. After creating the fenestration as described below, the retractors are removed, the medial rectus is reattached to the globe with partial-thickness scleral bites using locking suture, and the conjunctiva is reapproximated.

20-2-2 *Lateral Approach*. DeWecker's original publication reported a lateral approach through a lower temporal conjunctival incision.[1] The surgeon would identify the optic nerve by palpation and incise the sheath blindly with a guarded knife. Then, Carter described a temporal transconjunctival approach that involved disinserting and retracting the lateral rectus to gain direct visualization before incising the sheath.[2,3] The next technical modifications attempted to improve exposure and gain a more perpendicular view of the retrobulbar optic nerve by performing a

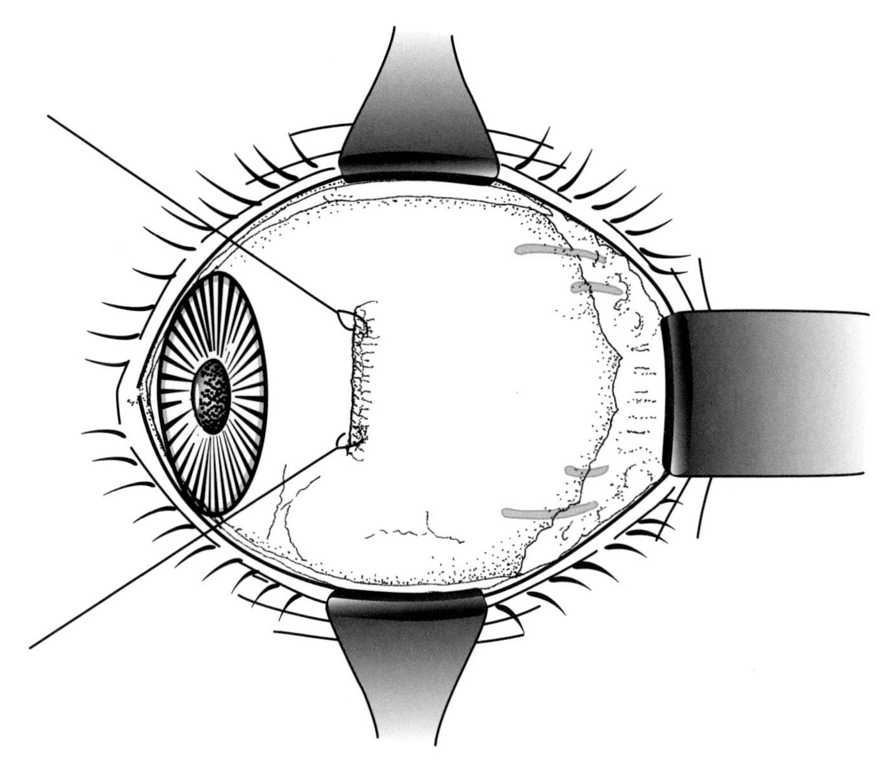

Figure 20-3 Exposure of optic nerve sheath by retracting globe laterally with two sutures and the medial rectus medially with malleable retractor. Optic nerve lies between long ciliary vessels.

cutaneous incision with a lateral bone window.[4,28–30] Adequate visualization without the need for a bone window through a lateral canthotomy incision has also been reported.[31]

For the bone window, a standard lateral skin incision is made, such as a Stallard-Wright or a Harris incision, to allow dissection to the lateral orbital rim. For the lateral canthotomy approach, an approximately 1-cm lateral canthotomy incision is made with straight scissors or a scalpel, which provides sufficient exposure to dissect down to the lateral orbital rim. For both techniques, the periosteum is then incised and then freed carefully from the lateral orbital wall with a periosteal elevator to approximately 2 cm posterior to the lateral orbital rim. To create a lateral bone window, the bone is removed in standard fashion between the zygomaticofrontal suture and a point just above the fusion of the zygomatic arch and the orbital rim, usually using an oscillating power saw.

A T-shaped incision is then made through the periorbita followed by blunt dissection to the lateral rectus muscle, which can be retracted inferiorly for exposure rather than disinserted. During dissection, half-inch cottonoids with Sewell retractors are helpful tools to keep the orbital fat from obscuring one's view. Blunt dissection through the intermuscular septum and intraconal fat to the optic nerve must safely bypass the vortex veins that lie within the orbital fat. With a lateral canthotomy approach, the dissection necessarily stays more anterior, adjacent to the posterior globe, making incision of the periosteum unnecessary. A traction suture can be placed transconjunctivally under the lateral rectus muscle; this allows the globe to be adducted, bringing the retrobulbar optic nerve closer to the incision site. The optic nerve can be isolated just as it exits the globe.

Once the fenestration is performed as described below, careful hemostasis is achieved and retractors are removed. The periorbital flaps can be reapproximated with polyglactin sutures. If a bone window was created, the bone is sewn or plated back into position. Lastly, the orbicularis oculi muscle and skin are closed in a layered fashion.

20-2-3 *Superomedial Approach.* The superomedial approach for ONSD is a relatively new approach that involves gaining access to the intraconal space via a medial upper eyelid crease incision, which does not require a bone window or disinsertion of any extraocular muscles.[32] The surgeon makes an incision through the medial third of the upper eyelid and sharply dissects through the orbital septum until the medial horn of the levator aponeurosis can be identified and retracted laterally. Then, blunt dissection is carried deeper into the orbit through the orbital fat in an inferior and lateral direction, moving toward the posterior aspect of the globe. The route passes above the medical rectus muscle and below the superior oblique muscle. Important landmarks to avoid damaging include the superior ophthalmic vein and, as stated previously, the vortex veins and the posterior ciliary vessels. The posterior ciliary vessels also provide a convenient way to identify the retrobulbar optic nerve. After creation of the optic nerve sheath window, the incision can be closed with a simple skin closure.

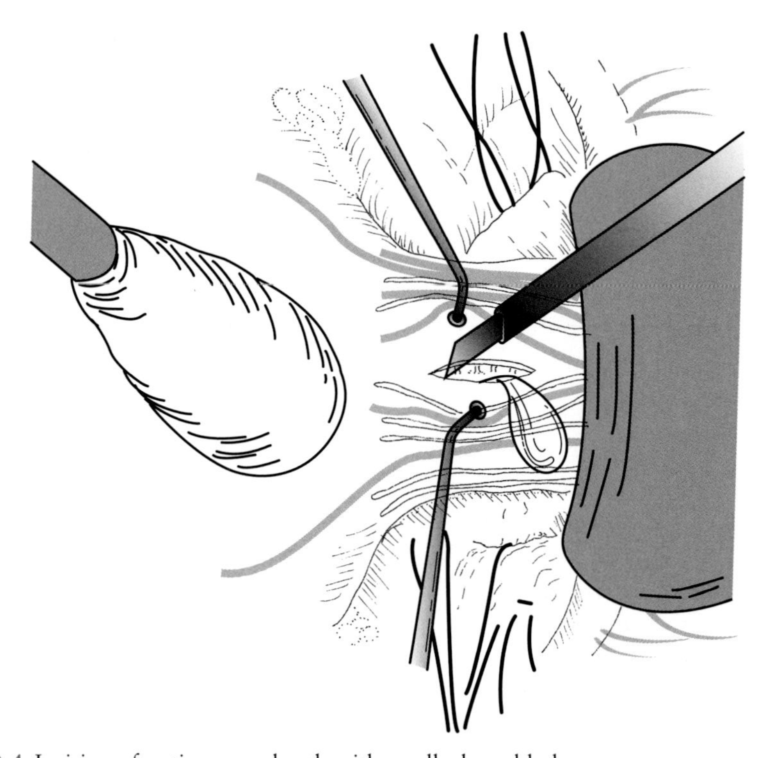

Figure 20-4 Incision of optic nerve sheath with small, sharp blade.

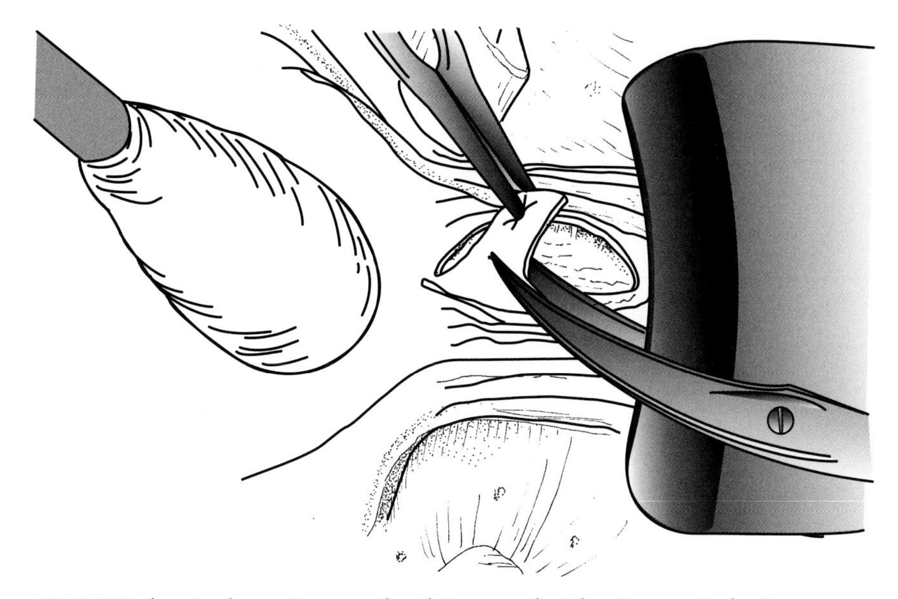

Figure 20-5 Window in the optic nerve sheath is created with microsurgical scissors.

20-2-4 *Fenestration of the Optic Nerve Sheath.* Once the retrobulbar optic nerve is reached, the fenestration is performed. The short ciliary nerve, the posterior ciliary arteries, and the vascular network from the ophthalmic artery that supply the more posterior optic nerve must all be identified and preserved. In an area that does not have any vessels, the dura can be grasped with microsurgery forceps and incised either with microsurgery scissors or a blade (Fig. 20-4). If the arachnoid was not adhered to the dura, it may remain intact and bulge through the dural incision. In such a case, this meningeal layer must be held and incised to create the window without damaging the underlying optic nerve of pial vasculature (Fig. 20-5). Various minor modifications have been proposed, mostly centering on creating windows, slits, or some combination through the nerve sheath. For example, Tse et al. reported making a 3 × 5-mm window, while Kersten and Kulwin described a larger 5 × 8-mm window.[29,30] Several reports also describe the intraoperative application of mitomycin C to the optic nerve sheath to inhibit fibrosis and fistula closure, although no controlled studies have specifically investigated its effectiveness.[33–35]

20-3 MECHANISM OF OPTIC NERVE SHEATH DECOMPRESSION

Although the mechanism of successful ONSD is unknown, two possibilities have been postulated. First, the operation may create a permanent fistula, draining CSF and reducing local subarachnoid pressure.[4,5,7,36] Second, incising the optic nerve sheath may incite scarring and glial proliferation in the subarachnoid space, protecting the optic nerve from high intracranial pressure.[27,28]

Supporting the drainage theory, Keltner, examining the optic nerve from a patient 39 days after ONSD, found no pathologic evidence for blockage of either the fistula or the subarachnoid space surrounding the optic nerve.[36] The patient was, however, treated with corticosteroids and immunosuppressive drugs, hindering his fibroblastic response. Postoperative observations, including relief of headaches, improvement of edema in the contralateral unoperated optic disc, and complete filling of the subarachnoid space without evidence of obstruction after instillation of intrathecal iopamidol, support fistulization as the probable mechanism of ONSD.[9–11] The use of topical mitomycin C as an adjunct to ONSD is based on this mechanism. In contrast, Davidson reported two pathologic studies demonstrating postoperative occlusion of the ONSD site and the subarachnoid space by early granulation tissue, consistent with creation of a barrier against the high ICP.[27,28] Hayreh described similar pathologic findings in a monkey model with balloon-induced papilledema that had previously undergone ONSD.[7] The possibility also exists that both play a role to varying degrees among individuals.

20-4 SURGICAL FAILURE AND REPEAT FENESTRATION

After successful ONSD, ICP may remain elevated despite resolution of the papilledema. Since the majority of patients undergoing ONSD have idiopathic intracranial hypertension, they have a chronic disease and often have elevated ICP for years regardless of treatment.[37] Spoor and McHenry reported progressive visual field deterioration in 15% of patients 6 months after surgery. The rate increased to 35% at 3 years and 50% at 5 years.[14] Therefore, all need to be followed routinely with formal visual field testing indefinitely.[14]

Persistent or recurrent papilledema and progressive visual field loss after optic nerve sheath fenestration suggest failure of the ONSD. Reoperation often demonstrates that the fenestration site is blocked by orbital fat. Spoor et al. reported that 11 of 13 patients who had repeat ONSD for progressive visual loss had improved visual function postoperatively.[13] However, repeat ONSD is technically more difficult because of excessive scarring and vascularization. For this reason, many clinicians would recommend VP or LP shunting over repeat ONSD.

20-5 COMPLICATIONS OF OPTIC NERVE SHEATH DECOMPRESSION

In terms of postoperative complications, the IONDT reported severe vision loss in 3 of 115 patients (2.6%), while another large study reported 3 of 200 patients (1.5%).[26,38] One study reported a rate of significant vision loss of 2 of 38 cases (5.2%).[39] The visually devastating complications usually result from ischemic events such as central retinal artery occlusions and optic nerve infarctions.[39,40] These occlusions result from vascular compromise, possibly by excessive, prolonged traction on the globe during the operation. Therefore, the traction sutures should be released periodically, permitting the eye to perfuse normally for a few moments. Other reported problems included temporary motility disorders (29%), pupillary dysfunction (11%), branched retinal artery occlusion (2.6%), and transient outer retinal ischemia (2.6%). Postoperative bleeding and infection causing vision loss have also been described.[41]

REFERENCES

1. DeWecker L. On incision of the optic nerve in cases of neuroretinitis. *Int Ophthalmol Congr Rep.* 1872;4:11–14.
2. Carter RB. On retrobulbar incision of the optic nerve in cases of swollen disc. *Brain.* 1887;10:199–209.
3. Carter RB. Operation of opening the sheath of the optic nerve for the relief of pressure. *Br Med J.* 1889;1:399–401.
4. Müller L. Die Trepanation der Optikusscheide: Eine neue Operation zur Heilung der Stauungspapille. *Wien Klin Wochenschr.* 1916;2:1001–1003.
5. Ingraham FD, Sears RA, Woods RP, et al. Further studies on the treatment of experimental hydrocephalus. *J Neurosurg.* 1949;6:207–215.
6. Matson DD. A new operation for the treatment of communicating hydrocephalus. *J Neurosurg.* 1949;6:238–247.
7. Hayreh SS. Pathogenesis of edema of the optic disc (papilloedema): a preliminary report. *Br J Ophthalmol.* 1964;48:522–542.
8. Smith JL, Hoyt WF, Newton TH. Optic nerve sheath decompression for relief of chronic monocular choked disc. *Am J Ophthalmol.* 1969;68:633–639.
9. Brourman ND, Spoor TC, Ramocki JM. Optic nerve sheath decompression for pseudotumor cerebri. *Arch Ophthalmol.* 1988;106:1378–1383.
10. Sergott RC, Savino PJ, Bosley TM. Modified optic nerve sheath decompression provides long-term visual improvement for pseudotumor cerebri. *Arch Ophthalmol.* 1988; 106:1384–1390.
11. Corbett JJ, Nerad JA, Tse DT, Anderson RL. Results of optic nerve sheath fenestration for pseudotumor cerebri: the lateral orbitotomy approach. *Arch Ophthalmol.* 1988;106:1391–1397.
12. Keltner JL. Optic nerve sheath decompression: how does it work? has its time come? *Arch Ophthalmol.* 1988;106:1365–1369.
13. Spoor TC, Ramocki JM, Madion MP, Wilkinson MJ. Treatment of pseudotumor cerebri by primary and secondary optic nerve sheath decompression. *Am J Ophthalmol.* 1991;112:177–185.
14. Spoor TC, McHenry JG. Long-term effectiveness of optic nerve sheath decompression for pseudotumor cerebri. *Arch Ophthalmol.* 1993;111:632–635.
15. Kelman SE, Sergott RC, Cioffi GA, et al. Modified optic nerve decompression in patients with functioning lumboperitoneal shunts and progressive visual loss. *Ophthalmology.* 1991;98:1449–1453.
16. Horton JC, Seiff SR, Pitts LH, et al. Decompression of the optic nerve sheath for vision-threatening papilledema caused by dural sinus occlusion. *Neurosurgery.* 1992; 31:203–212.
17. Garrity JA, Herman DC, Imes R, et al. Optic nerve sheath decompression for visual loss in patients with acquired immunodeficiency syndrome and cryptococcal meningitis with papilledema. *Am J Ophthalmol.* 1993;116(4):472–478.
18. Cremer PD, Johnston IH, Halmagyi GM. Pseudotumour cerebri syndrome due to cryptococcal meningitis. *J Neurol Neurosurg Psychiatry.* 1997;62(1):96–98.
19. Sergott RC, Cohen MS, Bosley TM, Savino PJ. Optic nerve decompression may improve the progressive form of nonarteritic ischemic optic neuropathy. *Arch Ophthalmol.* 1989;107:1743–1754.
20. Spoor TC, Wilkinson MJ, Ramocki JM. Optic nerve sheath decompression for the treatment of progressive nonarteritic ischemic optic neuropathy. *Am J Ophthalmol.* 1991;111:724–728.

21. Kelman SE, Elman MJ. Optic nerve sheath decompression for nonarteritic ischemic optic neuropathy improves multiple visual function measurements. *Arch Ophthalmol.* 1991;109:667–671.
22. Sergott RC, Anand R, Belmont JB, et al. Acute retinal necrosis neuropathy: clinical profile and surgical therapy. *Arch Ophthalmol.* 1989;107:692–696.
23. Dev S, Buckley EG. Optic nerve sheath decompression for progressive central retinal vein occlusion. *Ophthalmic Surg Lasers.* 1999;30(3):181–184.
24. Guy J, Sherwood M, Day AL. Surgical treatment of progressive visual loss in traumatic optic neuropathy. Report of two cases. *J Neurosurg.* 1989;70:799–801.
25. Hupp SL, Glaser JS, Frazier-Byrne S. Optic nerve sheath decompression. Review of 17 Cases. *Arch Ophthalmol.* 1987;105(3):386–389.
26. Optic nerve decompression surgery for nonarteritic anterior ischemic optic neuropathy (NAION) is not effective and may be harmful: The Ischemic Optic Neuropathy Decompression Trial Research Group. *JAMA.* 1995;273:625–632.
27. Galbraith JE, Sullivan JH. Decompression of the perioptic meninges for relief of papilledema. *Am J Ophthalmol.* 1973;76:687–692.
28. Davidson SI. A surgical approach to plerocephalic disc edema. *Eye.* 1969;89:669–690.
29. Davidson SI: The surgical relief of papilloedema. In: Cant JS, ed. *The Optic Nerve. Proceedings of Second William Mackenzie Memorial Symposium, Glasgow, 1971.* London: Kimpton; 1972;3:174–179.
30. Tse DT, Nerad JA, Anderson RL, et al. Optic nerve sheath fenestration in pseudotumor cerebri. A lateral orbitotomy approach. *Arch Ophthalmol.* 1988;106:1458–1462.
31. Kersten RC, Kulwin DR. Optic nerve sheath fenestration through a lateral canthotomy incision. *Arch Ophthalmol.* 1993;111(6):870–874.
32. Pelton RW, Patel BC. Superomedial lid crease approach to the medial intraconal space: a new technique for access to the optic nerve and central space. *Ophthal Plast Reconstr Surg.* 2001;17(4):241–253.
33. Spoor TC, McHenry JG, Shin DH. Long-term results using adjunctive mitomycin C in optic nerve sheath decompression for pseudotumor cerebri. *Ophthalmology.* 1995;102(12):2024–2028.
34. Kersten RC, Kulwin DR. MMC in ONS decompression. *Ophthalmology.* 1996; 103(6):864–865.
35. Taban M, Spoor TC, McHenry JG, Sadun AA. Histopathology and ultrastructural examination of optic nerve sheath biopsies after optic nerve sheath decompression with and without mitomycin. *Ophthal Plast Reconstr Surg.* 2001;17(5):332–337.
36. Keltner JL, Albert DM, Lubow M, et al. Optic nerve decompression: a clinical pathologic study. *Arch Ophthalmol.* 1977;95:97–104.
37. Corbett JJ, Savino PJ, Thompson HS, et al. Visual loss in pseudotumor cerebri: follow-up of 57 patients from five to 41 years and a profile of 14 patients with permanent severe visual loss. *Arch Neurol.* 1982;39:461–474.
38. Sergott RC. Optic nerve sheath decompression: History, techniques, and indications. *Int Ophthalmol Clin.* 1991;31:71–81.
39. Plotnik JL, Kosmorsky GS. Operative complications of optic nerve sheath decompression. *Ophthalmology.* 1993:100:683–690.
40. Rizzo JF, Lessell S. Choroidal infarction after optic nerve sheath fenestration. *Ophthalmology.* 1994;101:1622–1626.
41. Mauriello JA Jr, Shaderowfsky P, Gizzi M, et al. Management of visual loss after optic nerve sheath decompression in patients with pseudotumor cerebri. *Ophthalmology.* 1995;102(3):441–445.

21

Management of Orbital Cellulitis

THOMAS E. JOHNSON, MD, JENNIFER I. HUI, MD, ERIN M. SHRIVER, MD, AND CHRISFOUAD ALABIAD, MD

21-1 INTRODUCTION

Orbital cellulitis is an acute infectious inflammation of the post-septal orbital tissues. This chapter outlines the medical and surgical management of bacterial orbital cellulitis. The paranasal sinus complex is the most common source of orbital bacterial infection. Over 50% of orbital cellulitis cases result from secondary extension from the paranasal sinuses. Other causes of orbital cellulitis include spread from ocular and periocular infections such as dacryoadenitis, dacryocystitis,[1] and panophthalmitis; trauma,[2] insect bites, or surgery; or endogenous sources in immunocompromised or septic patients.

Orbital cellulitis resulting from sinusitis is believed to start with viral or allergic inflammation of the upper respiratory system. The inflammation decreases mucociliary clearance and causes obstruction of the sinus ostia. The sinus mucosa absorbs air, thereby creating negative pressure within the sinuses. Transudation occurs, creating a nutrient medium for bacteria. Aerobic and facultative organisms proliferate, and inflammatory products accumulate resulting in decreasing oxygen tension and pH. As inflammatory products are produced, sinus pressure increases, causing mucosal blood flow to decrease. A proliferation of obligate anaerobes occurs as aerobic bacteria consume the remaining oxygen.[3,4]

Young children are less likely to develop anaerobic conditions within their sinuses because their ratio of ostia size to sinus volume is much larger than that of adults. The sinus cavities enlarge markedly with age while the ostia remain approximately the same size. Thus, as children become adults, the decreased ratio of ostia size to total sinus volume increases the propensity for anaerobic sinus infections.[4]

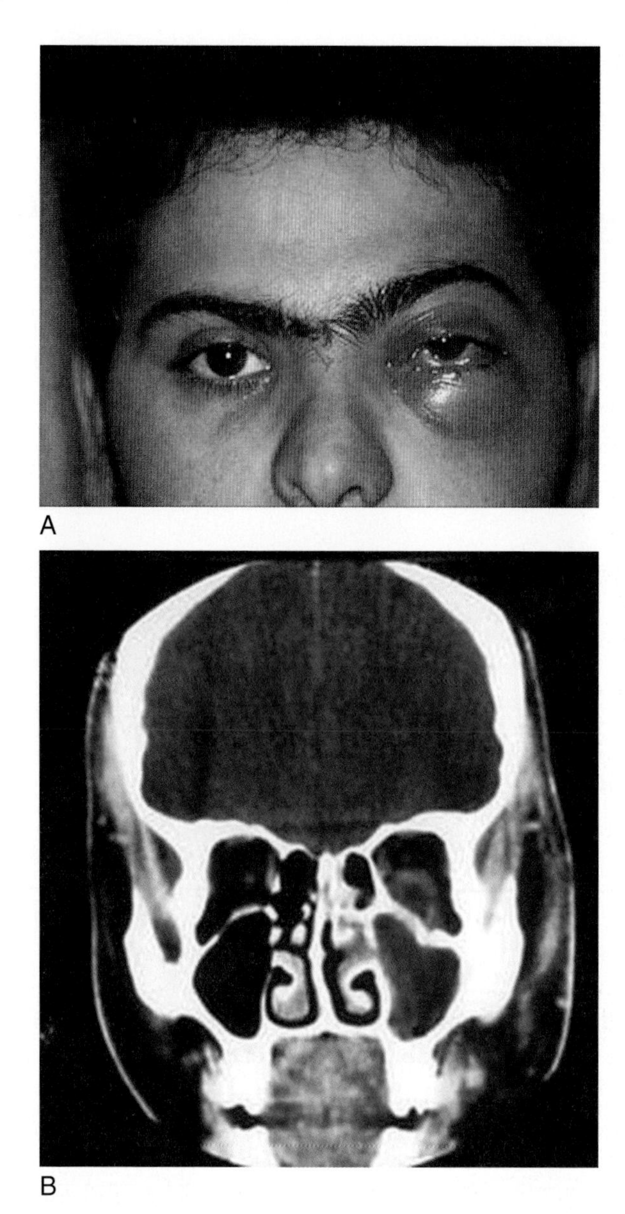

Figure 21-1 Orbital cellulitis from an odontogenic source. (A) External photo. (B) CT scan identifying infection traversing left maxillary sinus through orbital floor.

The bony walls shared by the orbit and sinuses account for approximately half of the orbital surface area.[3] Bacteria and inflammatory products from the sinuses may extend directly into the orbit through the neurovascular foramina, congenital bony dehiscences, anastomosing valveless venous channels, or compromised bony walls in cases of osteitis and necrosis secondary to sinusitis.[3] An abscess may form in the subperiosteal area, a relatively avascular potential space.

Subperiosteal abscesses most often involve the medial orbital wall, as it is the thinnest wall and is adjacent to the ethmoid sinuses. Infections may also enter the orbit inferiorly through the orbital floor, especially in patients with maxillary sinusitis or dental abscesses (Fig. 21-1). Frontal sinusitis rarely results in a superior subperiosteal abscess.

Antibiotic penetration into the subperiosteal space is minimal, and purulent material can rapidly accumulate. The resulting abscess may increase intraorbital pressure, decrease retinal perfusion, and compress the optic nerve. Delayed or inadequate treatment of orbital cellulitis can also lead to the development of an intraorbital abscess, or posterior propagation through the venous system, resulting in a cavernous sinus thrombosis. Other potential complications of a subperiosteal abscess include visual loss secondary to optic neuropathy, meningitis, or an intracranial abscess.

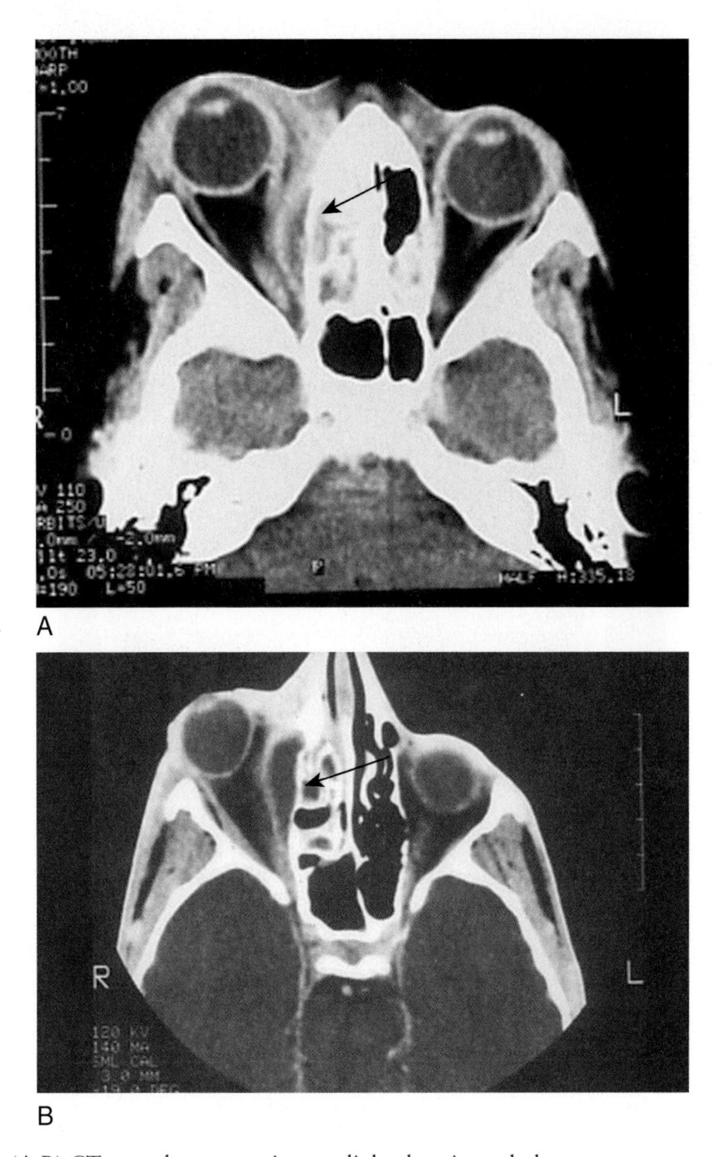

Figure 21-2 (A,B) CT scan demonstrating medial subperiosteal abscess.

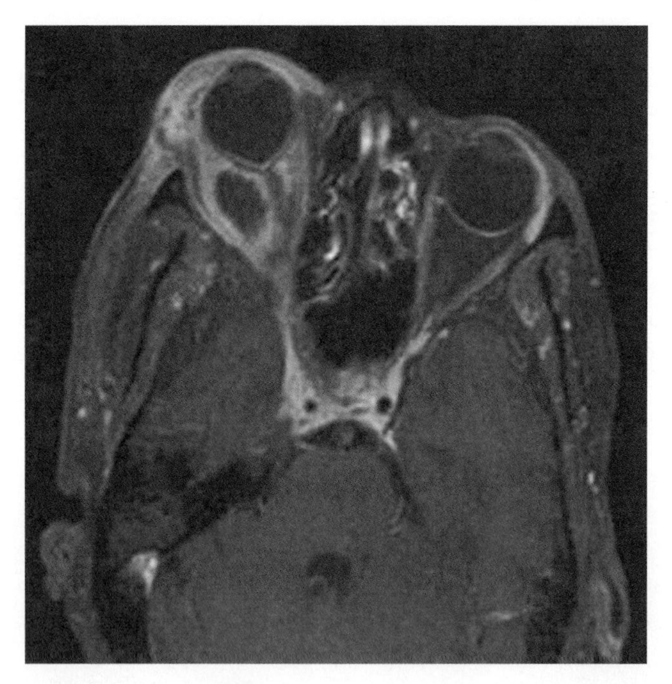

Figure 21-3 Intraorbital abscess on MRI.

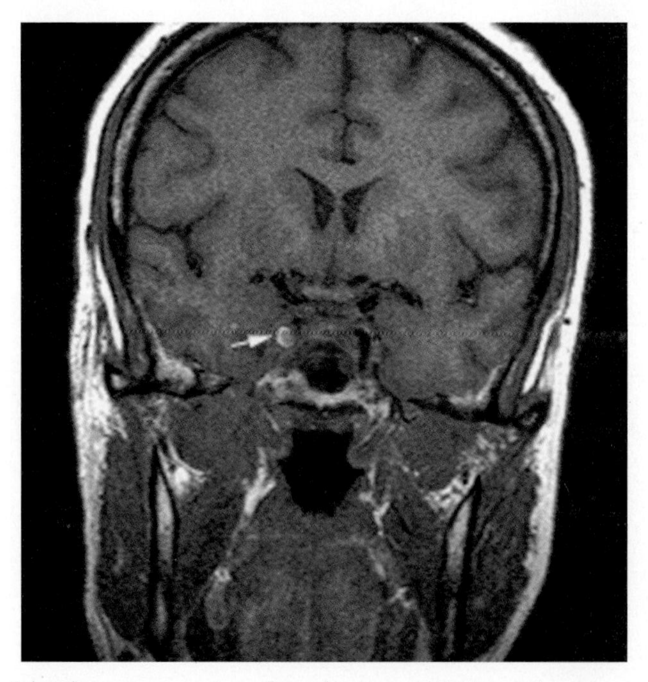

Figure 21-4 Partial right cavernous sinus thrombosis on MRI (*arrow*).

The Chandler classification describes five categories of orbital infection, not necessarily found in the following chronological order. Group I is preseptal cellulitis, when infection involves only the preseptal tissues. Group II is orbital cellulitis, with the infectious process extending posterior to the orbital septum. In group III, a subperiosteal abscess is present (Fig. 21-2) and surgical intervention is often required. Group IV is characterized by an intraorbital abscess (Fig. 21-3), and group V includes a cavernous sinus thrombosis (Fig. 21-4).[5]

21-2 EVALUATION

Prior to the examination of patients with orbital cellulitis, it is important to perform a thorough history. Past history of sinus disease, orbital trauma, periocular

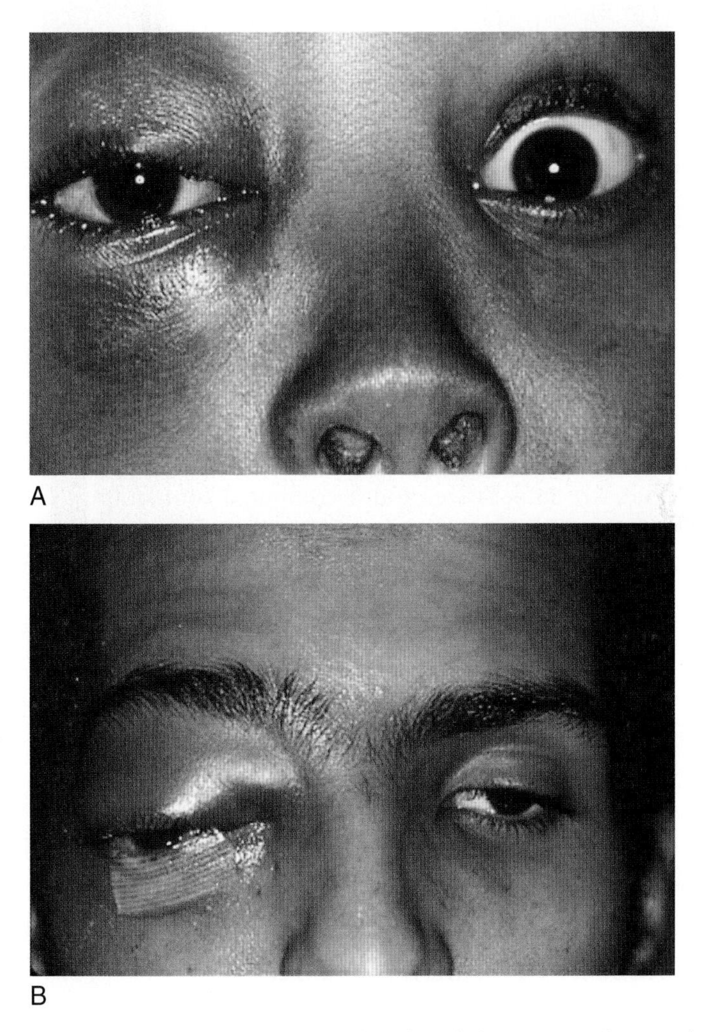

Figure 21-5 External photos. (A)Young boy with right-sided proptosis, decreased motility, and inflammation due to orbital cellulitis. (B) Adult with similar findings.

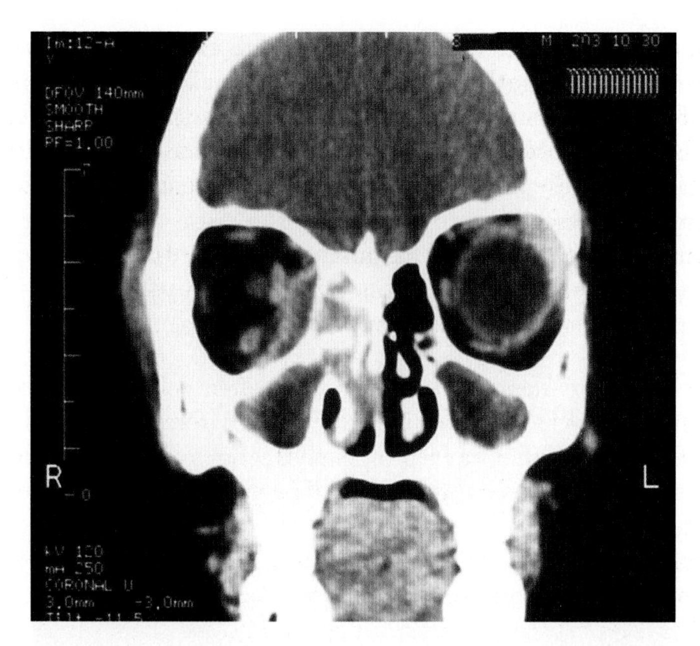

Figure 21-6 Pansinusitis on CT scan.

infections, insect bites, or previous ocular or periocular surgery should be identified. Special attention should be directed to the onset of symptoms, including fever, chills, pain, decreased vision, or bulging of the eye. Some patients may also have symptoms relating to sinusitis, including congestion, sinus pressure, or headache.

All patients with suspected orbital cellulitis require a thorough physical examination. Signs of orbital cellulitis include proptosis (Fig. 21-5), decreased ocular motility, decreased vision, conjunctival injection and chemosis, fever, and in severe cases, an afferent pupillary defect.

Imaging studies are imperative, and a computed tomography CT scan of the orbits (with/without contrast, axial/coronal views, thin cuts) is the method of choice. It is critical to carefully review the paranasal sinuses for sinusitis and the post-septal tissues for the presence of a subperiosteal or orbital abscess (Fig. 21-6). Coronal cuts are helpful in identifying and localizing an abscess and evaluating the frontal lobes for evidence of intracranial extension (Fig. 21-7). If clinical suspicion arises for cavernous sinus involvement, a magnetic resonance imaging MRI study with particular attention to this region is indicated.

Laboratory tests should include a complete blood count with differential, serum electrolytes, serum glucose, and urinalysis. Blood cultures have been shown to have a yield as high as 33% in children less than 4 years of age, but the utility of blood cultures is significantly less in those older than 4 years of age (<5%).[6]

21-3 MICROBIOLOGY OF ORBITAL CELLULITIS

Multiple organisms have been implicated in orbital cellulitis[4,7,8] (Table 21-1). Because orbital cellulitis can arise from sinusitis, bacteremia, infection of adjacent

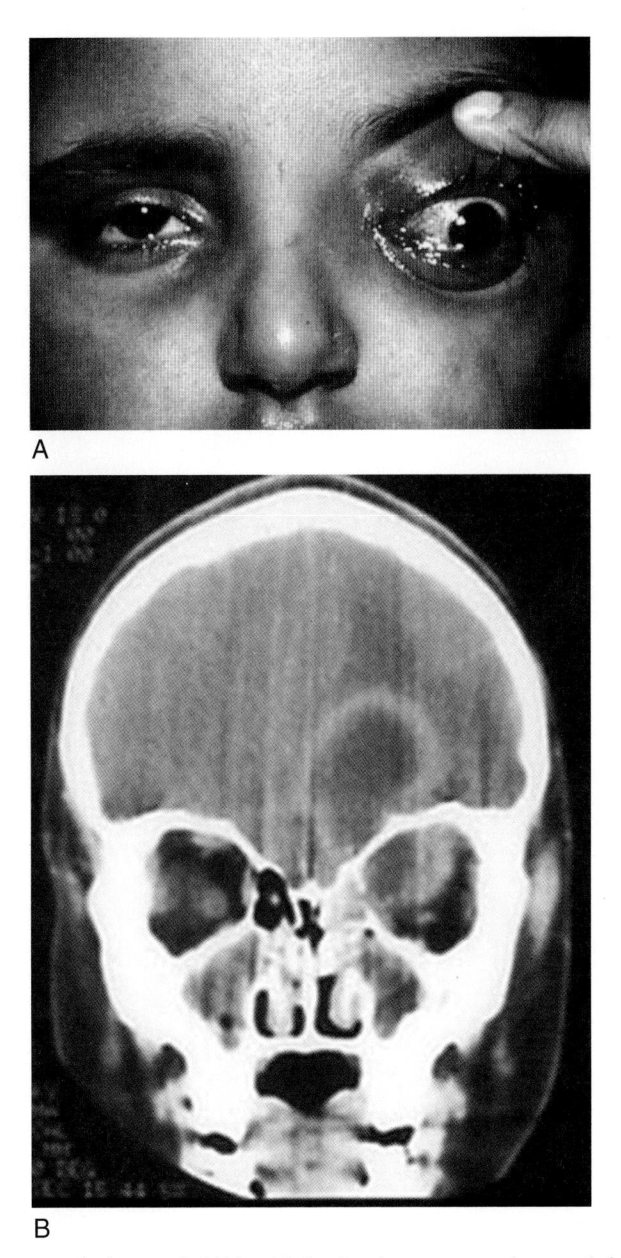

Figure 21-7 (A) External photo of child with brain abscess secondary to left orbital cellulitis. (B) CT scan demonstrating intraorbital abscess with intracranial extension involving the left frontal lobe.

structures, or penetrating trauma, the etiology of infection serves as a valuable clue to the responsible bacteria. Trauma patients are more likely to have orbital cellulitis from gram-negative organisms. Patients with sinusitis or recent dental procedures are commonly infected by anaerobes and gram-positive organisms.

Age is also a factor in the bacteriology of orbital cellulitis.[4] Children under the age of 9 are likely to have cultures positive for a single organism, typically

Table 21-1 Cultures from Subperiosteal Abscesses in Patients of all Ages with Orbital Cellulitis (123 Specimens from Three Centers)[2,8,9]

Organism	N = 234 (percent)
Gram-positive	124 (52.9)
Staphylococcus	53 (22.6)
Staphylococcus epidermidis and coagulase-negative	27 (11.5)
Staphylococcus aureus and coagulase-positive	26 (11.1)
Streptococcus	62 (27.3)
Streptococcus pneumoniae	11 (4.7)
Streptococcus viridans	10 (4.3)
Streptococcus milleri	9 (3.8)
Streptococcus pyogenes	5 (2.1)
Other	27 (11.5)
Enterococcus	6 (2.6)
Gemella morbillorum	3 (1.3)
Gram-negative	58 (24.8)
Bacteroides	13 (5.6)
Eikenella	8 (3.4)
Fusobacterium	8 (3.4)
Haemophilus	8 (3.4)
Pseudomonas	4 (1.7)
Escherichia coli	4 (1.7)
Other	13 (5.6)
Anaerobic	44 (18.8)
Peptostreptococcus	21 (9.0)
Propionibacteria	12 (5.1)
Veillonella	6 (2.6)
Other	5 (2.1)
Fungus	8 (3.4)

Staphylococcus or *Streptococcus* species. Patients over 9 years of age with orbital cellulitis more often exhibit a polymicrobial profile, including gram-positive, gram-negative, and anaerobic bacteria. Anatomic factors, particularly sinus development, seem to play a role in the differences with age. A recent study from Texas Children's Hospital in Houston revealed that 73% of *Staphylococcus* species cultured from pediatric orbital cellulitis patients were methicillin-resistant *Staphylococcus aureus* (MRSA).[9] *Haemophilus influenzae*, once a common offender, has become a rare cause of orbital infection since the inception of the Hib vaccine in 1985.[10]

Fungal infections, including mucormycosis, can occur in patients in diabetic ketoacidosis or those immunosuppressed after chemotherapy. Invasive aspergillosis also occurs in immunosuppressed patients and those with untreated acquired immunodeficiency syndrome (AIDS).

21-4 MEDICAL MANAGEMENT

All patients with orbital cellulitis should be admitted for intravenous antibiotic therapy, and therapy should be continued for 10 to 14 days. Empiric antibiotic therapy should correspond to the presumed etiology of the infection. In children 9 years of age or younger, infections resulting from sinusitis are usually due to one aerobic bacterium, and monotherapy with cefuroxime or ceftriaxone alone may be adequate.[4] In older children and adults, infections tend to be polymicrobial and often include anaerobic organisms. Clindamycin or metronidazole may be added to cefuroxime or ceftriaxone for anaerobic coverage. Gram-negative coverage should also be included in all patients with trauma-associated orbital cellulitis.

Many other antibiotic regimens have been described, including but not limited to nafcillin, choramphenicol, ticarcillin-clavulanic acid, cefoxatin, ampicillin/sulbactam, and vancomycin, either alone or in combination.[11] Ampicillin/sulbactam (Unasyn®) is commonly prescribed because it affords broad-spectrum coverage against most of the gram-positive, gram-negative, and anaerobic organisms implicated in orbital cellulitis, and may be used in all age groups. With the increasing incidence of MRSA, the empiric use of vancomycin is rising. Infectious disease consultation is helpful in choosing the appropriate antibiotic regimen for individual patients, taking into account their age, most likely source of infection, and resistance profiles of bacteria in the geographic region.

The use of corticosteroids as an adjunct to intravenous antibiotics to decrease orbital inflammation has also been described. Yen and Yen concluded that the concomitant use of intravenous corticosteroids with intravenous antibiotic therapy may be beneficial in the treatment of pediatric orbital cellulitis with subperiosteal abscess, and did not adversely affect clinical outcomes.[12] Steroids may be given once the patient has begun to show clinical improvement.

In sinusitis-related cases, nasal decongestants should be prescribed as well. An otorhinolaryngology consultation should be obtained for all patients with orbital cellulitis secondary to sinusitis, as some patients may benefit from surgical sinus drainage.

21-5 SURGICAL MANAGEMENT

Subperiosteal abscesses often require drainage. Factors that should be taken into account when considering surgical intervention include visual status, presence and location of an abscess, patient age, degree of sinusitis, and source of sinusitis. The visual status, including visual acuity and presence of a relative afferent pupillary defect, is the most important component.

Patients with a subperiosteal abscess fulfilling the following criteria generally require surgical intervention:[13]

1. Nine years of age or older
2. Presence of frontal sinusitis
3. Non-medial location of subperiosteal abscess
4. Large subperiosteal abscess
5. Suspicion of anaerobic subperiosteal infection (e.g., presence of gas within the abscess space as visualized on CT scan)
6. Recurrence of subperiosteal abscess after previous drainage
7. Evidence of chronic sinusitis (e.g., nasal polyps)
8. Acute optic nerve or retinal compromise
9. Infection of dental origin (suspected anaerobic infection)

Children under 9 years of age who develop orbital cellulitis often have negative cultures when drained. Positive cultures with a single aerobe may be seen if an abscess is drained within the first 3 days of treatment.[4] In young children, small abscesses can therefore be treated with antibiotics alone if there is no evidence of optic nerve or retinal compromise,[14] as these cases often resolve without drainage of the orbit or sinuses. Patients managed expectantly must be monitored closely for changes in visual acuity and pupillary reaction (every 6 hours for the first 48 hours), as these would suggest an immediate need for surgical intervention.

Harris specifically studied the behavior of subperiosteal abscesses in children. He found that in patients less than 9 years of age, 83% either cleared without drainage (25%) or had negative cultures at the time of drainage (58%). Children aged 9 to 14 years of age showed a transition to more complex infections. All patients 15 years of age or older had positive cultures after 3 days of intravenous antibiotics. They were found to have polymicrobial infections, and anaerobes were present in all cases. Harris concluded that patients 9 years of age or younger can be observed closely if there is no evidence of optic nerve compromise. Surgical drainage should be instituted if the patient develops a relative afferent pupillary defect or a fever that does not abate within 36 hours, if the patient continues to decline despite 48 hours of the appropriate intravenous antibiotics, or if the patient does not improve despite 72 hours of appropriate treatment with intravenous antibiotics. Most patients 9 years of age or older require drainage, and the urgency depends on the optic nerve status and the condition of the patient.[4]

The timing of surgical drainage of a subperiosteal abscess differs depending on the patient's presentation. Emergent drainage is indicated if a patient of any age has impaired optic nerve or retinal function or intracranial complications (meningitis, abscess). Urgent drainage should occur within 24 hours of presentation if a patient has a large subperiosteal abscess, a superior or inferior subperiosteal abscess, frontal sinusitis, evidence of chronic sinusitis including nasal polyps, or infection of dental origin, or if the patient is 9 years of age or older.[15]

The clinical examination is crucial in the decision process; the lack of improvement on serial CT scans should not be used as the sole indicator for surgical intervention. Patients with superior subperiosteal abscesses require urgent drainage. These occur in older children and young adults and are a more dangerous subset of abscess. Studies have demonstrated a correlation between frontal sinusitis, superior subperiosteal abscess, and intracranial abscess. In one study, three of six children with superior subperiosteal abscess had an associated intracranial abscess.[14]

Many patients will not need sinus surgery at the time of the subperiosteal abscess drainage.[16] However, if needed, the orbit and sinuses can usually be drained simultaneously. If simultaneous sinus surgery is pursued, the location of the abscess aids in surgical planning and determining whether external and/or endoscopic drainage should be attempted. Also, many medial subperiosteal abscesses can often be drained endoscopically. While surgeon preference sometimes dictates whether sinus surgery is performed concomitantly or at a later date, many surgeons recommend that the sinus infection be addressed at the time of the subperiosteal abscess drainage to prevent recurrence of orbital cellulitis and abscess formation.

The surgical approach to a subperiosteal abscess depends on its location and the preference and training of the surgeon. Approaches include the transcutaneous modified Lynch skin incision along the superomedial orbital rim, a lid crease incision, a sub-brow incision, an inferior orbital entry using either a transcutaneous or transconjunctival incision, a transcaruncular route, or an endoscopic endonasal approach. With abscesses located adjacent to the paranasal sinuses, a transcutaneous, transconjunctival, or transcaruncular external approach can be combined with an endoscopic sinus drainage technique.

21-5-1 *External Transcutaneous Approach.* Most subperiosteal abscesses occur along the medial orbital wall adjacent to the ethmoid sinus. A small skin incision can be made along the superomedial or medial orbital rim to gain access to this subperiosteal space. Care should be taken to avoid the supraorbital and supratrochlear neurovascular bundles, the trochlea, and the medial canthal tendon. Dissection is carried through the skin and muscle to reach the periosteum. The periosteum is incised with either a #15 scalpel blade or the sharp end of a Freer periosteal elevator. The periosteum is gently lifted from the bone and dissection is carried out in the potential subperiosteal space until the abscess is reached. Any purulent material (Fig. 21-8) encountered is cultured and then gently aspirated from the subperiosteal space with a suction tip. Antibiotic solution can be irrigated into the space, and a small Penrose drain left in place (Fig. 21-9). The wound is loosely closed around the drain. The drain is left in place for approximately 3 days and is slowly advanced on a daily basis. After the drain is removed, the small skin incision can be sutured closed if necessary. With careful closure, proper wound care, and sun avoidance, the site should heal well without a noticeable scar. This external transcutaneous approach can be combined with an external ethmoidectomy. Superior abscesses originating from the frontal sinus are usually drained through an incision at the superior rim, whereas inferior abscesses due to maxillary sinus infection can be drained through an inferior orbital rim or infraciliary incision.

21-5-2 *Endoscopic Ethmoidectomy and Drainage.* Another surgical option is the transnasal endoscopic ethmoidectomy with removal of a portion of the lamina papyracea and drainage of the abscess along the medial wall, as first reported by Manning in 1993.[17] One study described a clear trend toward shorter hospitalizations in patients

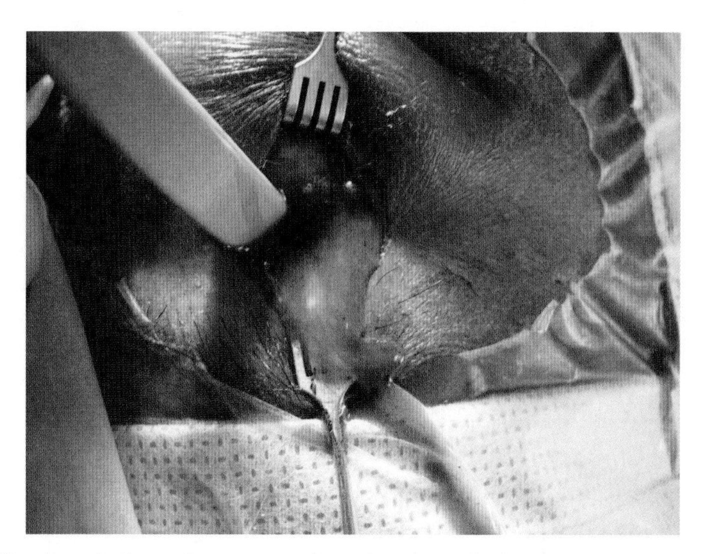

Figure 21-8 Purulent drainage from a superior subperiosteal abscess.

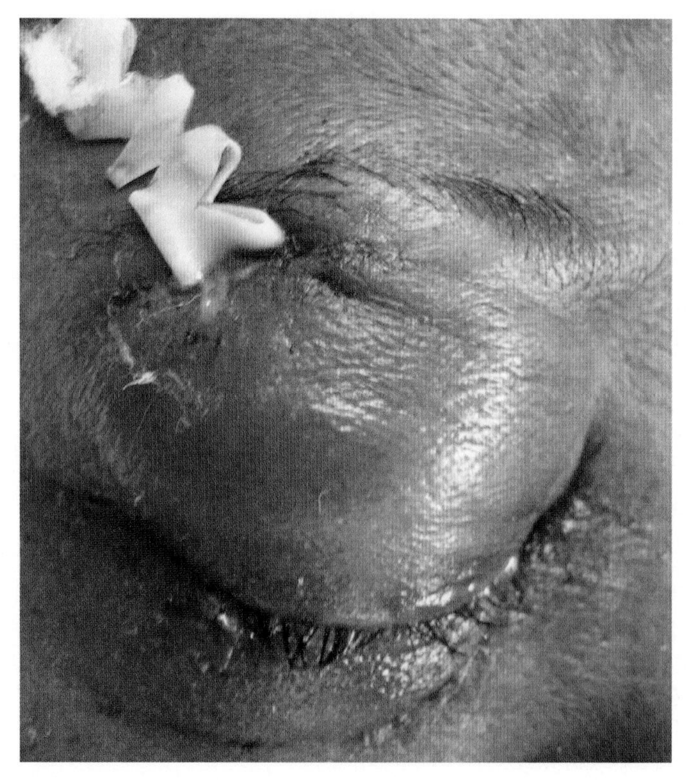

Figure 21-9 A Penrose drain is left in the subperiosteal space to allow continued drainage of purulent material postoperatively.

treated with endoscopic drainage of the abscess compared to those treated with external drainage, with or without sinus drainage. This trend did not reach statistical significance, however, due to the small number of patients in each group. Endoscopic ethmoidectomy and drainage should be performed by a surgeon experienced in this technique. Potential complications include avulsion of the medial rectus muscle, orbital hemorrhage, and damage to the optic nerve.[18]

21-5-3 *Minimal Endoscopic Approach with Drainage Only*. A limited endoscopic approach with endoscopic opening of the medial wall of the bulla ethmoidalis and lamina papyracea without concomitant ethmoidectomy has been used successfully to treat medial subperiosteal abscesses complicating acute sinusitis. One study revealed that minimal subperiosteal abscess drainage associated with antibiotic treatment enabled recovery in all of patients without the need for more extensive ethmoidectomy.[16]

21-5-4 *Transcaruncular Drainage*. The transcaruncular approach allows for the avoidance of a skin incision with subsequent scar.[19] An incision is made through the caruncle with small relaxing incisions in the conjunctiva superior and inferior to the caruncular incision. Stevens scissors are placed into the incision and directed to the posterior lacrimal crest. Spreading of the scissors will expose the periosteum of the medial wall posterior to the posterior lacrimal crest. The periosteum is opened, and drainage is performed in a fashion similar to that described in the transcutaneous approach. It is more difficult, however, to place a drain using this technique due to resulting contact with the cornea and concomitant ocular irritation.

A combined transcaruncular and transnasal endoscopic approach can be used to drain a medial subperiosteal abscess and perform a simultaneous ethmoidectomy.[20] The main advantage of this approach is improved visualization of the orbital contents. The inflamed tissues in acute sinusitis bleed easily, making endoscopic visualization of the orbital contents more difficult. This technique also allows confirmation of complete drainage of the abscess cavity. Finally, the lack of a cutaneous incision offers a cosmetic advantage.

REFERENCES

1. Kikkawa DO, Heinz GW, Martin RT, et al. Orbital cellulitis and abscess secondary to dacryocystitis. *Arch Ophthalmol*. 2002;120:1096–1099.
2. Ben Simon GJ, Bush S, Selva D, McNab AA. Orbital cellulitis: a rare complication after orbital blowout fracture. *Ophthalmology*. 2005;112:2030–2034.
3. Logani SC, Harris GJ. Bacterial orbital infections associated with sinus disease. *Ophthalmol Clin North Am*. 1996;9:629–643.
4. Harris GJ. Subperiosteal abscess of the orbit: age as a factor in the bacteriology and response to treatment. *Ophthalmology*. 1994;101:585–595.
5. Chandler JR, Langerbrunner DJ, Stevens ER. The pathogenesis of orbital complications in acute sinusitis. *Laryngoscope*. 1970;80:1414–1428.
6. Schramm VL, Curtin HD, Kennerdell JS. Evaluation of orbital cellulitis and results of treatment. *Laryngoscope*. 1982;92:732–738.

7. Brook I, Frazier EH. Microbiology of subperiosteal abscess and associated maxillary sinusitis. *Laryngoscope*. 1996;106:1010–1013.
8. Chaudhry IA, Shamsi FA, Elzaridi E, et al. Outcome of treated orbital cellulitis in a tertiary care hospital in the Middle East. *Ophthalmology*. 2007;114:345–354.
9. McKinley SH, Yen MT, Yen KG. Microbiology of pediatric orbital cellulitis. *Am J Ophthalmol*. 2007;144:497–501.
10. Ambati BK, Ambati, J, Azar N, et al. Periorbital and orbital cellulitis before and after the advent of the *Haemophilus influenzae* B vaccination. *Ophthalmology*. 2000;107:1450–1453.
11. Harris GJ. Subperiosteal inflammation of the orbit. A bacteriological analysis of 17 cases. *Arch Ophthalmol*. 1988;106: 947–952.
12. Yen MT, Yen KG. Effect of corticosteroids in the acute management of pediatric orbital cellulitis with subperiosteal abscess. *Ophthal Plast Reconstr Surg*. 2005;21:363–366.
13. Garcia G, Harris G. Criteria for nonsurgical management of subperiosteal abscess of the orbit. *Ophthalmology*. 2000;107:1454–1458.
14. Greenberg M, Pollard Z. Medical treatment of pediatric subperiosteal orbital abscess secondary to sinusitis. *J AAPOS* 1998;2:351–355.
15. Harris GJ, Bair RL. Anaerobic and aerobic isolates from a subperiosteal orbital abscess in 4-year-old. *Arch Ophthalmol*. 1996;114:98.
16. Froehlich P, Pransky SM, Fontaine P, et al. Minimal endoscopic approach to subperiosteal orbital abscess. *Arch Otolaryngol Head Neck Surg*. 1997;123:280–282.
17. Manning SC. Endoscopic management of medial subperiosteal orbital abscess. *Arch Ophthalmol*. 1993;119:789–791.
18. Page EL, Wiatrak BJ. Endoscopic vs external drainage of orbital subperiosteal abscess. *Arch Otolaryngol Head Neck Surg*. 1996;122: 737–740.
19. Shorr N, Baylis HI, Goldberg RA, Perry JD. Transcaruncular approach to the medial orbit and orbital apex. *Ophthalmology*. 2000;107:1459–1463.
20. Pelton RW, Smith ME, Patel BCK, Kelly SM. Cosmetic considerations in surgery for orbital subperiosteal abscess in children: experience with a combined transcaruncular and transnasal endoscopic approach. *Arch Otolaryngol Head Neck Surg*. 2003;129: 652–655.

22

Enucleation and Evisceration

DAVID R. JORDAN, MD, AND STEPHEN R. KLAPPER, MD

22-1 INTRODUCTION

Loss of an eye to tumor, trauma, or end-stage ocular disease is devastating. There is a loss of binocular vision with a reduced peripheral visual field and loss of depth perception. Job limitations are often a result of lost binocularity, and affected individuals may experience a sense of facial disfigurement. Since eye contact is such an essential part of human interaction, it is extremely important for the artificial eye patient to maintain a natural, normal-appearing prosthetic eye.

Characteristics of the ideal anophthalmic socket include:

1. A centrally placed, well-covered, buried implant of adequate volume, fabricated from a bioinert material
2. A socket lined with healthy conjunctiva and fornices deep enough to retain a prosthesis and to permit horizontal and vertical excursion of an artificial eye
3. Eyelids with normal position and appearance, as well as adequate tone to support a prosthesis
4. A supratarsal eyelid fold that is symmetric with the supratarsal fold of the contralateral eyelid
5. Normal position of the eyelashes and eyelid margin
6. Good transmission of motility from the implant to the overlying prosthesis
7. A comfortable ocular prosthesis that looks similar to the sighted, contralateral globe.

Currently, no surgical procedure satisfies all the above requirements, as evidenced by the variety of surgical techniques advocated over the years. Over the past few decades, however, there have been numerous developments and refinements in anophthalmic socket surgery with respect to implant material and design, implant wrapping, implant–prosthesis coupling, and socket volume considerations. It is now more possible than ever to provide the anophthalmic patient with an artificial eye that looks and moves almost as naturally as a normal eye.

22-2 ENUCLEATION AND ORBITAL IMPLANTS: A HISTORICAL PERSPECTIVE

As early as 500 b.c., Egyptian and Roman priests wore clay prostheses held in place with an adhesive substance or thong as external cosmetic coverings for disfigured and phthisical globes. Enucleation and evisceration techniques were not formally described in live patients until the late 16th century in Europe. Johannes Lange (1485–1565) made reference to removal of an eye, but George Bartisch in 1583 is credited with the first recorded description of removal of an eye for treatment of severe ocular disease.[1,2] A hook was passed through the globe, followed by sharp dissection to sever the globe from the orbit. The extirpation procedure, essentially subtotal exenteration, was performed without an anesthetic and considered dangerous and "dreadful" even by standards of that era.[2] The resulting socket deformity was not suitable for fitting with an ocular prosthesis. It was not until 1841 that the foundation for current enucleation techniques was established in separate reports by O'Ferrall (Dublin) and Bonnet (Paris).[1] The introduction of controlled general anesthesia in 1847 dramatically changed the field of surgery and certainly had an impact on advances in anophthalmic surgery. It was more than 40 years after O'Ferrall and Bonnet before orbital implants were introduced into what may now be considered "modern" anophthalmic surgery. P.H. Mules placed a glass spherical implant (the "Mules" sphere) into an eviscerated socket in 1885, and W.A. Frost, one year later, introduced a similar implant into Tenon's capsule following an enucleation procedure.[3,4] The Mules sphere revolutionized anophthalmic socket reconstructive surgery by replacing lost orbital volume and diminishing postoperative socket retraction. In 1906 Gallemaerts described the forerunner of postoperative conformers, now the standard of care more than 100 years later.[5]

While improved techniques reduced problems with Mules hollow glass sphere implants, complications, including migration, extrusion, and a tendency to shatter with sudden temperature changes, led to a search for improved implant materials.[4,6,7] Sponge, rubber, paraffin, ivory, wool, cork, cartilage, fat, bone, vitallium, platinum, aluminum, silver, and gold were some examples of substances tried as orbital implants.[5–7] By 1941, popular implants, in order of preference, included carbonized bone balls, ivory, decalcified bone, formalized cartilage, and the Mules glass sphere.[8] Prior to this time all implants were completely buried.

In 1945, Ruedemann described a combined motility implant and ocular prosthesis with a posteriorly oriented tantalum mesh for muscle and tissue attachment and an anteriorly exposed acrylic prosthetic eye.[9] A high rate of infection, inability to remove the prosthesis for hygiene and maintenance, and difficulties with alignment limited the acceptance of Ruedemann's combined implant. Numerous partially exposed, integrated implants with direct attachment to an overlying prosthesis to improve motility were subsequently developed by Cutler and others.[4,10] Use of these implants was also hindered by their high incidence of infection and extrusion.

By the 1950s completely buried implants were again the focus of orbital surgeons. A variety of implant designs were tried with an attempt to indirectly couple the buried implant to an overlying artificial eye by modifying the anterior surface of the implant as well as the posterior surface of the prosthesis. The Allen[11] and subsequently the Iowa[12,13] enucleation implants were the culmination of these investigations into buried-integrated (or, as they were initially described, "quasi-integrated") implants. The Iowa implant was made of methylmethacrylate resin and used four prominent mounds, which were coupled to concavities on the posterior surface of the prosthesis. Exposure of these implants often resulted over the surface of the mounds. These mounds were later reduced in size and convexity to create the Universal implant (1987), which is still used by some ophthalmologists in North America.[14,15] With the advent of porous, hydroxyapatite (HA) implants shortly after the introduction of the Universal implant, most orbital surgeons did not gain much experience with this implant.

Despite the initial acceptance of buried, quasi-integrated implants, surgical implantation, fitting, and exposure problems continued to plague these designs. Other implant designs continued to emerge (Troutman, Uribe, Iliff and Soll—1950s and 1960s), including the use of magnetic implants, but they also had a limited degree of acceptance.[4,16] Many ophthalmic surgeons gradually turned to simpler buried implants with fewer problems. By 1989, spherical implants made of silicone, glass, or polymethylmethacrylate (PMMA) were the implants most widely used by ophthalmic plastic surgeons.[17] Unwrapped spheres or those wrapped in donor sclera or fascia were the implants of choice in more than 80% of primary enucleations. Dermis fat grafts and the Iowa/Universal-type quasi-integrated implants represented the balance of implants placed at that time.[17] As porous implants (HA) emerged (1989), they became very popular and the implants of choice changed dramatically, ushering in a new era of anophthalmic orbital implant use.

22-3 CURRENT CLASSIFICATION OF IMPLANTS AND TERMINOLOGY

Orbital implants can be classified as porous or nonporous, and in either category the implants are nonintegrated, integrated, or quasi-integrated, depending on how the implant is connected to the overlying prosthetic eye (Table 22.1). Porous implants (HA, porous polyethylene, aluminum oxide) allow fibrovascular ingrowth, while nonporous implants (silicone, PMMA) do not. Nonintegrated implants have no connection with the prosthetic eye, whereas integrated implants can be directly coupled to the prosthetic eye through a peg system. Quasi-integrated (or indirectly integrated) implants may be porous or nonporous and because of their irregular anterior surface are partially coupled to the overlying prosthetic eye (e.g., Allen, Iowa, Universal, MEDPOR® Quad implant). These quasi-integrated implants remain buried. Extraocular muscles are attached to their surface by passing the muscles through tunnels in the implant (Allen implant) or through grooves in the

Table 22-1 Terminology in Anophthalmic Surgery

Anophthalmic implant: Material or substance used to replace an enucleated or eviscerated globe (e.g., polmethylmethacylate, silicone, hydroxyapatite, aluminum oxide, porous polyethylene)

Porous implant: Refers to an implant with numerous interconnected pores or channels throughout its structure that permit fibrovascular ingrowth (e.g., hydroxyapatite, aluminum oxide, porous polyethylene)

Nonporous implant: Refers to an implant that is solid and does not allow fibrovascular ingrowth (e.g., polymethylmethacrylate, silicone)

Conformer: A shell (typically acrylic) with or without holes placed over the closed bulbar conjunctival wound that extends into the conjunctival fornices behind the eyelids following implant placement in enucleation or evisceration surgery

Prosthesis (prosthetic eye, artificial eye)**:** A ceramic shell placed in the anophthalmic socket conjunctival fornices that is typically fabricated to look like the patient' contralateral healthy eye to provide a symmetric ocular appearance

Buried implant: An implant that has been placed within the anophthalmic socket with an overlying closed, smooth, uninterrupted conjunctival surface completely covering the anophthalmic implant

Exposed implant: An implant that does not have an overlying closed, smooth, uninterrupted surface completely covering it. An exposed implant is an unwanted complication postoperatively with any implant.

Nonintegrated implant: An implant that has been placed within the anophthalmic socket that has no connection with the overlying prosthetic eye. There is a closed, smooth, uninterrupted conjunctival surface completely covering the anophthalmic implant. Also known as a "buried nonintegrated implant."

Integrated implant: An implant that can be directly coupled to the overlying prosthetic eye with a peg system. As there is a small break in the overlying conjunctiva through which the peg protrudes, there is some debate whether this type of implant should also be known as a partially "exposed integrated implant."

Quasi-integrated implant: An implant that has been placed within the anophthalmic socket with a closed, uninterrupted conjunctival surface completely covering an anophthalmic implant that has an irregular anterior surface, allowing indirect coupling ("quasi-integration") of implant to overlying, modified prosthesis (e.g., Allen, Iowa, Universal, MEDPOR Quad implants). Also known as a "buried integrated implant" or an "indirectly integrated implant."

Peg: A motility coupling post, currently made of titanium, that permits direct coupling of the implant movement to an overlying prosthesis. Pegs may be inserted within sleeves that are drilled into the anterior aspect of the implant. Some implant–peg systems are designed for placement at the time of enucleation or evisceration, whereas others are inserted once implant fibrovascularizaton occurs, typically around 6 months postoperatively. There are also magnetic peg systems that remain within the implant and buried beneath the conjunctiva but coupled to the overlying prosthesis as a result of the magnetic components within the prosthetic eye and implant. An implant with a magnetic peg system in place would qualify as another type of quasi-integrated implant since the magnet within the implant remains covered by conjunctiva and does not directly couple to the overlying prosthesis, as occurs with a peg protruding through conjunctiva.

implant created by mounds on the anterior aspect (Iowa and Universal implants, MEDPOR Quad). The broad flat surface of the Allen implant or the protruding mounds of the Iowa/Universal/MEDPOR Quad, which have corresponding indentations on the posterior surface of the prosthetic eye, move the prosthesis because of this "quasi-integration." The movement is often better than a standard spherical implant, but may be as good as a porous integrated implant coupled to the overlying prosthesis through a peg system.

22-4 POROUS ORBITAL IMPLANTS

In the effort to design a biocompatible, integrated orbital implant Perry in 1985 introduced coralline (sea coral) HA spheres.[18] HA had been used for more than 10 years as a bone substitute in orthopedic surgery, but the Bio-Eye™ (Integrated Orbital Implants, San Diego, CA) did not receive U.S. Food and Drug Administration (FDA) approval until 1989. The HA orbital implants represented a new generation of buried, integrated spheres with a regular system of interconnecting pores that allowed host fibrovascular ingrowth.[18,19] Implant fibrovascularization potentially reduced the risk of migration, extrusion, and infection.[20] The HA implant also allowed secure attachment of the extraocular muscles, which may lead to improved implant motility and perhaps more rapid fibrovascular ingrowth.[18,19] By drilling into the HA implant, inserting a peg-sleeve system, and coupling the peg to the overlying prosthetic eye, an improved range of prosthetic movement as well as fine darting eye movements (commonly seen during close conversational speech) often resulted. This allowed a more life-like quality to the artificial eye.

Although HA implants represented a significant advance in anophthalmic surgery, experience over the past decade has expanded our understanding of their limitations. Reported complications are not uncommon and include implant exposure, conjunctival thinning, socket discharge, pyogenic granuloma formation, implant infection, and persistent pain or discomfort.[20–25] Implant exposure problems continue to deter some surgeons from using HA implants, but this complication appears to be related more to surgical implantation and wound closure techniques (including HA implant wrap selection) and host factors than to properties related to HA spherical implants.[20]

The introduction of HA as an orbital implant significantly raised the costs associated with enucleation, evisceration, and secondary orbital implant procedures. The Bio-Eye HA implant may cost over $650 (U.S.) more than traditional silicone or PMMA spherical implants ($15 to $50 U.S.). Additional expenses associated with HA placement include an implant wrap material, assessment of implant vascularization with a confirmatory magnetic resonance (MR) imaging study, a secondary drilling procedure with peg-sleeve placement, and prosthesis modification. In the search for porous orbital implants with a reduced complication profile and diminished surgical and postoperative costs, numerous alternative implant materials have been introduced around the world.

Synthetic HA implants developed by FCI (Issy-Les-Moulineaux, France) are currently in their third generation (FCI3). The FCI3 implant has an identical chemical composition to that of the Bio-Eye, although scanning electron microscopy has revealed decreased pore uniformity and interconnectivity and the presence of blind pouches.[26] Central implant fibrovascularization in a rabbit model still appears to occur in a similar manner in both the Bio-Eye and FCI3 implants.[27] The synthetic FCI3 implant has gained in popularity in many parts of the world over the past 10 years, but it is not yet available in the United States. The problems and complications associated with the synthetic FCI3 implant are similar to those of the Bio-Eye.[28] It is less expensive than the Bio-Eye (approximately $450 U.S.)

Other forms of HA implants in use around the world include the Chinese HA and the Brazilian HA.[29,30] Although less expensive than the Bio-Eye, these implants have impurities or poor porous structure that offer little advantage. Other implant designs continue to appear, some of which are of little added value,[31] while others have been in use for only a short time and their advantages and disadvantages are not yet apparent.[32]

Synthetic porous polyethylene (MEDPOR, Porex Surgical Inc., Newnan, GA) implants were introduced over a decade ago for use in the orbit and have been widely accepted as an alternative to the Bio-Eye HA.[33–36] Porous polyethylene implants, although less biocompatible than HA, are typically well tolerated by orbital soft tissue.[37] They have a smoother surface than HA implants, which permits easier implantation and potentially less irritation of the overlying conjunctiva following placement. These implants have a high tensile strength yet are malleable, which allows sculpting of the anterior surface of the implant. They may be used with or without a wrapping material and the extraocular muscles can be sutured directly onto the implant, although most surgeons may find this challenging without predrilled holes. Porous polyethylene implants are available in spherical, egg, conical, and mounded shapes (MEDPOR Quad implant).[34–36] The anterior surface can also be manufactured with a smooth, nonporous surface to prevent abrasion of the overlying tissue (e.g., MEDPOR smooth surface tunnel implant [SSTTM]) while retaining a larger pore size posteriorly to facilitate fibrovascular ingrowth. The MEDPOR implant costs approximately $200 (U.S.) less than the Bio-Eye HA sphere.

Aluminum oxide (Al_2O_3, Alumina, Bioceramic implant) is a ceramic implant biomaterial that has been used in orthopedic surgery and dentistry for more than 30 years. Spherical and egg-shaped Bioceramic Orbital Implants (FCI, Issy-Les-Moulineaux, France) were approved for use in the United States by the FDA in April 2000 and for use in Canada by Health and Welfare Canada in February 2001. Aluminum oxide is a porous, inert substance and has been suggested as a standard reference material in studies of implant biocompatibility.[38] These implants permit host fibrovascular ingrowth similar to the Bio-Eye.[39,40] Human fibroblasts and osteoblasts proliferate more rapidly on aluminum oxide than HA, suggesting it is a more biocompatible substance than HA.[37,38] The Bioceramic implant is lightweight and has a uniform pore structure and excellent pore interconnectivity (Fig. 22-1A,B).[26] The microcrystalline structure is smoother than the rough surfaced Bio-Eye (Fig. 22-1C). In our experience, anophthalmic sockets reconstructed with aluminum oxide implants appear to have less postoperative tissue inflammation than sockets in which HA implants have been placed.[40] Problems (e.g., exposure) encountered with its use are similar to those seen with the

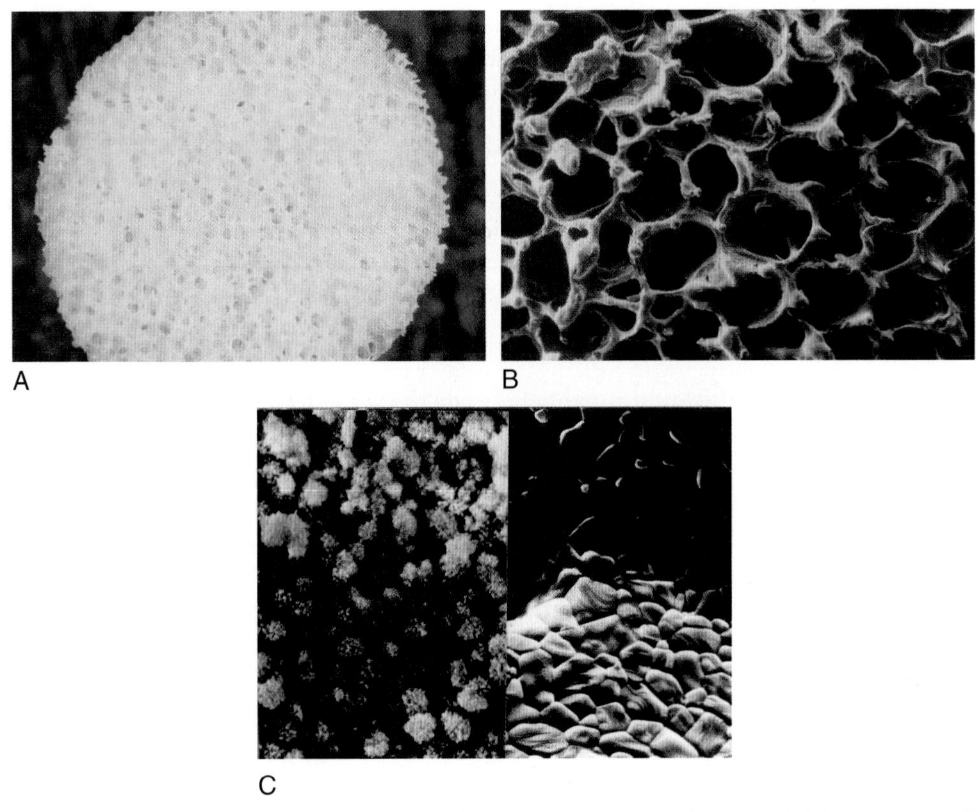

Figure 22-1 (A) The porous architecture of an aluminum oxide (Bioceramic) implant is well visualized. (B) Scanning electron microscopy illustrating the more uniform porous architecture of the aluminum oxide orbital implant (222 × 101). (C) On high-power scanning electron microscopy (230 × 103) the solid component of the Bio-Eye (left half of photo) has a rough-appearing microcrystalline structure compared to the smooth-appearing microcrystalline structure of the aluminum oxide (Bioceramic) implant (right half of photo).

Bio-Eye orbital implants.[40,41] As with other currently available porous orbital implants, aluminum oxide is less expensive than the Bio-Eye ($450 U.S. vs $650 U.S.).

22-5 ORBITAL IMPLANT SELECTION IN ADULTS

There continues to be little consensus regarding orbital implant material and design preference.[42] Surgeons have their own preferences regarding the use of spherical versus shaped implants, wrapped versus unwrapped implants, and pegged versus unpegged implants. Implant cost, insurance reimbursement, and marketing pressures also play a role in implant selection. In a 2004 survey of orbital surgeons, of 1,919 primary orbital implants used following enucleation, porous polyethylene was used in 42.7% of cases, followed by coralline HA (27.3%), nonporous alloplastic (PMMA, silicone) implants (19.9%), dermis–fat grafts (7.2%), Bioceramic (1.8%), synthetic HA (0.9%), and mammalian bone (0.2%).[42] The trends reported in this survey reflect a usage pattern in those responding to the survey (31.4% response rate) and do not suggest clinical superiority based on scientific evidence.[42]

When deciding which implant to use in an adult patient, we divide the various implants into three useful categories:

1. Porous spheres that may potentially be pegged (e.g. HA–coralline or synthetic, MEDPOR–porous polyethylene, Bioceramic–aluminum oxide)
2. Quasi-integrated implants (e.g., Universal implant–mounded PMMA, MEDPOR Quad–mounded porous polyethylene)
3. Traditional nonporous sphere (e.g., PMMA, silicone)

If the patient is healthy and roughly between the ages of 15 and 65 years a porous implant (aluminum oxide, HA) that can potentially be pegged is our first choice. The porous implant with a peg will be associated with the highest degree of movement.[42,43] If a peg is not being considered, the advantage of using a porous spherical implant is diminished, as the movement associated with a nonpegged porous spherical implant is equal to that of a wrapped nonporous spherical implant.[44–46] However, the advantages of fibrovascular ingrowth and the potentially diminished risk of implant migration remain substantial reasons to consider using a porous implant even when pegging is not contemplated.

A quasi-integrated implant such as the Universal (PMMA–mounded) or MEDPOR Quad implant (mounded) is an alternative consideration to the porous spherical implants if pegging is not a consideration but improved motility is desired. The mounded surface of the Universal or MEDPOR Quad implant offers improved motility over a standard sphere as a result of the coupling that occurs between the mounds on the implant and the posterior surface of the prosthesis. Proper placement and meticulous closure of Tenon's capsule and the conjunctiva are essential when using one of these mounded implants.

A nonporous sphere (e.g., PMMA, silicone), wrapped, centered within the muscle cone, and attached to each of the rectus muscles is another alternative if pegging is not a consideration. Although reasonable prosthetic movement occurs in most cases, excursion of the artificial eye is limited relative to that often observed following placement of a buried, mounded implant or a porous pegged implant. Because prosthetic movement is indirectly coupled to the buried sphere, the artificial eye may lag behind the contralateral normal eye on attempted horizontal or vertical gaze. A nonporous implant simply placed into the orbit, without a wrap and without connection to the rectus muscles, is the least desirable choice in our view as it offers little movement and the implants are prone to migrate over time, most commonly into the superotemporal space. A decentered implant can make fitting of a custom artificial eye problematic.

Nonporous spherical implants are frequently considered in elderly patients (roughly >65 years), debilitated or immunocompromised individuals, and patients with a history of poorly controlled diabetes or periorbital radiation therapy, as they would not be good candidates to consider a peg. A traditional nonporous sphere (e.g., PMMA, silicone) wrapped and centered in the muscle cone and connected to the rectus muscles is our typical approach. Older patients (roughly >65 years) in good health and seeking to maximize potential prosthesis motility may be candidates for a quasi-integrated (or buried-integrated) porous implant (e.g., Universal implant or MEDPOR Quad implant).

22-6 ORBITAL IMPLANT SELECTION IN CHILDREN

Adult orbital volume is believed to occur by 14 years of age.[47] It has also been shown in normal children that 80% of adult orbital volume is reached by 5 years of age.[48] Conventionally, enucleation early in childhood, as well as congenital anophthalmos or microphthalmos, is believed to contribute to underdevelopment of the involved orbital bone structure with secondary facial asymmetry.[49–52] More recent studies have indicated that obvious secondary cosmetic facial asymmetries may not always be a byproduct of pediatric enucleation, but rather a result of orbital irradiation early in life.[53–55] It is recognized, however, that orbital soft tissue volume is a critical determinant of orbital bone growth and that adequate volume replacement following enucleation is a critical factor in continued orbital growth.[47,56–58] The ocular prosthesis is also believed to be an important factor minimizing orbital growth retardation and preventing periorbital asymmetries.[47]

Our current approach in children less than 5 years of age undergoing enucleation surgery is to place a wrapped nonporous sphere implant (e.g., PMMA, silicone) centered within the muscle cone and connected to each of the rectus muscles and the inferior oblique muscle. Implant exchange, typically with a larger porous orbital implant, can be considered in the teenage years. Another option for volume replacement in children is autogenous dermis–fat grafts, as these grafts may undergo hypertrophy and perhaps contribute to orbital bone growth.[59,60]

In children between the ages of 5 to 15 years, we formerly advocated nonporous implants, either a PMMA mounded implant (e.g., Universal) or a wrapped sphere (e.g., PMMA, silicone). As with younger patients, implant exchange with a porous orbital implant was then considered at a later time. There is now an increasing trend to use porous implants in pediatric patients.[61,62] We have successfully placed porous spherical implants following childhood enucleation (5 to 15 years) and now consider the use of HA or aluminum oxide implants in many preteen and teenage patients undergoing enucleation surgery. Interestingly, the radiopaque nature of HA on imaging and potential limitations on postoperative external-beam irradiation are no longer significant concerns or strong contraindications to the use of HA following enucleation for retinoblastoma.[61,63,64]

22-7 VOLUME CONSIDERATIONS IN ORBITAL IMPLANT SELECTION

Removal of an eye following enucleation or evisceration creates an orbital soft tissue volume deficiency. Insufficient volume replacement results in a post-enucleation socket syndrome, which may consist of an abnormally deep superior sulcus, upper eyelid ptosis, enophthalmos, and lower eyelid malposition and may require a larger-than-desirable prosthesis.[65–69] Proper implant volume may be determined either preoperatively or intraoperatively (enucleation cases) from the axial length of the eye or by determining the volume of fluid the enucleated eye displaces in a graduated cyclinder.[67–69] Several authors have reported considerable interpatient variability of axial length and globe volume, with globe volumes varying between 6.9 and 9.0 mL.[67–69] Kaltreider has shown that the axial length minus 2 mm (or A-scan minus 1 mm) approximates the implant diameter for optimal volume replacement in emmetropic and myopic individuals.[67,68] Custer suggested a graduated cylinder be used to measure the volume of fluid displaced by an enucleated eye.[68]

Approximately 70% to 80% of the volume of an individual's normal globe should be replaced with an orbital implant.[67,68] This generally allows for a prosthetic volume that is ideally 2.0 to 2.5 mL.[65] While the upper limit of prosthetic volume is around 4.0 mL, larger prostheses often result in progressive lower eyelid laxity and malposition due to the weight of the prosthesis on the eyelid. Larger prostheses may also have limited socket excursion.[66] An 18-mm sphere has a volume of 3.1 mL, a 20-mm sphere has a volume of 4.2 mL, and a 22-mm sphere has a volume of 5.6 mL. Individualization of the implant size is important in optimizing orbital volume replacement and in achieving the best possible aesthetic result.[66–70] Theoretically, the volume of the enucleated globe minus 2.0 to 2.5 mL gives the ideal implant size to use.[68] Unfortunately, implants larger than 22 mm may have a higher exposure rate and if too large will hinder fitting of an acceptable custom prosthesis.[22,69] We typically use 20- to 22-mm spherical implants following enucleation and 18- to 20-mm implants after evisceration procedures. In pediatric patients slightly smaller implants may be required, depending on the patient's age and orbital development.

22-8 ORBITAL IMPLANT WRAPPING

Placement of a HA implant or Bioceramic implant within the soft tissue of the eye socket is facilitated by a smooth wrapping material, which diminishes tissue drag.[18] The wrap facilitates precise fixation of the extraocular muscles to the implant surface.[18] Implant wraps may also provide a barrier function over the spiculated porous implant surface,[18] although there is some debate among ophthalmic plastic surgeons as to whether covering the anterior surface of the implant with an avascular material is helpful in preventing implant exposure.[71,72] Several authors have questioned whether an implant wrap is advantageous.[72,73] In a 2003 survey, the majority of respondents (59%) preferred not to wrap.[42] Placement of an unwrapped implant may simplify the procedure, decrease operating room time, reduce the total cost of the procedure, avoid creating a second surgical site for harvesting autogenous wraps, and decrease the risk of disease transmission.[42,72,73]

Human donor sclera has traditionally been the first choice of implant wrapping material for most orbital surgeons.[18,19] The use of human donor material, however, has fallen out of favor with both surgeons and patients due to concerns of infectious disease transmission and the potential risk of human immunodeficiency virus

(HIV), hepatitis B or C, and prion transmission (Creutzfeldt-Jakob disease).[74] Although we are not aware of any reports of disease transmission from donor sclera, segments of the HIV-1 genome have been identified in preserved human sclera.[75] Creutzfeldt-Jakob disease transmission from dural and corneal transplants has been reported.[76–78] In addition, seronegative organ and tissue donors may transmit HIV.[79] Many eye banks charge a substantial fee to provide donor sclera.

Specially processed human donor pericardium, fascia lata, and sclera are marketed as safe alternatives to preserved human donor tissues implant wraps (Biodynamics International [U.S.], Inc., Tampa, FL). These wraps have the convenience of a long (up to 5 years) shelf life; however, they contribute significantly to the cost of the procedure.

Processed bovine pericardium (Peri-Guard® or Ocu-Guard™ Supple, Bio Vascular Inc., Saint Paul, MN) is FDA approved and also available as an implant wrap material.[80,81] Although there have been no reported cases of bovine spongiform encephalopathy (BSE) in American cattle to date, there have been reports of infected cattle in Alberta, Canada, and the potential for prion transmission and BSE remains a concern.[74]

Autologous temporalis fascia,[82] fascia lata,[83] rectus abdominis sheath,[84] and posterior auricular muscle complex graft[67] have been tried as orbital implant wrapping materials. Use of these tissues requires a second operative site, involves a prolonged operative time, and adds a potentially increased risk of morbidity.

Microporous expanded polytetrafluoroethylene (e-PTFE) (Gore-Tex, W.L. Gore & Associates, Flagstaff, AZ) has also been advocated as an implant wrapping material (Oculo-Plastik, Montreal, Quebec, Canada); however, complications with its use have made it undesirable.[85–88]

Undyed polyglactin 910 mesh (Vicryl mesh, Ethicon, Somerville, NJ) is a bioabsorbable synthetic material and is our preference as a wrapping material for porous orbital implants.[88,89] Vicryl mesh eliminates the risk of infectious disease transmission, does not require a second surgical site, is readily available, is simple to use, and is inexpensive. Vicryl mesh-wrapped HA implants have been shown to permit rapid implant fibrovascularization in an animal model[89,90] and may provide a potential advantage of permitting fibrovascular ingrowth over the entire implant surface, unlike implants wrapped in sclera.[91] We have reported a 2.1% incidence of implant exposure in 187 consecutive patients receiving Vicryl mesh-wrapped HA orbital implants.[92] Oestreicher et al.[24] also reported a low exposure incidence using a similar bioabsorbable wrapping material composed of polyglycolic acid (Dexon mesh style No. 8, non-stretch, medium-weight closed tricot, Davis & Geck, Manati, Puerto Rico). Despite our success with polyglactin 910 mesh as an implant wrap material, some surgeons continue to believe that it is associated with a higher rate of implant exposure.[93,94] We believe that high exposure rates with Vicryl mesh-wrapped implants is a technique-related problem that can be minimized with correct implant insertion and meticulous tension-free wound closure. However, as exposure can occur at anytime post enucleation or secondary implantation, the true incidence of implant exposure (with any wrap) may not be appreciated until large numbers of patients are followed for prolonged time intervals (e.g., 5–10 or more years).[95]

22-9 PREOPERATIVE PREPARATION FOR ANOPHTHALMIC SURGERY (ENUCLEATION/EVISCERATION)

1. Conduct a careful medical history and ophthalmic examination to diagnose or confirm the ocular disorder and to assess perioperative surgical risk.
2. Review the goals of anophthalmic surgery with the patient: removal of the diseased eye, restoration of orbital volume, and a cosmetically acceptable outcome, including the potential for prosthesis motility.
3. Review the surgical procedure with the patient, including the temporary use of a postoperative conformer and custom prosthesis fitting typically 6 to 7 weeks after surgery. Discuss monitored anesthesia care (MAC) versus general anesthesia, potential postoperative pain, anticipated time away from work, and follow-up visits required. Mention potential surgical complications, including implant infection, exposure, extrusion and migration, and the need for additional anophthalmic socket and/or eyelid procedures.
4. Discuss the relative advantages and disadvantages of enucleation versus evisceration surgery and select a technique that is most suitable for the clinical situation.
5. Select either a porous or a nonporous implant. Proper selection of implant volume helps minimize the potential for a superior sulcus deformity and enophthalmos of the prosthesis. In general, a 20- to 22-mm sphere will adequately restore volume following enucleation surgery in the adult, whereas 18 to 20 mm is typically sufficient for evisceration procedures.
6. If the implant is to be placed with a wrapping material during enucleation surgery, then select an implant wrap.

22-10 INDICATIONS FOR ENUCLEATION

Enucleation involves removal of the entire globe while preserving the remaining adnexal and orbital tissues. The primary indications for enucleation include:

1. Primary intraocular malignancies (e.g., uveal melanoma, retinoblastoma) not amenable to alternative modes of therapy such as external- or proton-beam irradiation or episcleral plaque brachytherapy
2. Blind, painful, and/or disfigured or deformed eyes where the past ophthalmic history is not entirely clear and an intraocular tumor cannot be ruled out
3. In severely traumatized eyes, with extensive prolapse of uveal tissue, enucleation within the first 10 to 14 days may be considered if the risk of sympathetic ophthalmia and disease in the remaining contralateral eye is judged to be greater than the likelihood of recovering useful vision in the traumatized eye. However, the infrequency of sympathetic ophthalmia, coupled with improved medical therapy for uveitis, has made early enucleation strictly for prophylaxis a debatable practice. The retained traumatic eye often becomes phthisical and acts as an excellent template for an overlying prosthetic eye. The psychological impact of retaining one's own blind (phthisical) eye is also less than having one's eye removed. Our current approach is to repair and retain the traumatized eye

whenever possible as we feel the benefits of retention out weigh the risks of sympathetic opthahlmia.

22-11 INDICATIONS FOR EVISCERATION

Evisceration involves removal of the entire intraocular contents of the eye, leaving the scleral shell behind. It is typically preformed with keratectomy. Since the sclera, Tenon's capsule, extraocular muscle attachments, orbital connective tissue framework, and suspensory ligaments are virtually undisturbed, evisceration is thought to be associated with better postoperative cosmesis and motility than enucleation (regardless of which implant is used). Evisceration also is simpler and quicker to perform than enucleation.

The primary indications for evisceration surgery include:

1. A blind, painful normotensive or hypertensive eye with a well-documented past ocular history, no suspected or verified intraocular tumor, and clear intraocular media permitting adequate visualization of the fundus. Ultrasonography with or without computed tomography is performed before evisceration is considered if the posterior pole cannot be visualized but the past history is known.
2. A blind, nonpainful, disfigured eye with no or mild contraction (phthisis) with a well-documented past ocular history, no suspected or verified intraocular tumor, and clear intraocular media permitting adequate visualization of the fundus. Ultrasonography with or without computed tomography is performed before evisceration is considered if the posterior pole cannot be visualized but the past history is known. If moderate to severe phthisis and globe contraction is present, a larger posterior sclerotomy may be required, or a complete sclerotomy where the scleral shell is bisected into two complete halves (from superotemporal quadrant to inferonasal quadrant). Occasionally one has to place the implant immediately behind the sclera (i.e., posterior to posterior Tenon's capsule in order to put in a large-diameter implant).

Blind, painful eyes and blind, nonpainful, disfigured eyes (with or without some phthisis) where the ophthalmic history is well known (e.g., following end-stage glaucoma, trauma, hypotony) and recent posterior segment examinations did not demonstrate any evidence of neoplasm can be managed by enucleation or evisceration. Dramatic relief from discomfort and improved cosmesis can be achieved with either technique. The choice between enucleation and evisceration is somewhat controversial and varies by surgeon's preference. Enucleation is required if a complete histopathologic examination of the globe is required.

22-12 ENUCLEATION SURGICAL TECHNIQUE

1. The surgeon must develop a presurgery routine to ensure that the correct eye is removed. The patient should identify the eye to be removed by pointing to or touching the correct side of surgery. Confirm that this eye corresponds to

the informed consent and to office chart notes. Large arrows using a sterile surgical marking pen should be placed within the visible surgical field around the eye to be removed. If there is a tumor in the eye, dilate the eye in the presurgery waiting area so that direct visualization of the mass can be performed when the patient arrives in the operating room.

2. Anesthesia: Local anesthesia with intravenous sedation (MAC) or general anesthesia can be used. If MAC is used, then the upper and lower eyelids are blocked with 2% lidocaine in combination with 1:100,000 epinephrine mixed 1:1 with bacteriostatic saline (approximately 1.5 to 2 mL in each eyelid and lateral canthal area). In all cases a retrobulbar, intraconal injection of 2% lidocaine in combination with 1:100,000 epinephrine, mixed 1:1 with 0.75% bupivacaine, is administered (5 to 7 mL), followed by pressure application to the orbit for 5 to 10 minutes.
3. Intravenous antibiotic therapy should be administered 30 to 60 minutes prior to incision in the presurgery preparation area. If this is missed, antibiotics should be administered at the time of surgery.
4. Prophylactic antiemetic therapy should be given intraoperatively.
5. Place an eyelid speculum (Lancaster or similar to protect surgical field from eyelashes).
6. Perform 360-degree conjunctival limbal peritomy using Westcott scissors.
7. Bluntly dissect Tenon's tissue away from the globe in each oblique quadrant using Stevens tenotomy scissors (Fig. 22-2A).
8. Localize each rectus muscle on a large muscle hook to ensure that the entire muscle is isolated.
9. Pass a double-armed 5-0 polyglactin (Vicryl) suture in whiplock fashion on either side of the muscle near its insertion (Fig. 22-2B).
10. Sever each rectus muscle from the globe. Leave a 1- to 2-mm stump of muscle tendon attached to the globe over the medial and lateral rectus insertions so that traction sutures can be applied later in the procedure.
11. Isolate the inferior oblique muscle in the inferotemporal quadrant with the tip of the muscle hook sweeping from posterior to anterior (staying adjacent to the globe) toward the inferior rectus muscle. The muscle is then held between two muscle hooks, clamped with a straight hemostat, cauterized in the clamped section, cut and recauterized if the muscle stumps are still bleeding. Secure the inferior oblique with a double-armed 5-0 polyglactin suture in a similar manner as described for the rectus muscles.
12. The superior oblique is located in the superonasal quadrant by sweeping the muscle hook form anterior to posterior (staying adjacent to the globe) toward the superior rectus muscle. The superior oblique is cut and left untagged.
13. Attach a 4-0 silk suture to the lateral and/or medial rectus insertion sites to allow traction of the globe anteriorly during removal.
14. Place the closed enucleation scissors behind the globe and localize the optic nerve by strumming the nerve with the closed scissors. Gentle blunt dissection is carried out on either side of the optic nerve and the open scissor tips are placed on either side of the optic nerve (Fig. 22-2C). To get as much optic nerve stump as possible, direct the scissor tips posteriorly for several millimeters. As the optic nerve is cut, posteriorly directed pressure prevents the scissor tips from sliding off the optic nerve. Once the nerve is transected, the entire globe should release forward. Cut the remaining Tenon's tissue away from the globe, staying as close as possible to the globe to avoid inadvertent

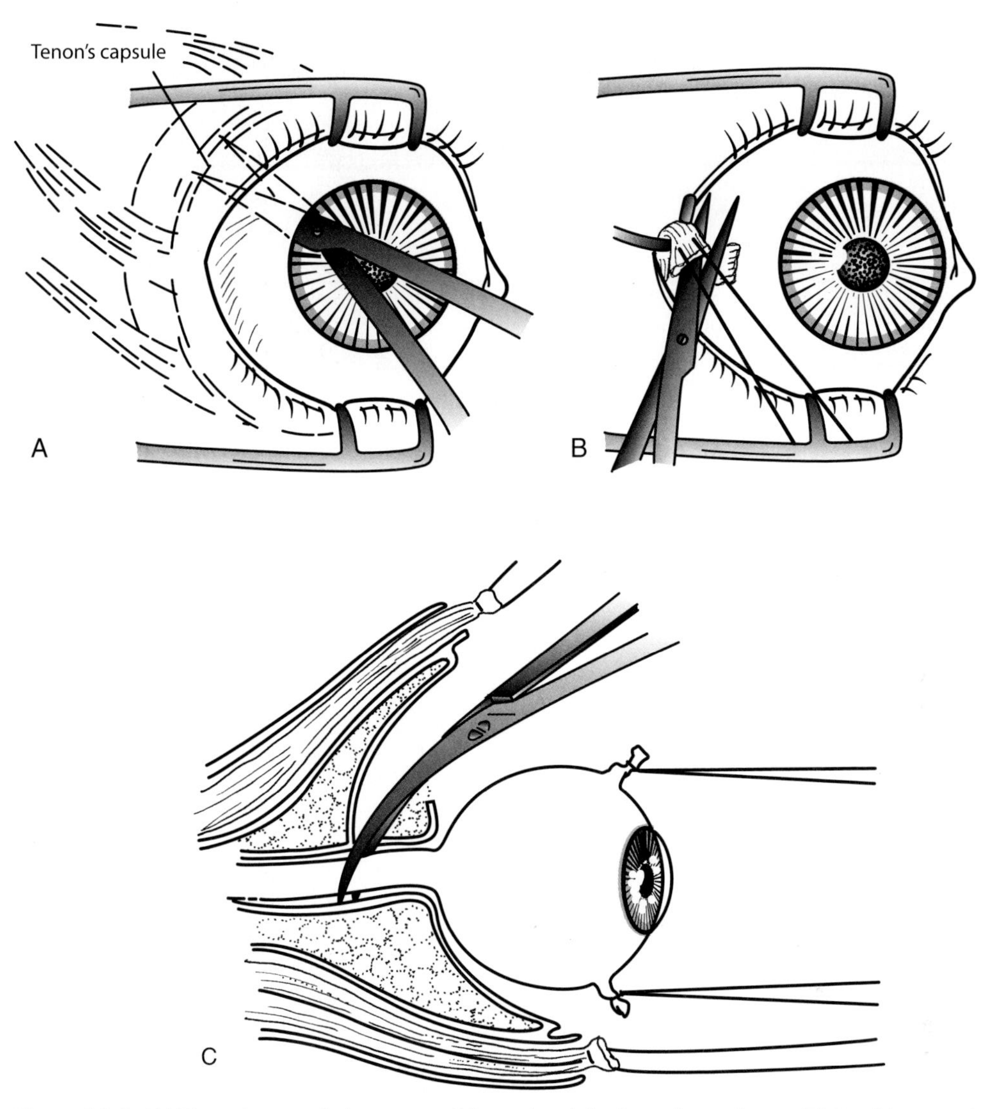

Figure 22-2 (A) Tenon's capsule is separated from the globe in each quadrant. (B) Double-armed 5-0 polyglactin suture is passed through muscle insertions and muscle is disinserted from the globe. (C) Enucleation scissors are shown cutting optic nerve as posterior as possible, leaving a significant amount attached to globe. (D) Additional pressure is applied to the wrapped implant with a cotton-tipped applicator while pulling anteriorly on Tenon's to seat the implant properly. (E) The extraocular muscles have been attached to the Vicryl mesh-wrapped implant. (F) Closure of anterior Tenon's with 4-0 or 5-0 polyglactin interupted sutures.

soft tissue or muscle injury and to avoid cutting the preplaced polyglactin sutures.

15. Once the globe has been removed, apply pressure to the socket with cotton sponges soaked in thrombin, 4% cocaine, or saline for 5 minutes to assist in hemostasis.
16. If active bleeding occurs following socket tamponade, then malleable ribbon or orbit retractors may used to gently retract orbital fat away from the optic

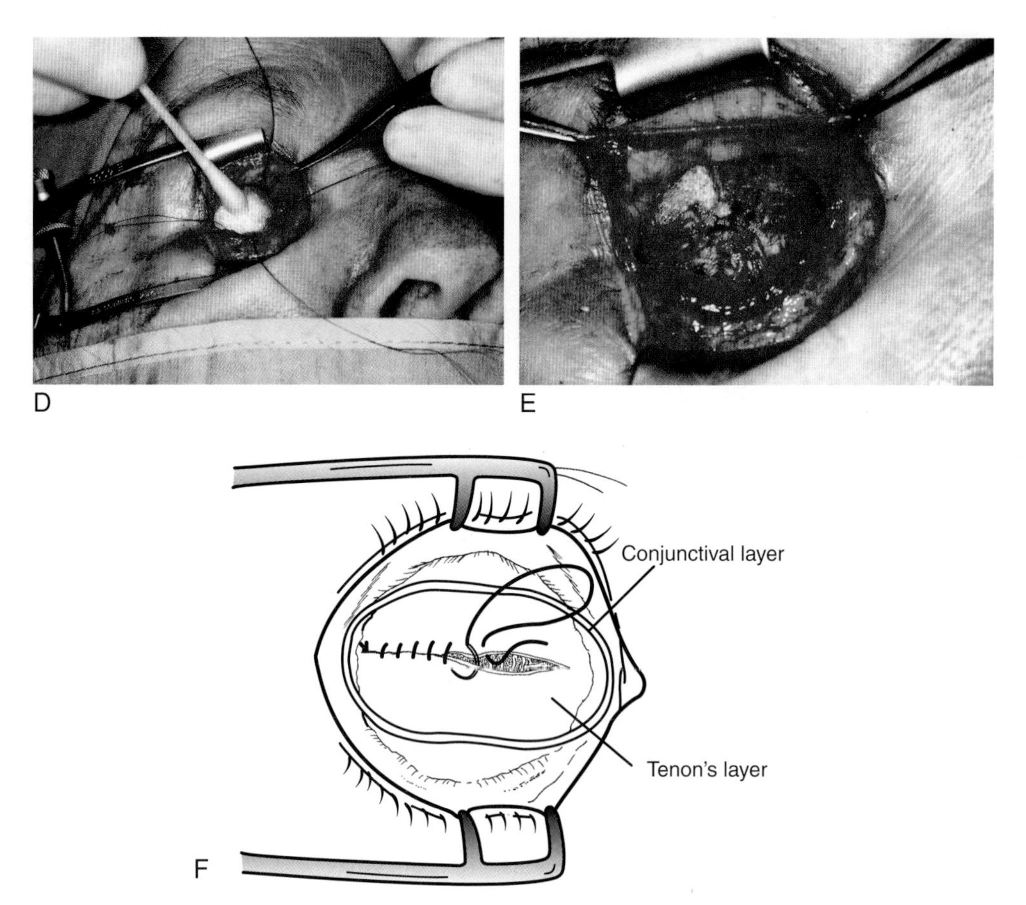

Figure 22-2 (Continued)

nerve stump. Bipolar cautery can then be performed in this area under direct visualization

17. Prior to insertion of a porous implant, the implant is immersed in an antibiotic solution (e.g., 500 mg cefazolin or bacitracin in 500 mL normal saline) within a 60-mL syringe, and an air–fluid exchange is performed.
18. An 18-gauge needle is used to place drill holes to the core of the implant around the equator of the implant near where the anterior rectus muscle bellies will contact the implant. A drill hole is also placed posteriorly. These holes in the implant facilitate implant fibrovascular ingrowth.
19. Vicryl mesh (or other wrap; surgeon's preference) is placed around the implant, twisting the excess mesh around the posterior aspect of the implant and securing the mesh to the implant with a 4-0 polyglactin suture tied around the twisted mesh. The excess mesh is then cut.
20. The wrapped implant is placed within a Carter sphere introducer or similar plunger-like mechanism, with the anterior aspect of the implant appropriately oriented. We recommend placing the orbital implant partly within Tenon's capsule and partly within the intraconal space. Other surgeons prefer placing the implant entirely within the intraconal space. Anterior Tenon's capsule should be retracted by a surgical assistant to avoid dragging

anterior Tenon's tissue posteriorly with implant placement (a common problem with porous orbital implants). Once the implant is placed into the orbit, we routinely "seat" the implant. Gentle posterior pressure is applied to the anterior implant surface using a cotton-tipped applicator while an Adson toothed forceps is used to unravel any rolled Tenon's edges for 360 degrees. Additional posterior pressure is applied to the implant with a cotton-tipped applicator while pulling anteriorly on Tenon's if the surgeon would like to place the implant deeper within the orbital cavity (Fig. 22-2D).

21. Secure the rectus muscle sutures to the anterior portion of the wrapped implant, just anterior to their normal anatomic insertion sites (Fig. 22-2E).
22. Meticulously close anterior Tenon's tissue with a buried 4-0 or 5-0 polyglactin suture in an interrupted fashion. It is extremely important that Tenon's tissue not be closed under tension (Fig. 22-2F).
23. Tension-free closure of the conjunctiva is performed with a running suture (6-0 plain gut suture) in a locking or nonlocking fashion. Rapid-absorbing 6-0 plain gut suture is avoided due to the risk of early wound dehiscence.
24. Apply antibiotic ointment to the eye socket, and insert a small, medium, or large acrylic conformer with holes, depending upon the forniceal volume. A temporary suture tarsorrhaphy is often helpful to maintain the conformer during the first 1 to 2 weeks following surgery. A single, simple suture using the remaining 6-0 plain can be placed through the upper and lower lid margin and left in place until it dissolves over 7 to 10 days. Alternatively, a double-armed suture (e.g., 4-0 silk) can be passed over a cotton or red rubber bolster to secure the eyelids.
25. Tightly apply two eye patches, which are generally left in place for 3 to 5 days.

22-13 EVISCERATION SURGICAL TECHNIQUE (WITH KERATECTOMY)

1–6. See "Enucleation Surgical Technique."

7. Undermine the conjunctiva by approximately 5 mm for 360 degrees.
8. Enter the anterior chamber with a #11 scalpel blade passed horizontally through the limbus. A 360-degree keratectomy with the scalpel blade and curved Westcott scissors is performed (Fig. 22-3A).
9. Place an evisceration spoon into the potential space between the choroid and sclera and attempt to remove the intraocular contents en bloc. Once the intraocular contents have been completely removed, maintain hemostasis with suction and bipolar cautery (Fig. 22-3B).
10. Wipe (débride) the entire internal scleral surface with cotton-tipped applicators soaked with absolute alcohol.
11. With a straight Stevens tenotomy scissors, remove a V-shaped piece of sclera 3 to 6 mm in length at the 3 o'clock and 9 o'clock positions; these sclerectomies can be increased in length as required up to the insertions of the medial and lateral rectus muscles to accommodate a large implant (Fig. 22-3C).
12. Use a #11 scalpel blade to create a posterior sclerotomy about 5 to 10 mm away from the optic nerve head. Incise the posterior sclera for 360 degrees around the nerve head with the #11 blade or Stevens scissors. Prolapse the

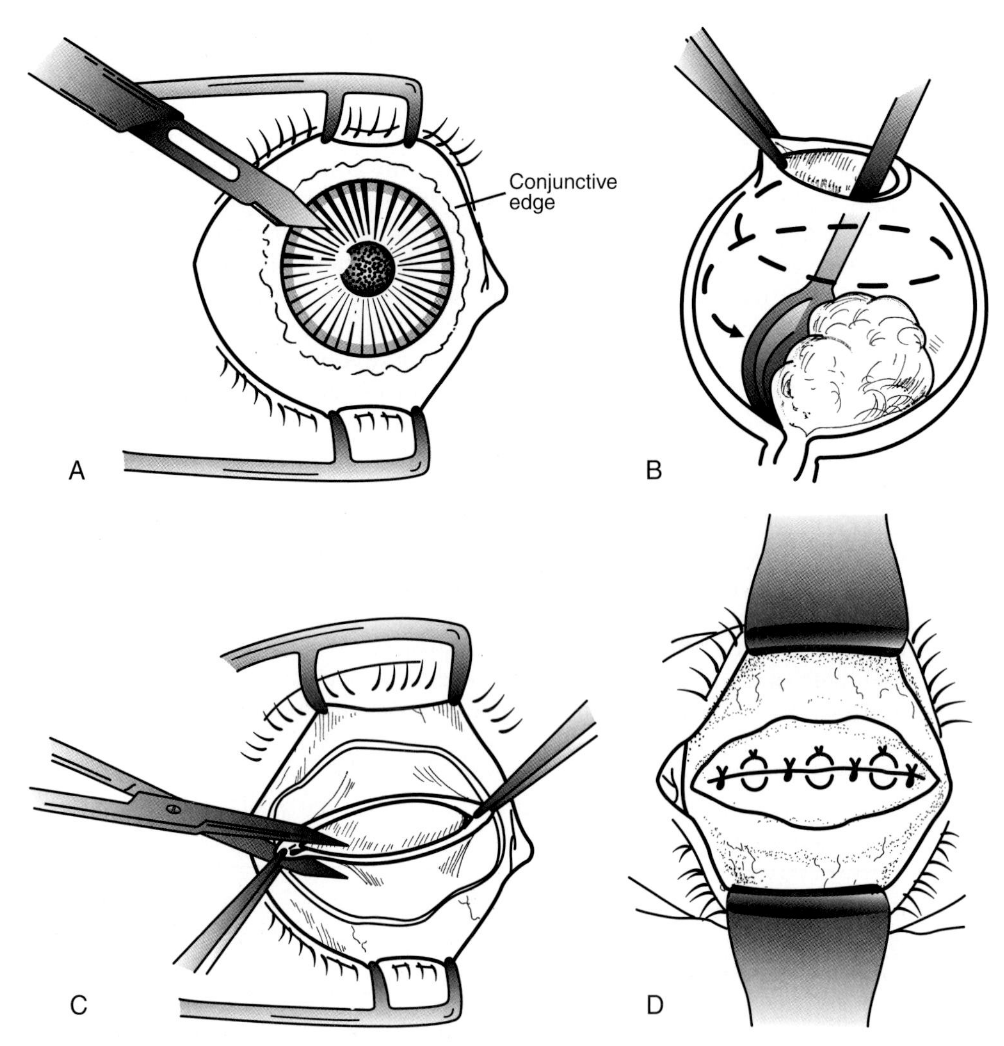

Figure 22-3 (A) A #11 scalpel blade is used to enter the limbus at the 11 o'clock position. (B) Evisceration spoon is used to remove the contents of the globe. (C) V-shaped pieces of sclera are removed at 3 o'clock and 9 o'clock to open the anterior entrance. (D) The anterior scleral edges are overlapped by 5 to 7 mm and closed with three equally spaced 5-0 polyglactin 910 sutures in a horizontal mattress suture. In between these are 4-0 polyglactin 910 sutures placed in as a simple stitch.

posterior sclera (with attached optic nerve) into the retrobulbar space with a cotton-tipped applicator.

13. Make 10-mm to 15-mm radial scleral incisions with the #11 scalpel blade or Stevens scissors in the four oblique quadrants, avoiding the rectus muscle insertions. The radial sclerotomies allow placement of a larger implant (e.g., a 20-mm sphere) and facilitate fibrovascularization of the posterior surface of the implant. Alternatively, a complete posterior sclerotomy can be performed. The sclera is transected from the superior nasal scleral edge posteriorly toward the optic nerve and from the inferior temporal scleral edge posteriorly toward the optic nerve. Sclera is then trimmed away from the optic nerve and

the optic nerve is gently moved posteriorly with a cotton-tipped applicator. This technique will allow placement of even larger orbital implants (e.g., 21- or 22-mm spheres).

14. Place an implant into a Carter sphere introducer (or similar plunger device) and insert the implant into the scleral cavity while a surgical assistant retracts the sclera. If the anterior scleral opening is too small to allow entry of the implant, the V-shaped sclerotomies are opened further using a scissors or a #11 scalpel blade to incise the sclera immediately beneath the medial and lateral rectus insertion sites. An unwrapped, moistened porous implant often sticks to the scleral walls as it is being injected into the scleral shell and may not completely enter the shell. To seat the implant within the scleral shell so that the anterior scleral edges can be apposed anteriorly without tension, an Adson toothed forceps is used to retract the anterior scleral lip while pressure is applied to the implant with a cotton-tipped applicator. The implant is not pushed posterior to the posterior sclerotomy. Any pieces of cotton fluff are removed from the surface of the implant and the surface is irrigated with an antibiotic solution.
15. Close the anterior scleral wound with three equally spaced double-armed 5-0 polyglactin sutures passed in horizontal mattress fashion so that the scleral edges are overlapped by 5 to 7 mm and are under no tension. Between each 5-0 polyglactin suture, additional 4-0 or 5-0 polyglactin sutures are placed in interrupted fashion through the apposing edges of sclera to reinforce the closure (Fig. 22-3D).
16. Meticulously close anterior Tenon's tissue with several buried 6-0 polyglactin sutures passed in an interrupted fashion. It is extremely important that Tenon's not be closed under tension.
17. Tension-free closure of the conjunctiva is performed with a running suture (6-0 plain gut suture) in a locking or nonlocking fashion. Rapid-absorbing 6-0 plain gut suture is avoided due to the risk of early wound dehiscence.
18. Apply antibiotic ointment to the eye socket, and insert a small, medium, or large acrylic conformer with holes, depending upon the forniceal volume. A temporary tarsorrhaphy is often helpful to maintain the conformer during the first 1 to 2 weeks following surgery. A single, simple suture using the remaining 6-0 plain can be placed through the upper and lower lid margin and left in place until it dissolves over 7 to 10 days. Alternatively, a double-armed suture (e.g., 4-0 silk) can be passed over a cotton or red rubber bolster to secure the eyelids.

22-14 POSTOPERATIVE CARE FOLLOWING ENUCLEATION/ EVISCERATION SURGERY

Pain is typically managed with moderate analgesics (acetaminophen with or without codeine, hydrocodone). Severe pain not adequately managed by moderate analgesia may require more intensive oral or intramuscular pain medication administration. Up to one third of anophthalmic surgery patients experience significant postoperative nausea. If intraoperative and recovery area antiemetic therapies do not relieve postoperative nausea, then oral or suppository medications should be prescribed prior to discharge.

Once the eye patches are removed, there is no special cleaning required. Showering and gentle face washing are acceptable. A broad-spectrum oral antibiotic is recommended for 5 days in most patients. Topical antibiotic–steroid eye drops or ointment (i.e., tobramycin-dexamethasone) are started four times daily for 2 to 3 weeks after surgery.

Cool compresses are applied for 15 to 20 minutes four times daily for a few days following patch removal. The temporary acrylic conformer is left in the socket until the patient is fitted with an "impression-fitted" custom prosthesis once the conjunctival chemosis has adequately resolved, typically 6 to 7 weeks after surgery. If the conformer falls out prematurely, it can be easily replaced by the patient or in the surgeon's office after the application of a lubricating eye ointment to the interior surface of the conformer. If the conjunctival chemosis prolapses out of the lid fissure, it must be kept moist with a lubricating ophthalmic ointment applied every 1 to 2 hours while awake. Prolonged edema may require replacement of the temporary tarsorrhaphy.

The following intervals are general recommendations for postoperative follow-up: 1 to 2 weeks, 4 to 6 weeks just prior to the initial visit with an ocularist, 3 months, 6 months, and annually thereafter.

22-15 COMPLICATIONS

22-15-1 *Implant Infection.* Infection is unusual in the immediate postoperative period. If infection is suspected, topical and systemic antibiotics are required. Removal of the implant becomes necessary if the infection is refractory or extrusion appears likely. A secondary implant can be placed once the infection has completely resolved.

22-15-2 *Implant Exposure.* Exposure of the implant is uncommon in the first few weeks following surgery. If it does occur, it is most commonly due to improper wound closure, placement of an oversized implant, or infection. Provided that there is no infection, additional surgery with reclosure or a patch graft (e.g., sclera, temporalis fascia) is required as soon as possible, whether a porous or nonporous implant is used. Do not wait for spontaneous closure when a porous implant is in place, as they are quite vulnerable to infection in this early phase. If infection is suspected, topical and systemic antibiotics are required.

Late exposures (months to years) can occur at any time postoperatively and with any type of orbital implant. If an acrylic implant exposes, extrusion is inevitable and a secondary orbital implant is required. If a porous orbital implant exposes and the exposure is small, vaulting the posterior surface of the artificial eye may take some pressure off the area, allowing it to heal. If the exposure does not spontaneously close by 8 weeks, a patch graft is recommend (e.g., temporalis fascia, sclera) to close the defect. If the exposure is larger (>6 mm), the chance of spontaneous closure is remote and a patch graft should be scheduled without delay. Topical antibiotic drops are recommended when any exposure is identified until surgical closure of the defect is achieved.

22-15-3 *Implant Migration*. Migration of the anophthalmic implant following enucleation surgery occurs less frequently with porous spherical implants than with acrylic or silicone implants. If the implant is decentered in the socket, the posterior surface of the prosthesis can be modified to accommodate the shifted implant. If prosthesis movement is compromised or a satisfactory prosthetic fit cannot be obtained because of the migrated implant position, an implant exchange is indicated, with centering of the secondary orbital implant within the muscle cone of the anophthalmic socket.

22-16 PEG PLACEMENT IN POROUS IMPLANTS

A recent infrared oculography study demonstrated significant objective improvement in horizontal gaze after motility peg placement.[43] Despite the improved motility, many surgeons and patients still elect to avoid peg placement due to the satisfactory results without pegging and the possibility of post-pegging complications (increased discharge, recurrent pyogenic granulomas, exposure of implant around peg, implant infection, tissue overgrowth, clicking).[96–101]

Although the use of pegging has declined dramatically over the past few years, a precise and meticulous technique under local anesthesia with intravenous sedation in the appropriately selected patient can still be a successful outpatient procedure.[102]

It is important to be selective in deciding which patients receive a peg. Proper care of the artificial eye and regular follow-up visits with the ocularist and ophthalmic plastic surgeon are important to be sure the peg system remains free of problems. If the patient is unlikely, unable, or unwilling to have adequate postoperative care, then pegging should be avoided. Children (under 15 years of age), adults over the age of 65 years, or individuals of any age with a chronic illness (e.g., a collagen vascular disease, sarcoidosis, diabetes mellitus, immunosuppressive therapy, prior orbital radiation therapy) should not be considered for pegging.

Peg and sleeve implant–prosthesis coupling systems were generally designed for peg/sleeve placement once fibrovascularization of the implant has been completed. Implant fibrovascularization is believed to diminish the risks of implant infection, exposure, and migration.[38,91] Drilling into an avascular area of the implant may predispose the implant to infection.[103] Gadolinium-enhanced MR imaging is currently the recommended method of assessing the extent of implant vascularization.[104] Fibrovascular ingrowth may occur at varying rates in different patients. Implant drilling and peg placement is generally deferred until 5 to 6 months after porous implant insertion.

Several titanium peg systems are currently available for use with porous orbital implants. Titanium is more biocompatible and better tolerated by human soft tissue than the original peg systems made of polycarbonate.[105] Complications associated with peg placement have also been reduced with the introduction of titanium pegs.[102] The FCI (Issy-Les-Moulineaux, France) peg-sleeve coupling system uses a HA-coated titanium sleeve.[102] The HA coating potentially allows for stronger interface bonding with the orbital fibroblasts than the uncoated P-K system supplied for use with the Bio-Eye. The MEDPOR Motility Coupling Post (MCP) (Porex Surgical, College

Park, GA) is a titanium screw that can be screwed directly into porous polyethylene implants.[106,107] Some authors have advocated primary placement of the MCP at the time of implant insertion.[108,109] This practice, however, remains controversial, and most North American oculoplastic surgeons defer implant pegging for more than 6 months after implant placement.

22-17 SECONDARY ORBITAL IMPLANTS

In North America and most developed countries an orbital implant is placed into the socket after enucleation or evisceration in almost all cases. In rare patients with severe endophthalmitis, implant placement may be delayed until the tissue swelling settles or a gross infection resolves. In individuals without an orbital implant, the term "secondary implant" is used when the implant is placed into the socket at a time other than the initial enucleation or evisceration procedure.

An attempt should be made to localize the extraocular muscles so that the secondary implant can be placed within the muscle cone (the ideal anatomic position) to allow some implant motility. A common misconception is that the extraocular muscles once transected (in an earlier enucleation procedure) from the globe retract into the orbit, precluding their later localization. Fortunately, the fibrous connective tissue framework remains intact and prevents the extraocular muscles from retracting into the posterior eye socket. The extraocular muscles are straightforward to localize in the majority of anophthalmic sockets without an implant.[110]

22-17-1 *Secondary Orbital Implant Placement Surgical Technique*

1. General anesthesia is preferred, but surgery may be done under local injection with intravenous sedation. Prior to administering any anesthesia, a topical anesthetic as well as a vasoconstrictor (topical 2.5% Neo-Synephrine) is applied to the conjunctiva.
2. The patient is asked to look in the direction of each rectus muscle. The surgeon puts a gentian violet mark on the conjunctiva over the area of strongest conjunctival retraction (Fig. 22-4A).
3. After injecting 3 mL of lidocaine 2% with epinephrine into the muscle cone and waiting for 5 minutes to allow for vasoconstriction, a horizontal incision is made in the conjunctiva and Tenon's capsule. The conjunctival edges are placed on traction and the surgeon uses cotton-tipped applicators to gently dissect into the area previously marked with gentian violet (Fig. 22-4B,C).
4. Once the rectus muscle is identified, it is dissected from the surrounding tissue and tagged with a 5-0 polyglactin suture passed in whiplock fashion. Once all four rectus muscles have been tagged, a central pocket is created and a secondary implant is placed into the muscle cone using a Carter sphere introducer as previously described.
5. For patients who have had an evisceration without an implant, there are two options. First, the shrunken eviscerated scleral remnant can be enucleated after identifying and tagging the extraocular muscles; a secondary implant is then put in place and attached to the extraocular muscles. Second, the scleral remnant can be opened by incising it from the superonasal quadrant to the

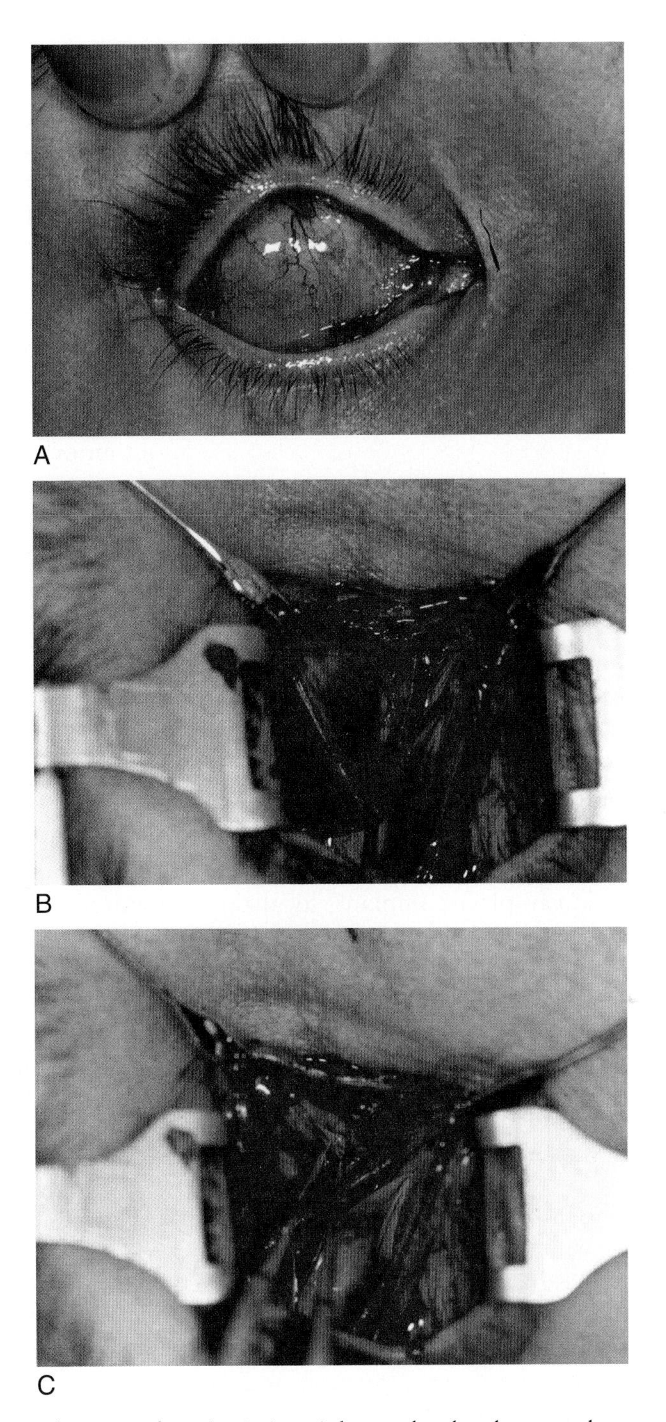

Figure 22-4 (A) Right eye socket. A gentian violet marker has been used to mark the areas on the conjunctiva where the recti muscles are pulling. (B) Right eye socket, looking toward caruncle. The conjunctiva is elevated with double-pronged rake retractors and the fibrous connective framework tunnels are visualized. (C) The medial rectus muscle is seen. A Castoveijo toothed forcep is used to grasp it and a double-armed 5-0 polyglactin 910 suture is passed through its distal end.

inferotemporal quadrant and from the superotemporal quadrant to the inferonasal quadrant.[111] A 5-0 polyglactin suture is attached to each of these scleral remnants (as if they represented extended muscle tendons on the rectus muscles). Transecting the sclera like this allows exposure to the muscle cone. A wrapped nonporous or porous implant can be placed into the muscle cone posterior to the four scleral remnants that have been created. The scleral remnant pieces can then be reattached to the wrapped implant 4 to 5 mm anterior to the normal extraocular muscle attachment sites, or in some cases they may be reconnected to their counterparts, creating a barrier of sclera over the implant.

6. Tenon's capsule and conjunctiva are closed in layered fashion without tension as described previously for enucleation/evisceration cases.

22-18 ORBITAL IMPLANT EXCHANGE

Four clinical scenarios exist where an implant exchange might be considered:

1. To improve motility
2. To reposition a migrated implant
3. To replace an exposed implant
4. To increase orbital volume

Prior to the widespread use of porous orbital implants (early 1990s), orbital implants were often placed into the socket without any wrap or any attachment to the extraocular muscles. Improvement in prosthetic motility may be possible by removing the previously placed implant, localizing the extraocular muscles, and reattaching them to one of the current porous orbital implants (aluminum oxide, HA, porous polyethylene). Similarly, if an implant migrates or rotates into a position that does not allow custom fitting of a prosthesis, the original implant can be removed and a new one placed. For large exposures that have failed previous free graft (i.e., scleral or temporalis fascia) or local tarsoconjunctival flap repair, an implant exchange may be required.

22-19 DERMIS–FAT GRAFTS

Dermis–fat grafts have traditionally been used most frequently after extrusion of an orbital implant or removal of a migrated implant where there is some loss of conjunctival tissues and shortened fornices. Conjunctival epithelium will migrate over the anterior surface of the dermis–fat graft and expand the conjunctival surface area. Dermis–fat grafts have also been used for the following indications: to expand orbital volume, to treat partially contracted eye sockets, to augment socket volume after enucleation without an implant, to repair extrusion of an evisceration implant, and to augment superior sulcus deformities in anophthalmic patients, and are occasionally used as a primary implant.[112–117] More recently, surgeons have reported good success with autogenous dermis–fat grafts in young children. These grafts may continue to grow and stimulate orbital expansion.[59,60]

Disadvantages of dermis–fat grafts include an unpredictable rate of absorption with a resulting superior sulcus deformity and orbital volume deficiency. In addition, there is little or no transfer of eye socket movement to the overlying prosthesis, resulting in an artificial eye with little natural motility.

22-20 FABRICATION, CARE, AND MAINTENANCE OF THE ARTIFICIAL EYE

Following enucleation, evisceration, or secondary implantation surgery, an acrylic (PMMA) conformer is placed in the conjunctival fornices to maintain the conjunctival space during the early postoperative healing phase. An anophthalmic socket without a conformer may contract within several days, compromising placement of an adequately sized prosthesis. The conformer is replaced with a custom-made ocular prosthesis typically fashioned 6 to 8 weeks following an enucleation, evisceration, or secondary orbital implant once the postoperative socket edema has subsided. Premade or "stock eyes" are unsatisfactory in developed countries as they are less than satisfactory cosmetically, limit prosthetic motility, may trap secretions between the socket and prosthesis, and not uncommonly rotate or fall out.

The ideal prosthesis is custom-fit to the exact dimensions of the orbit using the "modified impression technique." An impression of the socket is taken in a similar fashion to that of impressions taken while fitting dentures. The initial impression material is made of a highly refined alginate mixed with water. This paste-like material is placed into the socket. Once the impression material sets to a firm consistency, it is removed and the shape is copied into a wax mold. A prepared iris–cornea piece is positioned on the front surface of the wax pattern. The wax mold is placed into the socket and modified (reshaped) for comfort and to improve cosmesis. The wax shape is then translated (using additional molds) into fine-quality acrylic (from methylmethacrylate resin), painted, cured, and polished. The patient's remaining eye is used as a template to match the size and shape of the pupil and iris color, as well as the fine superficial vascular network on the sclera, episclera, and conjunctiva.

22-20-1 *Care and Handling of Artificial Eye.* Most patients become accustomed to wearing an artificial eye within a few days and eventually are unaware of its presence. Patients are asked to carry on with their normal facial hygiene and to try to ignore the presence of the prosthesis, including leaving the prosthesis in the socket while sleeping. Regular removal and manipulation of the artificial eye roughens the fine polished surface of the prosthesis and may lead to microtrauma of the conjunctiva and socket irritation. The patient should return to his or her ocularist at least once per year to have the artificial eye polished and adjusted. A smoother surface not only looks better but also allows for smoother movement of the eyelids over the prosthesis, decreasing the chance of conjunctival irritation with subsequent mucus production. Progressive changes to the eye socket such as fat atrophy and laxity of the upper and lower eyelids may cause rotation or malposition of the prosthetic eye. Minor adjustments in the shape or thickness of the artificial eye may provide the patient with a more comfortable fit and natural appearance.

If the prosthetic eye has to be removed, proper handling of it is important. A mild, nonirritating soap (e.g., Dove®, Ivory®, or baby shampoo) can be used to clean the prosthesis by gently rubbing soapsuds on the artificial eye surface, followed by rinsing with warm water. Alternatively, daily soft contact lens cleaner can be used instead of the mild soap along with contact lens rinsing solution for a final rinse. The prosthetic eye is gently dried with a nonabrasive soft cloth or soft facial tissue. Abrasive cloth materials will wear away the polished surface, creating a dull appearance. Similarly, solvents such as alcohol will damage the acrylic surface.

If the artificial eye has to be left out overnight or longer, it is best stored in contact lens soaking or rinsing solution made for soft contact lens wearers. If these are not available, it can be stored in water with a bit of salt (1/4 teaspoon to a cup of water). If the prosthesis is allowed to dry out, the layers may separate at the painted surface.

22-20-2 *Common Prosthesis Problems*

22-20-2-1 *Dryness*. A dry eye socket can often be corrected with artificial tear drops or gel applied throughout the day. If tear supplements do not relieve dry eye symptoms, then a drop of "light" mineral oil (a laxative purchased at any pharmacy) can be used on the artificial eye surface to allow the eyelids to glide over it smoothly. Topical silicone oil (Sil-Ophtho; Stony Brook, Inc., Davenport, Iowa) may also be used and is often available through the ocularist's office.

22-20-2-2 *Discharge*. A mild amount of mucoid discharge is common in the healthy anophthalmic socket. Some discharge may be due to the goblet cells of the conjunctiva producing mucus in response to the presence of a foreign body (the artificial eye). Discharge may worsen in the presence of an upper respiratory tract infection. One drop of a mild corticosteroid (i.e., FML) or an antibiotic–corticosteroid (i.e., tobramycin–dexamethasone) once or twice daily often diminishes the discharge in these situations. Eyelashes trapped behind the artificial eye can cause irritation and increase mucus production.

A poorly fitting prosthesis may result in a dead space between the posterior aspect of the ocular prosthesis and the conjunctival surface. This can be a site for accumulation of conjunctival and mucoid debris, which may cause further irritation and often leads patients to believe they have an infection. Most patients require polishing of the prosthesis annually, but some sockets require semiannual polishing of the artificial eye to smooth the surface and remove protein build-up ("biofilm") on the surface of the prosthesis. The average life of an artificial eye is about 5 to 7 years, but this varies based on how well it is been maintained. An older prosthesis loses its smooth surface and may irritate the conjunctival surface, resulting in increased mucoid discharge. It is important to involve the ocularist in the management of all patients with symptomatic socket discharge.

With moderate discharge, conjunctival infection (viral or bacterial conjunctivitis) is always a possibility. Usually there are accompanying signs of acute or chronic conjunctivitis, including edematous eyelids, conjunctival hyperemia, and mucopurulent discharge in the conjunctival fornices. A conjunctival culture should be performed if significant mucopurulence is present.

A pyogenic granuloma is another etiology of recurrent discharge (as well as some bleeding) and is typically present along the conjunctival closure site or around a peg. Pyogenic granulomas are a sign of irritation or microtrauma and may also indicate an underlying implant infection.[118]

Recurrent discharge may also be seen in patients who have developed giant papillary conjunctivitis (GPC). The etiology of GPC is not known, but it is believed to be an immunologic reaction to an antigen on the surface of the prosthesis. Giant papillae (>1 mm) on the tarsal conjunctiva of the upper eyelid are hallmarks of GPC. Treatment is difficult and may involve corticosteroid eye drops in conjunction with allergy drops and frequent enzymatic cleaning of the prosthesis. Removing the artificial eye at bedtime, cleaning it with a soft contact lens daily cleaner, and soaking it overnight in a denture-cleaning product (e.g., Polydent, Efferdent, Bufferdent) may provide some relief and permit continued wear of the artificial eye. Topical cyclosporine eye drops may also be helpful. As a last resort, carbon dioxide laser or cryoablation of the giant papillae can be attempted. In severe cases GPC may limit the amount of time the patient can wear the prosthetic eye. Rarely, a prosthesis made of a different material (e.g., glass) may be considered.

22-20-2-3 *Lagophthalmos with Dried Matter on the Prosthesis Surface.* Some individuals with nocturnal lagophthalmos may develop unsightly and irritating dried matter on the anterior surface of the prosthesis. Sometimes this debris can be cleaned without removing the prosthesis by rinsing the surface of the prosthetic eye with an irrigating solution (eye wash or saline). If this is not successful, the artificial eye should be removed and the debris washed off with mild soap and warm water. Light mineral oil or lubricating eye ointment may be used at bedtime on the anterior surface of the prosthesis if prosthetic debris is a chronic problem.

22-20-3 *Living With a Prosthetic Eye.* It is important for patients to learn not to focus on the presence of their prosthesis. An unhealthy level of self-consciousness can lead to chronic anxiety. The ocularist has a critical role in helping patients to cope with their disability by keeping their prosthetic eye and socket natural-appearing and comfortable. The patient's primary care physician and/or a psychologist or psychiatrist may also play a role in helping the monocular patient to learn to live with an artificial eye.

All ocular prostheses entail some form of limited motility. The patient should learn to turn the head and shoulders in the direction of gaze. Maintaining the primary gaze with both eyes will minimize ocular asymmetries. Facial expressions, such as smiling, animate the periorbital muscles and distract attention from the artificial eye.

Polycarbonate safety lenses are important to protect the remaining, functioning eye. Ideally, safety spectacles should be worn at all times. This is essential when the patient is involved in sports, using machinery or high-speed drills, and so forth. Spectacles with a light tint may also help minimize imperfections in the artificial eye, as well as camouflage asymmetries of the superior sulcus and eyelids. Cosmetic optics, involving plus (magnification) or minus (minification) lenses, are useful in altering the apparent size of the prosthesis and palpebral fissure. In addition, prisms in the spectacles may be used to adjust the perceived position of the prosthesis.

22-21 SUMMARY

Anophthalmic surgery is no longer simply about replacing a diseased eye with an orbital implant. Ophthalmic surgeons, working closely with qualified ocularists, must focus on restoring a patient's appearance and prosthetic motility to as near normal as possible. Although evisceration surgery has recently increased in popularity and is favored by many oculoplastic surgeons,[119,120] enucleation is still required in patients with known or potentially occult ocular malignancies as well as blind, painful, and/or unsightly eyes with opaque media and incomplete past ocular histories.

REFERENCES

1. Luce CM. A short history of enucleation. *Int Ophthalmol Clin.* 1970;10:681–687.
2. Grinsdale H. Note on early case of Mules' operation. *Br J Ophthalmol.* 1919;8:452–456.
3. Mules PH. Evisceration of the globe, with artificial vitreous. *Trans Ophthalmol Soc UK.* 1885;5:200–206.
4. Gougelmann HP. The evolution of the ocular motility implant. *Int Ophthalmol Clin.* 1976;10:689–711.
5. Kelley JJ. History of ocular prosthesis. *Int Ophthalmol Clin.* 1970;10:713–719.
6. Allen TD. Guist's bone spheres. *Am J Ophthalmol.* 1930;13:226–230.
7. McCoy LL. Guist bone spheres. *Am J Ophthalmol.* 1932;15:960–963.
8. Spaeth EB. *The Principles and Practices of Ophthalmic Surgery.* Malvern, PA: Lea and Febiger, 1941:127–142.
9. Ruedemann AD. Plastic eye implants. *Am J Ophthalmol.* 1946;29:947–951.
10. Cutler NL. A Universal type integrated implant. *Am J Ophthalmol.* 1949;32:253–258.
11. Allen JH, Allen L. A buried muscle cone implant: I. Development of a tunneled hemispherical type. *Arch Ophthalmol.* 1950;43:879–890.
12. Allen LH, Ferguson III EC, Braley AE. A quasi-integrated buried muscle cone implant with good motility and advantages for prosthetic filling. *Trans Am Acad Ophthalmol Otolaryngol.* 1960;64:272–278.
13. Spivey BE, Allen LH, Burns CA. The Iowa enucleation implant: a ten-year evaluation of techniques and results. *Am J Ophthalmol.* 1969;67:171–181.
14. Jordan DR, Anderson RL, Nerad JA, et al. A preliminary report on the Universal implant. *Arch Ophthalmol.* 1987;105:1726–1731.
15. Jordan DR, Anderson RL. The Universal implant as an evisceration implant. *Ophthalmic Plast Reconstr Surg.* 1997;13:1–7.
16. Soll, DB. Expandable orbital implants. In: Turtz A, ed. *Proceedings of Cent. Symposium, Manhattan Eye, Ear, and Throat Hosp, Vol. I: Ophthalmology.* St Louis: Mosby, 1969:197–202.
17. Hornblass A, Biesman BS, Eviatar JA. Current techniques of enucleation: a survey of 5,439 intraorbital implants and a review of the literature. *Ophthalmic Plast Reconstr Surg.* 1995;11:77–88.
18. Perry AC. Advances in enucleation. *Ophthalmic Plast Reconstr Surg.* 1991;4:173–182.
19. Dutton JJ. Coralline hydroxyapatite as an ocular implant. *Ophthalmology.* 1991;98: 370–377.
20. Nunery WR, Heinz GW, Bonnin JM, et al. Exposure rate of hydroxyapatite spheres in the anophthalmic socket: histopathologic correlation and comparison with silicone sphere implants. *Ophthalmic Plast Reconstr Surg.* 1993;9:96–104.

21. Goldberg RA, Holds JB, Ebrahimpour J. Exposed hydroxyapatite orbital implants: report of six cases. *Ophthalmology*. 1992;99:831–836.
22. Kim YD, Goldberg RA, Shorr N, et al. Management of exposed hydroxyapatite orbital implants. *Ophthalmology*. 1994;101:1709–1715.
23. Remulla HD, Rubin PAD, Shore JW, et al. Complications of porous spherical orbital implants. *Ophthalmology*. 1995;102:586–593.
24. Oestreicher JH, Liu E, Berkowitz M. Complications of hydroxyapatite orbital implants: a review of 100 consecutive cases and a comparison of Dexon mesh (polyglycolic acid) with scleral wrapping. *Ophthalmology*. 1997;104:324–329.
25. Jordan DR, Brownstein S, Jolly SS. Abscessed hydroxyapatite orbital implants: a report of two cases. *Ophthalmology*. 1996;103:1784–1787.
26. Mawn L, Jordan DR, Gilberg S. Scanning electron microscopic examination of porous orbital implants. *Can J Ophthalmol*. 1998;33:203–209.
27. Jordan DR, Munro SM, Brownstein S, et al. A synthetic hydroxyapatite implant: the so-called counterfeit implant. *Ophthalmic Plast Reconstr Surg*. 1998; 14:4:244–249.
28. Jordan DR, Bawazeer A. Experience with 120 synthetic hydroxyapatite implants (FCI3). *Ophthalmic Plast Reconstr Surg*. 2001;17:184–190.
29. Jordan DR, Pelletier C, Gilberg SM, et al. A new variety of hydroxyapatite: The Chinese Implant. *Ophthalmic Plast Reconstr Surg*. 1999;15(6): 420–424.
30. Jordan DR, Hwang I, McEachren TM, et al. Brazilian hydroxyapatite implant. *Ophthalmic Plast Reconstr Surg*. 2000;16:363–369.
31. Jordan DR, Brownstein S, Gilberg S, et al. Investigation of a bioresorbable orbital implant. *Ophthalmic Plast Reconstr Surg*. 2002;18:342–348.
32. Klett A, Guthoff R. Deckung von Orbitaimplantaten mit muskelgestielter autologer sklera. *Ophthalmologe*. 2003;100:449–452.
33. Blaydon SM, Shepler TR, Neuhaus RW, et al. The porous polyethylene (Medpor) spherical orbital implant: a retrospective study of 136 cases. *Ophthalmic Plast Reconstr Surg*. 2003;19:364–374.
34. Karesh JW, Dresner SC. High-density porous polyethylene (Medpor) as a successful anophthalmic implant. *Ophthalmology*. 1994;101:1688–1696.
35. Rubin PAD, Popham J, Rumeldts S, et al. Enhancement of the cosmetic and functional outcomes of enucleation with the conical orbital implant. *Ophthalmology*. 1998;105: 919–925.
36. Anderson RL, Yen MT, Lucci LM, et al. The quasi-integrated porous polyethylene orbital implant. *Ophthalmic Plast Reconstr Surg*. 2002;18:50–55.
37. Mawn LA, Jordan DR, Gilberg S. Proliferation of human fibroblasts in vitro after exposure to orbital implants. *Can J Ophthalmol*. 2001;36:245–251.
38. Christel P. Biocompatibility of alumina. *Clin Orthop Relat Res*. 1992;282:10–18.
39. Jordan DR, Mawn L, Brownstein S, et al. The bioceramic orbital implant: a new generation of porous implants. *Ophthalmic Plast Reconstr Surg*. 2000;16:347–355.
40. Jordan DR, Gilberg S, Mawn LA. The bioceramic orbital implant: experience with 107 implants. *Ophthalmic Plast Reconstr Surg*. 2003;19:128–135.
41. Jordan DR, Gilberg SM, Bawazeer A. The coralline hydroxyapatite orbital implant (Bio-EyeTM): experience with 170 patients. *Ophthalmic Plast Reconstr Surg*. 2004; 20(1):69–71.
42. Su GW, Yen MT. Current trends in managing the anophthalmic socket after primary enucleation and evisceration. *Ophthalmic Plast Reconstr Surg*. 2004;20(4):274–280.
43. Guillinta P, Vasani SN, Granet DB, et al. Prosthetic motility in pegged versus unpegged integrated porous orbital implants. *Ophthalmic Plast Reconstr Surg*. 2000;19: 119–122.

44. Custer PL, Kennedy RH, Woog JJ, et al. Orbital implants in enucleation surgery, a report by the American Academy of Ophthalmology. *Ophthalmology.* 2003;110: 2054–2061.
45. Custer PL, Trinkaus KM, Fornoff J. Comparative motility of hydroxyapatite and alloplastic enucleation implants. *Ophthalmology.* 1999;106:513–516.
46. Colen TP, Paridaens DA, Lemij HG, et al. Comparison of artificial eye amplitudes with acrylic and hydroxyapatite spherical enucleation implants. *Ophthalmology.* 2000; 107:1889–1894.
47. Yago K, Furuta M. Orbital growth after unilateral enucleation in infancy without an orbital implant. *Jpn J Ophthalmol.* 2001;45:848–852.
48. Bentley RP, Sgouros S, Natarujan K. Normal changes in orbital volume during childhood. *J Neurosurg.* 2002;96:742–746.
49. Apt L, Isenberg S. Changes in orbital dimensions following enucleation. *Arch Ophthalmol.* 1978;90:893–895.
50. Kennedy RE. The effect of early enucleation on the orbit in animals and humans. *Trans Am Ophthalmol Soc* 1964;62:460–509.
51. Pfieffer RL. The effect of enucleation on the orbit. *Trans Am Acad Ophthalmol.* 1945;49:236–239.
52. Taylor W. Effect of enucleation of one eye in childhood upon subsequent development of the face. *Trans Ophthalm Soc UK.* 1939;59:368–373.
53. Hintschich C, Zonneveld F, Baldeschi L. Bony orbital development after early enucleation in humans. *Br J Ophthalmol.* 2001;85:205–208.
54. Howard GM, Kinder RS, MacMillan AS Jr. Orbital growth after unilateral enucleation in childhood. *Arch Ophthalmol.* 1965;73:80–83.
55. Imhof SM, Mourits MP, Hofman P. Quantification of orbital and mid-facial growth retardation after megavoltage external beam irradiation in children with retinoblastoma. *Ophthalmology.* 1996;103:263–268.
56. Cepala MA, Nunnery WR, Martin RT. Stimulation of orbital growth by the use of expandable implants in the anophthalmic cat orbit. *Ophthalmic Plast Reconstr Surg.* 1992;8:157–169.
57. Kaste SC, Chen G, Fontaesi J. Orbital development in long-term survivors of retinoblastoma. *J Clin Oncol.* 1997;15:1183–1189.
58. Fountain TR, Goldberg S, Murphree AL. Orbital development after enucleation in early childhood. *Ophthalmic Plast Reconstr Surg.* 1999;15;32–36.
59. Heher KI, Katowitz JA, Low JE. Unilateral dermis-fat graft implantation in the pediatric orbit. *Ophthalmic Plast Reconstr Surg.* 1998;14:81–88.
60. Mitchell KT, Hollstein DA, White WL. The autogenous dermis-fat orbital implant in children. *J AAPOS.* 2001;5:367–369.
61. DePotter P, Shields CL, Shields JA. Use of the hydroxyapatite ocular implant in the pediatric population. *Arch Ophthalmol.* 1994;112:208–212.
62. Jordanidou V, DePotter P. Porous polyethylene orbital implant in the pediatric population. *Am J Ophthalmol.* 2004;138:425–429.
63. DePotter P, Shields CL, Shields JA, et al. Role of magnetic resonance imaging in the evaluation of hydroxyapatite orbital implant. *Ophthalmology.* 1992;99:824–830.
64. Arora W, Weeks K, Halpern EC, et al. Influence of corralline hydroxyapatite used as an ocular implant on the dose of external beam photon radiation therapy. *Ophthalmology.* 1992;99:380–382.
65. Kaltreider SA. The ideal ocular prosthesis. Analysis of prosthetic volume. *Ophthalmic Plast Reconstr Surg.* 2000;16:5:388–392.

66. Kaltreider SA. The ideal ocular prosthesis: analysis of prosthetic volume. *Ophthalmic Plast Reconstr Surg.* 2000;16:388–392.
67. Kaltreider SA, Lucarelli MJ. A simple algorithm for selection of implant size for enucleation and evisceration. *Ophthalmic Plast Reconstr Surg.* 2002;18:336–341.
68. Custer PL, Trinkaus KM. Volumetric determination of enucleation implant size. *Am J Ophthalmol.* 1999;128:489–494.
69. Thaller VT. Enucleation volume measurement. *Ophthalmic Plast Reconstr Surg.* 1997;13:18–20.
70. Kaltreider SA, Jacobs JL, Hughes MO. Predicting the ideal implant size before enucleation. *Ophthalmic Plast Reconstr Surg.* 1999;15:3:37–43.
71. Perry JD. Hydroxyapatite implants [letter]. *Ophthalmology.* 2003;110:1281.
72. Long JA, Tann TM, Bearden WH, Callahan MA. Enucleation: is wrapping the implant necessary for optimal motility? *Ophthalmic Plast Reconstr Surg.* 2003;19(3): 194–197.
73. Suter AJ, Molteno AC, Becin TH, et al. Long-term follow-up of bone derived hydroxyapatite orbital implants. *Br J Ophthalmol.* 2002;86:1287–1992.
74. Nunery WR. Risk of prion transmission with the use of xenografts and allografts in surgery. *Ophthalmic Plast Reconstr Surg.* 2003;17:389–394.
75. Seiff SR, Chang Jr. JS, Hurt MH, et al. Polymerase chain reaction identification of human immunodeficiency virus-1 in preserved human sclera. *Am J Ophthalmol.* 1994;118:528–529.
76. Long CJ, Heckman JG, Neunderfer B. Creutzfeldt-Jakob disease via dural and corneal transplants. *J Neurol Sci.* 1998;160:128–139.
77. Hogan RN, Brown P, Heck E, et al. Risk of prion disease transmission from ocular donor tissue transplantation. *Cornea.* 1999;18:2–11.
78. Heckman JG, Lang CJ, Petruch F, et al. Transmission of Creutzfeldt-Jakob disease via a corneal transplant. *J Neurol Neurosurg Psychiatry.* 1997;63:388–390.
79. Simonds RJ, Holmberg SD, Hurwitz RL, et al. Transmission of human immunodeficiency virus type 1 from a seronegative organ and tissue donor. *N Engl J Med.* 1992;326:726–732.
80. Arat YO, Shetlar DJ, Boniuk M. Bovine pericardium versus homologous sclera as a wrapping for hydroxyapatite orbital implants. *Ophthalmic Plast Reconstr Surg.* 2003; 19:189–193.
81. Gayre GS, DeBacker CM, Lipham W, et al. Bovine pericardium as a wrapping for orbital implants. *Ophthalmic Plast Reconstr Surg.* 2001; 17:381–387.
82. Pelletier C, Gilberg S, Jordan DR. Use of temporalis fascia for management of exposed hydroxyapatite implants. *Ophthalmic Plast Reconstr Surg.* 1998;14:198–203.
83. Naugle Jr TC, Fry CL, Sabatier RE, Elliot LF. High leg incision fascia lata harvesting. *Ophthalmology.* 1997;104:1480–1488.
84. Kao SCS, Chen S. The use of rectus abdominis sheath for wrapping of the hydroxyapatite orbital implants. *Ophthalmic Surg Lasers.* 1999;30:69–71.
85. Naugle Jr TC, Lee AM, Haik BG, et al. Wrapping hydroxyapatite orbital implants with posterior auricular muscle complex grafts. *Am J Ophthalmol* 1999; 128:495–501.
86. Karesh JW. Polytetrafluoroethylene as a graft material in ophthalmic plastic and reconstructive surgery: an experimental and clinical study. *Ophthalmic Plast Reconstr Surg.* 1987;3:179–185.
87. Choo PH, Carter SR, Crawford JB, et al. Exposure of expanded polytetrafluoroethylene-wrapped hydroxyapatite orbital implant: a report of two patients. *Ophthalmic Plast Reconstr Surg.* 1999;15:77–78.

88. Kao L. Polytetrafluoroethylene as a wrapping material for a hydroxyapatite orbital implant. *Ophthalmic Plast Reconstr Surg.* 2000;16:286–288.
89. Jordan DR, Allen LH, Ells A, et al. The use of Vicryl mesh (polyglactin 910) for implantation of hydroxyapatite orbital implants. *Ophthalmic Plast Reconstr Surg.* 1995;11:95–99.
90. Jordan DR, Ells A, Brownstein S, et al. Vicryl-mesh wrap for the implantation of hydroxyapatite orbital implants: an animal model. *Can J Ophthalmol.* 1995;30: 241–246.
91. Klapper SR, Jordan DR, Punja K, et al. Hydroxyapatite implant wrapping materials: analysis of fibrovascular ingrowth in an animal model. *Ophthalmic Plast Reconstr Surg.* 2000;16:278–285.
92. Gayre GS, Lipham W, Dutton JJ. A comparison of rates of fibrovascular ingrowth in wrapped versus unwrapped hydroxyapatite spheres in a rabbit model. *Ophthalmic Plast Reconstr Surg.* 2002;18:275–228.
93. Jordan DR, Klapper SR, Gilberg SM. The use of Vicryl mesh in 200 porous orbital implants. *Ophthalmic Plast Reconstr Surg.* 2003;19:53–61.
94. Custer PL. Enucleation: past, present, and future. *Ophthalmic Plast Reconstr Surg.* 2000;16:316–321.
95. Jordan DR, Klapper SK, Gilberg SM, et al. The bioceramic implant: evaluation of exposures in 419 implants. *Ophthal Plast Reconstr Surg.* 2010; 26:2:80-85.
96. Custer PL. Reply to Dr. D. R. Jordan's letter on polyglactin mesh wrapping of hydroxyapatite implants. *Ophthalmic Plast Reconstr Surg.* 2001;17:222–223.
97. Jordan DR, Chan S, Mawn L, et al. Complications associated with pegging hydroxyapatite orbital implants. *Ophthalmology.* 1999;106: 505–512.
98. Edelstein C, Shields CL, DePotter P, et al. Complications of motility peg placement for the hydroxyapatite orbital implant. *Ophthalmology.* 1997;104:1616–1621.
99. Lin CJ, Lio SL, Jou JR, et al. Complications of motility peg placement for porous hydroxyapatite orbital implants. *Br J Ophthalmol.* 2002;86: 394–396.
100. Jordan DR. Spontaneous loosening of hydroxyapatite peg sleeves. *Ophthalmology.* 2001;108: 2041–2044.
101. Cheng MS, Lio SL, Lin L. Late porous polyethylene implant exposure after motility coupling post placement. *Am J Ophthalmol.* 2004;138:420–424.
102. Lee SY, Jang JW, Lew H, et al. Complications in motility peg placement for hydroxyapatite orbital implants in anophthalmic socket. *Jpn J Ophthalmol.* 2002;46: 103–107.
103. Jordan DR, Klapper SR. A new titanium peg system for hydroxyapatite orbital implants. *Ophthalmic Plast Reconstr Surg.* 2000;16:380–387.
104. Ainbinder DJ, Haik BG, Tellado M. Hydroxyapatite orbital implant abscess: histopathologic correlation of an infected implant following evisceration. *Ophthalmic Plast Reconstr Surg.* 1994;10:267–270.
105. Klapper SR, Jordan DR, Ells A, et al. Hydroxyapatite orbital implant vascularization assessed by magnetic resonance imaging. *Ophthalmic Plast Reconstr Surg.* 2003;19: 46–45.
106. Cook S, Dalton J. Biocompatibility and biofunctionality of implanted materials. *Alpha Omegan.* 1992;85:41–47.
107. Choi JC, Iwamoto MA, Bstandig S, et al. Medpore motility coupling post: a rabbit model. *Ophthalmic Plast Reconstr Surg.* 1999;15:190–201.
108. Rubin PAD, Fay AM, Remulla HD. Primary placement of motility coupling post in porous polyethylene orbit implants. *Arch Ophthalmol.* 2000;118:826–832.

109. Hsu WC, Green JP, Spilker MH, et al. Primary placement of a titanium motility post in a porous polyethylene orbital implant. *Ophthalmic Plast Reconstr Surg.* 2003; 16:370–379.
110. Tawfik HA, Dutton JJ. Primary peg placement in evisceration with the spherical porous polyethylene orbital implant. *Ophthalmology.* 2004;111:1401–1406.
111. Jordan DR. Localization of extraocular muscles during secondary orbital implantation surgery: the tunnel technique. Experience in 100 patients. *Ophthalmology.* 2004; 111:1048–1054.
112. Jordan DJ, Parisi J. The scleral filet technique. *Can J Ophthalmol.* 1996;31(7):357–361.
113. Archer KF, Hurwitz JJ. Dermis-fat grafts and evisceration. *Ophthalmology.* 1989: 96:170–174.
114. Borodic GE, Townsend DJ, Beyer-Machule CK. Dermis fat graft in eviscerated sockets. *Ophthalmic Plast Reconstr Surg.* 1989;5:144–149.
115. Nunery WR, Hetzler KJ. Dermal-fat graft as a primary enucleation technique. *Ophthalmology.* 1985:92:1256–1261.
116. Migliori ME, Petterman AM. The domed dermis-fat graft orbital implant. *Ophthalmic Plast Reconstr Surg.* 1991;7:23–30.
117. Lisman RD, Smith BC. Dermis-fat grafting. In: Smith BC, ed. *Ophthalmic Plastic and Reconstructive Surgery.* St. Louis: CV Mosby Co., 1987:1308–1320.
118. Saunders CK, Garber PF, Della Rocca RC. Socket reconstruction. In: Levine MR, ed. *Manual of Oculoplastic Surgery.* Philadelphia: Butterworth Heinmann, 2003:314–316.
119. Jordan DR, Brownstein S, Dorey MW. Clinicopathologic analysis of 15 explanted hydroxyapatite implants. *Ophthalmic Plast Reconstr Surg.* 2004;20(4):285–290.
120. Timothy NH, Feilich DE, Linberg JV. Perspective: evisceration versus enucleation, the ocularist's standpoint. *Ophthalmic Plast Reconstr Surg.* 2003;19(6):417–420.

23

Orbital Exenteration

ADAM HSU, MD, AND BITA ESMAELI, MD

Orbital exenteration is a surgical procedure that removes varying degrees of the orbital contents and periorbital soft tissue, including periorbital skin, the globe, extraocular muscles, optic nerve, the periorbita, and the orbital fat. In some instances, the disease process may necessitate removal of the bony orbital walls as well.

23-1 INDICATIONS FOR ORBITAL EXENTERATION

Orbital exenteration is reserved for highly malignant and potentially fatal neoplasms originating from the ocular adnexal structures; ocular tumors with extension to the orbital soft tissue; orbital extension of tumors of the paranasal sinuses or nasal cavity; and orbital extension from intracranial processes.[1–8] Tumors necessitating orbital exenteration may include squamous cell carcinoma, basal cell carcinoma, sebaceous carcinoma, melanoma of the conjunctiva, uveal melanoma with extrascleral or orbital extension, epithelial cancers such as adenoid cystic carcinoma of the lacrimal gland, rhabdomyosarcoma, and other rare tumors. The indications for orbital exenteration in a number of previously published series are summarized in Table 23-1.

In addition to cancers, nonmalignant neoplasms—such as neurofibromatosis causing severe orbital displacement, immobility, and blindness or extensive lymphangioma compromising function and cosmesis—may also lead to orbital exenteration. Nonneoplastic diseases of rapidly infiltrative nature, either inflammatory or infectious, and nonneoplastic diseases associated with refractory orbital pain may also be indications for orbital exenteration. Examples include invasive fungal infections of the orbit such as mucormycosis; orbital socket contracture

Table 23-1 Indications for Orbital Exenteration in Previously Published Series

Series	No. of patients	Squamous Cell Carcinoma	Basal Cell Carcinoma	Sebaceous Cell Carcinoma	Malignant Melanoma (any site)	Other Epithelial Tumor	Sarcoma	Infection	Other
Levin[1] 1969–1988	99	32	8	6	18	15	4	6	10
Mohr[2] 1974–1995	74	13	6	—	13	16	12	—	14
Nssab[3] 1975–1995	32	3	17	4	6	1	1	—	—
Shields[4] 1979–1999	56	5	4	3	36	3	1	1	3
Goldberg[5] 1983–1999	25	7	2	3	6	3	2	—	2
Rahman[6] 1991–2004	69	6	28	9	10	4	2	—	10
Ben Simon[7] 1999–2003	34	9	6	3	9	5	1	1	—
Total	389	75	71	28	98	47	23	8	39

after enucleation causing severe pain; and extreme cases of Graves orbitopathy unresponsive to other treatment modalities.

23-2 PREOPERATIVE EVALUATION

Orbital exenteration results in complete loss of vision in the affected eye as well as significant disfigurement of the upper face; thus, counseling of the patient prior to surgery and understanding of the patient's expectations are important to minimize the patient's distress.

During the preoperative interview, the patient's past medical and surgical history, current medications, coagulation status, and allergies should be ascertained; there should also be a review of systems, with a focus on symptoms of cancer and metastasis. The physical examination should include careful inspection for signs of local or regional extension of disease. Regional lymph node and distant-organ metastasis must be ruled out prior to the decision to proceed with an orbital exenteration. Imaging studies are an integral part of the preoperative evaluation, providing information about the gross anatomic extent of cancer.

Histopathologic review of the previous surgical resection specimens is critical to identify high-risk features or extent of disease that may justify orbital exenteration. In some cases, most commonly with extensive recurrent eyelid or conjunctival cancers, the full extent of cancer involvement of orbital soft tissue may be difficult to determine on the basis of preoperative physical examination and radiographic assessment. In such cases, the decision whether to do an orbital exenteration may depend on the findings on intraoperative frozen-section evaluation of the margins of resection. For example, in patients with locally advanced eyelid or adnexal squamous cell carcinoma or basal cell carcinoma, the patient should be fully informed of the possibility of an orbital exenteration prior to the planned surgery to remove the adnexal cancer.

The workup for systemic disease should be tailored to the cancer type and should be completed prior to the decision to do an orbital exenteration. In patients with widespread metastatic disease, especially elderly patients or those with a short life expectancy, palliative radiation therapy or various degrees of debulking procedures may offer a better quality of life than orbital exenteration.

General endotracheal anesthesia is necessary for orbital exenteration; thus, a preoperative visit with anesthesiology to rule out any cardiac or pulmonary contraindications to general anesthesia is a good idea.

A general discussion about the types of reconstructive procedures available for the orbital cavity is also a good idea. It is important to find out whether the patient is interested in wearing an orbital prosthesis after exenteration as this may affect the choice of reconstructive procedures (see sections 23-4 and 23-6 below).

23-3 SURGICAL TECHNIQUES

We have subdivided the types of orbital exenteration into three general categories based on the extent of tissue resection: standard anterior, eyelid-sparing, and orbital exenteration plus removal of one or more of the bony orbital walls.

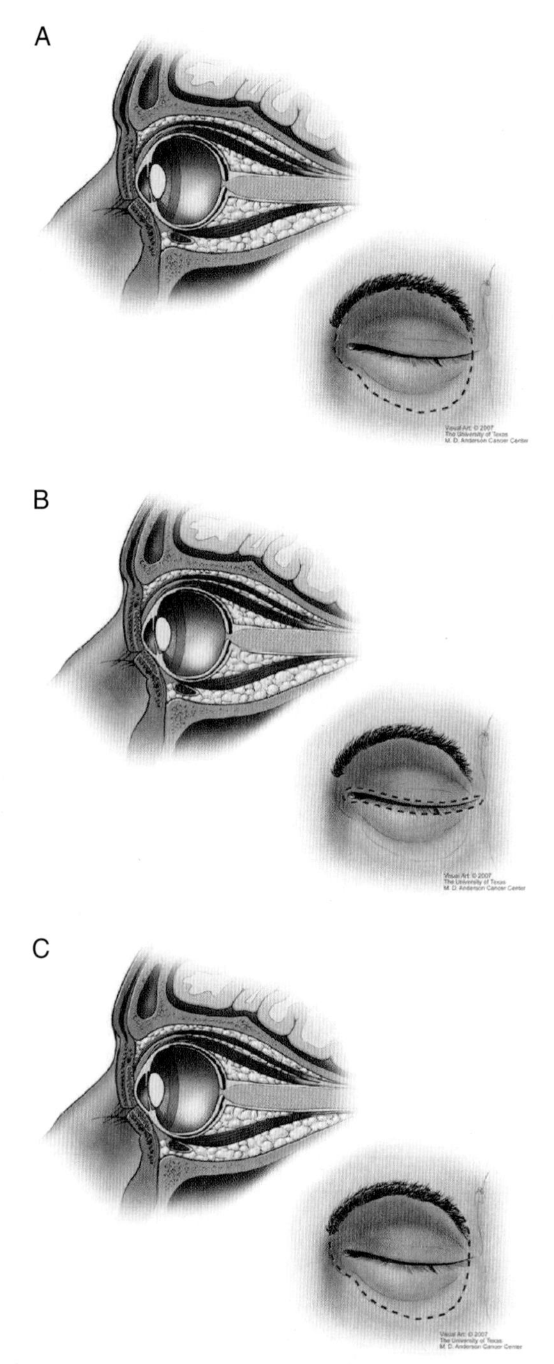

Figure 23-1 (A) Skin incision for standard orbital exenteration includes some of the skin of the upper and lower eyelids. The blue-shaded area contains the orbital soft tissue that are removed during a standard exenteration. (B) In the "eyelid-sparing" technique the skin of the upper and lower eyelid is spared; all other components of the eyelids are otherwise removed as in the standard exenteration. (C) Occasionally it is necessary to include the bony walls of the orbit in the surgical specimen.

23-3-1 *Standard Anterior Orbital Exenteration.* The standard technique is useful for the majority of adnexal cancers, particularly those involving a significant part of the upper or lower eyelid skin, in which case the eyelid-sparing technique would not adequately address the eyelid soft tissue involved with cancer.

The procedure begins by outlining the amount of skin to be removed in the upper and lower eyelids (Fig. 23-1A). The upper and lower eyelids are secured at the eyelid margin with 4-0 silk suture for traction and to maintain the integrity of the ocular-surface structures. The planned incision is marked and is designed to create an appropriate disease-free margin around the lesion. To achieve hemostasis, 1:100,000 epinephrine is infiltrated along the marked incision line. Scalpel or monopolar cutting electrocautery is used to carry out the dissection down to the orbital rim, and the periosteum is incised. With a periosteal elevator, the periosteum is dissected away from orbital bone posteriorly toward the orbital apex. Firm attachment of periosteum to orbital walls—for example, orbital fissures, lateral tubercle, medial canthal tendon insertion—may necessitate scalpel and electrocautery. The nasolacrimal duct is cut just distal to the lacrimal sac. To avoid formation of a sino-orbital fistula, care is taken not to violate the orbital walls adjacent to the paranasal sinuses, especially medially and inferiorly, where they are thin. Bipolar electrocautery is used to maintain hemostasis during the periorbital dissection. Once adequate dissection is accomplished to the orbital apex, a curved clamp is used to clamp the orbital contents at the apex. The orbital contents within the periorbita are cut just above the curved clamp with a pair of heavy scissors. Hemostasis is achieved using bipolar cautery. The specimen is clearly oriented with placement of sutures and is taken to the pathology lab for evaluation of margin status, which is accomplished by frozen-section analysis. The orbital cavity is inspected for any residual disease that may require further excision. The results of frozen-section examination dictate whether further resection is required. The discovery of perineural invasion or deep orbital, possibly intracranial, extension indicates that complete surgical eradication is improbable. In such cases, adjuvant postoperative radiation therapy may be used to decrease the likelihood of locoregional recurrence.

The orbital cavity is packed with cottonoid or gauze soaked with thrombin. Any remaining bleeding can be controlled with bipolar cautery or, in the case of bone-perforating vessels, bone wax.

23-3-2 *Eyelid-Sparing Orbital Exenteration.* In an eyelid-sparing procedure, the skin incision is made just a few millimeters above the upper eyelid lash line and a few millimeters below the lower eyelid lash line. This modification of the standard technique is most appropriate for cancers involving the conjunctiva or limited to the palpebral conjunctiva or anterior-orbit soft tissue and sparing the skin and orbicularis layer of the eyelid.

After the skin incision is made (Fig. 23-1B), a plane of dissection is established between the skin and orbicularis muscle with blunt-tipped scissors to the area around the orbital rim. Scalpel or electrocautery is then used to deepen the incision to the periosteum. From this point, the procedure is carried out like standard exenteration. The skin flaps are sutured together once hemostasis is achieved. A drain may be inserted, but it is not always necessary. An additional skin graft may be necessary to adequately line the orbital socket, particularly for a deep orbital exenteration where the orbital contents are removed to the apex and there may not be enough eyelid skin to adequately cover the cavity.

23-3-3 *Orbital Exenteration plus Removal of One or More of the Orbital Bony Walls.* Cancers of the paranasal sinuses or nasal cavity may secondarily involve the orbit (Fig. 23-1C). In these cases, the bony walls of the orbit may have to be removed in addition to the orbital soft tissue. In addition, primary orbital cancers may involve the bony walls. For example, adenoid cystic carcinoma of the lacrimal gland tends to be associated with gross or microscopic involvement of the lateral wall and the orbital

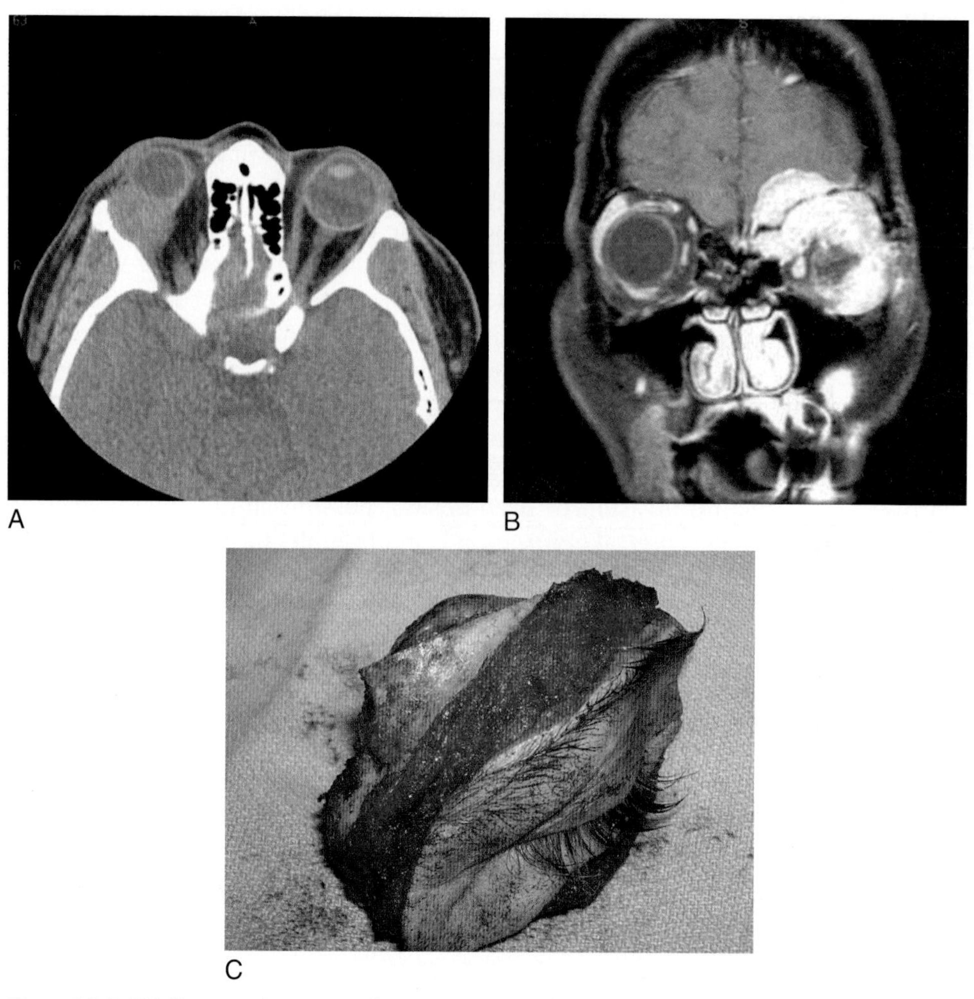

Figure 23-2 (A) Computed tomography in a patient with adenoid cystic carcinoma of the lacrimal gland with involvement of the lateral wall of the orbit. (B) Magnetic resonance imaging in another patient with adenoid cystic carcinoma of the lacrimal gland with extension into the intracranial cavity and erosion of the orbital roof. (C) Orbital exenteration specimen includes en bloc excision of the superolateral bony walls.

roof (Fig. 23-2). In such cases, a multidisciplinary surgical approach with planned removal of the involved bony walls may be required to achieve the best outcome.

23-3-4 *Other Modifications of the Standard Technique.* Depending on the extent of disease within the orbit, there are many modifications of the standard orbital exenteration technique that can be used. For example, in some cases only the anterior orbital soft tissue are resected; the posterior orbital soft tissues are left behind.[5] In contrast, for tumors that extend only to the posterior orbital soft tissues, eyelid- and conjunctiva-sparing procedures can be considered to improve overall cosmesis.[8]

An individualized approach to surgical removal of involved structures and selective sparing of structures that are unlikely to be involved can lead to enhanced cosmesis and less overall morbidity.[5,7] However, the desire to preserve tissues has to be weighed against the potentially increased risk of locoregional recurrence associated with tissue-sparing approaches for aggressive cancers of the orbit and periorbita.

23-4 RECONSTRUCTION OF THE ORBITAL CAVITY

The primary goal of reconstruction of the orbital cavity is to provide durable coverage of the orbit, and to protect the brain if there is a cranial defect. In many instances, the reconstructed orbital cavity has to withstand postoperative adjuvant radiation therapy as well as accommodate a prosthesis if the patient desires one. Numerous reconstructive methods that attempt to fulfill these goals have been described.[9–13]

Table 23-2 Method of Reconstruction after Orbital Exenteration for 79 Consecutive Patients Who Underwent Orbital Exenteration at M.D. Anderson Cancer Center Between 1999 and 2007

Procedure	OE	EOE	OM	Total (%)
Skin graft only				
Split-thickness skin graft	3	4	0	7 (8.9)
Full-thickness skin graft	9	2	0	11 (13.9)
Vascularized regional pedicled flap				
Temporoparietal fascia	0	2	0	2 (2.5)
Temporalis muscle	0	4	0	4 (5.0)
Microvascular free flap				
Radial forearm	2	2	0	4 (5.0)
Rectus abdominis muscle plus:				
Split-thickness skin graft	1	2	0	3 (3.8)
Rectus abdominis myocutaneous	4	14	2	20 (25.3)
Anterolateral thigh	5	18	5	28 (35.4)
Total	24	48	7	79 (100)

OE, orbital exenteration; EOE, extended orbital exenteration; OM, orbital exenteration with total maxillectomy (personal communication from Dr. Mattew Hanosono)[14]

A recent review of 79 consecutive patients who underwent orbital exenteration at The University of Texas M. D. Anderson Cancer Center identified a variety of reconstructive procedures used in cancer patients after orbital exenteration (Table 23-2).[14]

Reconstructive options depend on the extent of the orbital defect and whether the patient plans to use an orbital prosthesis postoperatively. Split- or full-thickness skin grafts are selected when an open (concave) cavity is desired to allow for future fitting of an orbital prosthesis (Fig. 23-3A), when there is no need to isolate the orbital cavity from the sinonasal, oral, or intracranial cavities, and when there is no anticipated need for postoperative radiation therapy.[14] Vascularized regional pedicled flaps (temporoparietal fascial flap or temporalis muscle flap) or microvascular free flaps are usually the most appropriate reconstructive choice when orbital exenteration is combined with removal of the orbital bony walls, when orbital exenteration is combined with removal of paranasal sinuses, when high-dose postoperative radiation therapy is planned, and when the patient has already undergone irradiation of

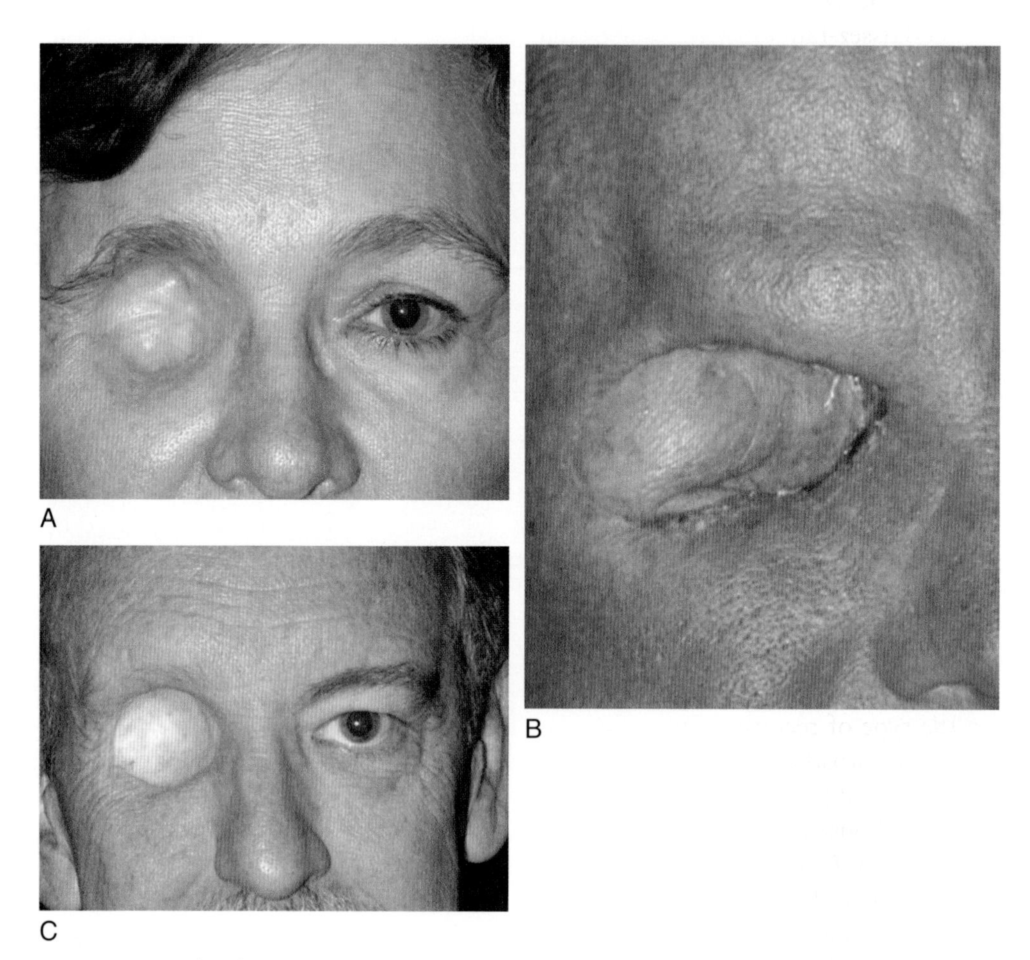

Figure 23-3 Orbital exenteration cavity lined with (A) a full-thickness skin graft, (B) a microvascular free flap, and (C) a temporoparietal fascia flap covered by a skin graft.

the orbital area. Preoperative or postoperative radiation therapy is a relative contraindication to skin-graft reconstruction because of the risk of poor engraftment or subsequent graft loss in patients who have undergone or will undergo irradiation of the orbit; vascularized flaps are preferred in this situation. Vascularized regional flaps or microvascular flaps also decrease the likelihood of osteoradionecrosis after radiation therapy. However, the use of microvascular free flaps for reconstruction of the orbital cavity after exenteration is associated with a lower success rate for orbital prosthesis wear compared to success rates with full-thickness or split-thickness skin grafts or regional flaps (Fig. 23-3B). Other disadvantages of microvascular free flaps include the longer length of surgery, the need for hospital admission and intensive care monitoring, and associated donor-site morbidities. Another relative disadvantage may be the inability to fully inspect the orbital cavity after reconstruction with complex bulky flaps. An immediate postoperative baseline imaging study may facilitate monitoring of the orbital area for cancer recurrence. Vascularized regional flaps such as temporalis muscle or fascia flaps are compatible with good prosthesis fit (Fig. 23-3C) but are associated with the minor disadvantage of donor-site bony depression in the temple.

The laissez-faire method of allowing granulation of the orbital cavity with no reconstruction has been advocated in some situations, especially when there is concern about early recurrence. In these cases, the orbital cavity is allowed to heal by secondary intention. During healing, which usually takes at least 8 to 12 weeks, daily wound care consisting of irrigation with 2% hydrogen peroxide and wet-to-dry dressings is critical.

23-5 POSTOPERATIVE COMPLICATIONS

The most common postoperative complications of orbital exenteration are skin graft failure or partial slough, infections of the orbital cavity or donor site, sino-orbital fistula, donor site morbidities, and inability of the reconstructed orbit.[7,15,16]

Monocular precautions should be stressed in patients after orbital exenteration; protection of the remaining eye is a top priority.

23-6 ORBITAL PROSTHESIS

Rehabilitation of the orbital cavity after reconstruction is an important step. As mentioned in Section 23-4, the success of orbital prosthesis fitting heavily depends on the type of reconstruction chosen for the orbital cavity. Another factor in the success of prosthesis fit and wear is patient motivation. If a patient intends not to use an orbital prosthesis, an eye patch can be used to cover the orbital defect. Some patients choose to wear only a patch because of the simplicity of use and care and the low cost. Oculofacial prostheses, custom-made of polymethylmethacrylate, are more aesthetically pleasing and can produce considerable facial symmetry (Fig. 23-4). Osteo-integrated oculofacial prostheses can be secured to previously implanted magnetic anchors for better stability and eliminate the need for gluing of the prosthesis to surrounding skin.[17–19]

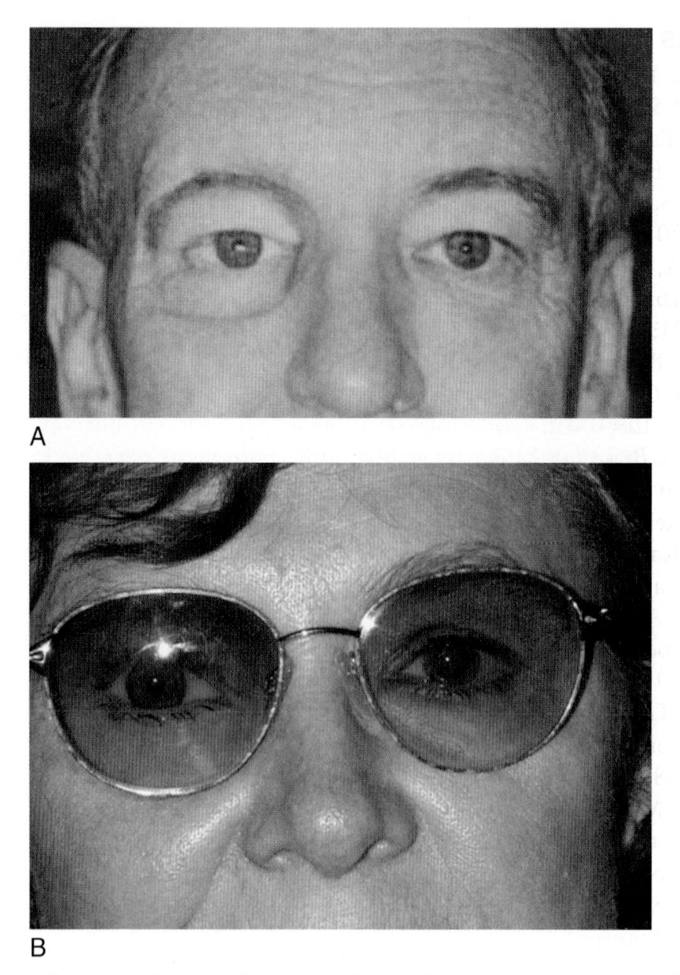

Figure 23-4 (A) Orbital prosthesis in the patient depicted in Figure 23-3C. (B) Orbital prosthesis and glasses in the patient depicted in Figure 23-3A.

23-7 PSYCHOSOCIAL CONSIDERATIONS AFTER ORBITAL EXENTERATION

A recent study suggests that patients who undergo orbital exenteration experience social and psychological problems because of their facial disfigurement.[20] Patients and their family members should be warned about the occurrence of possible difficulties when interacting in large and small groups alike. In this study that was based on in-depth interviews with patients and family members of patients with cancer who had an orbital exenteration, the investigators found that, in particular, spouses should be the subjects of counseling programs. Additionally, it was suggested in this study that interacting groups with the patient should be sensitized about the patterns of stigmatization toward the patients after orbital exenteration identified in this study. The study suggested that additional educational programs for physicians and other health care providers may help alleviate this problem at various levels.

REFERENCES

1. Levin PS, Dutton JJ. A 20-year series of orbital exenteration. *Am J Ophthalmol.* 1991;112(5):496–501.
2. Mohr C, Esser J. Orbital exenteration: surgical and reconstructive strategies. *Graefe's Arch Clin Exp Ophthalmol.* 1997:235:288–295.
3. Nassab RS, Thomas SS, Murray D. Orbital exenteration for advanced periorbital skin cancers: 20 years' experience. *J Plast Reconstr Aesthet Surg.* 2007, April 12 (Epub).
4. Shields JA, Shields CL, Demirci H, Honavar SG, Singh AD. Experience with eyelid-sparing orbital exenteration: the 2001 Tullos L. Coston Lecture. *Ophthal Plast Reconstr Surg.* 2001;17(5):355–361.
5. Goldberg RA, Kim JW, Shorr N. Orbital exenteration: results of an individualized approach. *Ophthal Plast Reconstr Surg.* 2003;19(3):229–236.
6. Rahman I, Cook AE, Leatherbarrow B. Orbital exenteration: a 13-year Manchester experience. *Br J Ophthalmol.* 2005;89(10):1335–1340.
7. Ben Simon GJ, Schwarcz RM, Douglas R, Fiaschetti D, McCann JD, Goldberg RA. Orbital exenteration: one size does not fit all. *Am J Ophthalmol.* 2005;139(1):11–17.
8. Looi A, Kazim M, Cortes M, Rootman J. Orbital reconstruction after eyelid- and conjunctiva-sparing orbital exenteration. *Ophthal Plast Recontr Surg.* 2006;22(1):1–6.
9. Atabay K, Atabay C, Yavuzer R, Kermikan F, Latifoglu O. One-stage reconstruction of the eye socket and eyelids in orbital exenteration patients. *Plast Reconstr Surg.* 1998;101:1463–1470.
10. Menon NG, Girotto JA, Goldberg NH, Silverman RP. Orbital reconstruction after exenteration: use of a transorbital temporal muscle flap. *Ann Plast Surg.* 2003;50:38–42.
11. Pryor SG, Moore EJ, Kasperbauer JL. Orbital exenteration reconstruction with rectus abdominis microvascular free flap. *Laryngoscope.* 2005;115:1912–1916.
12. Reese A. Exenteration of the orbit with transplantation of the temporalis muscle. *Am J Ophthalmol.* 1958;45:386–390.
13. Taylan G, Yildirim S, Akoz T. Reconstruction of large orbital exenteration defects after resection of periorbital tumors of advanced stage. *J Reconstr Microsurg.* 2006;22: 583–589.
14. Hanasono MM, Lee J, Yang J, Skoracki RJ, Reece GP, Esmaeli B. An algorithmic approach to reconstructive surgery and prosthetic rehabilitation after orbital exenteration. *Plast Reconstr Surg.* 2009;123(1):98–1105.
15. Limawararut V, Leibovitch I, Davis G, Rees G, Goldberg RA, Selva D. Sino-orbital fistula: a complication of exenteration. *Ophthalmology.* 2007;114(2):355–361.
16. Taylor A, Roberts F, Kemp EG. Orbital exenterations: a retrospective study over an 11-year period analyzing all cases from a single unit. *Orbit.* 2006;25(3):185–193.
17. Nerad JA, Carter KD, LaVelle WE, Fyler A, Branemark PI. The osseointegration techniques for the rehabilitation of the exenterated orbit. *Arch Ophthalmol.* 1991;109(7):1032–1038.
18. Moran WJ, Toljanic JA, Panje WR. Implant-retained prosthetic rehabilitation of orbital defects. *Arch Otolaryngol Head Neck Surg.* 1996;122(1):46–50.
19. Schoen PJ, Raghoebar GM, van Oort RP, et al. Treatment outcome of bone-anchored craniofacial prostheses after tumor surgery. *Cancer.* 2001;92:3045–3050.
20. Bonanno A, Esmaeli B, Fingeret MC, Nelson D, Weber R. Social Challenges of Cancer Patients with Orbitofacial Disfigurement. Ophthalmic Plastic Reconstructive Surgery 26(1):18–22, 2010.

24

Complications of the Anophthalmic Socket

JOHN D. McCANN MD, PHD, AND CHUN CHENG LIN YANG MD, MSC

The anophthalmic socket is subject to four major deformities: enophthalmos, exposure, eyelid malposition, and socket contraction. Enophthalmos occurs when there is a lack of soft tissue volume, creating a sunken or hollow appearance. Exposure occurs when a previously placed orbital implant erodes through the ocular surface. Eyelid malposition occurs largely as a consequence of wearing of a prosthesis. Socket contraction occurs when there is insufficient ocular surface area and fornix depth to accommodate a mobile prosthesis. Understanding these disfigurements and their treatments is the goal of this chapter.

24-1 ENOPHTHALMOS

Anopththalmic enophthalmos is an acquired condition that occurs when there is a lack of orbit volume after removal of the eye. In a typical case 6 mL of volume is lost with removal of the eye. An orbital implant will replace 2 to 4 mL of volume, and a prosthesis will replace 1 to 2 mL of volume. This leaves a volume deficit of 1 to 3 mL. This typical volume deficit can be exacerbated by fat and muscle atrophy secondary to surgery or antecedent trauma. In cases of eyes removed secondary to orbital trauma, unrepaired orbital fractures expand the bony orbit, further exacerbating the lack of orbital soft tissue.

After removal of the eye the orbital implant and the inadequate volume of orbital soft tissue tend to settle toward the orbital floor, creating more of a volume deficit in the superior orbit. The orbital fat is somewhat liquid and much of the preaponeurotic fat in the upper eyelid flows posterior and inferior, creating the hollow appearance in the superior fornix of the anophthalmic socket. This deformity is referred to as the

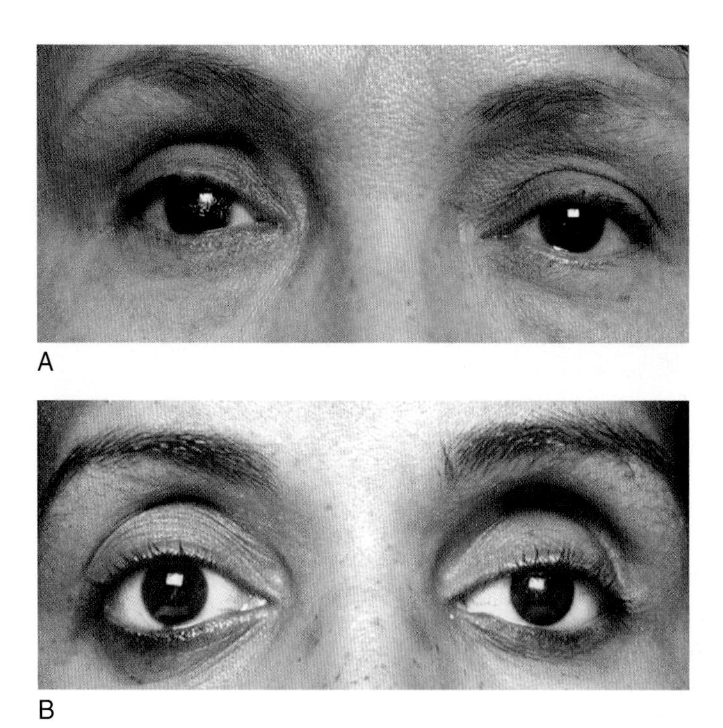

Figure 24-1 Superior sulcus defect. (A) Patient with superior sulcus defect on OD, 36 months after evisceration. (B) Patient with pronounced superior sulcus defect on OS, 18 months after evisceration.

superior sulcus deformity (Fig. 24-1) and is present in some degree in the majority of anophthalmic sockets.

24-1-1 *Diagnosis*. History-taking should direct the ophthalmologist toward the cause of the patient's anophthalmos. If the eye was lost to trauma, the possibility of orbital fractures expanding the orbital volume and exacerbating the condition should be considered. If the socket was radiated, the possibility of radiation-induced orbital soft tissue atrophy should be considered. It is useful to review the operative note to determine the size of implant that was placed. Placement of an implant of less than 18 mm will nearly always result in enophthalmos. It is important to elicit the volume, frequency, color, and odor of socket discharge.

The ophthalmologist often recognizes enophthalmos by observing the patient from below, and en face, comparing the prosthesis with the fellow globe. If the lateral orbital rims are normal, the examiner can use a Hertel-type exophthalmometer. If the rims are not normal, a Naugle exophthalmometer can be used to quantitate the disparity in anterior projection between the globe and the prosthesis. In the ideal situation, the vertex of the prosthesis will sit 1 to 2 mm posterior to the vertex of the fellow cornea. It is not desirable to have the prosthesis project anterior to the cornea or to sit more than 2 mm posterior to the cornea, as this draws attention to the anophthalmic socket. Note the conformation of the tissue in the superior fornix.

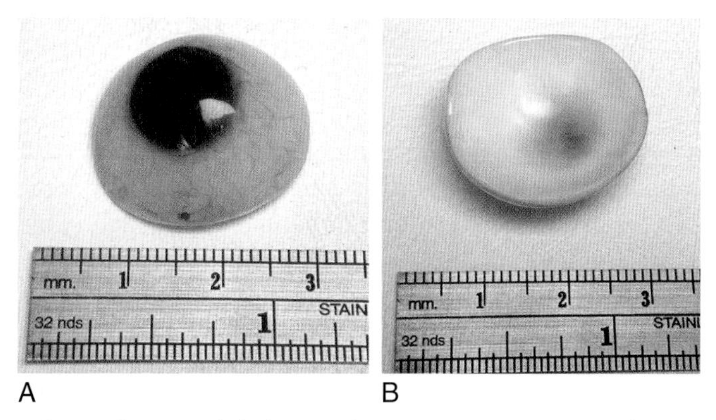

Figure 24-2 Prosthesis of an anophthalmic socket. (A) Anterior view and (B) posterior view of the prosthesis.

A sulcus that is sunken relative to the fellow eye is evidence of a lack of orbital volume. The location of the implant within the socket also should be noted. Sometimes implants will migrate out of the muscle cone, which causes volume problems and great difficulty in fitting a prosthesis. The examiner must also identify bony abnormalities of the orbit or facial bones and inferior globe or prosthesis displacement (hypo-ophthalmos).

Much can be gained by removing the prosthesis and examining it (Fig. 24-2). A thick prosthesis is evidence of the ocularist attempting to make up for lack of orbital volume by increasing prosthesis volume. Unfortunately, a thick prosthesis has greater inertia, so it is not as mobile as a thin prosthesis. A large prosthesis also weights down the lower eyelid, resulting in more frequent ectropion of the lower eyelids. Finally, a large prosthesis may cause more friction between the conjunctiva and prosthesis, causing chronic conjunctivitis and socket discharge.

Anytime a patient complains of chronic discharge from the socket, the prosthesis should be removed and the socket carefully examined for evidence of implant exposure. If there is mucus in the socket at the time of examination, the socket should be irrigated clean, as the mucus will often cover over areas of implant exposure. If only one region of the socket is inflamed, the examiner should suspect an abnormal interaction of the prosthesis with the socket.

24-1-2 *Treatment*. Treatment of anophthalmic enophthalmos may be surgical or nonsurgical. Nonsurgical management includes revision of the prosthetic eye in an anophthalmic patient or the placement of a cosmetic shell overlying a small or phthisic eye to add volume and improve appearance. Ocular prostheses can be designed with a superior shelf-like edge; these can restore some superior volume and lift the upper eyelid outward and upward, which helps camouflage the superior sulcus deformity. Trying to correct a significant lack of orbital volume by fitting a large thick prosthesis often fails for the reasons mentioned previously. Magnifying lenses before a nonfunctioning eye or a prosthesis may make a narrow palpebral fissure look larger. Minifying or astigmatic lenses, as well as prisms, may also be useful.

24-1-3 *Surgical Correction of Anophthalmic Enophthalmos.* The goal of surgery to correct the anophthalmic enophthalmos is to restore orbital volume so that when a patient wears a prosthesis, the volume appears the same as the fellow orbit. It is important that any surgery performed to augment socket volume is done in a fashion that maintains adequate implant motility and fornix depth to facilitate a mobile prosthesis. In adding volume to the anophthalmic socket, the surgeon has many options, including implant exchange, placement of an extraconal implant, and injection of alloplastic materials to augment volume.

24-1-3-1 *Implant Exchange.* A common cause of anophthalmic enophthalmos is placement of a small prosthesis. In addition, migration of an orbital implant out of the muscle cone is a common cause of a poorly fitting prosthesis. Both of these problems can be remedied by removal of the existing implant and placement of an implant of adequate volume in the muscle cone. Prior to deciding on surgery, it is useful to review the operative report and determine what type of implant material was used in the prior procedure. Porous implants develop tissue ingrowth, which makes removal substantially more difficult. There are many options for augmenting orbital volume in the anophthalmic socket, so implant exchange should be moved down on the list of possibilities if a porous implant is in place. Most often it is nonporous implants that migrate out of the muscle cone as these are not held in place by tissue ingrowth.

When performing implant exchange, the surgeon should use the same conjunctival incision used to place the initial implant. The implant should be dissected out of the encasing tissue with minimal trauma to adjacent tissue. Given that nonporous implants are more likely to migrate out of the muscle cone, it is reasonable to place a porous implant when correcting this problem. Picking implant size is important. We agree with Kaltreider et al. that the implant should have a diameter 2 to 3 mm less than the axial length of the fellow eye. Often there is not enough conjunctiva and Tenon's capsule to facilitate an implant of this volume without collapsing the conjunctival fornices. In these cases placement of a dermal graft can expand the ocular surface area and facilitate an implant of adequate volume, as explained later in this chapter.

24-1-3-2 *Placement of an Extraconal Implant.* Lack of orbital volume is nearly always most evident when looking at the hollow superior sulcus defect. Adding volume in the form of an extraconal implant placed along the posterior orbital floor or posterior lateral orbital wall can assist in shifting the implant anterior and shifting fat into the superior sulcus defect. There are many options for alloplastic implants to be placed in these areas.

Alloplastic materials are artificial implants used in the orbit to replace volume loss or bony defects by providing framework. These materials have qualities such as availability, biocompatibility, and lack of immunogenic activity. The most commonly used alloplastic materials for orbital repair are cyanoacrylate, nylon mesh or sheets (Supramid), solid silicone, curable methylmethacrylate (Cranioplastic), calcium phosphate derivatives, polymethylmethacrylate (PMMA), polytetrafluoroethylene

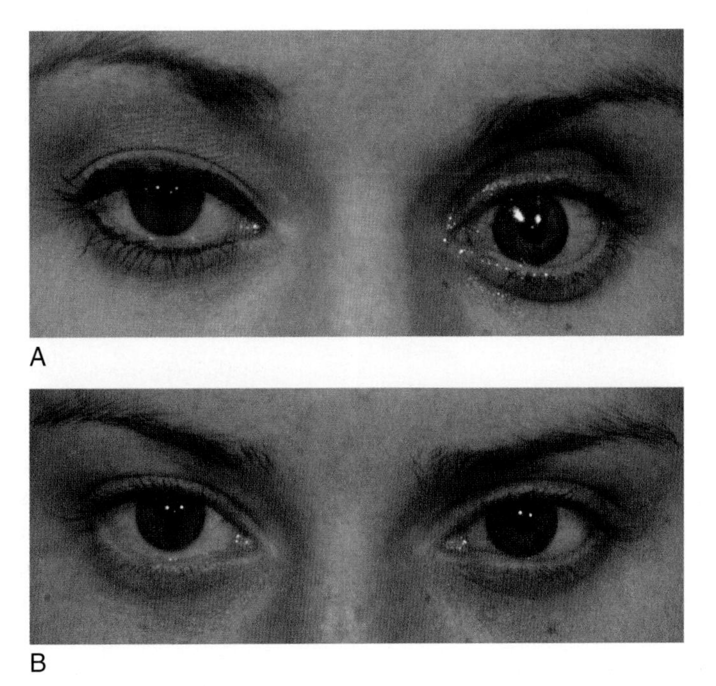

Figure 24-3 Pre- and postoperative clinical appearance of anophthalmic enophthalmos treated with Medpor floor implant. (A) Anophthalmic patient demonstrating superior sulcus deformity OS. (B) One month after Medpor floor implant, patient shows improvement of superior sulcus deformity and enophthalmos.

(PTFE or Teflon), porous or expanded polytetrafluoroethylene (ePTFE or Gore-Tex), particulate hydroxyapatite (HA), and porous polyethylene (Medpor).

We have greatest experience using polyethylene (Medpor), which is available in blocks that can be cut to need, or preshaped enophthalmos wedges. We typically approach the orbital floor via a swinging eyelid incision. A disadvantage of this approach is that it requires a conjunctival incision. If shortening of the fornix is present, this can be deleterious. Typically, in these cases, we approach the subperiosteal space of the lateral orbital wall via an upper eyelid crease incision, which has the advantage of granting surgical access without violating the conjunctiva, not risking further shortening the fornix (Fig. 24-3).

24-1-3-3 *Injection of Alloplastic Material to Augment Volume.* Many patients who have undergone either enucleation or evisceration have a mild to moderate volume loss that is bothersome. In the past this was often not addressed because it requires orbitotomy. In this group of patients volume can be augmented using an office-based procedure performed with local anesthesia.

The senior author's initial attempt to improve volume deficit in enophthalmos using an office-based procedure was the use of hydrogel pellets, self-expanding and hydrophilic osmotic expanders. The use of hydrogel orbital expanders started in Europe during the late 1990s. Recently these have been introduced and marketed in the United States (Osmed GmbH, Illmenau, Germany, distributed in the United

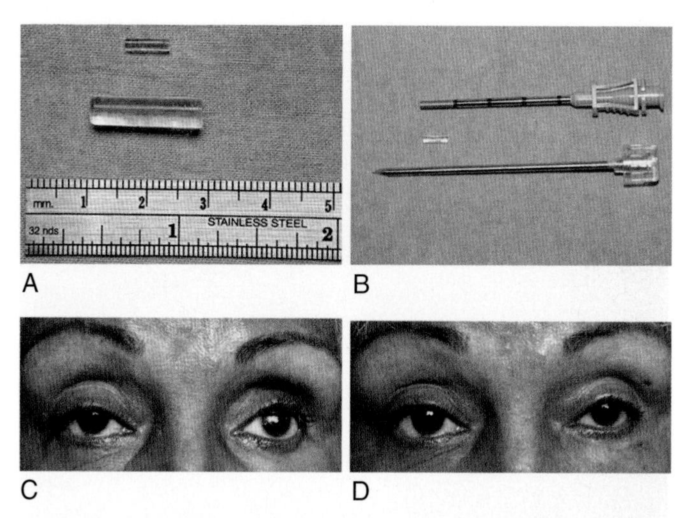

Figure 24-4 Hydrogel pellets and pre- and postoperative clinical appearance of anophthalmic orbit treated with hydrogel pellets. (A) Expander hydrogel pellets before (*above*) and after (*below*) in vitro swelling in 0.9% sodium chloride. (B) Hydrogel pellet injector with the guidance trocar for transcutaneous injection. (C) A patient with anophthalmic enophthalmos demonstrating superior sulcus deformity OS. (D) Patient underwent placement of hydrogel pellets to the left orbit, showing improved enophthalmos and correction of superior sulcus deformity.

States by IOP, Inc., Costa Mesa, CA). The pellet expander is made of a highly hydrophilic hydrogel consisting of N-vinyl pyrrolidone and methylmethacrylate. These augment in size by osmotic hydration. In the dry state the pellet expander is 8 mm in length and 2 mm in diameter, with a volume of 0.025 mL. The swelling capacity of the pellet is approximately eightfold (Fig. 24-4). The pellets can be injected via a cutaneous approach using a transcutaneous 13-gauge trocar directed into the extraconal space. Li et al. reported at the 2003 ASOPRS meeting positive experiences using this method for orbital volume augmentation. It is important to place the implants in the mid-orbit, as placing them too anterior can lead to extrusion, and placing them too posterior can elicit orbital pain and nausea lasting 2 to 5 days.

The newest concept in addressing anophthalmic enophthalmos is a minimally invasive technique to restore orbital volume that has proven to be effective in the senior author's experience. This innovative technique consist of injecting an FDA-approved dermal filler, Radiesse® (Bioform Medical, Inc., San Mateo, CA), into the medial, inferior, and lateral extraconal orbital space to help restore volume. The material is injected at about the equator of the implant. Radiesse is made of 30% HA microspheres (25 to 45 μm) in a carrying vehicle (1.3% sodium carboxymethylcellulose, 6.4% glycerin, and 36.6% sterile water for injection) (Fig. 24-5).

We obtained encouraging enophthalmos correction of 3 mm for every 1.3 mL of Radiesse application, with no major complications (Fig. 24-6); however, it is uncertain how frequently patients will require reinjection. In addition to the minimally invasive nature, this procedure offers another advantage of not violating the conjunctiva. In our experience these noninvasive treatments to expand orbital volume fail if there is significant shortening of the fornices, or if the implant is scarred or fibrosed into the posterior socket.

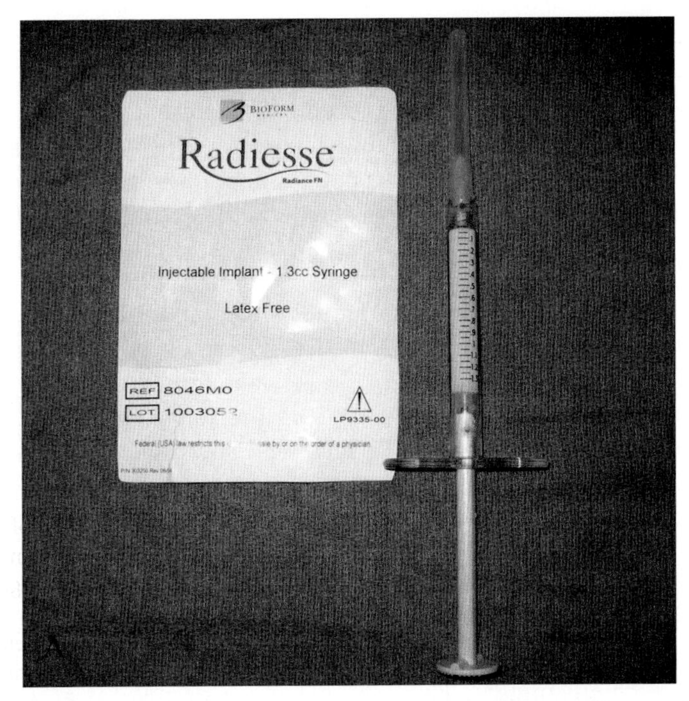

Figure 24-5 Injectable calcium hydroxyapatite FDA-approved dermal filler, Radiesse (Bioform Medical, Inc., San Mateo, CA). Radiesse is made of 30% hydroxyapatite microspheres (25 to 45 μm) in a carrying vehicle (1.3% sodium carboxymethylcellulose, 6.4% glycerin, and 36.6% sterile water for injection).

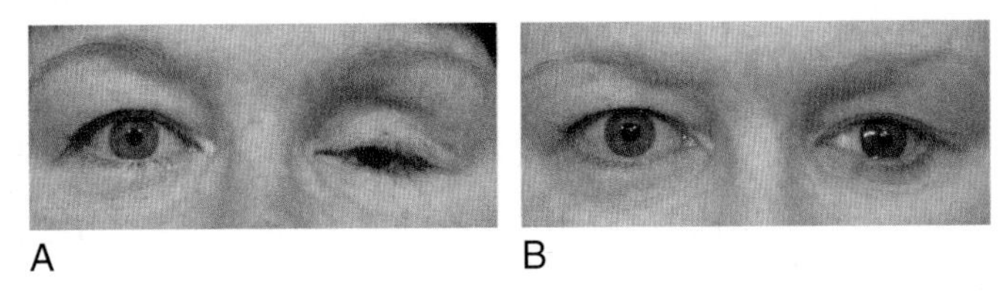

Figure 24-6 Pre- and postoperative clinical appearance of anophthalmic orbit. (A) A 51-year-old woman preoperatively demonstrated 7 mm of anophthalmic enophthalmos, blepharoptosis, and superior sulcus deformity OS. (B) Patient received 2 vials (2.6 mL) of injectable calcium hydroxyapatite with correction of 5 mm of enophthalmos that has persisted at 71 weeks, without surgical correction of ptosis.

24-2 EXPOSURE

Exposure of orbital implants occurs in roughly 10% of patients after enucleation and 5% of patients after evisceration. Sometimes exposure occurs as a postoperative complication. If the exposure is discovered early and the patient has been covered with topical antibiotics, the implant can often be spared. In our experience, attempting to undermine the conjunctiva and close the defect almost never resolves the problem. In cases of early postoperative exposure, we undermine the defect and place an autologous graft of dermis beneath the defect.

24-2-1 *Diagnosis.* More commonly patients present years after placement of an implant with complaints of mucopurulent discharge from the socket. After irrigating the discharge out of the socket, the exposed implant usually is visible. In most of these late cases the implant is colonized with bacteria. The surgeon may attempt to patch the defect with dermis. If the graft sloughs or pyogenic granulomas repeatedly grow where the graft was placed, this is evidence of an implant that is colonized with bacteria.

24-2-2 *Treatment.* In our experience systemic or topical antibiotics cannot sterilize a colonized implant; it must be partly or totally removed. In the case of plastic implants, we remove the entire implant. In the case of a HA implant, the anterior quarter of the implant and the avascular core are removed until bleeding tissue within the implant is encountered. We have had success in leaving this vascular portion of HA implants in place.

We often do not place an alloplastic implant back in the socket at the time of removal of the infected implant because the risk of the new implant becoming infected is felt to be too high. One option is to leave the patient without an implant and let the socket heal prior to returning to the operating room for placement of a secondary implant. Another option is to place a dermis–fat graft. This procedure offers a couple of advantages. First, the placing a dermis–fat graft can prevent socket contraction, which may occur if the socket is left to heal without an implant. Second, the dermis–fat graft can expand the ocular surface area if chronic conjunctivitis has already led to some shrinkage. Disadvantages of a dermis fat–graft include unpredictable absorption of fat, leading to a potential volume deficit and greater difficulty in fitting a prosthesis.

24-2-3 *Dermis–Fat Graft Procedure.* The graft may be harvested from the left lower quadrant of the abdomen or the buttocks. We drape the dermis donor area with a transparent adhesive drape. An ellipse of dermis measuring about 3 by 1.5 cm is harvested. The drape, epidermis, and dermis are incised with a #15 blade. The epidermis is sharply dissected away from the dermis. We have found that leaving the adhesive drape attached to the epidermis facilitates this dissection (Fig. 24-7).

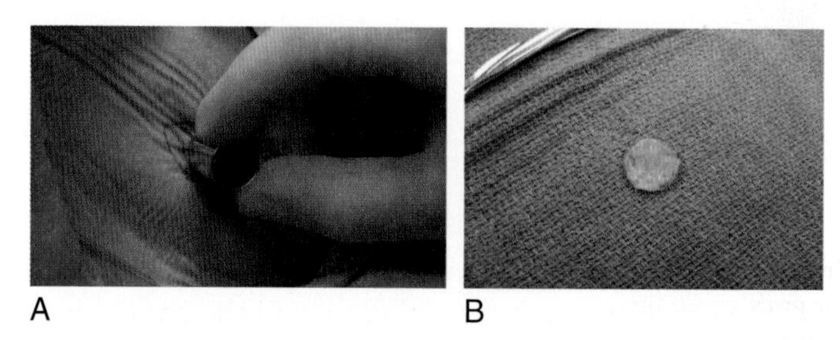

Figure 24-7 Dermis–fat graft procedure. (A) Harvesting of dermis–fat graft. Transparent adhesive drape over an ellipse on the dermis donor area. The drape, epidermis, and dermis are incised using a 14-mm corneal trephine (Katena, Denville, NJ). (B) Dermis graft with the epidermis and subcutaneous fat trimmed from the dermis.

The dermis and subcutaneous fat is then excised with scissors. The abdomen or buttocks is closed in three layers. The socket is overfilled with fat, as loss of at least one fourth of the fat grafted is anticipated. We have never encountered a case of overcorrection of volume by placing a dermis–fat graft in an adult. Tenon's capsule is sutured to the edge of the dermis ellipse with 4-0 chromic gut suture. No attempt

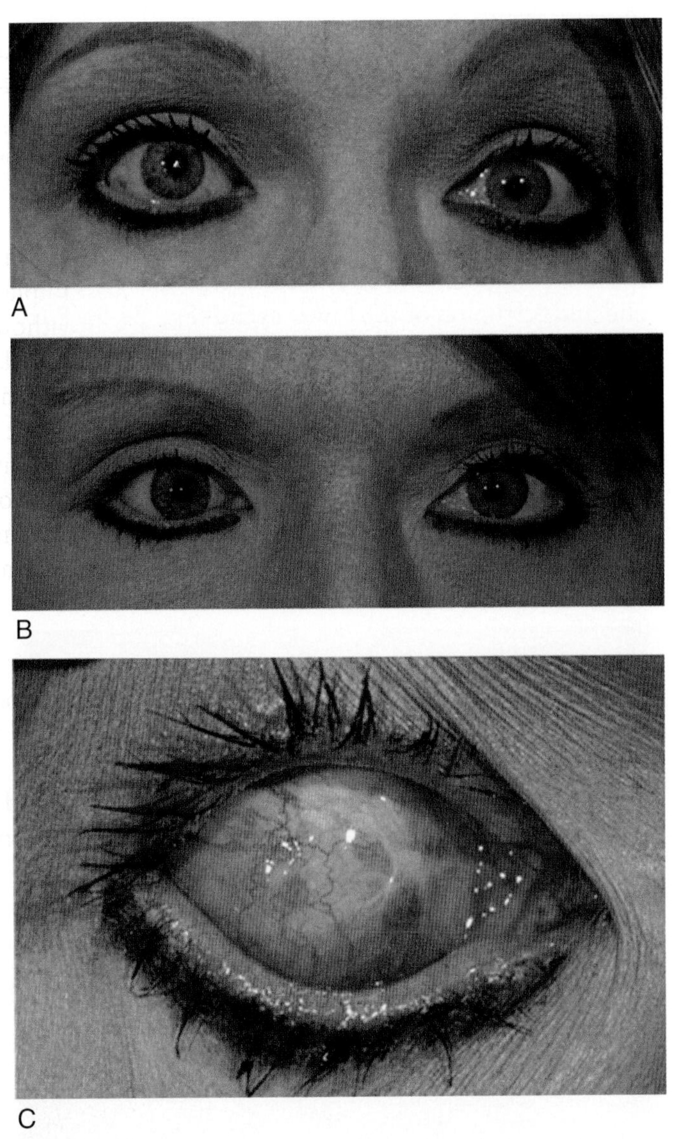

Figure 24-8 Pre- and postoperative clinical appearance of anophthalmic enophthalmos treated with dermis–fat graft procedure. (A) Patient with a scleral shell over a nonfunctional phthisical eye, showing poor lower eyelid position and instability due to excessive weight and size of the scleral shell on OD. (B) Fifteen months after dermis–fat graft procedure, patient shows good contour of eyelid position and fitting of the prosthesis in OD. (C) Aspect of anophthalmic socket after dermis–fat graft procedure, showing good vascularization of the conjunctiva over the dermis graft and good surface area in the socket for prosthesis fitting.

is made to primarily close the conjunctival edges, as this would not facilitate placement of large enough dermis–fat graft. The conjunctiva is sutured to the anterior surface of the dermis graft with 6-0 chromic suture. At the end of surgery, a conformer is placed, and the wound is dressed with an occlusive dressing.

Four to 6 days after surgery, the dressing and the conformer are removed. Both the conformer and topical corticosteroids slow vascularization and conjunctival overgrowth of the dermis. Therefore, the conformer is typically left out for 2 to 3 weeks while the graft begins to vascularize, and topical medications containing corticosteroids are avoided until the dermis graft is completely covered with conjunctiva. In most cases the dermis graft will be vascularized, covered with conjunctiva, and awaiting fitting of a new prosthesis by 10 weeks after surgery (Fig. 24-8).

24-3 EYELID MALPOSITION

Eyelid malposition in the anophthalmic socket consists primarily of ptosis or entropion of the upper eyelid and ectropion of the lower eyelid (Fig. 24-9). Ptosis of the upper eyelid is typically caused by stretching or disinsertion of the levator aponeurosis. It can also be caused by a lack of orbital volume to support the superior rectus levator complex. If the patient has a deep superior sulcus, the lack of orbital volume should be addressed prior to correcting the ptosis. Ptosis surgery is typically done via an anterior approach to avoid unnecessary incision of the conjunctiva. Entropion of the upper eyelid is typically caused by overly aggressive use of a ptosis ledge on the

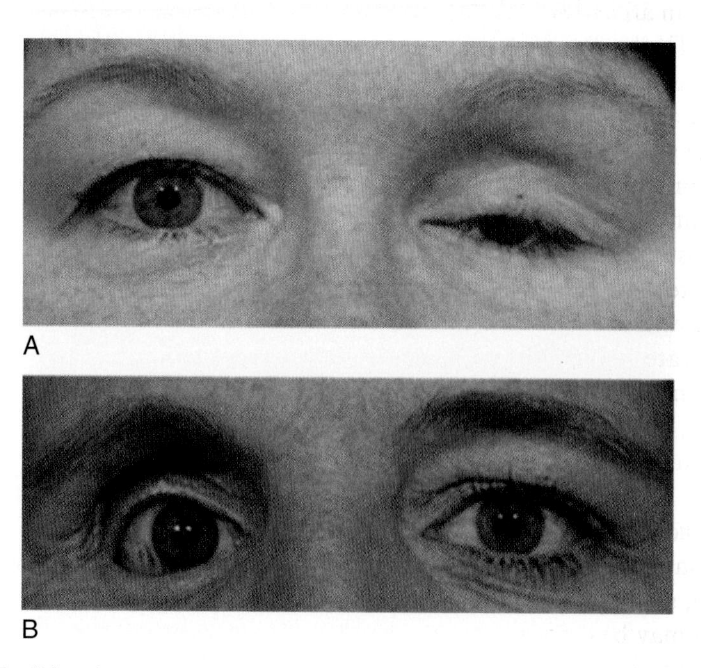

Figure 24-9 Eyelid malposition in an anophthalmic patient. (A) Patient with blepharoptosis in the left anophthalmic socket. (B) Patient with lower eyelid entropion in the right anophthalmic socket.

prosthesis or contraction of the socket. Surgical correction of the ptosis, combined with reducing the size of the ptosis ledge on the prosthesis, often resolves the former problem. Correction of socket contraction is addressed later in this chapter. Ectropion of the lower eyelid is typically caused by the weight of the prosthesis stretching out the lower lid. This can be resolved with a procedure that horizontally shortens the lower eyelid, such as a lateral tarsal strip.

24-4 SOCKET CONTRACTURE

A contracted anophthalmic socket does not have enough ocular surface area for maintenance of the conjunctival fornices. Mild shortening of the conjunctival fornices contributes to poor prosthesis mobility and comfort. Severe shortening of the conjunctival fornices results in the inability to maintain a prosthesis. This condition may occur immediately or years after removal of the eye. The pathogenesis of socket contracture is incompletely understood and varied. The primary factors that predispose a socket to contracture are poor vascularization of the ocular surface, scarring of the ocular surface, iatrogenic removal or shrinkage of the ocular surface, and placement of an implant too large to be covered with available ocular surface.

Clinical presentations associated with poor vascularization include prior radiation or chemical burn of the socket. Trauma, cicatrizing conjunctival disease, and chronic conjunctivitis are clinical entities associated with scarring of the conjunctiva. Chronic conjunctivitis from an exposed implant or poorly fitting prosthesis should be treated before it leads to contracture of the socket. When an eye is enucleated or eviscerated, an area of ocular surface equal to or greater than the area of the cornea is removed. The loss of the corneoscleral cap decreases the amount of ocular surface area. Many eyes undergo multiple intraocular surgeries prior to removal. In each surgery that a conjunctival incision is made, there is some shrinkage of the ocular surface. The size of the orbital implant that can be placed is nearly always limited by the amount of conjunctiva and Tenon's capsule available to cover the implant. If an implant with greater size than can be covered by available conjunctiva and Tenon's capsule is placed, wound closure under tension results. Consequently, this contributes to both implant exposure and shortening of the conjunctival fornices and socket contraction.

We advocate reducing the chance of socket contraction by primarily placing a circular dermis graft, autograft or allograft (Dermamatrix Acellular Dermis®, Synthes Inc., West Chester, PA) at the time of all enucleations and eviscerations to replace the surface area lost in the corneoscleral cap.

24-4-1 *Diagnosis.* In overt cases of socket contraction there is loss of the inferior or superior conjunctival fornix, or both. Depending on the mechanism of socket contraction, symblepharon or adhesions of the eyelids to the conjunctiva covering the implant may be evident. The conjunctiva may appear noninflamed due to poor blood supply. Subconjunctival fibrosis may be evident in cases of cicatricial conjunctivitis. Discharge and papillary reaction indicate chronic conjunctivitis. It is also useful to look at the prosthesis. The patient may not be wearing it because it does not fit. There may be a very small white area of the prosthesis as the ocularist might have made adjustments for collapse of the fornices.

24-4-2 *Treatment.* The goal of treating a contracted socket is to expand the fornices to allow the patient to wear an ocular prosthesis. Medical treatment has the greatest role in treating cases of chronic conjunctivitis. This often responds to a course of topical antibiotic steroid drops and a consult with the ocularist to improve fitting of the prosthesis. Polishing of the prosthesis once or twice yearly will maintain a smooth surface, and this limits giant papillary conjunctivitis and inflammation. A socket conformer, however small, should be placed if possible when the patient's prosthesis is lost or falls out of the socket. This can assist in preventing worsening of the situation while other treatments are used.

24-4-3 *Surgery.* If there is evidence of exposure of the implant leading to chronic conjunctivitis, then the implant will need to be removed as previously described. Mild contraction may be treated with fornix reconstruction, while more severe contraction requires grafting of tissue. Surgery should be restricted to noninflamed and noninfected sockets. Because scarring can normally progress over 6 months after trauma, whether accidental or surgical, the surgeon should wait at least that long after the previous event before deciding to intervene surgically.

Rebuilding the superior or inferior fornix in cases of mild contraction may simply involve placing sutures to deepen the fornix. This technique works well if there is no symblepharon, and the fornix is present but shallow. The surgeon may place three or four double-armed 4-0 chromic sutures, full-thickness through the eyelid from the conjunctival fornix exiting the skin. These sutures create an adhesion to maintain the fornix. This deepening may be modified by passing the sutures through the dense fibrous tissue of the arcus marginalis. A conformer should be placed immediately to keep the conjunctiva on stretch. A temporary tarsorrhaphy can assist in maintaining the conformer.

In more severe cases of contracture, it is necessary to expand the ocular surface by placing free grafts. Grafts take better in the region of the bulbar conjunctiva than in the fornices. Different tissues have been used for grafting over the implant, including sclera, buccal mucosa, and palatal grafts. We have found that an autograft of dermis works best.

In moderate to severe cases of socket contraction, a transverse incision is made across the middle of the socket. The incision is then undermined toward the superior and inferior fornix to free the conjunctiva from underlying scar tissue. A free graft is then placed over the top of the implant. Double-armed 4-0 chromic gut sutures are then attached from the free edge of the undermined conjunctiva to the free edge of the graft and then placed in full thickness through the eyelid. These sutures anchor the conjunctiva and the graft into the superior and inferior fornices. A large conformer and temporary tarsorrhaphy are then placed at the end of the procedure. Steroid-containing topical medications are avoided to facilitate vascularization of the graft. In some cases temporary removal of the conformer will also encourage vascularization of the dermis graft. A new prosthesis can typically be fitted 10 weeks after the procedure.

24-4-4 *Postoperative Complications*. Grafts may fail to take, or they may initially appear to take only to contract. Cases of poor vascular supply caused by prior radiation or chemical burn are the most difficult to correct. The surgeon should recognize that reoperation will not benefit certain patients with contracted sockets that have failed multiple prior attempts at reconstruction. Such patients should be referred to an ocularist who specializes in orbitofacial prostheses. A facial prosthesis, placed behind a spectacle lens, can be a cosmetic improvement over a patch for the patient who is not a surgical candidate.

SUGGESTED READINGS

Amato MM, Blaydon SM, Scribbick FW. Use of Bioglass for orbital volume augmentation in enophthalmos: a rabbit model (Oryctolagus Cuniculus). *Ophthal Plast Reconstr Surg*. 2003;19:455–465.

Bacskulin A, Vogel M, Wiese KG, et al. New osmotically active hydrogel expander for enlargement of the contracted anophthalmic socket. *Graefes Arch Clin Exp Ophthalmol*. 2000;238:24–27.

Blaydon SM, Shepler TR, Neuhaus RW, et al. The porous polyethylene (Medpor) spherical orbital implant: a retrospective study of 136 cases. *Ophthal Plast Reconstr Surg*. 2003;19:364–371.

Chen D, Heher K. Management of the anophthalmic socket in pediatric patients. *Curr Opin Ophthalmol*. 2004;15:449–453.

Custer PL, Kennedy RH, Woog JJ, et al. Orbital implants in enucleation surgery: a report by the American Academy of Ophthalmology. *Ophthalmology*. 2003;110:2054–2061.

Detorakis ET, Engstrom RE, Straatsma BR, Demer JL. Functional anatomy of the anophthalmic socket: insights from magnetic resonance imaging. *Invest Ophthalmol Vis Sci*. 2003;44:4307–4313.

Hornblass A, Biesman BS, Eviatar JA. Current techniques of enucleation: a survey of 5,439 intraorbital implants and review of the literature. *Ophthal Plast Reconstr Surg*. 1995; 11:77–86.

Huang ZL, Ma L. Restoration of enophthalmos in anophthalmic socket by HTR polymer. *Ophthal Plast Reconstr Surg*. 2005;21:318–321.

Jordan DR. Problems after evisceration surgery with porous orbital implants: experience with 86 patients. *Ophthal Plast Reconstr Surg*. 2004;20:374–380.

Jordan DR, Klapper SR. Surgical techniques in enucleation: the role of various types of implants and the efficacy of pegged and nonpegged approaches. *Int Ophthalmol Clin*. 2006;46:109–132.

Kaltreider SA, Jacobs JL, Hughes MO. Predicting the ideal implant size before enucleation. *Ophthal Plast Reconstr Surg*. 1999;15:37–43.

Kim YD, Goldberg RA, Shorr N, Steinsapir KD. Management of exposed hydroxyapatite orbital implants. *Ophthalmology*. 1994; 101:1709–1715.

Li GT, McCann JD, Goldberg RA. Orbital volume augmentation in anophthalmic patients using injectable hydrogel implant. *ASOPRS Abstracts*. 2003:91.

Li T, Shen J, Duffy MT. Exposure rates of wrapped and unwrapped orbital implants following enucleation. *Ophthal Plast Reconstr Surg*. 2001;17:431–435.

Mazzoli RA, Raymond WR, Ainbinder DJ, Hansen EA. Use of self-expanding, hydrophilic osmotic expanders (hydrogel) in the reconstruction of congenital clinical anophthalmos. *Curr Opin Ophthalmol*. 2004;15:426–431.

Remulla HD, Rubin PA, Shore JW, et al. Complications of porous spherical orbital implants. *Ophthalmology*. 1995;102:586–593.

Rubin PA. Enucleation, evisceration, and exenteration. *Curr Opin Ophthalmol*. 1993;4: 39–448.

Schittkowski MP, Guthoff RF. Injectable self-inflating hydrogel pellet expanders for the treatment of orbital volume deficiency in congenital microphthalmos: preliminary results with a therapeutic approach. *Br J Ophthalmol*. 2006;90:1173–1177.

Su GW, Yen MT. Current trends in managing the anophthalmic socket after primary enucleation and evisceration. *Ophthal Plast Reconstr Surg*. 2004;20:274–280.

Trichopoulos N, Augsburger JJ. Enucleation with unwrapped porous and nonporous orbital implant: a 15-year experience. *Ophthal Plast Reconstr Surg*. 2005;21:331–336.

Tse DT, Pinchuk L, Davis S, et al. Evaluation of an integrated orbital tissue expander in an anophthalmic feline model. *Am J Ophthalmol*. 2007;143:317–327.

Vagefi MR, McMullan T, Burroughs JR, et al. Autologous dermis graft at the time of evisceration or enucleation. *Br J Ophthalmol*. 2007;91:1528–1531.

Vagefi MR, McMullen TFW, Burroughs JR, et al. Injectable hydroxyapatite for orbital volume augmentation. *Arch Facial Plast Surg*. 2007;9:439–442.

V

Aesthetic Surgery of the Eyelids and Face

25

Rejuvenation of the Forehead and Eyebrows

STUART SEIFF, MD, AND BRYAN SEIFF, MD

The eyes and upper face impart more emotion than any other part of the human body and can communicate temperament through a variety of complex movements and expressions. The influence of the eyebrow on facial anatomy is subtle but critical in establishing mood as determined by facial expression. Upward-slanting eyebrows suggest surprise or sadness, downward-slanting eyebrows denote anger, flat eyebrows hanging over the eyes suggest fatigue, and eyebrows with a proper arch suggest happiness.[1]

Concepts of facial beauty continue to evolve over time, yet certain aesthetic principles invariably define the youthful brow and upper face. The head of the brow should begin at a point directly above the alae of the nose, and the tail of the brow should end on a line drawn from the alae of the nose through the lateral canthus. Classical aesthetic principles held that women have eyebrows with a high, graceful arch, accompanied by a deep superior sulcus and well-defined lid crease. The head of the brow began 1 to 2 mm above the supraorbital rim and the lateral third was elevated up to 1 cm above the rim, with the high point of the arch directly above the lateral aspect of the limbus. Current fashion seems to prefer flatter brows with a subtle upward slanting of the brow tail, rather than a high, accentuated arch. The tail of the brow thins as it elevates laterally. Fullness of the brow tissue and a less shallow superior sulcus has also become en vogue, reflecting the overall trend toward facial fullness as a sign of youthfulness. Men tend to have a straighter brow that lies at or slightly above the orbital rim, with a shallow superior sulcus and a more subtle lid crease.

As the face ages, thinning skin and tissue laxity diminish the youthful appearance of the brow and upper eyelid. The eyebrows become ptotic, resulting in vertical redundancy of the upper lid skin. The drooping brow and inelastic skin combine to cause upper eyelid tissue to drape over the lid margin, often obstructing the superior visual field. This is most pronounced laterally, where the brow support is weakest, forming hoods of skin in the lateral canthal areas[2]. Patients must elevate the brows with the frontalis muscle, resulting in deep forehead wrinkles. Vertical creases in the glabellar area and deep horizontal furrows crossing the bridge of the nose may also become more pronounced with aging. Addressing these issues and rejuvenating the upper face requires that the forehead, brows, and upper eyelids be evaluated not individually, but as interlacing components of a larger unit. Simply excising upper eyelid and lateral canthal skin may produce further ptosis of the brows and canthal webbing. The eyebrows may appear to be sutured to the eyelashes, as the thicker eyebrow skin is pulled inferiorly into the eyelid. Eyebrow and forehead elevation, however, will raise the brows and greatly reduce lateral hooding and medial canthal redundancy, as well as obliterate forehead wrinkles. Often after eyebrow elevation an upper eyelid blepharoplasty becomes unnecessary, or at most becomes a straightforward cosmetic procedure addressing modest skin excess with normal structural position. Recognition and correction of eyebrow laxity and ptosis is therefore an integral step in treatment and rejuvenation of the upper face, and should take place prior to or in conjunction with any upper eyelid surgery. A multitude of surgical techniques are available to enhance the appearance of the brow and upper face, and may be combined with upper eyelid surgery for a stable, lasting, and natural result. Recognizing the underlying structural problems and matching them to the ideal rejuvenation techniques will allow for maximum aesthetic benefit and patient satisfaction.

25-1 FOREHEAD AND EYEBROW ANATOMY

Understanding the anatomy of the forehead and brow, including the temporal region, will facilitate the selection and successful execution of brow elevation procedures. Knowledge of fascial planes allows for the safe and effective dissection of tissues while avoiding important nerves and vascular structures, most notably the frontal branch of the facial nerve. Understanding the structure and function of the brow musculature facilitates targeted muscle resection or ablation, resulting in a smoother and more effective brow lift.

25-1-1 *Fascial Anatomy.* The forehead consists of five structural layers, which may be delineated using the acronym SCALP: *s*kin, sub*c*utaneous tissue, *a*poneurosis, *l*oose areolar tissue, and *p*ericranium. The skin is the most superficial layer, and tends to be quite thick. Just below the skin is the superficial fascia or subcutaneous tissue, which is a fibrofatty layer adherent to the skin as well as the underlying muscle and aponeurosis. The third layer consists of the epicranial aponeurosis (galea aponeurotica), which gives rise to and ensheaths the occipitofrontalis muscle. The frontalis and galea together function as part of a larger fascial and muscular system that extends to the temporoparietal fascia laterally and continues as the superficial musculo-aponeurotic system (SMAS) below the level of the zygomatic arch. The fourth layer is composed of loose areolar tissue, which occupies the sub-aponeurotic space. This tissue is surgically important because it is a fibrillar and avascular plane, facilitating dissection in such procedures as the mid-forehead brow lift and the coronal brow lift. The deepest layer is the periosteum of the skull, or pericranium. The avascular subperiosteal plane becomes important in dissection and fixation when performing endoscopic forehead and brow procedures.

The paired temporalis muscles are located laterally in each infratemporal fossa, where they originate along the temporal line, pass deep to the zygomatic arch, and insert on the coronoid process of the mandible. The importance of these muscles during upper facial rejuvenation pertains to their overlying fascia, which can be used to delineate surgical planes and aid in fixation (Fig. 25-1). The temporalis fascia proper is dense and firmly adherent to the underlying muscle, and is easily identified during dissection by its characteristic glistening white appearance. In the lower half of the fossa, at the level of the superior orbital rim, the temporalis fascia proper splits into a superficial and deep layer to ensheath the superficial temporal fat pad. This fat pad extends to the level of the zygomatic arch. A deep temporal fat pad lies beneath the deep temporal fascia 2 cm above the zygomatic arch and overlies the temporalis muscle and tendon; it is an extension of the buccal fat pad through the zygomatic arch. The spongy temporoparietal fascia lies superficial to the temporalis fascia and bridges the SMAS of the lower face to the galea aponeurosis of the upper face. The temporal branch of the facial nerve courses through the deep surface of this fascia, and is therefore avoided during dissection within the loose avascular plane that separates the temporal and temporoparietal fascia. Fixation during lateral brow elevation can be achieved by suturing the overlying loose temporoparietal fascia to the dense, adherent temporalis fascia proper.

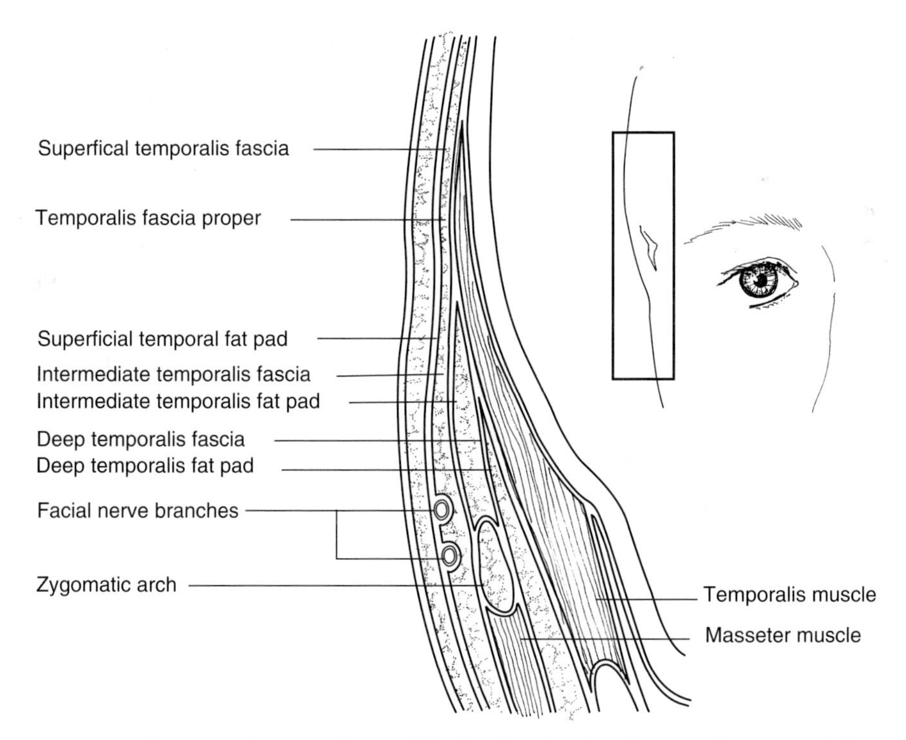

Figure 25-1 Familiarity with tissue planes of the forehead and scalp can aid in surgical dissection and fixation.

The temporoparietal fascia is contiguous with the galea aponeurotica, while the temporalis fascia proper is continuous with the periosteum of the skull. The confluence of these fascial planes occurs just medial to the temporal fusion line of the skull, where the deep layers of the temporoparietal fascia and galea are bonded to the periosteum and fixed to the bone. This zone is termed the conjoined tendon, and it demarcates the frontal and temporal optical cavities during endoscopic brow procedures. The anterior extent of the conjoined tendon at the orbital rim is known as the orbital ligament. This ligament is an important release point during lateral brow procedures, as it effectively tethers the lateral eyebrow to the orbital rim and can limit movement of the temporoparietal fascia.

25-1-2 *Vessel and Nerve Anatomy.* The upper face has an abundant blood supply composed of branches of both the external and internal carotid artery. Branches of the external carotid artery include the superficial temporal artery and the facial artery. These give rise to the blood supply in the medial canthal region via the angular artery and in the lateral canthal region by way of the anterior branch of the superficial temporal artery. The first major branch of the internal carotid artery is the ophthalmic artery, which gives rise to the supraorbital and supratrochlear arteries. These exit their respective foramina and supply the majority of the forehead and midscalp.

Venous drainage of the upper face mirrors the arterial supply, with some variability. Of particular importance is the medial zygomaticotemporal vein, or sentinel vein, which runs perpendicular through the temporalis fascia in the area of the intermediate fat pad and connects the superficial and middle temporal veins. Identification and avoidance of this vein during endoscopic dissection will prevent significant bleeding and bruising and impaired visualization.

The facial nerve innervates the majority of the facial musculature. It emerges from the stylomastoid foramen and enters the anteromedial surface of the parotid gland. It passes forward within the gland superficial to the retromandibular vein and external carotid artery. The nerve then divides into five terminal branches (temporal, zygomatic, buccal, mandibular, and cervical), although anatomic variations are frequent (Fig. 25-2).

The temporal branch emerges from the upper border of the parotid gland and supplies the anterior and superior auricular muscles, the frontal belly of the occipitofrontalis, the orbicularis oculi, and the corrugator supercilii.[3,4] It lies along a line running from the earlobe to a point along the zygoma below the anterior temporal hairline, and continues through a point 1.5 cm lateral to the eyebrow.[5–8] The temporal branch travels superiorly in the temporoparietal fascia, and lies just medial to the superficial temporal vessels. It can be avoided by dissection within the loose avascular plane that separates the temporalis fascia proper and the temporoparietal fascia.

The zygomatic branch emerges from the anterior border of the parotid gland and supplies the inferior orbicularis.[3,4] The buccal branch leaves the anterior border of the gland below the parotid duct and runs near the lower border of the zygoma. It supplies the buccinator, the procerus, and the muscles of the upper lip and nostril.[3–5] The mandibular and cervical branches emerge from the anterior and lower borders of the gland, respectively.[3,4]

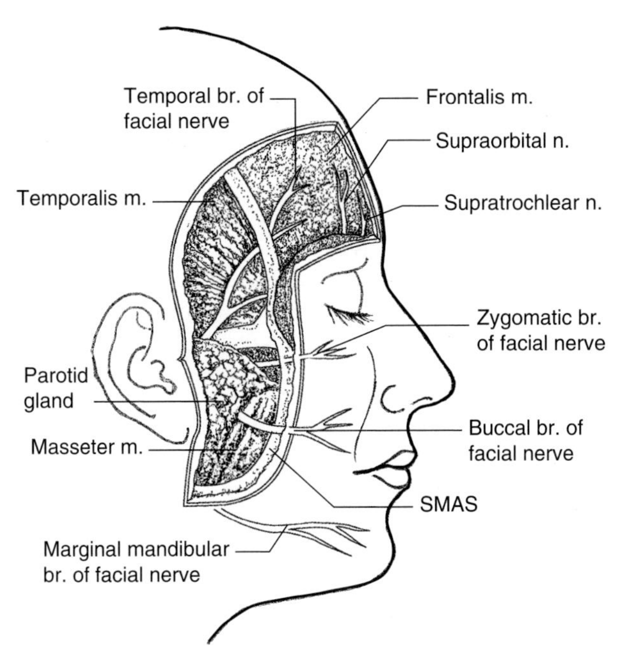

Figure 25-2 Anatomy of the facial nerve as it divides into its terminal branches (temporal, zygomatic, buccal, mandibular, and cervical). Cervical branch not shown in this figure.

Sensory innervation of the brow is derived from the supraorbital and supratrochlear branches of the ophthalmic (V_1) division of the trigeminal nerve. The ophthalmic division of the trigeminal nerve enters the orbit through the superior orbital fissure and gives off a frontal branch, which runs along the superior aspect of the orbit and divides into the supraorbital and supratrochlear nerves. The supraorbital nerve exits the orbit at the junction of the medial and central thirds of the superior orbital rim through the supraorbital notch. It innervates the scalp, lateral forehead, and lateral upper eyelid. The supratrochlear nerve emerges from the medial aspect of the superior orbital rim and penetrates the corrugator muscle to provide sensation to the glabella, medial forehead, and medial upper eyelid. These nerves cross the orbital rim anterior to the periosteum and course superiorly within the superficial (superficial branch) or deep (deep branch) frontalis fascia. Dissection deep to the frontalis in a subgaleal or subperiosteal plane will avoid all sensory nerves, as well as the frontal branch of the facial nerve.

25-1-3 *Muscular Anatomy.* The four major muscles of the forehead and eyebrow are the occipitofrontalis, orbicularis oculi, corrugator supercilii, and procerus. The occipitofrontalis consists of four bellies (two occipital and two frontal) connected by the epicranial aponeurosis, or galea aponeurotica. Each occipital belly arises from the highest nuchal line on the occipital bone and passes forward and inserts on the galea. The frontal bellies arise from the galea aponeurotica, which splits into a superficial and deep layer to ensheath the muscle. This occurs approximately midway between the coronal suture and brow. The frontalis muscle inserts onto the skin and superficial fascia of the eyebrow, where it interdigitates with the orbicularis oculi and corrugator supercilii muscles. The action of the occipitofrontalis allows the scalp to move anteriorly and posteriorly. The frontal bellies are used to elevate the brows. They are supplied by the temporal branch of the facial nerve; the occipital bellies are supplied by the posterior auricular branch of the facial nerve.

There are three concentric parts of the orbicularis oculi: the orbital, preseptal, and pretarsal orbicularis. The orbital portion overlies the orbital rim and arises from the anterior limb of the medial canthal tendon and the surrounding periosteum. The fibers sweep superiorly and inferiorly around the eye and meet laterally over the zygoma. The preseptal portion has superficial heads from the medial canthal tendon and deep heads from the posterior lacrimal crest. The fibers sweep laterally and form the lateral palpebral raphe. The pretarsal fibers arise from the medial canthal tendon and tensor tarsi (Horner's) muscle.[9] The fibers pass laterally to unite at the lateral canthal tendon. The orbicularis closes the eyelids. The superior portions are innervated by the temporal branch of the facial nerve, while the inferior portions are supplied by the zygomatic branch.

The corrugator supercilii has its origin in the periosteum of the nasal process of the frontal bone. The corrugator fibers blend with the deeper portions of the frontalis and orbital orbicularis. The fibers insert into the skin of the medial eyebrow. The action of this muscle pulls the medial eyebrow inferiorly and medially, producing vertical glabellar wrinkles. It is supplied by the temporal branch of the facial nerve.

The procerus is continuous with the inferior medial margin of the frontalis. Its origin is from the lower part of the nasal bone. The muscle pulls the medial end of the eyebrow inferiorly and produces horizontal wrinkles at the bridge of the nose. It is innervated by the buccal branch of the facial nerve. Together the paired procerus and corrugator muscles are the main depressors of the medial brow and produce horizontal and vertical glabellar furrows, respectively. They are commonly treated with Botulinum toxin type A to help alleviate these glabellar lines.

Posterior to the brow musculature at the level of the eyebrow, the deep galea aponeurotica splits and encloses a layer of fat, the retro-orbicularis oculi fat (ROOF), or brow fat pad. The musculature forms the anterior boundary of the eyebrow fat pad. The posterior boundary of the eyebrow fat pad continues into the eyelid as the superior orbital septum. The brow fat pad continues into the upper eyelid as the areolar posterior orbicularis fascia. In the Caucasian eyelid, this layer maintains little of its fatty differentiation into the upper eyelid. In the Asian eyelid, significant fatty differentiation is maintained, creating the typical full appearance of the Asian eyelid.

The eyebrow is anchored to the frontal bone periosteum by firm attachments along the posterior aspect of the brow fat pad. These attachments primarily extend over the medial half to two thirds of the orbit along the supraorbital rim. Weaker connections exist laterally. The attachments provide fixation and support for the deeper tissues, while the fat anterior to these bony attachment sites permits vertical sliding of the overlying skin and muscle. The relative paucity of lateral attachments is responsible for the earlier and greater ptosis of this portion of the eyebrow.

Medial eyebrow ptosis may follow due to atrophy of the eyebrow fat, which allows the overlying skin and muscle layer to sag inferiorly. When eyebrow ptosis occurs, the frontalis muscle is used to help elevate the brow, resulting in deep forehead furrows. However, due to the lack of frontalis fibers temporally, lateral eyebrow ptosis persists in spite of frontalis contraction. This causes drooping of the thin upper eyelid skin, giving the appearance of dermatochalasis. This is the reason eyebrow position must be evaluated prior to undertaking any rejuvenation procedure involving the upper eyelids and face.

A small percentage of the youthful population appears to have medial eyebrow ptosis with otherwise good structure. This is likely an inherited characteristic and may be difficult to correct with eyebrow elevation.

25-2 PREOPERATIVE EVALUATION

Patients must be carefully evaluated preoperatively to identify factors that may increase the risk of potential complications. A general preoperative evaluation should elicit any medical conditions that pose an anesthesia risk, or a history of previous anesthetic complications. Coagulation disorders should be addressed to avoid intraoperative bleeding complications, and a review of all medications and vitamins will allow identification of any agent that maintains the patient in a hypocoagulable state. Information of specific interest in upper face and eyelid surgery includes a history of dysthyroid ophthalmopathy, proptosis, keratitis sicca, or seventh-nerve paresis, as these may place the patient at increased risk for postoperative exposure problems. Contact lens wear should also be discussed, as this may affect corneal sensitivity and cause a propensity toward corneal dryness. Baseline best-corrected vision must be obtained, and assessment of tear production and corneal sensation should be documented. The anterior segment of the eye should be examined to identify conjunctival or corneal disease.

After the general medical and ophthalmic information has been gathered to determine whether the patient is an appropriate surgical candidate, attention can be turned to an aesthetic evaluation and discussion regarding surgical planning and expectations. The structural position of the forehead and hairline, the eyebrows (arch and position), eyelids (function, position, and redundancy), lateral and medial canthi (position and laxity), and upper lid crease (position and symmetry) are examined. Notation is made of areas of herniating orbital fat and redundant or hypertrophic orbicularis muscle. Skin type and quality are also evaluated with respect to scarring. Abnormalities and asymmetries are discussed with the patient. Photographs or a mirror are useful in this regard. Patients are then asked to delineate their aesthetic and surgical goals. The surgeon should explain the variety of surgical techniques available to address these goals, explaining the limits of each and educating the patient on what can realistically be achieved with each procedure. The majority of patients with brow ptosis and secondary dermatochalasis expect simple removal of upper eyelid skin, without understanding the underlying brow and forehead pathology contributing to their condition. The patient needs to understand that the forehead, brows, and upper eyelids do not function individually but as interlacing components of a larger unit and need to be addressed as such. Simply excising upper eyelid and lateral canthal skin may produce further ptosis of the brows and pull the thicker eyebrow skin inferiorly into the eyelid. Lateral canthal hooding may not be eliminated with skin excision alone. Eyebrow elevation, however, will raise the brows and greatly reduce lateral hooding and medial canthal redundancy, as well as obliterate forehead wrinkles. An upper eyelid blepharoplasty may then become unnecessary, or at most becomes a straightforward cosmetic procedure requiring modest skin excision. Having this discussion with the patient allows selection of the appropriate surgical procedure necessary to obtain maximum aesthetic benefit and patient satisfaction.

If the patient understands the limits of upper lid blepharoplasty alone in the setting of brow ptosis but still wishes to proceed with lid surgery only, a conservative blepharoplasty may be performed. If the patient recognizes the benefit of brow ptosis correction and agrees to proceed, the most appropriate procedure can be selected from a multitude of brow elevation techniques. This selection is based on multiple factors, including the degree and position (medial, lateral, or diffuse) of brow ptosis, density and location of hairline, medical conditions affecting the patient's ability to tolerate straight local or intravenous sedation, and aesthetic and functional goals (improvement of visual fields alone or additional aesthetic benefits, including smoothing of glabellar and forehead wrinkles). As part of the consent process, likely and rare complications of each procedure should always be discussed.

25-3 DIRECT BROW ELEVATION

Direct eyebrow elevation affords the most lift per millimeter of excised tissue. It is excellent for lateral segmental brow elevation but is less effective in elevating the medial brow and in reducing horizontal glabellar or forehead folds. It is useful for patients with small to moderate eyebrow ptosis, especially men in whom coronal or temporal lifts are not advised because of a tendency toward male pattern baldness. It is also useful in elderly patients who cannot tolerate more extensive surgery, as it is a simple procedure that can be performed under local anesthesia. The main disadvantage is a faint scar that may persist above the brow.

The proposed incision site should be marked out with the patient in the sitting position. The lower border should lie just within the most superior row of eyebrow hairs. The brow is then elevated to the desired level with the fingers. The marking pen is placed over, but does not touch, the superior brow border (Fig. 25-3A). When the brow is released, the marking pen overlies what will be a point on the superior incision line. This point is marked and the procedure repeated serially along the brow until the entire incision line is constructed. Less arching of the brow can be achieved by excising more tissue over the medial and lateral brow than over the central portion (Fig. 25-3B).

The procedure is readily performed under local anesthesia. The incision is carried out using a #15 blade. Along the inferior margin of the incision an attempt is made to bevel the blade in order to preserve the brow hair follicles.[10] The incision need only be carried to the level of the frontalis muscle, especially in the region of the

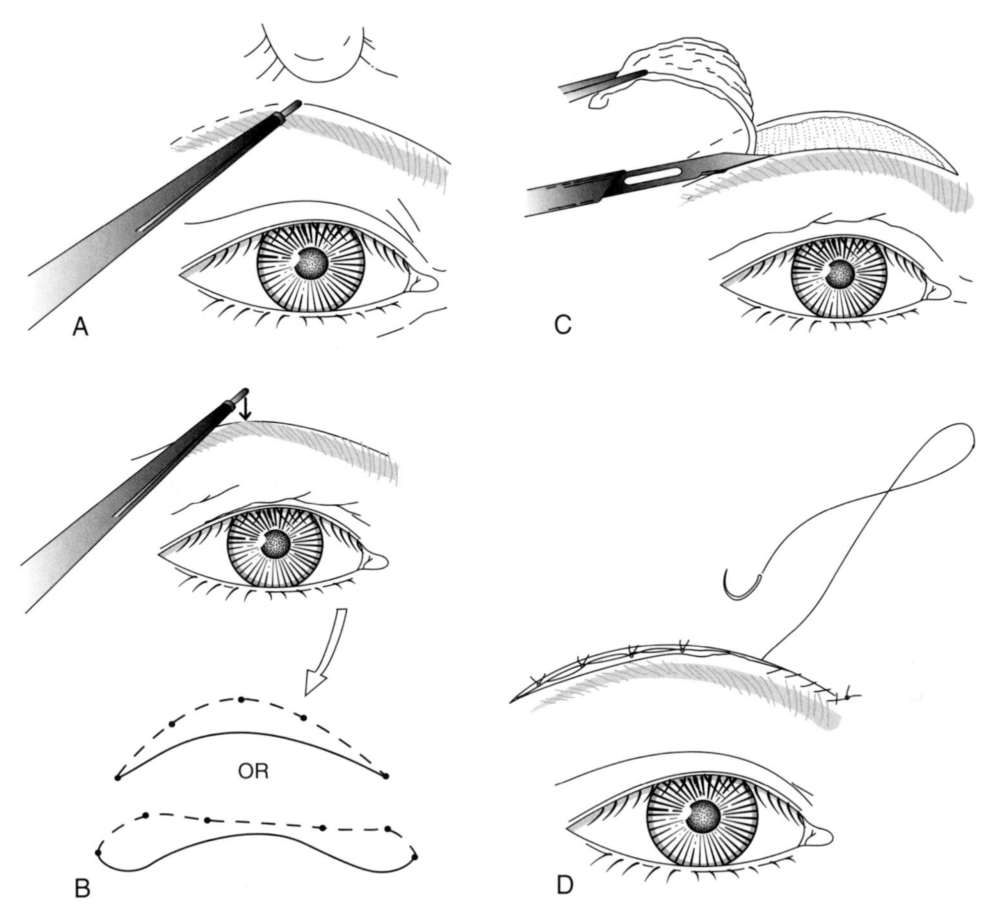

Figure 25-3 Direct brow lift. (A) The eyebrow is elevated and the marking pen is placed over, but does not touch, the superior brow border. (B) When the brow is released, the marking pen overlies what will be a point on the superior incision line. (C) The demarcated tissue is excised. (D) The wound is closed in layers.

supraorbital nerve. Scissors are used to remove the ellipse of tissue (Fig. 25-3C). Meticulous punctate hemostasis is maintained.

The wound is closed in layers. The deepest tissues are approximated with interrupted 4-0 polyglactin sutures. The subcutaneous layer is closed with interrupted 5-0 polyglactin sutures to reduce tension on the wound. The skin is closed with a continuous 6-0 nylon, taking care to evert the wound edges to minimize scarring (Fig. 25-3D). The wound should be dressed with antibiotic ointment and ice packs applied four times a day for 4 days. The sutures may be removed after 5 to 7 days.

In general, fixation of the brow to the underlying periosteum is to be avoided, as this will inhibit brow movement and diminish facial animation. However, in patients who require additional brow stability, such as those with longstanding facial nerve palsy, permanently buried 4-0 nylon sutures can be placed between the elevated brow tissue and the periosteum of the frontal bone. These will counteract the effect of gravity following the brow ptosis repair. Additional variations of the internal browpexy procedure are discussed below.

25-4 INTERNAL BROWPEXY

Browpexy is most useful in stabilizing the eyebrow after elevation, usually in conjunction with the direct eyebrow lift or as an adjunctive procedure to upper lid blepharoplasty. It is not effective by itself in cases of severe brow ptosis.

The patient is anesthetized according to the surgeon's protocol for blepharoplasty or direct eyebrow elevation. Supraorbital nerve blocks may be used to enhance anesthesia. The redundant tissue to be excised with blepharoplasty is marked with the brow held in the post-browpexy position. The supraorbital notch is identified and marked inferior to the brow. This will serve as the medial limit to the dissection. An additional mark may be made just below the tail of the brow laterally, where greatest elevation is desired.

The redundant eyelid tissue is removed in standard blepharoplasty fashion. Care is taken to remove the orbicularis muscle underlying the temporal skin incision. This enhances temporal brow elevation by weakening the depressor action of the lateral orbicularis. Superior dissection is then undertaken in a plane posterior to the orbicularis and carried to a level 1 to 2 cm above the superior orbital rim. At this point, the dissection plane lies between frontalis muscle and brow fat. The anterior leaf of the deep galea overlies the brow fat pad and contributes to the orbital ligament laterally. This tissue should be incised to release its periosteal attachments along the superolateral orbit and allow adequate brow elevation. The brow fat can be thinned or sculpted as desired. Oversculpting should be avoided, as a fuller lateral brow gives a more youthful appearance than a pronounced bony rim.

A 4-0 nylon or other nonabsorbable suture is passed through frontal bone periosteum at the desired brow height. The suture is then passed through the anterior flap at the level of the lowest brow hairs, through the retro-orbicularis fat and orbicularis muscle. It is important that this bite not be too superficial, as it may dimple the skin or limit brow mobility. The knot is tied firmly, and similar sutures are passed medially and laterally to stabilize the elevated brow. The blepharoplasty is then completed in standard fashion. The wound should be dressed with antibiotic ointment and ice packs applied four times a day for 4 days. After the fourth day warm compresses may be beneficial in the resolution of edema and ecchymosis. The sutures may be removed after 5 to 7 days.

An alternative method of internal browpexy involves placement of an absorbable transblepharoplasty endotine (Coapt Systems Inc, Palo Alto, CA) placed subperiosteally on the frontal bone. Following the excision of upper lid tissue, the periosteum of the superior orbital rim is incised along the central and lateral thirds using the cutting cautery. Care is taken not to extend the incision medially across the supraorbital neurovascular bundle. A periosteal elevator is then used to dissect the frontal flap off the underlying bone to allow adequate exposure for endotine placement. Some surgeons may prefer to complete the frontal subperiosteal dissection to allow movement of the flap superiorly after insertion of the endotine. An anchoring hole is drilled into the frontal bone at the junction of the central and lateral thirds of the eyebrow, approximately 1 cm from the orbital rim. It is important to place the hole far enough from the rim to prevent the implant from lying directly under the thin eyelid skin. The implant can then be seated into position using the accompanying inserter. An audible "pop" should be heard when the device is fully engaged. The flap is then advanced superiorly and engaged on the implant tines using digital pressure. A double-armed suture may be passed through platform holes in the device prior to implantation to aid in subcutaneous tissue fixation. The goal is brow symmetry with slight overcorrection, as the brows will settle during the postoperative period. The blepharoplasty is then completed in standard fashion. The endotines are resorbed over 6 to 12 months.

Postoperative stability following endotine fixation may be enhanced by administration of Botox to the glabella preoperatively to limit brow movement and depression during the immediate healing phase. In addition, the patient is instructed to wear a snugly fitting headband while at home for 2 weeks postoperatively to encourage periosteal reattachment to bone in its newly elevated position.

25-5 MID-FOREHEAD BROW LIFT

The mid-forehead brow lift is particularly effective in correcting eyebrow ptosis with horizontal glabellar folds and forehead creases. This technique lowers the hairline by shortening the forehead, unlike the coronal lift, which raises the hairline. Thus, the mid-forehead lift is often more appropriate than the coronal lift for men with high or sparse frontal hairlines and deep horizontal rhytides. Patients with unfurrowed foreheads are poor candidates, as the mid-forehead lift can produce a prominent hyperemic scar that may persist for many months. The mid-forehead lift provides more brow elevation medially than laterally, and is less effective in patients with lateral brow ptosis and functional hooding with visual field deficits. A shortened mid-forehead approach may be combined with the direct brow approach to minimize the length of the scar and achieve both medial and lateral brow elevation.

The superior incision is marked along a central forehead crease. If a large resection is anticipated, the incision line should be carried across the majority of the forehead to facilitate wound closure. In some patients, breaking up the incision may be helpful in allowing better camouflage of the scar. Different forehead rhytides can be used to make the incisions, producing smaller scars at different levels on the forehead.

This procedure is easily performed under local anesthesia. The initial incision is made through the full thickness of the skin and through the galea aponeurotica. The inferior flap is elevated in a subgaleal plane, taking care to avoid the supraorbital nerves (Fig. 25-4A). This allows access to and dissection of the corrugator and procerus muscles to eliminate glabellar furrows, if indicated. Redundant forehead skin is then elevated and excised as appropriate to eliminate the eyebrow ptosis (Fig. 25-4B). The amount of tissue excised can be fashioned as an ellipse or "figure of eight" to correct medial or lateral brow ptosis, respectively.[11,12]

The incision is closed in two layers. The deep layer is closed with 5-0 polyglactin. The superficial layer is closed with a running 5-0 nylon stitch (Fig. 25-4C). Antibiotic ointment is applied and the wound is dressed with a head wrap. Ice compresses are used over the eyes four times a day for 4 days to reduce edema and ecchymosis. Sutures are removed after 5 to 7 days.

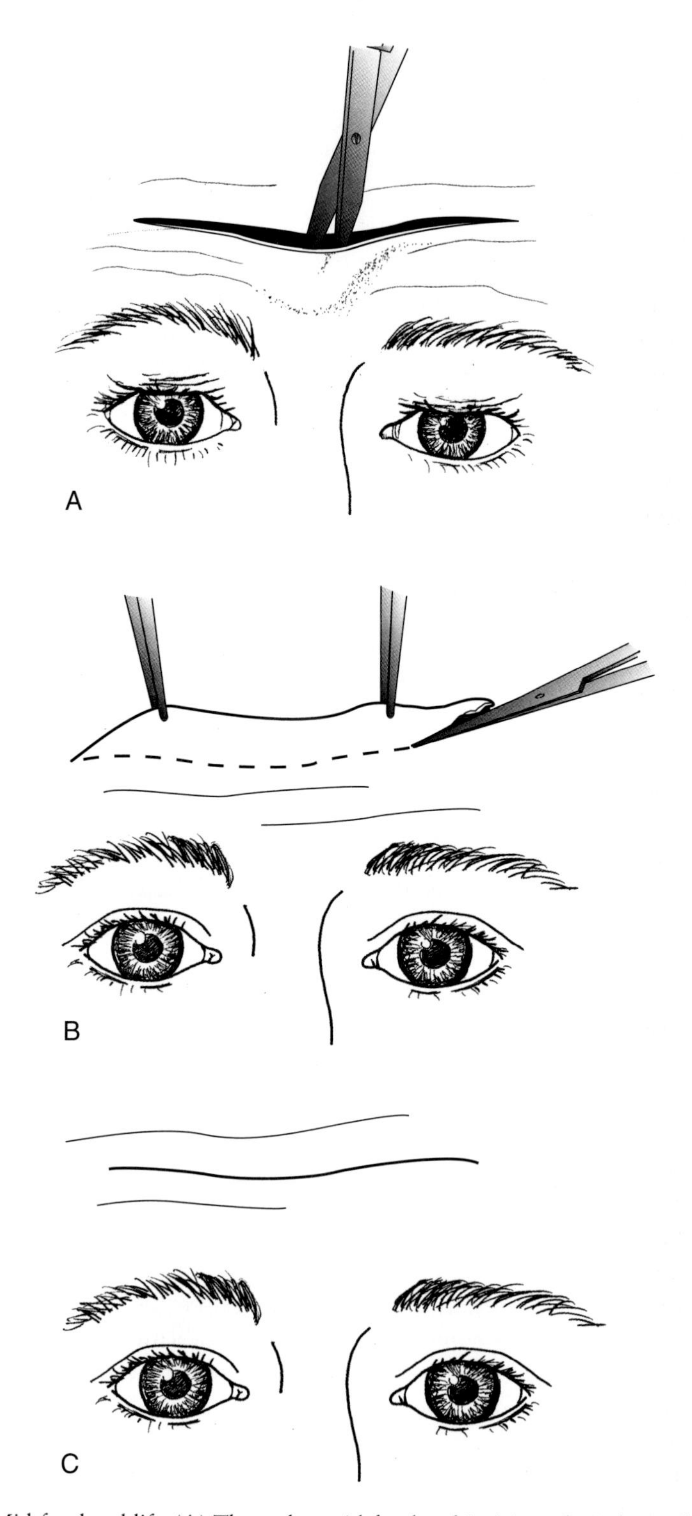

Figure 25-4 Mid-forehead lift. (A) Through a mid-forehead incision, the inferior flap is elevated in a subgaleal plane, taking care to avoid the supraorbital nerves. (B) Redundant forehead skin is then elevated and excised as appropriate to eliminate the eyebrow ptosis. (C) The incision is closed in layers, leaving a forehead incision that mimics a forehead rhytid.

25-6 TEMPORAL BROW LIFT

The temporal lift procedure for brow elevation is especially useful in patients with elevation of the medial brow and slight elevation of the temporal hairline, which may be undesirable in some patients.

The procedure may be performed under local anesthesia, although some intravenous sedation may be useful. Prior to injection the hair is parted along a line perpendicular to the alar–canthal line, just above and anterior to each ear. Local anesthetic is infiltrated along the part line. Supraorbital nerve blocks are performed with 0.5% bupivacaine. An incision approximately 12 cm long is then made along the part line through the skin to the level of the temporalis fascia proper (Fig. 25-5A).

Blunt dissection using either a finger or a large scissors is performed along the temporalis fascia proper toward the eyebrow (Fig. 25-5B). The temporal flap is undermined to just below the level of the brow and lateral canthus. The flap is then advanced, and redundant tissue is excised. A single-layer closure using skin staples is performed (Fig. 25-5C). Occasionally, this approach may be used in combination with a facial rhytidectomy. In this case, the flap can be started as described above, but above the hairline, a transition may be made to the level of the temporoparietal fascia. The dissection can be continued in this subcutaneous plane to join the rhytidectomy flap. Care must be exercised as the temporal branch of the facial nerve is below the superficial flap.

Antibiotic ointment is placed on the wound, and a light head wrap is applied. Ice compresses are placed over the eyes and forehead four times a day for 4 days. The staples are removed after 7 to 10 days.

25-7 CORONAL FOREHEAD AND BROW LIFT

The coronal eyebrow and forehead lift is a more aesthetically pleasing approach to the brow lift than the direct and mid-forehead methods. It effectively raises the brows medially and laterally, reduces glabellar furrows, and smoothes the forehead. It is a relatively easy dissection and provides excellent exposure. The incision is entirely within the hair-bearing scalp, which covers the scar. This technique is used primarily in women, as men may have a tendency toward male pattern baldness. It is discouraged in patients with a naturally high hairline because it may further elevate the hairline significantly.

In the operating room, the hair is parted along the proposed coronal incision line with the use of water-based jelly as needed. The incision line extends from the most superior point where one the ear touches the scalp to the most superior point where the other ear touches the scalp. In the midline, the incision is approximately 5 cm posterior to the hairline.

Additional markings are made before anesthetic is injected. A line is drawn from the midline of the nose (M) to the midpoint of the incision (M′). A line is drawn from the lateral limbus on each side (L) to a point (L′) along the incision line, generally 4 cm from M′. A line is then drawn bilaterally from the temporal portion of the brow (T) to a point 6 cm along the incision from L′ (T′). These lines will form the

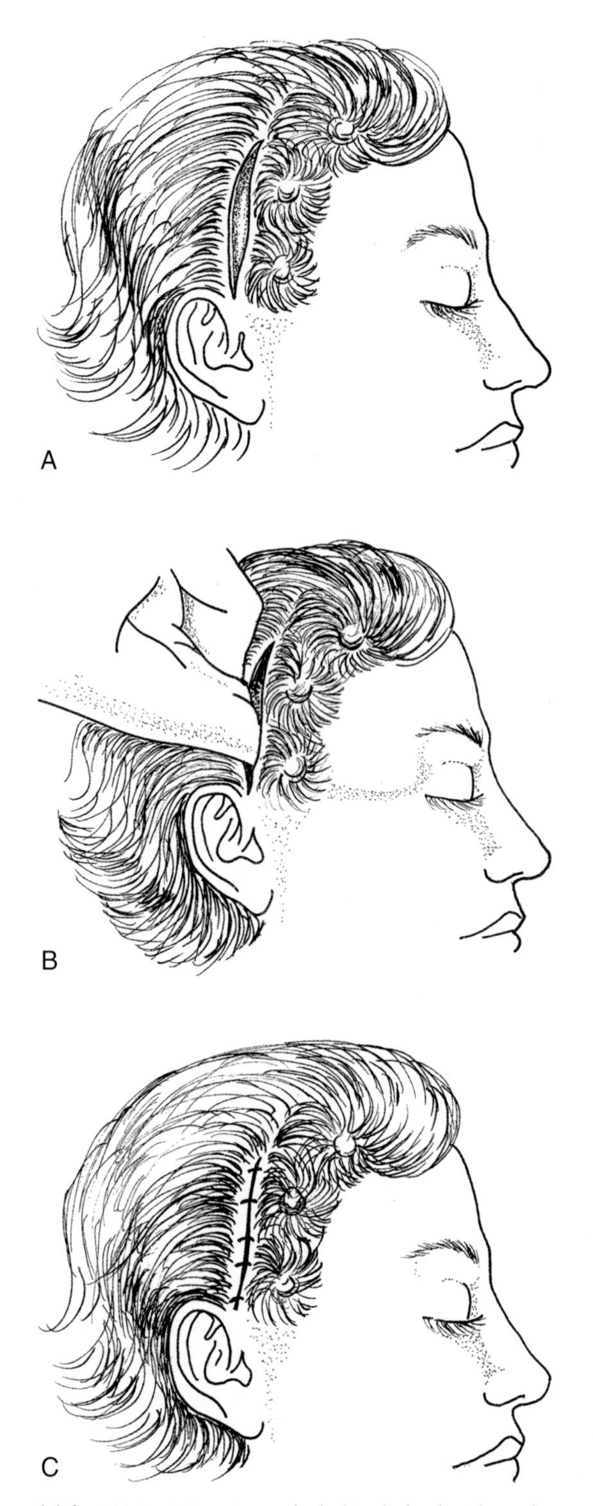

Figure 25-5 Temporal lift. (A) Incision is made behind the hairline down to the level of the temporalis fascia proper. (B) Blunt dissection using either a finger or a large scissors is performed along the temporalis fascia proper toward the eyebrow. (C) The flap is then advanced, redundant tissue is excised, and a single-layer closure using skin staples is performed.

lines of traction for elevating the brow. The hair is then bundled within the areas formed by the marking lines and clipped short just anterior to the incision line.

The coronal eyebrow lift is ideally performed under local anesthesia with intravenous sedation. It may be done under general anesthesia, but hemorrhage can be increased in this setting due to a vasodilatory effect. The local anesthetic solution consists of 40 cc of 0.5% lidocaine with 1:200,000 epinephrine with hyaluronidase and 10 cc of 0.5% bupivacaine. Care should be taken to avoid lidocaine toxicity; thus, 0.5% lidocaine is used. Bilateral supraorbital nerve blocks are performed with the 0.5% bupivacaine. Lidocaine 10 cc is then injected along the right incision line, 10 cc along the left incision line, 10 cc across the right brow, and 10 cc across the left brow. This effectively forms a "vascular tourniquet," and excellent hemostasis is obtained.

The incision is made to the level of periosteum with a #15 blade. Dissection between the periosteum and the galea is performed with a combination of sharp and blunt techniques. The conjoined tendon is released and dissection is continued temporally over the temporalis fascia proper on each side. The coronal flap is elevated to the superior orbital rims. The temporal branch of the facial nerve lies in this flap. Care should be taken to avoid excess trauma to the nerve through traction or cautery, as injury may cause temporary or permanent paralysis of the eyebrow and forehead. Care should also be taken to preserve the supraorbital neurovascular bundles. A subperiosteal plane is then established 1 to 2 cm superior to the orbital rims. The periosteum is elevated inferiorly across the orbital rims and onto the nasal bridge. This allows for maximum elevation of the brows.

Superior traction on the scalp will lift the brows but will not remove creases and furrows between the brows or in the forehead. Therefore, the procerus–corrugator muscle complex should be selectively relaxed to help smooth the glabellar area. Also, several horizontal relaxing incisions should be made in the posterior muscle layer of the forehead flap to allow the posterior lamella to relax, thereby stretching and smoothing forehead furrows. This procedure, done with cutting cautery, will interrupt motor innervation superior to the incisions. The incisions should therefore be placed at least 3 cm superior to the lateral orbital rims (approximately the second forehead crease) to preserve the brow animation necessary for a natural appearance.

Using a D'Assumpcao clamp, the forehead flap is advanced over the posterior scalp wound margin in the midline until the flap is moderately tight. A cut is made anteriorly into the flap, indicating the desired extent of excision. A staple is placed to fix this point. This procedure is repeated along each of the previously marked lines. The redundant segments of flap are then excised with scissors. Excision of the temporal segment is gradually tapered toward the ear. Additional staples are placed to close the wound with the edges everted. Drains are typically not needed.

The hair is then rinsed with 1.5% hydrogen peroxide to remove accumulated blood, shampooed, conditioned, and gently dried. Antibiotic ointment is applied to the wound. A head dressing is placed at the end of the procedure. Ice compresses are applied to the eyes and forehead to minimize edema. Patients are instructed to shampoo and rinse their hair in the shower with warm water daily, beginning 24 hours after surgery. Hair should be towel-dried on postoperative day 1, as complete sensation may not have returned. A hair dryer can be used with caution on postoperative day 2. Patients may gently brush their hair, taking care to avoid their skin staples. Staples are removed after 7 to 10 days.

25-8 ENDOSCOPIC FOREHEAD AND BROW LIFT

Over the past decade, the endoscopic forehead and brow lift procedure has become for many the state-of-the-art technique for upper facial rejuvenation. The original concept of the endoscopic brow lift was to relax the depressors of the brow and allow them to passively rise.[13] With advancements in fixation materials and techniques, we can now achieve better brow elevation and symmetry and meet all of the goals of upper facial rejuvenation. The most noted benefits of the endoscopic technique are the smaller scars hidden in the hairline, the selective brow elevation without the need for removal of any hair or skin, the excellent control of both the glabellar region and temporal brow, and the rapid recovery time. The subperiosteal plane used in this approach is ideal due to the ease of dissection, reduced bleeding, and easy identification of neurovascular landmarks. The endoscopic brow lift is also a versatile procedure that can be performed in combination with many other facial rejuvenation techniques and procedures. It does require a significant investment in equipment and has a steep learning curve. Like the coronal technique, it also raises the hairline.

The endoscopic brow lift involves several incisions placed strategically behind the hairline to gain access for the endoscope and dissecting tools such as periosteal elevators, electrocautery, lasers, tissue graspers, and suction instruments. The placement and number of incision sites varies among surgeons. It is important to remember that fixation points will be placed at the incision sites; therefore, their placement should correlate to the vector of maximally desired lift. The authors prefer four separately placed incisions posterior to the hairline. The two central incisions are marked in the parasagittal plane above the head of the brow in a vertical alignment, approximately 2 to 3 cm posterior to the hairline if possible. Higher or thinning hairlines may require more anterior placement of the incision with a horizontal orientation to hide the scar in a brow furrow, although scar exposure remains a risk. Alternatively, incisions may be placed further posteriorly in an effort to hide them, but this may increase the difficulty of visualization and dissection. Two temporal incisions are also marked, one on each side of the head, for direct access to the thick temporalis fascia and ultimately elevation of the tail of the brow. These incisions are placed posterior to the hairline at the intersection of the alar–lateral canthal line and the coronal plane. The hair at each of these incision sites is clipped short, and the surrounding hairs are bundled along the proposed incision lines with the use of water-based jelly as needed.

The endoscopic eyebrow lift is ideally performed under local anesthesia with intravenous sedation, as described for the coronal lift. In addition, tumescent solution will be used to irrigate under the flap during direct endoscopic visualization. This solution is composed of 1 liter of lactated Ringer's solution with 1 mg of epinephrine, 40 mg of triamcinalone, 10 cc of 8.4% sodium bicarbonate, and 50 cc of 0.5% lidocaine.

A #15 blade is used to incise the full thickness of the scalp in the area of the parasagittal incisions. These incisions are carried through the periosteum and down to bone. Dissection can be carried out after reaching the subperiosteal plane using a straight periosteal elevator to lift the tissue anteriorly to a point 1 cm above the orbital rim. Posteriorly the dissection should continue at least 5 to 10 cm but can extend as far back as the lambdoid suture to prevent folding and redundancy when the forehead and scalp are advanced posteriorly. Laterally the dissection should be carried up to but not through the conjoined tendon.

The surgical blade is then used to carefully incise the scalp at the temporal incision sites. A blunt tenotomy scissors can be used to dissect down to the glistening temporalis fascia proper, avoiding unnecessary injury to the underlying temporalis muscle. The endoscope is inserted through the temporal incisions. Dissection is carried inferiorly to the intermediate fat pad and sentinel vein under direct endoscopic visualization. It is then continued superiorly and medially to the conjoined tendon. A connection can now be made from the temporal optical space to the central subperiosteal optical space under direct visualization. The conjoined tendon is opened bluntly in a lateral to medial direction, then extended superiorly and inferiorly. Endoscope-guided dissection becomes critical during release of the more inferior portion of the tendon, as this is where the temporal branch of the facial nerve travels. Tissue elevation should be performed firmly against the periosteum and the temporalis fascia when connecting the optical spaces. After careful release along the inferior conjoined tendon and orbital ligament, the lateral orbital rim should be exposed in the subperiosteal plane down to the zygomaticofrontal suture line. Posteriorly, blunt dissection should be completed to release all tissue superficial to the temporalis fascia proper.

The endoscope is then inserted through each of the parasagittal incisions. Inferior dissection over the nasofrontal suture and around the superior orbital rims is performed under direct endoscopic visualization. Careful dissection will avoid inadvertent tearing of the periosteum. Once the entire edge of the orbital rim is visualized, the periosteum can be incised from lateral to medial, taking care to remain below the lowest brow hairs to provide maximum lift. This relaxing incision may be performed with endoscopic scissors, cautery, or laser. The supraorbital nerves and vessels, which lie at the junction of the medial and central thirds of the superior orbital rim, should be identified. Palpation of the supraorbital notch will aid in their localization. Meticulous dissection under direct visualization in this area will avoid injury to these structures during periosteal release. Good periosteal release is the key to good elevation and control of brow height and contour.

Once the periosteum has been adequately incised, the corrugator supercilii and procerus can be visualized. Vertical and horizontal rhytides in the glabella can be improved greatly by transection and weakening of these muscles. A CO_2 laser or cautery unit can be used for transection. Weakening of the procerus is first performed in the midline at the level of the superior orbital rim. Dissection then proceeds laterally with weakening of both corrugators. The supraorbital neurovascular bundles pass through the corrugators and should be identified and spared. Overly aggressive removal of these muscles should be avoided, as it may lead to postoperative irregularities, including a glabellar depression.

Once the forehead and temporal scalp are adequately released and the periosteum and brow depressors relaxed, the dissection for the standard endoscopic brow lift is complete. However, one of the many advantages of the endoscopic brow lift is its versatility and the ease with which additional procedures can be performed concurrently to enhance facial rejuvenation,[14] including mid- and lower face procedures. The reader is encouraged to explore these procedures in greater detail.

After dissection is complete, good brow elevation and control will be achieved with appropriate fixation. Elevation of the brow head to approximately 1 cm above the supraorbital rim typically allows for a natural elevation and contour.

Fixation of galeal tissue and the periosteum at the parasagittal incision sites can be accomplished using a myriad of techniques, including temporary and permanent surgical screws, resorbable endotines, bone tunnels, and tissue glue.[15] Permanent or resorbable surgical screws anchored into or bone tunnels created through the calvarium can be used to fix sutures passed through periosteum and galeal tissue. Temporary screws can also be anchored in the skull and traverse all layers of the scalp, allowing closure of the incision posterior to the screw following brow elevation. These screws may be removed after 10 to 14 days. Resorbable endotines are fixed to bone via burr holes placed in the calvarium. The overlying tissue layers are advanced posteriorly and seated onto the tines, which resorb over a period of 6 to 12 months. Tissue adhesives can be inserted into the optical cavity to fixate the periosteum in the desired position. Each technique has its advantages and disadvantages. Maximum control of the brow is achieved when fixation includes the anterior layers of the scalp. Sutures and endotines are therefore beneficial due to the incorporation of all layers of the scalp during fixation, unlike adhesive, which fixates only periosteum. Sutures may, however, lose their effectiveness due to "cheese wiring" through soft tissues, and any implanted device carries with it the risk of foreign body complications. The selection of fixation technique should take into account surgeon and patient preference, as well as cost. Recent evidence suggests that at least 6 weeks of fixation may be necessary to allow the periosteum to adhere to its new location on the frontal bone cortex.[16,17] Although no direct studies in humans have been performed, clinical experiences corroborate these findings.

Fixation of the lateral tail of the brow is performed at each temporal incision. Two 3-0 polydioxanone sutures are used on each side to anchor the anterior scalp flap to the thick, immobile temporalis fascia. An enlarged ellipse of tissue may be excised if additional lift is desired, but this is usually unnecessary and can increase wound complications.

Closure of the scalp incisions can be performed with skin staples only, as no skin has been excised and no pressure exists at the incision sites. Redundant forehead tissue created by brow elevation is distributed over the posterior elevated scalp, occasionally causing a posterior "hump." This tends to redistribute over several days.

The hair is then rinsed with 1.5% hydrogen peroxide to remove accumulated blood, shampooed, conditioned, and gently dried. Antibiotic ointment is applied to the wound. A head dressing is placed at the end of the procedure. Ice compresses are applied to the eyes and forehead to minimize edema. Patients are instructed to shampoo and rinse their hair in the shower with warm water daily, beginning 24 hours after surgery. Hair should be towel-dried on postoperative day 1, as complete sensation may not have returned. A hair dryer can be used with caution on postoperative day 2. Patients may gently brush their hair, taking care to avoid their skin staples. Staples are removed after 7 to 10 days.

The brow position remains very stable following this early recovery period, and very little relapse occurs with proper technique. Stability will be enhanced by administration of Botulinum A toxin to the glabella preoperatively to limit brow movement and depression during the immediate healing phase. In addition, the patient is instructed to wear a snugly fitting headband while at home and during exercise for 2 to 4 weeks postoperatively, again to limit periosteal slippage during the healing phase.

25-9 TRICHOPHYTIC FOREHEAD AND BROW LIFT

The trichophytic eyebrow and forehead lift offers advantages similar to those of the coronal lift. It is a relatively easy dissection and provides excellent exposure. It effectively raises the brows medially and laterally, reduces glabellar furrows, and smoothes the forehead. The incision in this procedure is placed at the hairline and involves excision of bare forehead skin, allowing lowering of a high forehead. It is ideal in patients with both brow ptosis and a high hairline or thinning in the temporoparietal area by allowing excision of areas of hair loss and advancement of dense hair-bearing scalp.

The trichophytic eyebrow lift is ideally performed under local anesthesia with intravenous sedation, as described for the coronal lift. The proposed incision site is marked approximately 1 to 2 mm posterior to the anterior hairline in the frontal region, and moves posteriorly into the temporal scalp. Following the hairline creates a more natural postoperative appearance when compared with a straight scar. Depth of incision and plane of dissection vary among surgeons. Subcutaneous, subgaleal, and subperiosteal dissections have all been described. Subcutaneous dissection has the advantage of breaking the dermal insertions of the frontalis that create deep horizontal rhytides and has a role for patients who do not need to rejuvenate their entire brow–forehead complex. Deeper dissections, however, allow greater and more extensive release and elevation of brow tissues, less bleeding in the plane of dissection, and easier access to the glabella and brow depressors for resection. Subperiosteal dissections may be combined with an endoscopic approach, reaping the benefits of endoscopic lifting while still lowering the hairline.[18] This is the preferred approach of the authors.

The hairline incision is made with a #15 blade down to bone, taking care to bevel the incision in a posterior to anterior direction. This preserves the follicles at the leading edge of the posterior flap, allowing them to grow hair anterior to the incision and camouflage the scar.[19] Undulation of the incision also aids in camouflage. Injudicious use of cautery for hemostasis should be avoided, as it can damage hair follicles and increase the risk of alopecia.

Dissection is then performed in the subperiosteal plane using a straight periosteal elevator to lift the tissue anteriorly to a point 1 cm above the orbital rim.

Laterally the dissection should be carried up to but not through the conjoined tendon. The incisions and dissection for the endoscopic lift are then performed as previously described.

A #15 blade is used to incise the full thickness of the scalp down to bone in the area of the parasagittal incisions. These incisions are placed several centimeters posterior to the trichophytic incision to allow placement of the fixation device and prevent distortion of the trichophytic wound. Dissection is performed in the subperiosteal plane anteriorly to connect this dissection to the trichophytic incision. Dissection is also carried posteriorly. The amount of posterior dissection performed depends upon the amount of hairline lowering desired. More lowering equates to more posterior release. If the hairline is to remain at its natural level, limited or no posterior dissection can be performed.

The surgical blade is then used to carefully incise the scalp at the temporal incision sites. A blunt tenotomy scissors can be used to dissect down to the glistening temporalis fascia proper, avoiding unnecessary injury to the underlying temporalis muscle. The endoscope is inserted through the temporal incisions. Dissection is carried inferiorly to the intermediate fat pad and sentinel vein under direct endoscopic visualization. It is then continued superiorly and medially to the conjoined tendon. A connection can now be made from the temporal optical space to the central subperiosteal optical space under direct visualization as described for the endoscopic lift. After careful release along the inferior conjoined tendon and orbital ligament, the lateral orbital rim should be exposed in the subperiosteal plane down to the zygomaticofrontal suture line. Posteriorly, blunt dissection should be completed to release all tissue superficial to the temporalis fascia proper.

The endoscope is then inserted anterior to the trichophytic incision. Inferior dissection over the nasofrontal suture and around the superior orbital rims is performed under direct endoscopic visualization. Once the entire edge of the orbital rim is visualized, the periosteum can be incised from lateral to medial, taking care to remain below the lowest brow hairs to provide maximum lift. The supraorbital nerves and vessels, which lie at the junction of the medial and central thirds of the superior orbital rim, should be identified. Meticulous dissection under direct visualization in this area will avoid injury to these structures during periosteal release. Good periosteal release is the key to good elevation and control of brow height and contour.

Once the periosteum has been adequately incised, the corrugator supercilii and procerus can be visualized. Vertical and horizontal rhytides in the glabella can be improved greatly by transection and weakening of these muscles. Weakening of the procerus is first performed in the midline at the level of the superior orbital rim. Dissection then proceeds laterally with weakening of both corrugators. The supraorbital neurovascular bundles pass through the corrugators and should be identified and spared.

The posterior scalp is advanced forward from the vertex, and the frontal flap is grasped with the D'Assumpcao clamp and elevated to the level of the desired hairline. The amount of excess tissue is determined, and cutbacks are made. Excess tissue is trimmed using the same posterior-to-anterior beveled incision to allow anterior hair growth and camouflage the scar. The deep layers are closed with 4-0 polyglactin sutures. The scalp skin is closed with running 5-0 nylon in the frontal region and staples in the hair-bearing region.

Fixation of the periosteum and galeal tissue may now be performed between the trichophytic incision and the parasagittal incisions by any of the previously discussed techniques: temporary and permanent surgical screws, resorbable endotines, bone tunnels, and tissue glue. The selection of fixation technique should once again take into account surgeon and patient preference, as well as cost. Fixation of the lateral tail of the brow is performed at each temporal incision using two 3-0 polydioxanone sutures on each side to anchor the anterior scalp flap to the thick, immobile temporalis fascia. Closure of the endoscopic scalp incisions can be performed with skin staples.

The hair is then rinsed with 1.5% hydrogen peroxide to remove accumulated blood, shampooed, conditioned, and gently dried. Antibiotic ointment is applied to the wound. A head dressing is placed at the end of the procedure. Ice compresses are applied to the eyes and forehead to minimize edema. Patients are instructed to shampoo and rinse their hair in the shower with warm water daily, beginning 24 hours after surgery. Hair should be towel-dried on postoperative day 1, as complete sensation may not have returned. A hair dryer can be used with caution on postoperative day 2. Patients may gently brush their hair, taking care to avoid their skin staples. Sutures and staples are removed after 7 to 10 days.

25-10 BOTULINUM TOXIN/DERMAL FILLER-ASSISTED BROW LIFT

Botulinum toxin has been used for nearly two decades to improve the esthetic appearance of the upper third of the face by reducing wrinkles of the forehead (horizontal lines), glabella (frown and bunny lines), and lateral orbital crow's feet (laugh lines).[20] In patients with mild brow ptosis who are not yet candidates or do not wish to undergo surgery, Botulinum toxin may be used to obtain a "chemical brow lift."[21] Treatment of the corrugator and procerus muscles, in addition to effectively smoothing glabellar frown lines, allows elevation of the medial brow through the unopposed action of the frontalis muscle. The lateral brow is elevated by treating the orbital portion of the orbicularis oculi muscle immediately below the temporal third of the brow, decreasing the tone and downward pull of this muscle. The amount of both medial and lateral elevation can be substantial, but it is less precise and less predictable than that achieved with surgery.[22] In patients who seek improvement in brow position without undergoing surgery, Botulinum toxin is an effective alternative.

Botulinum toxin dilution varies with individual surgeons. The authors currently use a dilution of 5.0 units/0.1 cc, with 0.1 cc as the typical volume used per injection site. The muscles of the glabella (procerus and corrugators) are identified by asking the patient to frown, causing these muscles to contract and become more prominent. It is important to remember that Botulinum toxin is not a filler; it is a paralytic agent. Injections should therefore be placed in the muscle causing a rhytid, not in the rhytid itself. A single midline injection of 0.1 cc is placed in the procerus muscle between the eyebrows, just above the nasal bridge. Two injections are then placed in each corrugator, one at the superomedial aspect of the eyebrow and a second just lateral to it, along the superior aspect of the brow. These muscles lie just anterior to the periosteum; thus, the Botulinum toxin should be placed deep for maximum effect. Appropriate dosage in the glabella is highly variable, but the area usually requires 10 to 30 units for an effective result. Treatment of the lateral brow consists of one or two injections into the superotemporal portion of the orbicularis oculi below the lateral third of each brow, totaling 2.5 to 10 units. The toxin is placed intradermally, in close proximity to the orbicularis muscle, and should raise a superficial bleb upon injection. Injections should be placed at least 1 cm from the lateral orbital rim to reduce the risk of intraorbital diffusion and complications.[23] Management of horizontal forehead lines typically requires between 15 and 25 units administered in a series of four to six injections spaced evenly along the forehead in intervals of approximately 3 to 4 cm. Treatment of the frontalis to reduce horizontal forehead lines may increase brow ptosis or at least offset brow elevation that otherwise may have been created by Botulinum toxin treatment of the brow depressor muscles.

Current aesthetic constructs are based on the principle that cutaneous fullness is a sign of youthfulness and beauty. It therefore follows that increasing the fullness of the temporal brow with a dermal filler enhances rejuvenation of the upper face, especially when combined with the brow elevation generated by Botulinum toxin injection. Both hyaluronic acid and calcium hydroxyapatite fillers can be used in this area, but hyaluronic acid should be tried first as it is technically more forgiving. In either case, 0.2 to 0.4 cc of the filler is placed on each side along the superior orbital rim just below the brow at the level of the periosteum. The material should be injected slowly, in a fanning pattern. Directing the bevel of the needle posteriorly will help ensure deep placement. Correct placement of the filler will support and raise the tail of the brow while adding fullness and softness to the lateral orbital rim.

25-11 COMPLICATIONS OF EYEBROW PTOSIS REPAIR

Scarring of the incision line is a universal side effect of all brow surgery. The scars from direct and mid-forehead lifts are at first prominent, but tend to fade with time. Meticulous surgical technique should minimize noticeable scarring. The scars can also be concealed to some extent in the brow hairs in direct lifts or in a forehead crease in mid-forehead lifts. Recalcitrant scars may be treated with dermabrasion to improve scar camouflage. Beveling of the incision can aid in concealing scars in direct and trichophytic lifts by preserving follicles at the leading edge of the posterior flap and allowing hair to grow anterior to the incision. Coronal, endoscopic, and temporal lifts have the advantage of hiding scars in the hair, but suffer the disadvantages of elevation of the hairline and possible alopecia along the incision sites.

Alopecia can be caused by excessive tension on the flaps, rough handling of wound margins, or excessive use of cautery near hair follicles. Hair may return after a 4- to 8-month period of dormancy for the follicle, but hair loss can occasionally be permanent. Atraumatic tissue handling and careful cautery protects hair follicles and minimizes this complication.

Transient anesthesia of the forehead and scalp is not uncommon following brow lifting procedures. This frequently results from manipulation of the supraorbital neurovascular bundle at the superior orbital rim. It usually disappears after several months, but may occasionally be permanent. These symptoms are more common following coronal and trichophytic techniques than following endoscopic, mid-forehead, or direct brow lift procedures.

Postoperative hemorrhage is uncommon, especially when the dissection plane is subgaleal or subperiosteal. Dissection in a more superficial plane can lead to some blood accumulation. Hematoma formation can represent a significant problem when large flaps have been created, as in the mid-forehead, temporal, and coronal lifts, and may compromise the vascular supply to the flaps and cause them to necrose. Some surgeons have used drains in these procedures. However, most have abandoned them because of the discomfort encountered in removal and the possibility of forming a groove in the forehead along the drain tract. Further, removal of the drain may initiate bleeding under the flap. Meticulous hemostasis at the time of surgery usually suffices to prevent hematoma formation.

Paresis of the forehead and brow is of particular concern in more extensive brow lifting procedures. Surgical dissection in the frontal region should be carried out in a subgaleal or subperiosteal plane, below the plane of the facial nerve and its branches. Similarly, dissection in the temporal region should be confined to the subtemporoparietal plane, also below the plane of the facial nerve. In the isolated temporal lift, the dissection may be in a plane anterior to the facial nerve branches, and extra caution should be exercised. Avoidance of improper or excessive retraction and the overzealous use of cautery in the region of the nerve will minimize the risk of brow and forehead weakness postoperatively.

Lagophthalmos may result after a brow lift, causing severe corneal exposure. This is particularly likely in patients who have previously undergone upper lid blepharoplasty. Careful attention to the extent of brow elevation and corneal lubrication will minimize serious consequences. One to 2 mm of lagophthalmos immediately after brow elevation is not uncommon and may be desirable for a maximum result. In such instances proper corneal lubrication during the postoperative period is critical.

Wound infection is a possible problem but has not been common. The scalp, brow, and eyelids are extremely vascular, thus helping to minimize the incidence of infections in this area. The prophylactic use of antibiotics may still be beneficial, especially if fixation devices have been implanted.

Most asymmetry in the postoperative period relates to preexisting facial asymmetry. A thorough evaluation of the patient's face preoperatively with photographic documentation of the preoperative state, as well as a candid discussion of facial and brow asymmetries, will allow the patient to set realistic goals regarding surgical results. Postoperative over- or undercorrection can be minimized by forming and meticulously executing a precise surgical plan based on the preoperative evaluation and discussion. Preoperative assessment and markings should be carried out with the patient in the sitting position.

REFERENCES

1. Ellenbogen R. Transcoronal eyebrow lift with concomitant upper blepharoplasty. *Plast Reconstruc Surg*. 1983;71:490–495.

2. Lemke BN, Stasior OG. The anatomy of eyebrow ptosis. *Arch Ophthalmol.* 1982;100:981–986.
3. Snell RS. *Clinical Anatomy for Medical Students.* Boston: Little, Brown & Co., 1973:613–809.
4. Warwick R, Williams PL. *Gray's Anatomy*, Br Ed 35. Philadelphia: W.B. Saunders Co., 1973:496–497.
5. Furnas DW. Landmarks for the trunk and the temporofacial division of the facial nerve. *Br J Surg.* 1965;52:694–696.
6. Correia P, Zani R. Surgical anantomy of the facial nerve, as related to the ancillary operations and rhytidoplasty. *Plast Reconstruc Surg.* 1973;52:549–552.
7. Loeb R. Technique for preservation of the temporal branches of the facial nerve during face lift operations. *Br J Plast Surg.* 1970;23:390–394.
8. Pitanguy I, Ramos AS. The frontal branch of the facial nerve: The importance of its variations in face lifting. *Plast Reconstruc Surg.* 1966;38:352–356.
9. Beard C, Quickert M. *Anatomy of the Orbit.* Ed 2. Birmingham, AL: Aesculapius Publishing Co., 1977:4–11, 18–21.
10. Tardy ME, Tom LWC: Aesthetic correction of the ptotic brow. In: Putterman A, ed. *Cosmetic Oculoplastic Surgery.* New York: Grune & Stratton, 1982:147–176.
11. Johnson CM, Waldman SR. Mid-forehead lift. *Arch Otolaryngology* 1983;109:155–159.
12. Brennan HG, Rafaty FM. Mid-forehead incisions in treatment of the aging face. *Arch Otolanyngology.* 1982;108:732–734.
13. Vasconez LO, Gore GB, Gamboa-Bobadilla M, et al. Endoscopic techniques in coronal brow lifting. *Plast Reconstr Surg.* 1994;94:788.
14. Cuzalina A. *Facial Esthetic Surgery: Forehead and Brow Procedures.* In: Miloro M, Ghali GE, et al., *Peterson's Principles of Oral and Maxillofacial Surgery.* Ed 2. Vol 2, Part 9, Sect 67. Philadelphia: BC Decker Inc. 2004:13831406.
15. Loomis MG. Endocsopic brow fixation without bolsters or miniscrews. *Plast Reconstr Surg*, 1996;98:373.
16. Dyer WK, Yung RT. Botulinum toxin-associated brow lift. In: Larrabee WF, Thomas JR, eds. *Facial Plastic Surgery Clinics of North America: Rejuvenation of the Upper Face.* Vol 8, Number 3. Philadelphia: W.B. Saunders Co., 2000:343–354.
17. Sciafani AP, Fozo MS, Romo T III, McCormick SA. Strength and histological characteristics of periosteal fixation to bone after elevation. *Arch Facial Plas Surg.* 2003;5:63–66.
18. Tower RN, Dailey RA. Endoscopic pretrichial brow lift: Surgical indications, technique and outcomes. *Ophthal Plast Reconstr Surg.* 2004;20:268–273.
19. Holcomb JD, McCollugh EG. Trichophytic incisional approaches to upper facial rejuvenation. *Arch Facial Plast Surg.* 2001;3:48–53.
20. Keen MS, Khosh MM. The role of botulinum toxin A in facial plastic surgery. In: Willet JM, ed. *Facial Plastic Surgery.* Upper Saddle River, NJ: Prentice Hall, 1997: 323–329.
21. Frankel AS, Kamer FM. Chemical browlift. *Arch Otolaryngol Head Neck Surg.* 1998;124:321.
22. Ahn MS, Catten M, Maas CS. Temporal brow lift using botulinum toxin A. *Plast Reconstr Surg.* 2000;105(3): 1129–1139.
23. Petrus GM, Lewis D, Maas CS. Anatomic considerations for treatment with Botulinum toxin. *Facial Plastic Surg Clin North Am.* 2007;15(1):1–9.

26

Upper Eyelid Blepharoplasty

JED POLL, MD, AND MICHAEL T. YEN, MD

The purpose of this chapter on blepharoplasty is to familiarize the reader with relevant eyelid anatomy, appropriate preoperative evaluation, and the surgical fundamentals of upper eyelid blepharoplasty. In addition, modern modifications of blepharoplasty will be presented, with special attention to aesthetic blepharoplasty and surgical considerations in the Asian eyelid.

Blepharoplasty defines a group of surgical procedures by which excess skin, orbicularis muscle, and orbital fat are removed from the upper eyelids (Fig. 26-1). The ideal goal of blepharoplasty is to rejuvenate the eyelid and restore a youthful eyelid position without compromising eyelid function. A postoperative taut upper eyelid resulting in lagophthalmos and ocular surface compromise equates to an unsatisfied patient and surgeon. Likewise, excessive orbital fat excision can create a sunken superior sulcus and an eyelid contour with an undesirable cosmetic appearance. Similar to many other oculoplastic procedures, many variations in surgical technique in blepharoplasty have been employed over the years. Despite the differences, all these modifications rely upon the same underlying fundamental principles.

Key steps in successful blepharoplasty surgery occur before the first skin incision is made. The eyelids are not islands unto themselves; rather, they are intimately connected to other facial structures, most notably the brow and forehead for upper lid blepharoplasty and the midface complex for lower lid blepharoplasty. Failure to preoperatively address pertinent nearby structures can yield unwanted postsurgical results. In addition to the assessment of facial structure, a preoperative blepharoplasty evaluation should include a proper medical and ocular history. Patients with a bleeding diathesis or a history of anticoagulation should be counseled and anticoagulation medications withheld if medically appropriate. A history of ocular surface

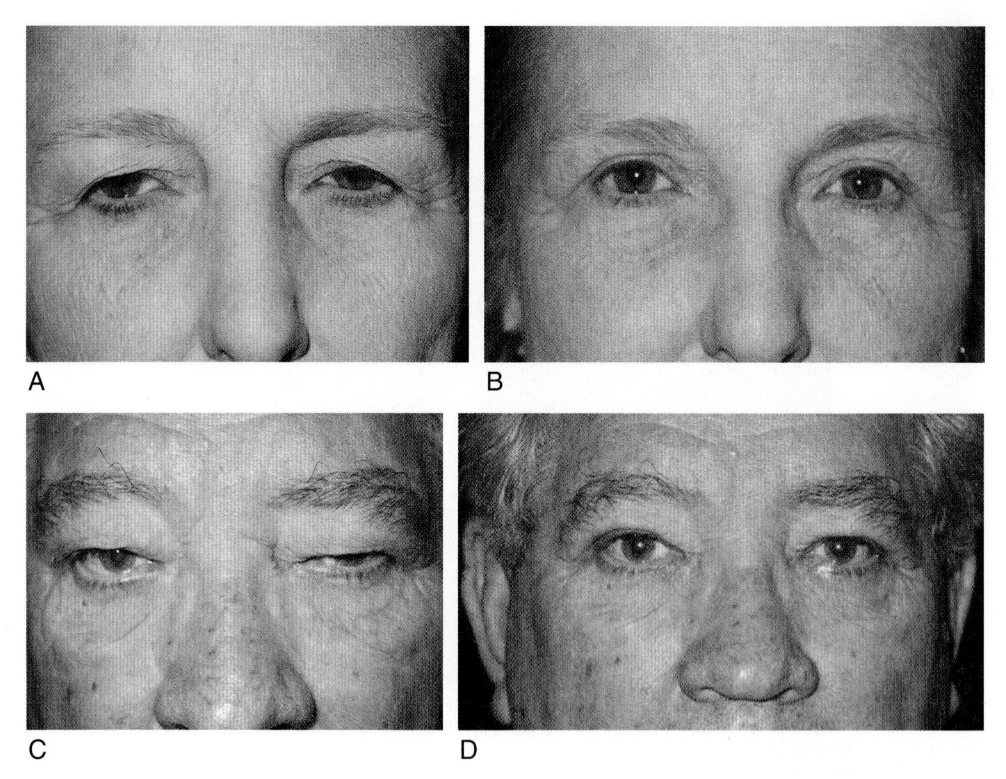

Figure 26-1 (A) A female patient with excessive upper eyelid skin obscuring the view of the eyelashes and eyelid margin. (B) After blepharoplasty, the upper eyelids have less redundancy and the eyelid margin and eyelashes are visualized. (C) A male patient with excessive upper eyelid skin and fullness from fat prolapse. (D) After blepharoplasty only, the eyelids appear more open and with less fullness.

issues or previous anterior segment surgery should be investigated and a slit-lamp examination performed to assess for dryness and corneal pathology. Conditions that can affect eyelid position, such as myasthenia gravis and thyroid-related orbitopathy, should be stable for a minimum of 6 months prior to blepharoplasty.

26-1 BROW ASSESSMENT

Assessing brow position and function is essential when considering a patient for upper eyelid blepharoplasty. Normal brow position in males is along the superior orbital rim, and in females normal brow position is about 1 cm superior to the orbital rim. Brow contour and symmetry are equally important variables that should be attended to by the surgeon. Detailed history and examination are needed to determine proper brow position for each individual patient. Often review of old photographs can aid in determining prior brow position and can guide the surgeon in surgical management. Assessment of forehead appearance and function is equally important. Deep, furrowed rhytids in the brow could indicate sustained frontalis effort to aid eyelid and brow elevation, while an abnormally flat, expressionless brow should alert the surgeon to possible facial nerve weakness.

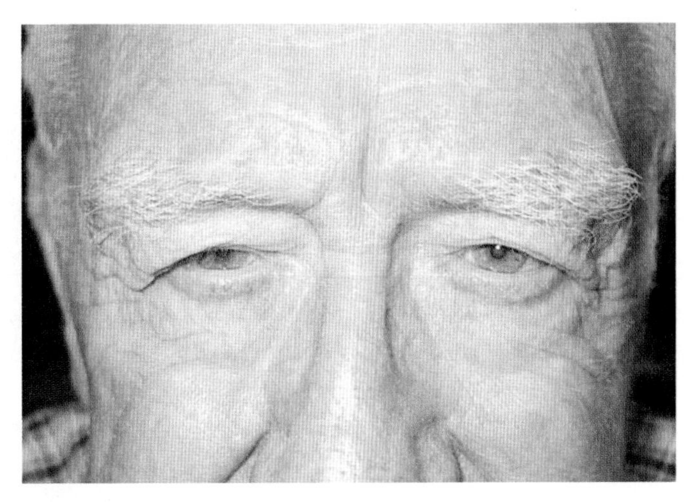

Figure 26-2 A patient with eyebrow ptosis may present with the appearance of eyelid droopiness and excess skin on the eyelids.

When evaluating the upper eyelids, the surgeon must first neutralize the effect of the brow. If the patient is using excess frontalis effort to keep the eyelids open, the amount of dermatochalasis on the eyelids will appear reduced or minimal. When, however, the frontalis effort is neutralized, the full amount of dermatochalasis can be assessed (Fig. 26-2). This is done by the surgeon placing a hand along the forehead to stabilize the brow position. Patients with significant brow ptosis can have the appearance of extensive dermatochalasis. However, upon elevating the brow back to its proper anatomic position, this redundancy can be significantly reduced. Often these patients seeking blepharoplasty will be better served by a brow lift procedure.

Neglecting to recognize and address brow malposition can result in an abnormal lid position after surgery in which the upper lid and brow are "sewn together." This oversight can create a relatively static lid position and yield significant lagophthalmos. Moreover, the patient's underlying issue of brow ptosis has not been corrected, but rather exacerbated by the blepharoplasty. In many patients combining blepharoplasty with a brow elevation procedure is necessary to achieve the desired surgical outcome.

26-2 UPPER EYELID ANATOMY

Understanding the anatomy of the upper eyelids and nearby bony structures and soft tissues is critical to successful, uncomplicated blepharoplasty. As discussed previously, assessment of brow position and function is a fundamental element of the blepharoplasty evaluation. Prior to blepharoplasty, the surgeon should be familiar with normal eyelid position and contour in addition to pertinent anatomic landmarks.

The upper eyelid stretches 28 to 30 mm across the globe, with a gentle curvature peaking just nasal to the center of the pupil and smoothly descending to form the canthal angles. Normally, the lateral canthus forms an acute 30- to 40-degree angle and is located 5 mm medial to the lateral orbital rim and approximately 2 mm higher than the medial canthus. An important landmark in upper eyelid blepharoplasty is the eyelid crease. The lid crease forms from anterior projections of the levator aponeurosis to the skin and superior tarsus. The upper eyelid crease in women is well defined and about 10 to 11 mm superior to the lid margin. In men, a more subtle lid crease is found 8 to 9 mm superior to the lid margin.

The upper eyelid can be divided into two zones, above and below the superior tarsal plate. Visualizing the normal lid crease approximates the superior border of the tarsus, but this assumption can be misleading, as in cases of blepharoptosis with levator dehiscence. In the inferior division near the lid margin, the layers of the eyelid from superficial to deep include eyelid skin, orbicularis muscle, tarsus, and palpebral conjunctiva. Superiorly, above the tarsal plate the layers are eyelid skin, orbicularis muscle, orbital septum, preaponeurotic fat, levator aponeurosis, Müller's muscle, and palpebral conjunctiva.

Eyelid skin is very thin, in fact the thinnest skin on the body. Beneath the skin is minimal subcuticular tissue and fat, especially so in the pretarsal skin. Deep to the skin is the orbicularis oculi muscle. The orbicularis is divided into three parts: pretarsal, preseptal, and orbital. Orbital orbicularis encircles the orbit and is responsible for forced lid closure. Preseptal orbicularis overlies the orbital septum and is involved in voluntary lid closure and blinking. The pretarsal orbicularis is intimately connected to the tarsus and helps contribute to the medial and lateral canthal tendons. The orbicularis receives a rich vascular supply and is innervated by the facial nerve.

The orbital septum is an important landmark in eyelid surgery as it separates the orbital contents from the preseptal eyelid structures. While a majority of excised tissue, orbicularis and skin, lies anterior to the septum, the orbital septum is frequently interrupted during blepharoplasty to allow the surgeon to sculpt and contour protruding orbital fat. In the upper eyelid, orbital fat is divided into a larger central fat pad and a paler nasal fat pat. Temporally is the lacrimal gland, which should not be confused with orbital fat and should be avoided in blepharoplasty. Caution must be exercised when manipulating and trimming orbital fat as the levator aponeurosis lies just deep to this and can be damaged or even transected by an aggressive surgeon wishing to debulk excess fat.

Deep to the orbital septum are the levator aponeurosis, Müller's muscle, and palpebral conjunctiva. In straightforward blepharoplasty these structures lie deep to the surgeon's working area; however, understanding the relationship between these structures is nonetheless important. When combining blepharoptosis repair with blepharoplasty, it is beneficial to elevate the lid initially by securing the levator to the superior tarsus before determining the amount of excess skin and orbicularis that is to be excised.

Aging and environmental influences produce structural changes in the eyelid skin, resulting in the clinical picture of dermatochalasis. Loss of elastic fibers, connective tissue weakening, and gravitational forces yield redundant eyelid skin that descends over the lash follicles, creating a heavy eyelid and possible superior visual field obstruction. Aging changes accumulate over the years until the patient develops a functional or aesthetic complaint and seeks surgical intervention.

The amount of dermatochalasis contributes to but does not define functional loss related to blepharoplasty. With blepharoplasty, the determination of aesthetic versus functional is predicated upon the functional visual impairment of the patient. Insurance reimbursement for blepharoplasty is typically limited to dermatochalasis with skin resting upon the upper lashes with demonstrable impairment of vision. Visual impairment is documented by two perimetric visual fields, one with the eyelids in their natural position and one with the eyelids taped and eyes held open. Tested visual field usually must increase by 20% from untaped to taped for the blepharoplasty to be considered functional. Detailed preoperative evaluation and counseling is necessary prior to blepharoplasty, especially in patients desiring cosmetic blepharoplasty.

26-3 SURGICAL PROCEDURE

Upper eyelid blepharoplasty can be performed in office-based procedure rooms or in outpatient surgery centers, as usually little to no sedation is required for the procedure. An awake patient with the ability to sit up and open and close his or her eyes is preferred as this will assist the surgeon in achieving proper height and symmetry of the eyelids.

A critical step in blepharoplasty occurs before anesthetic injection or skin incisions are made; this is the marking of the eyelid. Typically the natural eyelid crease is marked, representing the inferior incision location; however, there are exceptions to this when the surgeon and patient wish to create an alternate lid crease position. When the eyelid creases are asymmetric, as a general rule it is easier to raise rather than lower a lid crease. Normally, the lid crease can readily be identified by having the patient look down. Gentle superior retraction of redundant skin folded over the crease is often necessary to fully visualize and delineate the lid crease. Care must be exercised to extend the inferior marking laterally beyond the lateral canthus to incorporate excess skin creating temporal hooding. The appearance of temporal rhytids or crow's feet can be softened by extending the blepharoplasty temporal to the lateral canthus. However, this effect is variable and the patient's expectations should be appropriately guided by the surgeon. A gentle upward deflection at the medial and lateral ends of the marking will facilitate a more tapered excision and allow for easier skin closure.

Once the inferior marking is made, the surgeon must determine the amount of eyelid skin to remove and make the superior marking. Various techniques exist for how to determine the height of the superior marking and thus the amount of skin to remove. A maximum of 15 mm of skin may be removed; however, every patient is different and caution must be exercised when removing large amounts of skin as this may yield lagophthalmos. As a general rule, there should be at least 10 to 12 mm of skin separating the superior marking from the brow. Excising skin beyond this failsafe may complicate skin closure and pull the brow inferiorly, creating an eyelid that is tethered to the brow. Also, be mindful of preexisting ocular surface disease, as excess skin excision may exacerbate these conditions.

Local anesthesia is achieved in an infiltrative manner using 2% lidocaine with 1:100,000 epinephrine in a small-gauge needle. The entire length of the incisions should be infiltrated with as little anesthetic as possible to achieve adequate pain control and promote vasoconstriction. Ballooning the eyelid with larger volumes of anesthetic distorts the eyelid architecture and can make accurate scoring of the initial skin incisions problematic. In addition, excess anesthetic can diffuse past the septum and interfere with levator function, thus inhibiting the surgeon's ability to accurately gauge eyelid height intraoperatively.

Following administration of the anesthetic, a full face skin preparation and draping is performed. A full face prep is preferred as it allows the surgeon to simultaneously assess and compare both upper eyelids intraoperatively. The patient is also more comfortable without confining drapes over the nose and mouth.

Skin incisions are made along the premarked lines using a #15 blade. Typically the inferior incision is made first, as this represents the critical lid crease position. Putting the eyelid on stretch, using the non-incising hand, an assistant, or tractional suture, facilitates placement of the primary incisions. Medial-temporal traction, parallel to the skin incision, is preferred as it does not distort the wound during incision. Superior-inferior traction puts the eyelid on stretch perpendicular to the incision path and can create scalloping of the wound edge. The skin incision is meant to score the skin, not excise tissue. The surgeon must be mindful to keep this initial incision superficial. This will prevent complications of disturbing underlying structures but will not inhibit excision of redundant tissue.

Once both the superior and inferior incisions are completed, the surgeon is ready to remove the excess tissue. Most commonly, both skin and orbicularis are removed together (Fig. 26-3). Alternatively, skin can be excised initially and limited orbicularis removed as appropriate. Using toothed forceps and Stevens scissors, the skin and orbicularis is excised starting temporally and advancing toward the medial canthus. Removal is facilitated if the surgeon can enter into a dissection plane deep to the orbicularis and superficial to the orbital septum. Medial retraction of the skin–orbicularis flap, keeping the excised tissue on constant stretch, will help maintain the appropriate plane of dissection. When making the cuts along the incision line, keeping the scissor blades vertical will facilitate a sharp, vertical skin edge. Tapered edges, produced when the blades are not vertical, can leave a thin ribbon of orbicularis near the wound edge that when sutured can create bunching of the wound. Often a small amount of orbicularis remains in the temporal aspect of the wound prior to entering the suborbicular dissection plane. This should be removed prior to wound closure to prevent bunching of the wound edge.

With skin and orbicularis now removed, the surgeon is left to determine whether excess orbital fat should be excised. Fat excision requires opening the orbital septum to expose the central and nasal fat pads. Remember, the septum is a multilaminar structure. If fat contouring is desired, the septum should be held with toothed forceps and traction applied, placing the septum on stretch and equally important creating distance between the surgeon's scissors and the levator aponeurosis. Sharp dissection creating a small, central full-thickness opening in the septum is preferred. Once preaponeurotic fat prolapses through this opening, the septal incision can be safely extended nasally and temporally, exposing the entire fat pads and underlying levator. Failure to meticulously open the septum in such a controlled fashion can create button holes, allowing visualization of some orbital fat but inhibiting more appropriate graded sculpting of the entire fat pads.

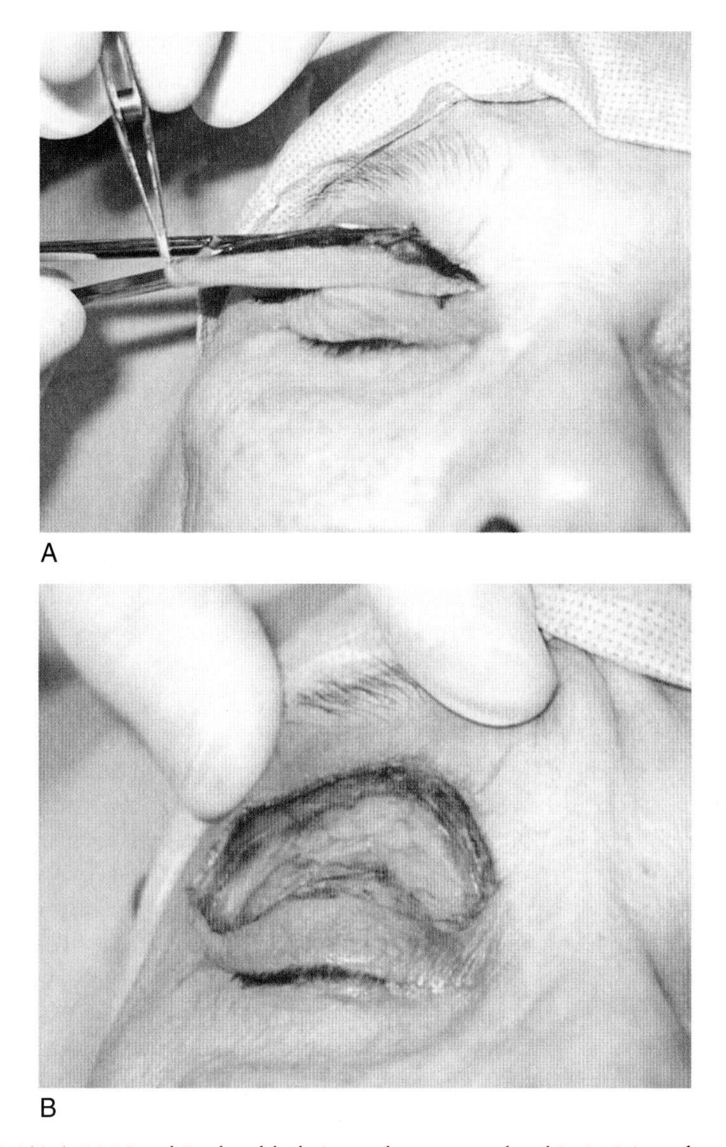

Figure 26-3 (A) A #15 Bard-Parker blade is used to create the skin incisions for upper eyelid blepharoplasty. The inferior edge of the skin excision should be placed in the eyelid crease. (B) Skin and orbicularis are removed en bloc down to the level of the orbital septum.

Gentle ballottement of the globe will prolapse orbital fat through the opening in the septum, promoting graded sculpting of the fat pads. Clamping, teasing forward, and Excised orbital fat that does not easily come forward with gentle posterior pressure is usually unnecessary and frequently uncomfortable for the patient. Excising orbital fat teased forward may continue to bleed further back in the orbit when released, even if cautery is applied. Furthermore, excess removal of orbital fat can yield a sunken appearance to the superior sulcus, creating an unwanted cosmetic outcome for the patient.

When performing bilateral upper eyelid blepharoplasty, following achievement of hemostasis in the first eyelid, attention should be directed to skin incision and skin–orbicularis excision on the contralateral eyelid. A damp gauze pad can be applied to the first eyelid to keep the wound clean and patient comfortable. With skin removed from both upper eyelids the surgeon can assess the lids for symmetry and make final adjustments prior to wound closure.

With excess skin and orbicularis excised, orbital fat contoured, and hemostasis achieved, the surgeon is then ready for closure. Deep sutures or suturing the septum closed is unnecessary, and if done the surgeon can inadvertently imbricate the levator and create a ptosis and/or eyelid retraction. A majority of the time closure is skin to skin using small dissolvable suture in an interrupted or running fashion. The location of greatest tension on wound closure is typically temporally, just supero-lateral to the lateral canthus. Placing the first suture at this location lines up the incisions nicely, and unless excess skin is removed the remainder of closure should be relatively tension-free. Interrupted fashion, while more time-consuming for the surgeon, is preferred as it leaves small gaps in the wound following closure. These small gaps allow for egress of serosanginous fluid that would otherwise be sequestered behind the closure and would contribute to eyelid swelling and bruising. Patients should be counseled regarding these gaps and instructed on how to blot away draining fluid without breaking the fine sutures holding the wound closed.

When eyelid crease position is being surgically altered, an extra step occurs in closure to create the new lid crease. Remember, the normal eyelid crease is formed from anterior projections from the levator as it approaches the superior tarsal edge. Similarly, when surgically altering the lid crease position, the levator must be involved in the closure. In creating the new eyelid crease, the surgeon will pass the suture through the inferior skin edge and imbricate the levator before exiting through the superior skin edge. Thus, the wound will be tacked down to and move with the levator. Having the patient look up and down intermittently during closure will ensure proper placement of the sutures and illustrate the new lid crease. Proper placement is crucial, as securing the skin to the levator too superiorly or inferiorly can interfere with levator function, producing lid ptosis or retraction.

Following closure, a combination ophthalmic steroid and antibiotic ointment is placed along the suture line. Typically no bandaging or patching is performed, although a small gauze pad placed at the temporal aspect of the wound can collect draining fluid in the early postoperative period. Owing to the rich vascular supply of the eyelids, postoperative infections following blepharoplasty are rare. As such, prophylactic systemic antibiotics are not frequently prescribed. Patients should be cautioned regarding postoperative swelling and encouraged to apply cold packs for the first 18 to 24 hours to help reduce edema and bruising. Reminding patients about the gaps in the suture closure and interconnections of the upper and lower eyelids can comfort the patients and avoid concerned phone calls and pages when the patient wakes to discover lower eyelid ecchymosis.

26-4 CONSIDERATIONS IN ASIAN UPPER BLEPHAROPLASTY

Comparisons of the characteristic Asian and Caucasian upper eyelids underscore significant variations in anatomy. Although in general the classical Asian eyelid is

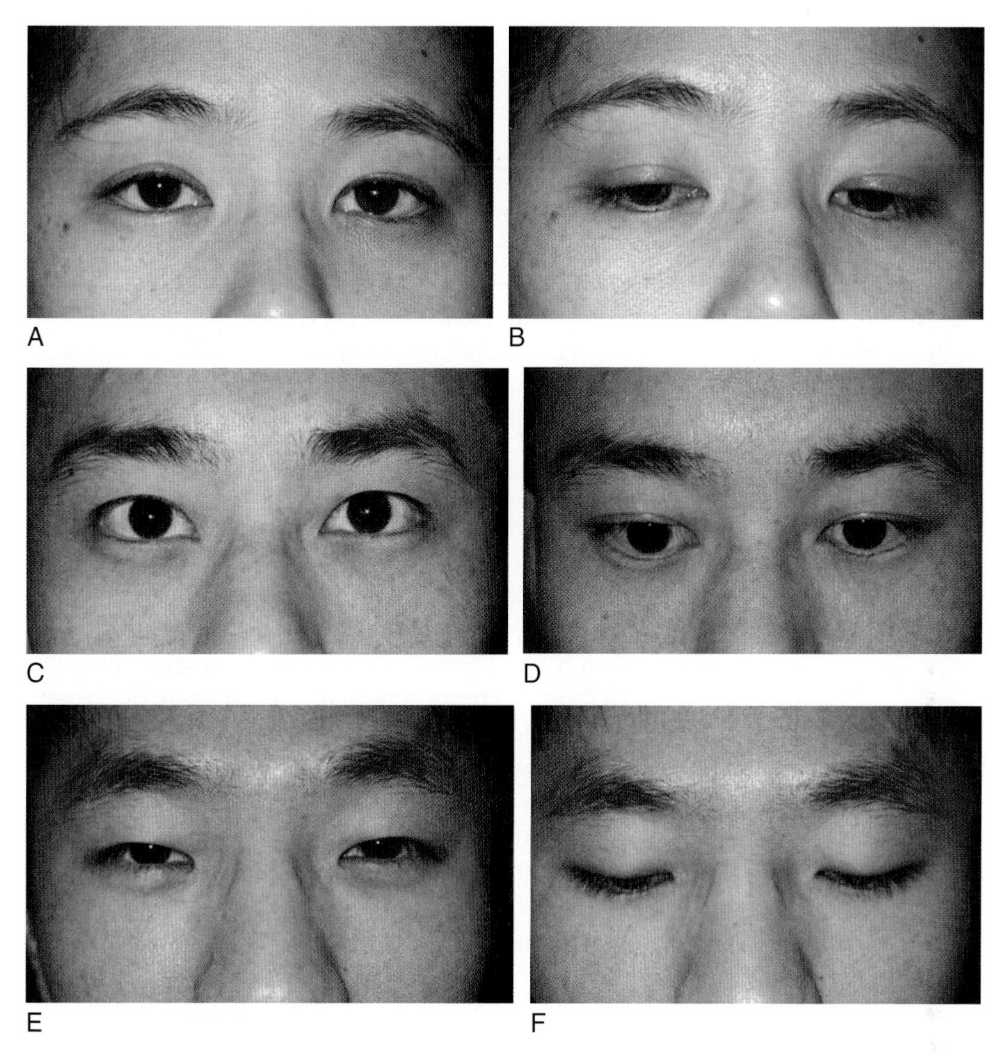

Figure 26-4 Three anatomic configurations of the Asian eyelid. (A) The Asian double eyelid with the pretarsal eyelid distinctly visible. (B) In down gaze, the eyelid crease is visible in the Asian double eyelid. (C) The Asian single eyelid with crease. The supratarsal fold extends down to the eyelid margin. (D) In down gaze, the eyelid crease is visible in the Asian single eyelid with crease. (E) The Asian single eyelid without crease. There is no supratarsal fold as the eyelid crease is nonexistent or very low toward the eyelid margin. (F) In down gaze, no eyelid crease is identifiable in the Asian single eyelid without crease.

fuller, with an absent or lower lid crease much closer to the eyelid margin, even among Asian patients there are different configurations to the eyelid anatomy (Fig. 26-4). This difference in appearance can be explained by examining the eyelid anatomy. In the Caucasian eyelid the levator aponeurosis and orbital septum intersect and insert on the superior aspect of the tarsus, some 8 to 10 mm above the lid margin. At a similar height, anterior projections of the levator attach to the overlying dermis, creating a well-defined lid crease. In the Asian eyelid, the levator likewise inserts on the superior aspect of the tarsus. The septum, however, inserts more inferiorly along the anterior surface of the tarsus. The anterior projections of the levator to the dermis are absent. Instead, preaponeurotic orbital fat is allowed to descend further inferiorly, creating a fuller eyelid appearance.

An additional feature of the Asian upper eyelid is a prominent epicanthal fold. The Asian epicanthal fold can override the medial canthus and caruncle and give the impression of a widened nasal bridge. Surgical modification, epicanthoplasty, can be an adjunct procedure during Asian blepharoplasty.

Prior to undertaking upper eyelid blepharoplasty in an Asian patient, the surgeon should obtain a clear understanding of the patient's expectations. The key determination is whether to create a more elevated and distinct lid crease. The creation of the so-called "Westernized" lid appearance is a popular surgery, especially in Asia, but most blepharoplasty patients will still desire to simply rejuvenate their natural lid position and contour.

If a new lid crease is preferred, the surgeon makes symmetric incisions at a suitable height above the lid margin on both eyelids. An incision height of 6 to 7 mm will create a skin fold about 2 to 3 mm above the lid margin. The blepharoplasty is performed with trimming of excess skin and graded fat sculpting. In younger patients only a minimal amount of skin is removed to allow the surgeon access to the preaponeurotic fat. Supratarsal fixation, incorporating the levator with wound closure, will complete the procedure, forming a new, more superior lid crease. If the lid crease is to be maintained, standard blepharoplasty is performed using the natural lid crease as the inferior incision.

A small amount of redundant skin is necessary for the eyelid to move appropriately. This skin drapes over the lid crease with the eyes open in primary position. With eye closure or down gaze, the redundant skin flattens out, enabling the eyelid to follow the eye downward. Patients and surgeons deciding to maintain a lower Asian lid crease should be conscious of this need for redundant skin over the lid crease. With a lid crease so close to the lid margin, even a small amount of redundancy can creep over the lid margin or obscure lash follicles and give the appearance of untreated dermatochalasis. Aggressively removing excess skin in this situation has the potential to produce significant lagophthalmos.

26-5 BLEPHAROPLASTY COMPLICATIONS

With upper eyelid blepharoplasty, the most serious complication is retrobulbar hemorrhage and vision loss. The source of hemorrhage is most often attributed to persistent bleeding from orbital fat that has been incompletely cauterized or allowed to retract back into the orbit before the bleeding could be adequately assessed. Significant bleeding can generate markedly elevated intraorbital pressure, elevated intraocular pressure, optic nerve compression, and compromise of the ocular vascular supply. On examination the orbit is tight and the globe frequently proptotic. Extraocular movements can be severely limited and often painful. Subconjunctival hemorrhage is common and intraocular pressure elevated.

Treatment is aimed at reducing intraocular and intraorbital pressure. Fortunately, the rise in pressure acts to tamponade the bleeding, which will have usually stopped before the surgeon assesses the patient and intervenes. Opening the surgical wound with or without a lateral cantholysis will often ameliorate the pressure escalation. Ocular hypotensive drops and oral acetazolamide will help with intraocular pressure. Infrequently further interventions, such as an anterior chamber paracentesis, are necessary to restore retinal blood flow.

Fortunately, postoperative hemorrhage is a rare complication from blepharoplasty, with significant vision loss occurring in roughly 1 in 40,000 cases. The presentation can be delayed, with significant bleeding occurring only after the patient has traveled home following surgery. As such, a patient calling the office complaining of significant pain following blepharoplasty should not be dismissed as normal postoperative discomfort, even if the surgeon noted an uncomplicated excision and closure.

The most common complications following upper eyelid blepharoplasty involve postoperative lid position and asymmetry. For each complication, management is fairly straightforward. However, careful surgical planning and technique are the best prevention.

A common problem following upper lid blepharoplasty is lagophthalmos. A small lagophthalmos following blepharoplasty can be anticipated, especially when combined with either lower lid blepharoplasty or blepharoptosis repair. Frequent lubrication will keep the ocular surface protected, and reassurance from the surgeon will help guide the patient through this period. More significant lagophthalmos usually results from excess skin and orbicularis excision. Alternatively, inadvertent imbrication of the inelastic septum during closure can produce a lagophthalmos. Elevating the lower eyelid via a horizontal tightening procedure can serve to narrow the palpebral fissure height and improve the exposure keratopathy induced by the lagophthalmos. Such an intervention is usually the procedure of choice. Skin grafting can improve the lagophthalmos but rarely provides an acceptable cosmetic result.

A secondary goal of upper lid blepharoplasty is achievement of bilaterally symmetric lid creases. The lid creases are the single most striking and important feature of the upper eyelids and a prominent focal point of a person's face. Even subtle differences in height or contour can attract the scrutiny of a postoperative patient. Again, the best treatment for asymmetric lid creases is prevention. Careful placement of the lid crease marking and incision are critical steps in maintaining proper lid crease position. Secondary to firm and broad adhesions of the levator to the skin, lysis and lowering of a lid crease is exceptionally difficult. If lid crease asymmetry is noted preoperatively, the lower crease can quite easily be elevated to match the contralateral lid by performing a supratarsal fixation. If significant asymmetry persists after blepharoplasty, a similar procedure can be performed to elevate the lower of the two lid creases. This is meant only to reform a new lid crease, not remove more skin and orbicularis. Excision of more tissue at this point could yield upper lid retraction and an equally displeased patient.

Ultimately, patient dissatisfaction ranks number one in blepharoplasty complications. Patient dissatisfaction occurs in the presence of a true complication or when the patient had different expectations than the surgeon. The frequency of the former can be remedied with increasing surgeon experience and vigilant surgical technique. Detailed preoperative discussion is vital in aligning the expectations of the surgeon and patient. Unrealistic expectations regarding anticipated postoperative appearance should prompt the surgeon to consider alternatives to surgery.

SUGGESTED READINGS

Becker DG, Kim S, Kallman JE. Aesthetic implications of surgical anatomy in blepharoplasty. *Facial Plastic Surg.* 1999;15(3):165–171.

Burroughs JR, Bearden WH, Anderson RL, McCann JD. Internal brow elevation at blepharoplasty. *Arch Facial Plastic Surg.* 2006;8(1):36–41.

Castro E, Foster JA. Upper lid blepharoplasty. *Facial Plastic Surg.* 1999;15(3):173–181.

Fagien S. Advanced rejuvenative upper blepharoplasty: enhancing aesthetics of the upper periorbita. *Plastic Reconstructive Surg.* 2002;110(1):278–291.

Fincher EF, Moy RL. Cosmetic blepharoplasty. *Dermatologic Clin.* 2005;23(3):431–442.

Gentile RD. Upper lid blepharoplasty. *Facial Plastic Surg* Clin North Am. 2005;13(4): 511–524.

Griffin RY, Sarici A, Ayyildizbayraktar A, Ozkan S. Upper lid blepharoplasty in patients with LASIK. *Orbit.* 2006;25(2):103–106.

Halvorson EG, Husni NR, Pandya SN, Seckel BR. Optimal parameters for marking upper blepharoplasty incisions: a 10-year experience. *Ann Plastic Surg.* 2006;56(5):569–572.

Ichinose A, Tahara S. Extended preseptal fat resection in Asian blepharoplasty. *Ann Plastic Surg.* 2008;60(2):121–126.

Jeong S, Lemke BN, Dortzbach RK, Park YG, Kang HK. The Asian upper eyelid: an anatomical study with comparison to the Caucasian eyelid. *Arch Ophthalmol.* 1999;117(7): 907–912.

Kim DW, Bhatki AM. Upper blepharoplasty in the Asian eyelid. *Facial Plastic Surg Clin North Am.* 2007;15(3):327–335.

Kim HH, De Paiva CS, Yen MT. Effects of upper eyelid blepharoplasty on ocular surface sensation and tear production. *Can J Ophthalmol.* 2007;42(5):739–742.

Li FC, Ma LH. Double eyelid blepharoplasty incorporating epicanthoplasty using Y-V advancement procedure. *J Plastic Reconstructive Aesthetic Surg.* 2008;61(8):901–905.

McCurdy JA Jr. Upper blepharoplasty in the Asian patient: the "double eyelid" operation. *Facial Plastic Surg Clin North Am.* 2005;13(1):47–64.

Morax S, Touitou V. Complications of blepharoplasty. *Orbit.* 2006;25(4):303–318.

Niamtu J 3rd. Radiowave surgery versus CO(2) laser for upper blepharoplasty incision: which modality produces the most aesthetic incision? *Dermatologic Survey.* 2008;34(7):912–921.

Purewal BK, Bosniak S. Theories of upper eyelid blepharoplasty. *Ophthalmol Clin North Am.* 2005;18(2):271–8.

Rohrich RJ, Coberly DM, Fagien S, Stuzin JM. Current concepts in aesthetic upper blepharoplasty. *Plastic Reconstructive Surg.* 2004;113(3):32e–42e.

Rokshar CK, Ciocon DH, Detweiler S, Fitzpatrick RE. The short pulse carbon dioxide laser versus the Colorado needle tip with electrocautery for upper and lower eyelid blepharoplasty. *Lasers in Surgery and Medicine.* 2008;40(2):159–164.

Ross AT, Neal JG. Rejuvenation of the aging eyelid. *Facial Plastic Surgery.* 2006;22(2): 97–104.

Seiff SR, Seiff BD. Anatomy of the Asian eyelid. *Facial Plastic Surgery Clin North Am.* 2007;15(3):309–314.

Trussler AP, Rohrich RJ. MOC-PSSM CME article: Blepharoplasty. *Plastic Reconstructive Surg.* 2008;121(1 Suppl):1–10.

van der Lei B, Timmerman IS, Cromheecke M, Hofer SO. Bipolar coagulation-assisted orbital (BICO) septoblepharoplasty: a retrospective analysis of a new fat-saving upper-eyelid blepharoplasty technique. *Ann Plastic Surg.* 2007;59(3):263–267.

Wolfort FG, Gee J, Pan D, Morris D. Nuances of aesthetic blepharoplasty. *Ann Plastic Surg.* 1997;38(3):257–262.

Yen MT, Jordan DR, Anderson RL. No-scar Asian epicanthoplasty: a subcutaneous approach. *Ophthalmic Plastic Reconstructive Surg.* 2002;18(1):40–44.

Zimbler MS, Prendiville S, Thomas JR. The "pinch and slide" blepharoplasty: safe and predictable aesthetic results. *Arch Facial Plastic Surg.* 2004;6(5):348–350.

27

Lower Eyelid and Midfacial Rejuvenation

CHUN CHENG LIN YANG, MD, MSC, M. REZA VAGEFI, MD, RICHARD L. ANDERSON, MD, FACS, AND JOHN D. MCCANN, MD, PHD

Over the past two and a half decades, techniques for midfacial rejuvenation have evolved. Midfacial rejuvenation has gained significant popularity among many aesthetic surgeons,[1] including the ophthalmic plastic surgeon. Yet rejuvenation of the midface remains a challenge for the aesthetic surgeon who seeks facial harmony. A variety of techniques and approaches are available,[2–26] yet no single approach is ideal for all patients. It is clear that the age-related anatomic alterations that cause patients to seek rejuvenation vary from patient to patient, and that many patients have more than one anatomic alteration that must be addressed to rejuvenate the lower lid.[1] The surgeon must address the individual needs of each patient for optimal results. It has also become clear that the lower eyelid and midface form a continuum that needs to be addressed in its entirety for optimal rejuvenation. To achieve this, the surgeon must understand the basic concepts important to lower eyelid and midface rejuvenation, which include an understanding of eyelid and midfacial anatomy, an understanding of aging changes of the lower eyelid and midface, and surgical approaches and nonincisional options.

27-1 AGING CHANGES OF THE MIDFACE

A full understanding of aging changes in the lower eyelid and midface is essential to successfully address midfacial rejuvenation. A harmonious facial appearance consists of a balanced relationship among all tissues of the face.[2] With age, disturbance of this harmony among midfacial tissues occurs. The aging process of the midface encompasses the lower eyelid, malar fat pad and associated structures, melolabial fold, and lateral perioral region.[3] Hester describes four important features of midfacial

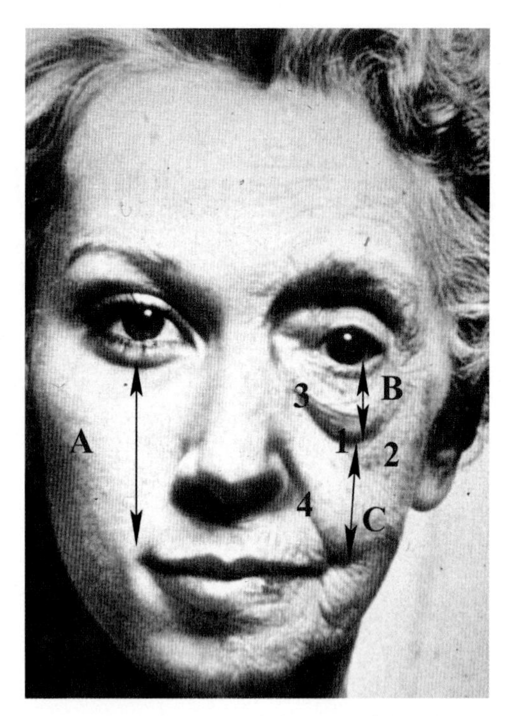

Figure 27-1 Split-face comparison of features of the youthful and aging face. The youthful side of the face has a single convex contour (A) with a short lower eyelid. The aged side of the face has a double convex contour (B, C) with a longer lower eyelid. Other features of the aging face are (1) baring of the inferior orbital rim with creation of a hollow valley at the junction of the lower eyelid and cheek; (2) descent of the malar fat pad, with loss of the malar prominence; (3) deepening of the tear trough deformity; and (4) exaggeration of the nasolabial fold.

aging: (1) baring of the inferior orbital rim with creation of a hollow valley at the junction of the lower eyelid and cheek; (2) descent of the malar fat pad, with loss of malar prominence; (3) deepening of the tear trough; and (4) exaggeration of the nasolabial fold (Fig. 27-1).[2]

27-2 ANATOMY OF THE MIDFACE

The midface represents a crucial aesthetic unit of the face. It is bordered by structures that play major roles in the overall appearances of the face. The lower eyelid and tear trough toward the nose and the lateral canthus and crow's feet at the superior lateral aspect frame the midface superiorly. The nasofacial angle of the nose and lateral nostril defines the medial extent. Laterally, the midface is bordered by the sideburns and pretragal skin. Inferiorly, the nasolabial fold and the corner of the mouth define the lower extent of the midface.[2] Important anatomic structures to consider in the midface region include periosteum, fascia, ligaments, muscles, nerves, suborbicularis oculi fat, temporal fat pad, malar fat pad, buccal fat pad, superficial muscular aponeurotic system (SMAS), tear trough, and nasolabial fold.

27-3 CLINICAL EVALUATION OF THE MIDFACIAL REJUVENATION PATIENT

In choosing the appropriate surgical approach to rejuvenate the midface, the surgeon must first listen carefully to the patient's concerns and then correctly define the problem or problems that underlie these concerns. A mirror or digital photograph of the patient allows the patient to better describe his or her concerns without having to use terminology more familiar to the surgeon.

The evaluation of age-induced alteration of the lower lid should progress through the various layers of tissue in the lower lid. Infoldings in the epidermis can cause fine wrinkles in the lower eyelids, while excessive sun exposure results in alterations in the dermis with loss of elasticity and deeper rhytides as well as pigment clumping. These changes are best addressed using nonincisional techniques such as a medium-depth chemical peel or laser skin resurfacing (Fig. 27-2). The most common mistake made in facial plastic surgery is to attempt to address texture changes of

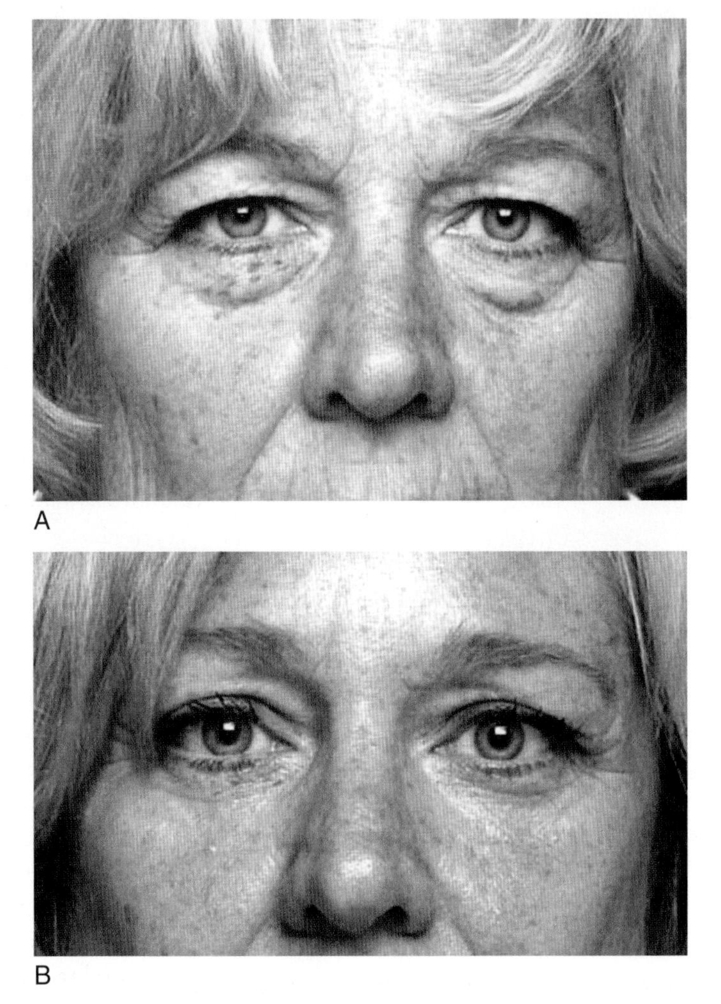

Figure 27-2 Patient before (A) and after (B) transconjunctival lower eyelid fat repositioning and a trichloroacetic acid peel. No skin was surgically excised from the lower eyelids.

the lower lids by removing skin from the infraciliary region. Most patients seeking rejuvenation of the lower lids do not have excess skin in the lower eyelids; they have texture changes in the lower eyelids. Removing skin from the lower eyelids to improve texture when there is no excess of skin will result in retraction of the lower lids. A minority of patients develop excess skin in the lower lids as part of the aging process, and in these cases removal of this excess skin is beneficial.

Just beneath the skin lies the orbicularis oculi muscle of the lower eyelids. Contraction of the orbicularis oculi muscle is responsible for the formation of the crow's feet wrinkles. Some develop scrolls of excess tissue in the pretarsal region when smiling. These changes of the muscle can be addressed with Botulinum toxin A injections (Fig. 27-3).

Deep to the muscle of the lower eyelids lies the fibrous supportive tissue of the lower lid. Loss of elasticity or laxity of these tissue results in sagging of tissue. Laxity of the lateral and medial canthal tendons results in the sclera being visible between

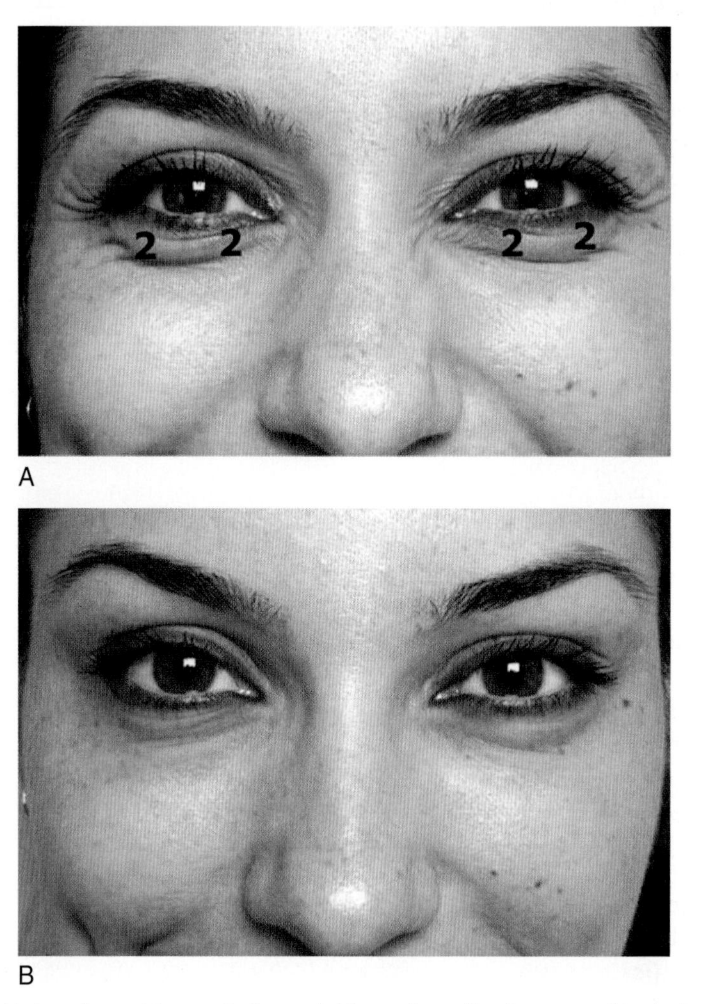

Figure 27-3 (A) A patient with crow's feet wrinkles and scrolls of excess orbicularis oculi muscle in the pretarsal region of the lower eyelid when smiling. (B) Patient after Botulinum toxin A injections into the crow's feet and the lower eyelid.

the lower lid margin and the inferior limbus. Laxity of the supporting tissue also results in the rhytides of the lower eyelid skin. This is why horizontal shortening of the lower lid is a common component of many lower eyelid rejuvenation procedures.[3]

A minority of patients actually have excess fat in the lower eyelid fat pads. Excess fat in the lower lids is typically not an aging change, but rather a familial trait present from youth. In these rare patients, performing a transconjunctival blepharoplasty and simply removing fat is a reasonable approach. For the vast majority of patients, however, performing a procedure where fat is simply removed from the lower lids results in a hollow, aged appearance.

The more common reason to develop a bulge in the lower lid with aging is descent of the midface. As the midface descends, a hollow or valley develops at the junction of the midface and lower eyelid. This valley converts the lower eyelid midface complex from a single convex contour of youth to a double convex contour (see Fig. 27-1). The first convex contour is formed by the eyelid and the second convex contour is formed by the cheek. In describing this aging change some patients will focus on the valley or "dark circle beneath the eyes" and others will focus on the convex contour of the lower eyelid or the "bag." Techniques to correct the double convex contour deformity focus on either elevating the sagging fat pads and associated fibrous support tissue or camouflaging the descent of the midface by repositioning eyelid fat into the valley along the inferior orbital rim.

The area of the midface just inferior to the malar prominence has the poorest lymphatic drainage on the face. Fluid tends to accumulate in this region of the face. The accumulation of fluid is more noticeable in the morning because of the formation of dependent edema, and this will improve throughout the day as the patient assumes the upright position. In some patients the edema never resolves during the day. This form of eyelid "bag" is quite difficult to treat and tends to worsen with any form of surgical treatment to the midface or upper face. If malar edema is a part of the patient's concerns, it is important to point out to the patient that surgery will not improve this area (Fig. 27-4).

27-4 CHOOSING THE BEST TECHNIQUE

Many techniques have been described to achieve midface rejuvenation.[2–26] Basically, the methods can be divided into surgical[2–22] and nonsurgical.[23–26] The choice of the appropriate approach depends on the clinical findings and the realistic expectations of the patient. The best-in-class methods of rejuvenating the lower eyelid and midface are currently in evolution, so no attempt will be made to describe the "best technique." Concepts that are important to addressing this area include surgical approach and dissection planes.

27-4-1 *Surgical Method*

27-4-1-1 *Lower Eyelid Blepharoplasty.* Traditionally, two techniques have been described to perform lower eyelid blepharoplasty, the anterior transcutaneous approach and the posterior transconjunctival approach.[5] The transcutaneous method involves removal of excess skin, muscle, and orbital fat through an infraciliary skin excision. This approach offers great exposure to the fat pads and little

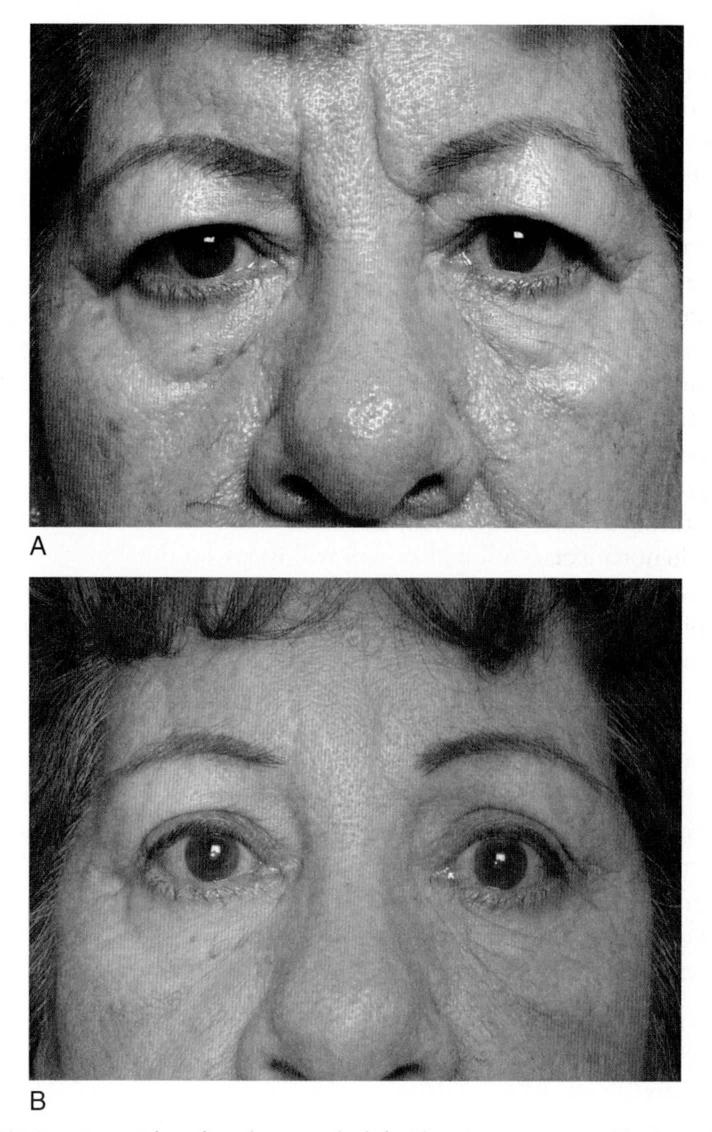

Figure 27-4 (A) A patient with malar edema on the left side prior to upper and lower eyelid blepharoplasty. (B) After upper and lower lid blepharoplasties, the malar edema is still present.

visible scar. However, the major drawback of this procedure is lower lid malposition, ranging from mild scleral show to frank ectropion. In some series, up to 20% of patients suffered this type of complication.[5] Lower lid malposition can occur from removal of too much skin, resulting in a cicatricial ectropion; removal of too much muscle, resulting in a weak or paralyzed lower lid; or scarring of the orbital septum and lower eyelid retractors to the inferior orbital rim. Due to the unsatisfying results of this technique, surgeons often avoid this approach when possible.

Over the past decade, transconjunctival lower eyelid blepharoplasty has gained great acceptance among surgeons.[5,6] The greatest advantages that this technique offers are hidden incision sites and reduced rates of lower eyelid retraction and ectropion when compared to the transcutaneous approach. Ideal candidates for the transconjunctival approach are the majority of patients who do not have excess skin in the lower eyelids. The transconjunctival blepharoplasty can be performed through two different approaches, preseptal and retroseptal. The last technique allows direct entry to the fat pads while maintaining an intact orbital septum.[5] The authors prefer to keep the orbital septum intact up to the orbital rim where it is lysed, as this encourages fat to displace inferior into the valley over the inferior orbital rim. In the minority of patients who are born with excess fat in the lower eyelids, it is a simple matter to conservatively remove fat from the lower eyelids via the transconjunctival approach. The more common procedure is to preserve all of the lower eyelid fat and to translocate it inferiorly through an opening in the orbital septum along the inferior orbital rim. Exposure of the inferior orbital rim via the transconjunctival approach also facilitates release of the orbicularis oculi muscle from its fibrous attachments to the lower eyelid at the level of the arcus marginalis (Fig. 27-5). Some authors have advocated suturing the lower eyelid fat into a subperiosteal or supraperiosteal pocket. The authors do not advocate this technique as it often results in lipogranuloma formation in the lower lids. In some patients there is little or no lower eyelid fat to translocate over the orbital rim. In these cases one should consider an alloplastic implant or nonsurgical options to add volume, as described later in the chapter.

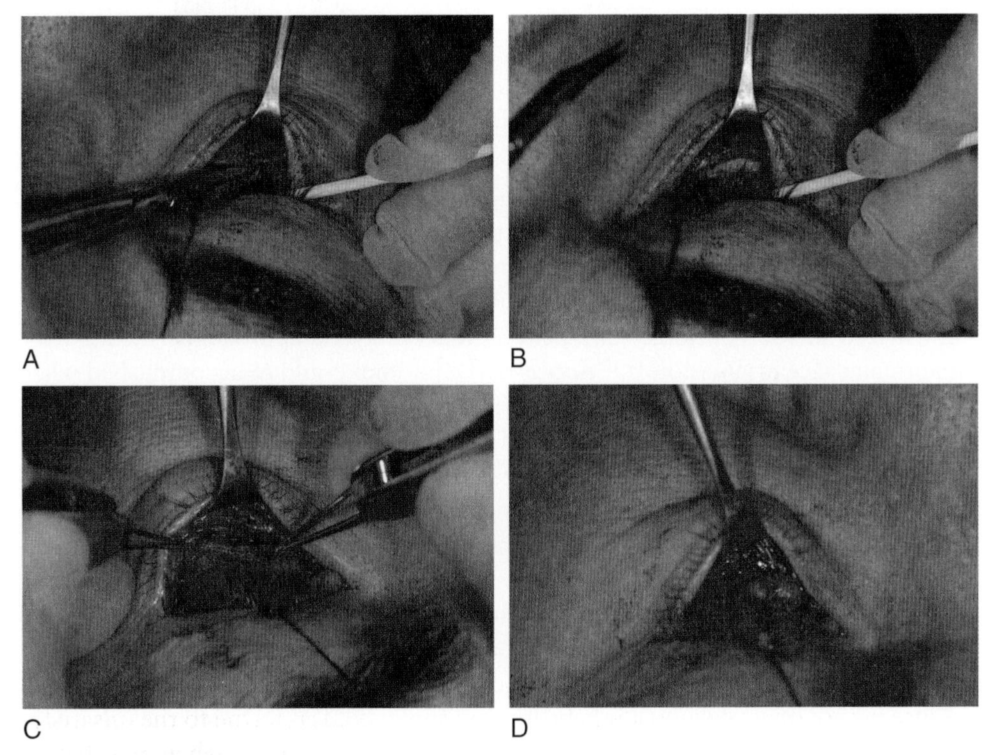

Figure 27-5 (A) Release of the fibrous attachments between the arcus marginalis of the lower eyelid and the orbicularis oculi muscle. (B) The bony inferior orbital rim is visible after completing release. (C) The lower eyelid orbital septum after release along the inferior orbital rim. (D) Prolapse of fat from the central fat pad of the lower eyelid beneath the orbital septum.

Horizontal tightening such as canthoplasty or a lateral tarsal strip may be employed at the time of lower lid blepharoplasty to address horizontal lower eyelid laxity. In selected patients who have texture changes in the skin of the lower eyelid, chemical peels or ablative laser resurfacing could be used as adjunct procedures for lower eyelid blepharoplasty. When patients have excess skin as opposed to texture changes in the lower eyelids, the authors address the bulging deeper tissues using a transconjunctival approach as described above, but use an infraciliary incision to conservatively excise the excess skin while leaving the orbicularis oculi muscle intact.

27-4-1-2 *Midface Lift.* Current surgical midface rejuvenation relies principally on elevation of the midface structures in a vertical vector.[2–4] When performing a midface lift, the surgeon must have complete knowledge of the dissection planes and understand the choices of the different surgical approach to address the midface anatomy.

There are two possible dissection planes allowed by the buccal branch of the facial nerve and zygomaticus major muscle. First, the surgeon may safely approach the midface superficial to the investing fascia of the zygomaticus major muscle. The retaining zygomatic cutaneous ligaments can then be divided, freeing the tissue overlying the body of the zygoma from the malar eminence. Dissection can then be carried inferomedially to free the malar fat pad, which is accomplished in a blunt fashion.

The second possible dissection plane involves the subperiosteal route. The periosteum can be lifted off the body of zygoma, releasing the origin of the zygomaticus major muscle. Dissection may be carried inferiorly over the masseteric fascia into the superior gingivobuccal sulcus. Carrying the dissection medially, the levator labii superioris alaeque nasi muscle may be detached from its origin adjacent to the inferior and medial rim. Caution must be taken to avoid damaging the infraorbital nerve and vascular package when dissecting over the mid-orbit in the subperiosteal plane. The periosteum of the midface is not compliant, so after releasing it from the bone it must be lysed horizontally to allow tissue to move superior.

Choices for the surgical incision to approach the midface for rejuvenation can be summarized in four options.[4] First, the midface may be approached through the preauricular face lift incision.[11–17] Access to the midface could be accomplished when performing either a subcutaneous face lift or a deep plane face lift. This method is effective, but it has limited durability and requires more extended recovery.

The second incision site that could lead to the midface is through a temporal approach. This is achieved when performing an endoscopic brow lift.[18–20] Through the temporal incision, the dissection can extend inferiorly on the plane immediately superficial to the deep temporalis fascia. At the level of the zygomatic arch, the dissection is transitioned to a subperiosteal plane. The branches of the facial nerve are avoided by keeping the dissection subperiosteal and over the anterior third of the zygomatic arch. Endoscopic guidance makes dissection of this plane safer. An endoscopic-assisted midface lift not only provides aesthetic improvement, but this technique has also been described to elevate the midface in patients with cicatricial and paralytic ectropion.[18] A very similar approach to the midface can be made via the upper eyelid blepharoplasty incision. This allows for a shorter dissection as well as direct fixation of elevated tissues to the dense periosteum over the superior lateral orbital rim.

A third approach to the midface is through the lower blepharoplasty incision. If the patient is undergoing lower eyelid blepharoplasty, the midface can be approached through the transconjunctival incision. Dissection can be carried out either in a superficial or subperiosteal plane. Complementary to this technique is lower eyelid fat repositioning. This approach is also used when lower eyelid retraction or malposition secondary to complicated blepharoplasties is corrected, using grafting material such as hard palate mucosa[8,9] or dermis graft.[9,10]

Finally, a less commonly used approach to the midface is the transoral, which consists of making a small incision in the gingival buccal sulcus to reach the subperiosteal plane of the midface. The transoral approach is typically combined with a second incision to facilitate fixation of the elevated tissues. This approach is often used when an alloplastic implant is to be used in conjunction to rejuvenate the midface.[4]

27-4-2 *Nonsurgical Technique*. Over the past few years, some nonincisional techniques to achieve lower eyelid and midfacial rejuvenation have been described, including injection of fat-dissolving agent to dissolve the lower eyelid fat[7] and injection of dermal filler to treat the aging midface.[23–26] These nonsurgical procedures share the main advantage of a short recovery period. However; some disadvantages and discomforts are also associated with these techniques, including transient burning and

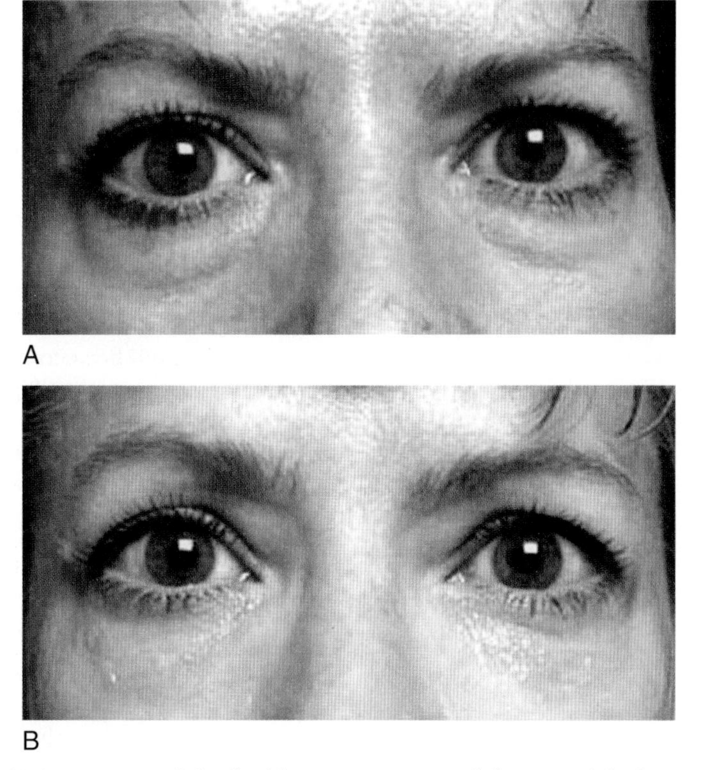

Figure 27-6 (A) Appearance of the double convex contour deformity of the lower eyelid before and (B) after injection of cross-linked hyaluronic acid into the valley where the lower eyelid and cheek meet.

erythema at the injection site; contour irregularities; bruising, swelling, and color change of the tissues; and the fact that the results are temporary, requiring reapplication of the treatment.

In reviewing Ablon and Rotunda's report on their experience with injecting phosphatidylcholine, a fat-dissolving agent, to treat lower eyelid fat pads, Weiss and Carraway[7] recommend a critical review of this technique, which has the potential risk of vascular injection, severe scarring of fat and scarring of muscle, and orbital injury. Nonincisional techniques for removing fat also suffer from the fact that the vast majority of patients do not have excess fat, but rather paucity or shifting of fat. In the majority of patients, removal of fat from the lower eyelids, whether performed with surgery or injections, will result in a hollow, aged appearance to the lower eyelids.

On the other hand, Kane,[23] Goldberg and Fiaschetti,[24] and Steinsapir and Steinsapir[26] report encouraging temporary aesthetic results using hyaluronic acid gel to add volume along the inferior orbital rim and to rejuvenate the midface, with effects lasting beyond 6 months (Fig. 27-6).[24]

At this point it would be useful for the reader to reconsider the anatomic alterations that define aging of the midface: (1) baring of the inferior orbital rim with creation of a hollow valley at the junction of the lower eyelid and cheek; (2) descent of the malar fat pad, with loss of malar prominence; (3) deepening of the tear trough; and (4) exaggeration of the nasolabial fold. Each of these changes is a result of volume loss or

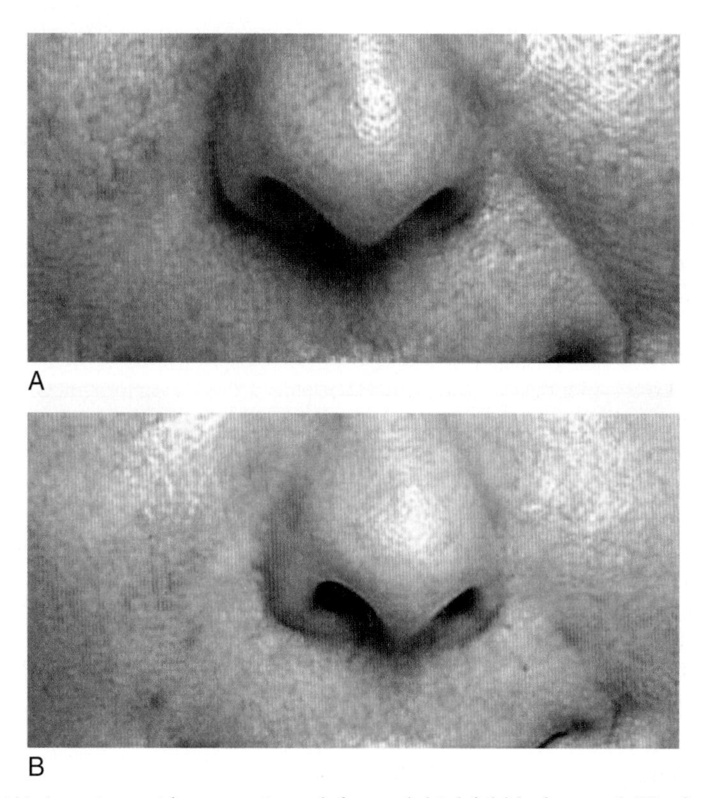

Figure 27-7 (A) A patient with a prominent left nasolabial fold before and (B) after injection of cross-linked hyaluronic acid filler into the nasolabial folds.

inferior shifting of facial volume with age. Each of these changes is potentially correctable by adding volume along the inferior orbital rim, over the malar prominence, over the tear trough, or in the nasolabial fold. The realization that most aging changes of the midface can be corrected by the addition of volume is no doubt why we see correction of these problems shifting more and more toward nonincisional techniques, such as filler and fat injections. The authors of this chapter commonly combine nonincisional techniques such as filler injections with incisional techniques such as fat repositioning to achieve optimal results (Fig. 27-7).

27-5 CONCLUSION

Lower eyelid and midfacial rejuvenation is a challenge for the aesthetic surgeon, and it involves a combination of procedures that must be tailored to the needs of the patient. The "best techniques" are currently in a state of evolution and no single technique is likely to address all of the varied changes that occur in the lower eyelid/midface complex with aging. The most important concepts driving evolution of rejuvenating procedures are (1) treatment of the lower eyelid and midface as a single complex; (2) preservation of lower eyelid fat; (3) addressing descent of the midface; and (4) addressing loss of volume and shifting of facial volume with volume augmentation.

REFERENCES

1. Goldberg RA, McCann JD, Fiaschetti D, Ben Simon GJ. What causes eyelid bags? Analysis of 114 consecutive patients. *Plast Reconstr Surg.* 2005;115(5):1395–1402.
2. Paul MD, Calvert JW, Evans GR. The evolution of the midface lift in aesthetic plastic surgery. *Plast Reconstr Surg.* 2006;117(6):1809–1827.
3. LaFerriere KA, Kilpatrick JK. Transblepharoplasty: subperiosteal approach to rejuvenation of the aging midface. *Facial Plast Surg.* 2003;19(2):157–170.
4. Finn JC. An overview of techniques, indications, and approaches to the midface lift. *Dermatol Clin North Am.* 2005; 23:505–514.
5. Kikkawa DO, Kim JW. Lower-eyelid blepharoplasty. *Int Ophthalmol Clin.* 1997;37(3):163–178.
6. Nessif PS. Lower blepharoplasty: transconjunctival fat repositioning. *Otolaryngol Clin North Am.* 2007;40:381–390.
7. Weiss DD, Carraway JH. Eyelid rejuvenation: a marriage of old and new. *Curr Opin Otolaryngol Head Neck Surg.* 2005;13:248–254.
8. Ben Simon GJ, Lee S, Schwarcz RM, McCann JD, et al. Subperiosteal midface lift with or without a hard palate mucosal graft for correction of lower eyelid retraction. *Ophthalmology.* 2006;113(10):1869–1873.
9. Li TG, Shorr N, Goldberg RA. Comparison of the efficacy of hard palate grafts with acellular human dermis grafts in lower eyelid surgery. *Plast Reconstr Surg.* 2005; 116(3):873–878.
10. Shorr N, Perry JD, Goldberg RA, et al. The safety and application of acellular human dermal allograft in ophthalmic plastic and reconstructive surgery. *Ophthal Plast Reconstr Surg.* 2000;16(3):223–230.
11. Hamra ST. A study of the long-term effect of malar fat repositioning in face lift surgery: short-term success but long-term failure. *Plast Reconstr Surg.* 2002;110(3):940–951.

12. Freeman MS. Rejuvenation of the midface. *Facial Plast Surg.* 2003;19(2):223–236.
13. Frankel AS. Midfacial rejuvenation: personal experience and philosophy. *Facial Plast Surg.* 2003;19(2):185–198.
14. Owsley JQ, Zweifler M. Midface lift of the malar fat pad: technical advances. *Plast Reconstr Surg.* 2002;110(2):674–685.
15. De Cordier BC, de la Torre IJ, Al-Hakeem MS, et al. Rejuvenation of the midface by elevating the malar fat pad: review of technique, cases, and complications. *Plast Reconstr Surg.* 2002;110(6):1526–1536.
16. Moelleken BR. Midfacial rejuvenation. *Facial Plast Surg.* 2003;19(2):209–221.
17. Ferreira LM, Horibe KE. Understanding the finger-assisted malar elevation technique in face lift. *Plast Reconstr Surg.* 2006;118(3):731–740.
18. Sullivan SA, Dailey RA. Endoscopic subperiosteal midface lift. Surgical technique with indications and outcomes. *Ophthal Plast Reconstr Surg.* 2002;18(5):319–330.
19. Williams EF, Lam SM. Midfacial rejuvenation via an endoscopic brow lift approach: a review of technique. *Facial Plast Surg.* 2003;19(2):147–156.
20. Quatela VC, Jacono AA. The extended centrolateral endoscopic midface lift. *Facial Plast Surg.* 2003;19(2):119–207.
21. Terino EO. Three-dimensional facial contouring: utilizing upper-midface suspension technology and alloplastic augmentation. *Facial Plast Surg.* 2003;19(2):171–184.
22. Monheit GD. Suspension for the aging face. *Dermatol Clin North Am.* 2005; 23:561573.
23. Kane MA. Treatment of tear trough deformity and lower lid bowing with injectable hyaluronic acid. *Aesth Plast Surg.* 2005;29:363–367.
24. Goldberg RA, Fiaschetti D. Filling the periorbital hollows with hyaluronic acid gel: initial experience with 244 injections. *Ophthalm Plast Reconstr Surg.* 2006;22(5): 335–341.
25. Kane MA. Commentary on "filling the periorbital hollows with hyaluronic acid gel: initial experience with 244 injections." *Ophthalm Plast Reconstr Surg.* 2006;22(5): 341–343.
26. Steinsapir KD, Steinsapir SM. Deep-fill hyaluronic acid for the temporary treatment of the naso-jugal groove: a report of 303 consecutive treatments. *Ophthalm Plast Reconstr Surg.* 2006;22(5):344–348.

28

Chemical and Laser Resurfacing of the Eyelids and Face

JOHN B. HOLDS, MD

28-1 INTRODUCTION

Chemical peels, mechanical abrasion, and more recently laser and electrosurgical devices are used to resurface eyelid and facial skin. The common feature in these techniques is the denaturation or removal of the skin surface. These techniques typically help to hide skin changes related to sun exposure and aging by evening the skin tone, decreasing dyschromia, and diminishing wrinkles. These techniques all require careful case selection and patient preparation with appropriate treatment and postoperative care. Recent interest has focused on less invasive therapy with techniques that leave the epithelium largely intact, shortening healing time and reducing the risk of complications.

28-2 INDICATIONS

Aging and sun damage induce a number of changes in skin, including wrinkling, the development of muscle- or gravity-related folds, irregular pigment or dyschromia, and the growth of benign and malignant skin lesions. Scars from acne, trauma, or surgery can also be indications for skin resurfacing. Potential benefit in all of these techniques must be balanced against risks and expected healing time.

28-3 PREOPERATIVE EVALUATION

A medical history must be obtained, looking for a history of immune dysfunction, prior acne, or a history of herpes simplex outbreaks. Prior treatment with radiation or isotretinoin (Accutane) may diminish the pilosebaceous units required for healing. Acne rosacea and cutaneous telangiectasia may be aggravated by skin resurfacing.

Cutaneous history must focus on scarring tendencies such as keloid formation, skin type, and ancestry. In particular, one must determine the patient's skin type, most commonly by assigning a Fitzpatrick's skin type[1] (Table 28-1). Patients with skin type III require careful topical preparation for skin resurfacing treatment in most cases, and patients with skin type IV or higher are more prone to scarring and pigment issues and are not treated with medium depth to deep skin resurfacing techniques by most clinicians.

Wrinkles may be graded by the Glogau classification scheme[2] (Table 28-2). This scale from "fine wrinkles" (type 1) to "only wrinkles" (type IV) will help to define

Table 28-1 Fitzpatrick Skin Type Classification[1]

Skin Type	Skin Color	Characteristics
I	White; very fair; red or blond hair; blue eyes; freckles	Always burns, never tans
II	White; fair; red or blond hair; blue, hazel, or green eyes	Usually burns, tans with difficulty
III	Cream white; fair with any eye or hair color; very common	Sometimes mild burn, gradually tans
IV	Brown; typical Mediterranean Caucasian skin	Rarely burns, tans with ease
V	Dark brown; Mid-Eastern skin types	Very rarely burns, tans very easily
VI	Black	Never burns, tans very easily

Table 28-2 Glogau Wrinkle Classification Scale[2]

Skin type	Age (years)	Findings	Treatment options
1, Mild	Early 20s or 30s	Early photoaging: early pigmentary changes, no keratoses, fine wrinkles. "Early wrinkles"	Topical retinoid (Retin-A, Avage) Alpha-hydroxy-acid creams/ peels Botulinum A toxin, nonablative lasers
2, Moderate	30s to 40s	Early to moderate photoaging: early senile lentigines, no visible keratoses. "Wrinkles in motion"	Type 1 treatment *plus* 15–25% TCA peels, microdermabrasion, injectable fillers; consider surgery
3, Advanced	50-plus	Advanced photoaging: dyschromia and telangiectasia, visible keratoses. "Wrinkles at rest"	Type 2 treatment *plus* 25–30% TCA peels, dermabrasion, laser skin resurfacing, surgery adjunctive
4, Severe	60s or 70s	Severe photoaging: dynamic and gravitational wrinkling, multiple actinic keratoses. "Only wrinkles"	Deep chemical peel or full-face ablative laser skin resurfacing; additional surgery to optimize result

the amount and type of treatment needed. These loose recommendations will generally hold true in determining effective therapy.

28-4 SKIN PREPARATION AND PROPHYLAXIS

The deeper and more invasive the treatment, the more important the role of skin preparation and prophylaxis. Patients are generally warned to avoid sun exposure for a month before and 2 months after treatment, at a minimum. The careful use of hats, sunblock, and sunglasses can aid skin preparation. Preoperative use of a topical retinoid (Retin-A, Avage) is beneficial in stimulating the basal cell layer and pilosebaceous units and appears to hasten healing and improve the final result with ablative skin resurfacing. Patients intolerant of these products may benefit from superficial therapies such as microdermabrasion, alpha-hydroxy-acid peels, and similar treatments.[3]

Botulinum A toxin therapy (Botox) may be administered in appropriate areas prior to skin resurfacing. Studies show that short- and long-term outcomes are enhanced after laser skin resurfacing with preceding Botulinum A toxin therapy.[4] A 4% hydroxyquinone bleaching cream should be started at least a month before treatment in any patient with residual tanning, chronic hyperpigmentation, or a Fitzpatrick III or higher skin type. Other bleaching creams such as Kojic acid may be employed in patients intolerant of 4% hydroxyquinone. The retinoids and bleaching creams may be resumed 4 to 8 weeks after an ablative skin resurfacing, as tolerated.

Antibiotic and antiviral prophylaxis is debated by clinicians. Routine antibiotic prophylaxis (ciprofloxacin [Cipro] 250 to 750 mg BID or TID for 5 to 10 days) can be argued against in healthy patients without risk factors undergoing uncomplicated procedures. Careful follow-up and excellent wound care are essential. Antiviral prophylaxis (valacyclovir [Valtrex] 500 mg BID for 5 to 10 days, beginning 2 days preoperatively) is prudent for full-face or lower-face treatments or in patients with a history of cold sores. Antiviral prophylaxis is probably unnecessary in most patients undergoing skin resurfacing limited to the periocular area.

28-5 ANESTHESIA AND PERIOPERATIVE CARE

Chemical peels are usually performed under topical, local, or even no anesthesia. Ablative laser skin resurfacing generally requires the injection of local anesthetic and conscious sedation or even a general anesthetic (especially for full-face laser resurfacing). Even for moderate-depth chemical peels, an anxiolytic such as diazepam (Valium) 5 to 10 mg orally is beneficial. Combinations of narcotics and benzodiazepines via oral or intravenous routes will aid patient comfort in more invasive therapies. The use of regional nerve blocks and a tumescent technique with dilute local anesthetic may be beneficial in treating large areas of the face.

Laser eye shields that cover the entire surface of the eye and cannot be readily dislodged are essential. Even with chemical peels it may be advisable to place laser eye shields and/or ointment into the eyes, in addition to careful monitoring of the placement of the peeling solutions.

28-6 CHEMICAL PEELS

The concept of chemical application to wound, burn, or coagulate the skin is an old one. Chemical peels run a gamut from light glycolic peels that only exfoliate the superficial epithelium to deep phenol peels that penetrate into the mid-reticular dermis as deep as any ablative skin resurfacing. A wide variety of techniques and reagents are possible. Individual skin characteristics or slight differences in preparation may yield widely different results. For this reason, the deeper chemical peels have largely been replaced by laser skin resurfacing.[5]

Light chemical peels use naturally occurring fruit acids such as alpha-hydroxy acids, or salicylic acid to injure the epidermis and exfoliate the skin surface. Often done in a series with increasing strength of peeling agents, recovery is generally quick and the risk of side effects is low. Improvement in fine wrinkles and dyschromia may be seen.

Medium-depth chemical peels attempt to injure into at least the upper reticular dermis. Common agents include 25% to 35% trichloroacetic acid (TCA) or Jessner's solution, a combination of salicylic and lactic acids and resorcinol. TCA peels require appropriate and careful patient selection and preparation. Depth of penetration is variable and dependent on a variety of individual factors. Penetration may be enhanced by a variety of means, including degreasing of the skin with acetone or other agents, multiple and wetter applications of the peeling agent, mechanical factors such as scrubbing the agent into the skin, and time before neutralization with or without occlusion. TCA produces a frost within 5 minutes when applied to the skin (Fig. 28-1). It is generally neutralized within 10 minutes using

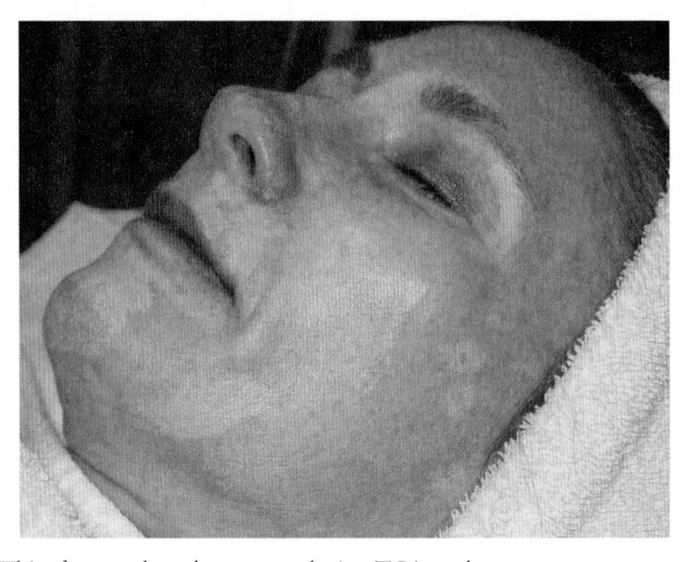

Figure 28-1 White frost and erythema seen during TCA peel.

wiping with wet gauze or towels to control the depth of burn. Cool compresses and head elevation with the application of an occlusive dressing or petrolatum aids healing.

Deep chemical peels using TCA in concentrations higher than 35% are unpredictable and are not performed by most clinicians. The classic deep peel is the Baker-Gordon phenol peel. Its use has declined markedly with the advent of predictable lasers for deep skin resurfacing.

28-7 DERMABRASION

Mechanical abrasion of the skin surface can be used to remove tissue into the papillary dermis. This time-honored treatment is commonly employed for acne scars, traumatic or surgical scars, photodamage, and perioral rhytides. A rotating fraize or wire brush is generally employed, although some surgeons even use sandpaper by hand to accomplish dermabrasion. Adequate anesthesia is required to accomplish this sort of treatment, and healing is variable depending on the site and depth of treatment. Postoperative care similar to that provided to patients undergoing ablative laser skin resurfacing is required. Laser skin resurfacing has replaced dermabrasion for many practitioners.

28-8 ABLATIVE LASER SKIN RESURFACING

Carbon dioxide (CO_2) and more recently Erbium-YAG (Er-YAG) lasers produce energy at infrared wavelengths strongly taken up by water. Delivered to the skin surface in a short pulse, these lasers have a largely ablative effect that removes superficial tissue and induces a variable amount of superficial thermal denaturation of collagen. Manipulation of the laser parameters allows for the appropriate clinical effect.

CO_2 lasers at 10,600 nm wavelength with a short pulse-width appropriate for skin resurfacing appeared first in the late 1980s. Strongly taken up by water, CO_2 laser energy above an energy fluence of 5 J/cm^2 will induce vaporization (Fig. 28-2). Early continuous-wave CO_2 lasers were unsuitable for laser skin resurfacing as they left behind a 200- to 1,000-μm zone of thermal damage. Limiting the pulse width to 1 ms or less maintains the pulse duration at less than the thermal relaxation time of the tissue (time in which the heated tissue loses 50% of its heat to surrounding tissue) with an acceptable 75 to 150 μm of surrounding thermal damage.[6] This is referred to as selective photothermolysis. Clinical treatments are generally performed in multiple passes, wiping char from the tissue before each successive pass. As water is the chromophore for photothermolysis, failure to wipe away char results in energy absorption rather than vaporization, with increased thermal damage. Likewise, progressively dehydrated dermal collagen left behind with subsequent laser passes absorbs more and more thermal energy with increasing depth of thermal damage. This effect may be desirable to a certain degree in inducing collagen contracture believed to aid rhytid reduction. Nonetheless, the potential for deeper thermal injury remains with CO_2 lasers, with the prospect of delayed healing, scarring, prolonged erythema, and permanent skin depigmentation (Fig. 28-3).

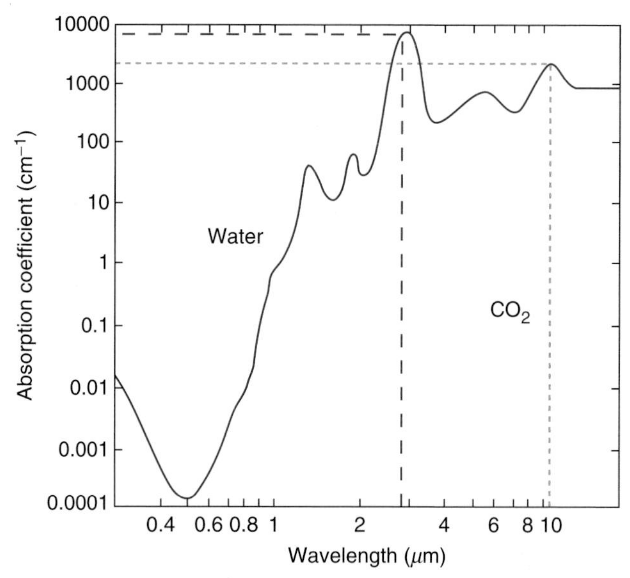

Figure 28-2 Graph of wavelength vs. absorption coefficient, showing stronger absorption of Erbium:YAG laser (2,940 nm) over CO_2 laser (10,600 nm).

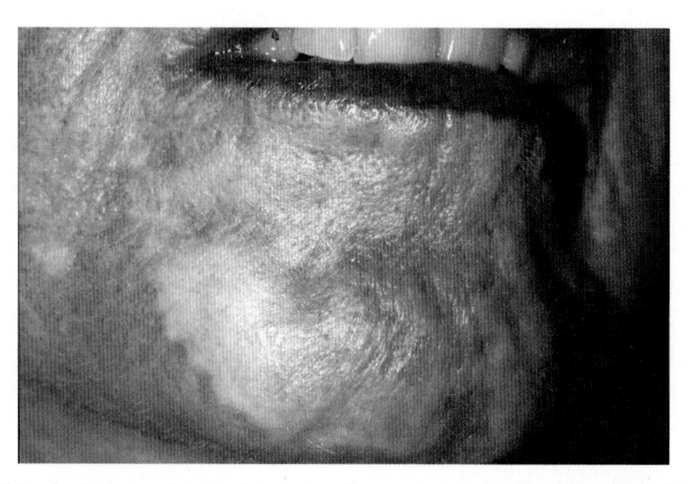

Figure 28-3 Skin depigmentation in the perioral area 6 years after CO_2 laser skin resurfacing. Skin depigmentation of this sort is generally permanent and much more common when skin resurfacing is performed with CO_2 laser than with erbium:YAG laser.

Medical Er:YAG lasers at 2,940 nm wavelength have appeared more recently. With an absorption coefficient in tissue 18 times that of CO_2 lasers, Er:YAG lasers produce a more purely ablative effect, with a 2- to 15-µm zone of thermal damage (Table 28-3), achieving ablation at fluences of 1.6 J/cm^2 and higher. Collagen also has a high absorption coefficient at this wavelength, so it serves as an excellent chromophore for Er:YAG lasers and vaporizes well. The depth of treatment will often be limited by pinpoint bleeding, and it is difficult in most situations to induce significant thermal injury in the skin. Complications generally relate purely to the

Table 28-3 CO_2 versus Erbium:YAG Laser Characteristics

	CO_2	Er:YAG
Wavelength (nm)	10,600	2,940
Pulse width (μs)	950	250
Ablation fluence (J/cm^2)	5	1.6
Tissue vaporization (μm)	20–70	5–200
Thermal damage (μm)	75–150	2–15*

*short pulse-width

depth of ablation. Clinically this translates into more rapid healing, generally shorter periods of erythema, and reduced risks of scarring or permanent skin depigmentation.

Enthusiasm for Er:YAG resurfacing was tempered early on because of a generally diminished clinical response noted with lesser rhytid reduction in comparison with CO_2 lasers. Early Er:YAG lasers were of generally low power, requiring numerous passes with prolonged treatment times. Treatment depths were not comparable to CO_2 lasers. Hughes'[7] study suggested that purely ablative Er:YAG laser skin resurfacing induced measurable skin contraction that was immediate and persistent. Further technological developments led to the production of long pulse-width Er:YAG lasers. The device that remains in production is the dual-mode Contour Er:YAG laser (Sciton Corp., Palo Alto, CA), which offers both a high-power (45W) ablative mode and multiplexing with 25 to 100 μm of controlled coagulative effect using a long pulse-width Er:YAG mode. Because of the reduced coagulative effect of even the dual-mode Er:YAG lasers in comparison with CO_2 lasers, the patient's appearance is fundamentally different early postoperatively, with much more oozing and pinpoint bleeding, but generally more rapid healing (Fig. 28-4) and similarly excellent long-term results.

28-9 POSTOPERATIVE CARE

Healing after chemical peeling, dermabrasion, or laser skin resurfacing requires the migration of epithelial cells with basal cell-like properties from remaining pilosebaceous units in the dermis. The high density of pilosebaceous units in the face explains the suitability of the face and general difficulty in other body sites in attempting to use these techniques. Likewise, the need to avoid irradiated areas or patients with permanent atrophy of the pilosebaceous units, as after oral isotretinoin (Accutane) treatment, is logical.

Immediately postoperatively the epithelium is absent and significant oozing, crusting, and scabbing occurs on the skin surface. Skin dressings such as 2nd Skin (Spenco), Vigilon (Delasco Corp.), or Flexan (Flexan Corp.) may be applied for 1 to 2 days to provide barrier function and lessen the patient's required care. The moist wound provides a fertile environment for bacterial, viral, or fungal colonization, and most patients are best served by switching to a bland petrolatum ointment with

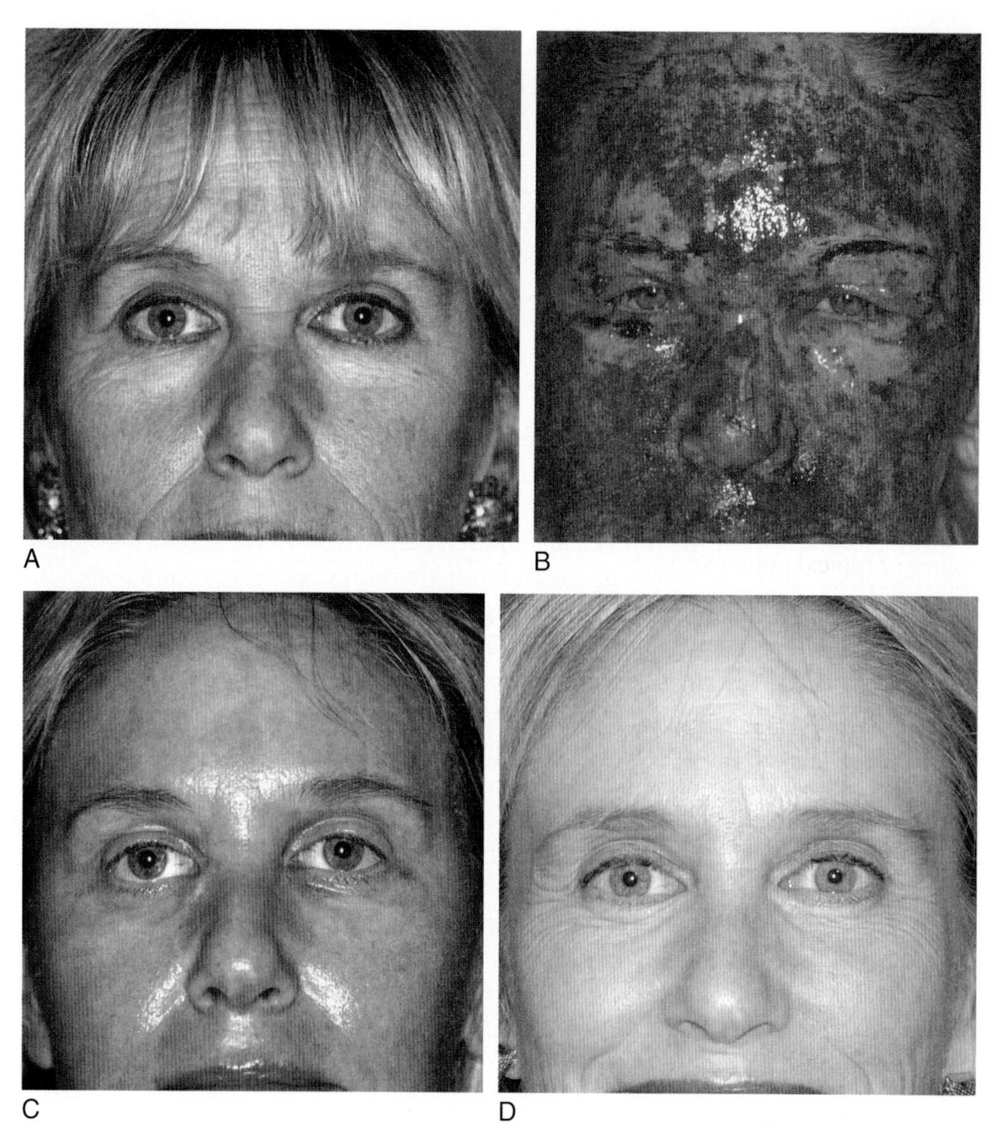

Figure 28-4 Er:YAG laser skin resurfacing and transconjunctival lower blepharoplasty patient shown with (A) prominent rhytides and dyschromia preoperatively, (B) 1 day postoperatively with serosanguinous oozing, (C) 9 days postoperatively with pink re-epithelialized skin, and (D) 18 months postoperatively showing excellent long-term results.

soaks of a cool dilute (1:50) white vinegar solution four to six times per day. Oral antibiotics and antivirals are continued, if prescribed.

The frequency of vinegar soaks and petrolatum reapplication can be gradually diminished as the skin epithelializes. Re-epithelialization is generally complete within 7 days after Er:YAG treatment, but requires up to 14 days after CO_2 laser resurfacing. Depending upon the depth of treatment, cosmetics can generally be resumed 3 to 7 days after medium-depth chemical peels and 8 to 14 days after laser skin resurfacing.

Prolonged erythema and potential post-inflammatory hyperpigmentation are ongoing concerns after skin resurfacing. These risks are dependent upon the depth of treatment and the patient's skin type. Appropriate treatment and wound care helps to diminish erythema somewhat. Topical steroid application and a number of vascular laser and other therapies are proposed to diminish erythema, although it is probably most dependent on the depth of thermal effect. Prolonged erythema does seem to correlate with risk of permanent hypopigmentation. Preoperative melanocyte stimulation and underlying Fitzpatrick skin type seem to correlate best with the risk of postinflammatory hyperpigmentation. This change will gradually respond to UV avoidance and bleaching cream application (4% hydroxyquinone or Kojic acid). Unlike hypopigmentation, which is generally permanent, hyperpigmentation resolves with time, although months of treatment may be required.

Hypertrophic or keloid scarring is uncommon. The first sign may be an area of itching with a thickened or raised area or web. This is most frequent in the perioral area or cheek or along the jawline. In most cases this will resolve with a short course of topical potent steroid (Temovate twice daily for 7 to 10 days) or the injection of triamcinolone (Kenalog) 5 mg/mL intralesionally in small amounts. Compressive silicone dressings may be helpful in persistent cases of scarring.

28-10 NONABLATIVE THERAPY AND NEW DEVELOPMENTS

A desire to achieve improvement in superficial skin characteristics or in facial wrinkling without the prolonged period of healing and erythema seen with ablative laser skin resurfacing has led to the development of a variety of devices using lasers, intense pulsed light, radiofrequency, or nitrogen plasma spray to injure and stimulate the dermis in hopes of evening skin tone and removing cutaneous dyschromia or fine wrinkles. These devices have their own list of risks and limitations, although they generally provide some level of improvement in aspects of facial aging with less risk and recovery time than that associated with the ablative laser skin resurfacing.[8]

Intense pulsed light therapy and a variety of visible light wavelength lasers are used to induce a nonablative injury to the epidermis and/or dermis, inducing a wound repair response with fibroblast stimulation and collagen reformation. A wide variety of equipment has been used with intense pulsed light to achieve improvements in skin tone, dyschromia, erythema, and fine vessels and wrinkles (Fig. 28-5). A variety of other devices are in clinical use for wrinkle reduction, including 1,320-nm and 1,064-nm Nd:YAG lasers, 1,540-nm Er:Glass, tunable dye lasers, and a long pulse-width He-Ne dye laser at 585 nm wavelength (N-lite). These devices have variable clinical indications, effect, and risks. Generally multiple treatment sessions are required, and no technology has emerged as a clear leader in this area.

Fractional laser resurfacing (photothermolysis) is emerging as a technology with potential indications in the treatment of dyschromia, rhytides, melasma, and acne scars. A variety of devices are available using nonablative laser energy versus ablative CO_2 or Er:YAG lasers.[9] Up to several thousand microscopic treatment zones are

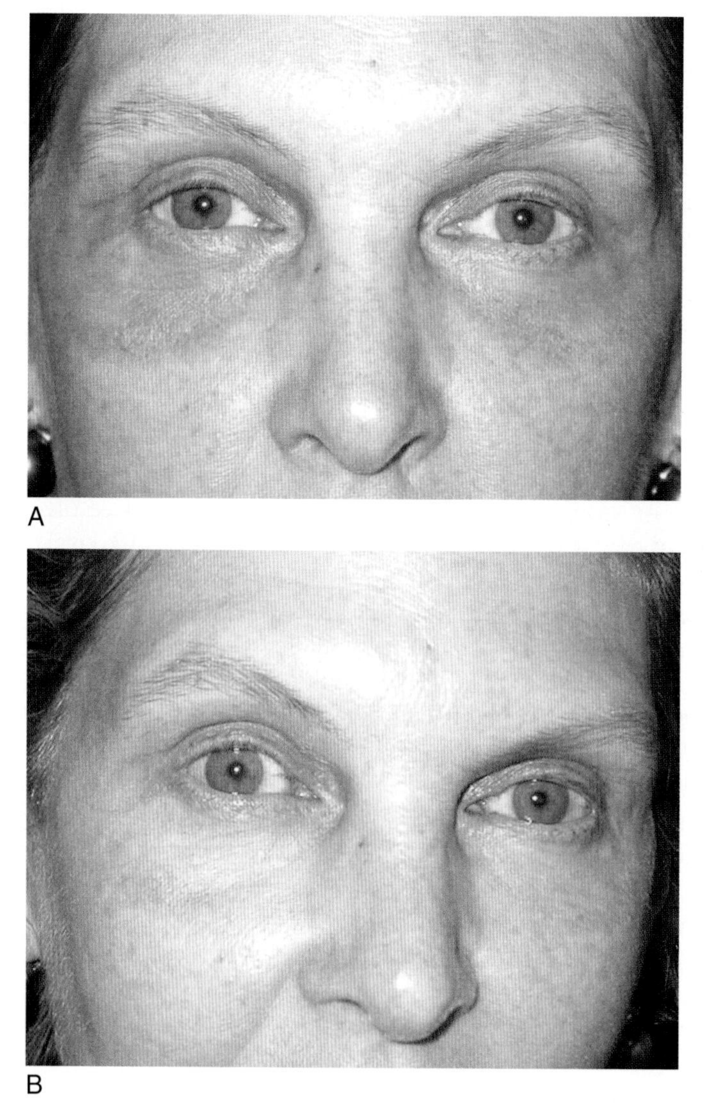

Figure 28-5 (A) Patient with persistent eyelid erythema 6 weeks after laser skin resurfacing. (B) Same patient 12 weeks postoperatively after three intense pulsed light therapy sessions, with marked improvement in erythema.

created per square centimeter of skin. This technology is evolving rapidly and offers the prospect of improved outcomes with markedly diminished recovery time.

28-11 SUMMARY

A variety of techniques exist to resurface the skin surface using mechanical, chemical, or laser abrasion to create an injury with a controlled depth. These techniques have varying equipment needs, benefits, and risks. Considerable improvement in skin tone, laxity, and rhytides is possible. Recent equipment developments focus on creating a dermal injury with lessened epithelial injury to lessen the time and risk during the healing phase. The optimal approaches with these new devices remain to be defined.

REFERENCES

1. Fitzpatrick RE, Goldman MP, Satur NM, Tope WD. Pulsed carbon dioxide laser resurfacing of photo-aged facial skin. *Arch Dermatol.* 1996;132:395–402.
2. Matarasso SL, Glogau RG. Chemical face peels. *Dermatol Clin.* 1991;9:131–150.
3. Draelos ZD, ed. Cosmeceuticals. In Dover JS, series ed. *Procedures in Cosmetic Dermatology*. Philadelphia: Elsevier-Saunders, 2005.
4. Zimbler MS, Holds JB, Kokoska MS, Glaser DA, Prendiville S, Hollenbeak CS, Thomas JR. Effect of botulinum toxin pretreatment on laser resurfacing results: a prospective, randomized, blinded trial. *Arch Facial Plast Surg*. 2001;3:165–169.
5. Roy D, Sadick NS. Ablative facial resurfacing. *Ophthalmol Clin North Am.* 2005;18: 259–270.
6. Kauvar AN, Geronemus RG. Histology of laser resurfacing. *Dermatol Clin.* 1997;15: 459–467.
7. Hughes PS. Skin contraction following erbium:YAG laser resurfacing. *Dermatol Surg.* 1998;24:109–111.
8. Shook BA, Hruza GJ. Periorbital ablative and nonablative resurfacing. *Facial Plast Surg Clin North Am.* 2005;13:571–582.
9. Tierney EP, Hanke CW. Recent advances in combination treatments for photoaging: review of the literature. *Dermatol Surg*. 2010;36:829-40.

29

Botulinum Toxin Injections for Facial Rhytides

MATTHEW P. OHR, MD, MARSHA C. KAVANAGH, MD,
AND JILL A. FOSTER, MD, FACS

29-1 INTRODUCTION

Once feared for its deadly properties, Botulinum toxin is now revered for its effectiveness as a treatment in minimally invasive facial rejuvenation. The injection of Botulinum toxin is the most frequently performed nonsurgical cosmetic procedure, with at least 4.8 million procedures in 2009.[1] First approved by the U.S. Food and Drug Administration (FDA) in 1979 for the treatment of strabismus, Botulinum toxin was shown to be both safe and effective for use to decrease muscle function. Botulinum toxin's cosmetic applications were first recognized when it was noted that facial rhytides improved in the areas of treatment with the toxin when it was used for noncosmetic applications in the late 1980s and early 1990s. FDA approval for cosmetic treatment of the glabellar furrows was announced in 2002, and off-label aesthetic indications have continued to evolve.

29-2 PHARMACOLOGY

Botulinum toxin is produced by the gram-positive, anaerobic *Clostridium botulinum*. The neurotoxin acts on the peripheral nervous system, where it inhibits release of acetylcholine from the presynaptic terminal at the neuromuscular junction.[2] There are seven distinct antigenic Botulinum toxins (BTX-A, B, C, D, E, F, and G) produced by different strains of *C. botulinum*.[3] The human nervous system is susceptible to only five of these serotypes (BTX-A, B, E, F, G),[4] and types A and B are currently available for human injection.

29-3 PREPARATIONS

In the United States, there are four commercially available Botulinum toxin preparations: three types of Botulinum toxin type A, OnabotulinumtoxinA or Botox Cosmetic® (Allergan, Inc., Irvine, CA), IncobotulinumtoxinA or Xeomin (Merz, Frankfort Germany), and abobotulinumtoxinA or Dysport (Medicis, Scottsdale, AZ). There is one preparation of Botulinum toxin type B, RimabotulinumtoxinB or Myobloc® (Elan Pharmaceuticals, San Diego, CA). Other Botulinum toxin type A products are anticipated to come to the U.S. market in the next decade as well. Different formulations of Botulinum toxin type A are biochemically unique and are not necessarily equivalent in dosing. The Botox unit is three times as potent as the Dysport unit,[5] but this conversion ratio does not take into consideration safety or antigenic potential.[6] Practically speaking, a range of 2.5 to 3 to one has been recommended to make Dysport dosing approximate the effects of Botox. For Xeomin, one may use the same dose as one would use for Botox. Botulinum toxins are measured in mouse units (MU) or (U). One mouse unit is defined as the median intraperitoneal dose required to kill 50% of a batch of 18- to 20-g female Swiss-Webster mice (LD50) over 3 to 4 days.[7–9]

In the United States, the Allergan formulation, Botox, is used for the majority of cosmetic treatments. Dysport use has been steadily increasing, and Xeomin is just recently introduced to the market. In the aesthetic realm, Botulinum type B is limited by its shorter duration. Myobloc does have a slightly faster onset, so it could be considered for a few selected indications of desire for rapid onset or failure to respond to type A toxin, but realistically the large majority of the treatments are done with type A. The rest of the chapter will refer to dosing applicable for Botox and Xeomin. For Dysport dosing, multiply the units by three unless otherwise stated.

Botox is a sterile, lyophilized (vacuum-dried) form of purified Botulinum toxin type A. Each vial of Botox contains 100 U of *C. botulinum* toxin type A, 0.5 mg of human albumin, and 0.9 mg of sodium chloride in a sterile, vacuum-dried form without a preservative. (Dysport is supplied in 300 unit bottles, xeomin in 100 unit vials.) The vials are stored in the freezer or refrigerator before reconstitution for clinical use. The recommended dilutant is nonpreserved or preserved normal saline. Whether use of preserved saline during reconstitution alters the dose, the response, discomfort at the time of injection, or the duration of the response is debated.[10–12] After reconstitution, the product may be stored in the refrigerator at 2° to 8°C.[13] Reports suggest that the material will retain potency beyond the manufacturer-recommended 4 hours, and that this effect may be prolonged by refrigeration of the solution.[14] Other studies show a loss of function with refrigeration.[15,16] Probably both are true, meaning that it is not necessary to discard the Botulinum toxin after 4 hours, but it is best to use it in a timely fashion to achieve the most predictable results. The concentration of the Botox solution is dependent on the volume of saline added and is typically described by how many units are present in 0.1 cc. For cosmetic uses, the reported concentrations of the solution vary from 1.0 U/0.1 cc to 10 U/0.1 cc. For most predictable results, control of diffusion, and diminished pain, we prefer concentrations of 10 U/0.1 cc to 2.5 U/0.1 cc. The reported volumes of solutions used for cosmetic indications vary from 0.025 cc to 1.0 cc per site. Since the vial of Dysport is 300 units, if one adopts the 3 to 1 ratio of dosing, it is easiest to just use the same volume of diluent in the Dysport vial that one would normally use for the 100U vial of Botox, and then inject the same amount of solution that one normally would have used with Botox. This makes the conversion seamless. It is also feasible to follow the package insert instructions for dilution and use the 2.5 to 1 conversion for Dysport, but this requires thought and calculation rather than the automatically familiar dosing pattern of Botox. The effect of Botulinum toxin type A is dependent on the location, concentration, and volume of solution that is injected. As described in the treatment section, we vary the concentration and volume to achieve the dose desired at a given location.

29-4 TREATMENT TECHNIQUES

Botulinum toxin is administered by injection into the target muscle. When treating wrinkles, the site of injection is chosen by asking the patient to squeeze and relax the muscles in the affected area. The surgeon then identifies the location of maximal skin displacement during the contraction of the muscle. The solution is injected at that site and into the muscle rather than into the crease line. Unlike "filler" techniques, the neurotoxin should be aimed at the muscle rather than the crease to be most effective. The injection should go into the muscle layer, or the subdermal tissue just above the muscle in the areas where the facial skin is thin. The muscles are relaxed prior to injection to decrease the pain of the injection. Patients can expect to experience the discomfort of the needle stick followed by a localized "stinging" as the solution is injected. There may also be some pressure sensation from the volume of the fluid injected. The onset of action varies from patient to patient and differs from one injection to another in the same patient, but most patients will notice alteration in muscle contraction within 24 to 48 hours. Onset may be more rapid with Dysport. In research studies, the maximal response in muscle weakness does not occur for 7 to 10 days. When describing the effects to patients, remember that the appearance of a skin wrinkle will continue to improve the entire time that the muscle relaxation is in place, so when treating wrinkles, the best effects are not seen until just before the muscle function begins to recover. The muscle-relaxing effects of Botulinum toxin are temporary and last 2 to 6 months after the injection. In subsequent injections, injections of the same volume, concentration, and location may have a different duration of effect in the same person.

Although it has been described in the therapeutic applications of Botulinum toxin, it does not appear that cosmetic patients will develop tachyphylaxis to Botulinum toxin. Where Botulinum toxin type A has been used for long-term treatment of dystonic muscle disorders, some reviews indicate that a "resistance" develops, while other reports show no long-term decrease in efficacy.[17] In contrast, anecdotal reports on the cosmetic use suggest that patients who have had multiple injections over a number of years may enjoy a lengthening of the duration of the effects. This is more likely to be the result of an increased improvement in the architecture of the skin that occurs as the overlying skin has the opportunity to remodel with repeated treatments rather than a true extension of the muscle weakening.

When the patient begins to notice the changes from Botox injection, there are two phases to the clinical response. The early alteration in the dynamic wrinkle lines stems from a relaxation of the resting tone to the muscle, decreased force of contraction, and a shift in the tissue fluids. This occurs during the first week. The second and more chronic process is remodeling of the dermis that occurs when the mechanical pressure of the contraction is relaxed. In addition to decreasing the wrinkle lines that are present, prolonged use of Botulinum toxin should prevent further deepening of the creases. This makes neurotoxin one of the few commodities that may prevent visible signs of aging. The most dramatic responses to treatment are seen in patients in the age ranges of 30 to 50. In these cases, the injections may obliterate the kinetic lines. With deeper wrinkles, treatment with Botulinum toxin will flatten the edges of the indentation, but additional filler techniques are usually necessary to make the area smooth. The neuromodulators may be used in association with hyaluronic acid gels, collagen, fat, polylactic acid solution, and other materials that mechanically elevate the depressed tissue of the wrinkle line. When considering simultaneous treatment, make sure that dilution and spread effects are not confounded by the filler material.

Preinjection counseling should cover the potential side effects and risks of the Botulinum toxin injections, as well as highlight the beneficial aspects of treatment. The side effects may be localized effects of the injection, or may occur when there is inadvertent spread of the material to the surrounding facial neuromuscular junctions. Small hematomas may occur when blood vessels are inadvertently injured by the injection needle. To help minimize this, digital pressure is placed on the injection site when the needle is withdrawn. Everyone experiences a small amount of transient redness at the injection site, as one might anticipate from an injection. This may last 30 to 60 minutes.

The incidence of unplanned spread of the neurotoxin in the cosmetic patients is low. The result of this spread depends on the area being treated and the amount of toxin used. Of these unplanned side effects, postinjection ptosis has been reported most frequently. Flu-like syndrome and headache have been noted. The albumin in Botox is a human product, and allergy to albumin is a contraindication to treatment. Although no teratogenic effects of Botulinum toxin have been reported, one might avoid planned injection of pregnant patients.

Botulinum toxin has been used for glabellar folds, lateral periocular rhytides, lower eyelid orbicularis ridges, mild ptosis, brow ptosis, horizontal forehead wrinkles, perioral lipstick lines, melolabial folds, and platysmal bands in the neck. It can be used as a single therapy, or in conjunction with other cosmetic surgical interventions. Botulinum toxin can be used to augment the results of laser resurfacing, chemical peels, wrinkle filler techniques, endoscopic rhytidectomy, and lower eyelid blepharoplasty.

29-5 INJECTION TECHNIQUE

Botox and Xeomin are supplied in bottles of 100 U and Dysport in vials of 300 units. The amount of saline added to the bottle determines the concentration of the solution. Some treatment techniques use the same concentration of solution at all locations, but other techniques vary the concentration at different locations. This may be accomplished by altering the dilution in the bottle, or by changing the concentration in the syringe. Altering the concentration in the syringe may theoretically result in uneven dilution, but this has not been found to be clinically troublesome. Injections may be given with a 1-cc syringe with a 30-gauge needle, or with a one-piece 1-cc insulin syringe. Insulin syringes have the advantage of less wasted material in the needle hub, but they have the disadvantage that the needle cannot be changed if it becomes dull or contaminated. Salvaging the last 5 U of Botox in the hub of the needle may be accomplished by drawing up 0.025 cc of air and tapping or shaking the solution into the head of the hub, using the air to push it through. Removing the top of the Botox bottle will allow the physician to retrieve an additional 0.05 cc of fluid.

Skin preparation varies from no prep to a 45-minute pretreatment with topical anesthetic and sterile cleansing techniques. For most cosmetic patients, the discomfort of the injections does not warrant the time necessary for the topical aesthetic to work, but for some it makes the injections more tolerable. Alcohol or iodine may be used to clean the skin. We use Betadine because it leaves a visible track of where the skin has been prepped that is helpful if the prep has been done by an assistant. A marking pen may be used to identify the locations of the injections. This helps the physician track the locations while injecting, assists the scribe in noting the locations in the chart, and also (with use of a mirror) allows the repeat patient to participate in location selection based on previous response. Many cosmetic patients are discriminating observers and will appreciate the opportunity to influence the design of their treatment pattern. Eyeliner pencil or dry erase markers make lines that are easily removed after treatment.

The dosing and concentration information given in the treatment techniques is based on Botox and Xeomin. This information can be altered to apply to Dysport or Myobloc once appropriate dosing ratios have been determined.

29-6 GLABELLAR FURROWS AND HORIZONTAL NASAL BRIDGE LINES

The glabellar complex was the first site targeted for aesthetic enhancement with Botulinum toxin. Even today, it continues to be one of the most common regions treated. Both the ubiquitous presence of glabellar lines and the ease of treatment in this area make it the most popular site for treatment. The first FDA-approved use of Botulinum toxin was granted for glabellar rhytides in 2002. Treatment of other anatomic areas at the time of this publication is considered off-label.

29-6-1 *Anatomy.* The glabella is typically defined as the region of smooth prominence between the eyebrows, just superior to the nasal bridge. Repeated contraction of the muscles of facial expression in this area leads to the development of vertical and horizontal rhytides. The vertical furrows that arise are secondary to the specific actions of the corrugator supercilii, depressor supercilii, and medial orbital orbicularis muscles that work together to depress the medial brow and adduct the soft tissue. Horizontal furrows at the nasal bridge develop as a result of the activity of the procerus and depressor supercilii muscles.

29-6-2 *Treatment Technique*. In general, when treating an area of the face, the physician starts with a plan for the total dose and has a preconceived map of what typical treatment patterns for that area might be. The physician then observes the particular patient for unique or asymmetric movement of facial expression. This is assessed by asking the patient to squeeze and relax the muscles acting in that area. For the glabellar complex, the locations of the anterior protrusions of the depressor muscles are noted about 5 to 7 mm above the brow cilia. These bulges are marked for injection. This is typically about 4 to 5 mm lateral to the vertical wrinkle lines. The patient may have two or more vertical wrinkle lines, resulting in a pattern of two to five injection sites. The two sides of the face may be asymmetric, and injection sites may be modified to accommodate for asymmetry.

Contraction of the procerus results in a horizontal line across the bridge of the nose. The injection site is marked 4 to 5 mm above the wrinkle line, typically in the midline. The procerus is usually injected centrally between the two brows, just above the bridge of the nose. A common treatment pattern involves two injections to each corrugator and one centrally targeted at the procerus (Fig. 29-1). Occasionally, the lateral extensions of the procerus muscles are injected with small doses of Botox to further efface the wrinkles on the sides of the nasal bridge.

29-6-3 *Dose*. In the glabella, the recommended total treatment dose, according to the Botox Cosmetic prescribing information, is 20 U.[13] However, starting doses from 10 to 80 U can be found throughout the literature and are based on individual considerations. The total dose is divided among the total number of injection sites. The units per injection are based on individual assessment of muscle function and goals of treatment. A typical concentration is 5 to 10 U/0.1 cc with a volume of injection of 0.05 to 0.1 cc per site. Compared to other facial locations, we use a higher concentration and lower volume in the glabellar area to achieve a higher dose with a smaller amount of injected liquid. This preference is to limit diffusion.

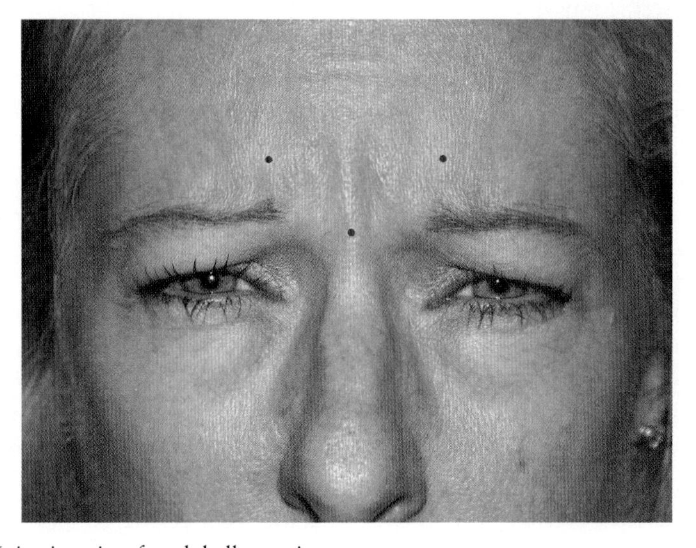

Figure 29-1 Injection sites for glabellar region.

29-6-4 *Special Considerations.* Women with thick sebaceous skin and highly mobile brows will require higher doses, and men may require doses in the 30- to 70-U range. Thin, female patients with relatively adynamic glabellar muscles are more likely to respond to lower doses.

Injection in the glabellar area may result in a low incidence of postinjection ptosis. This presumably occurs because of diffusion of the botulinum toxin into the levator muscle of the eyelid. Although no specific studies have been designed to investigate the factors that predispose the patient to developing ptosis, theoretically injection techniques that result in further diffusion of the toxin might seem to be also associated with ptosis—namely increased total dose, increased volume of injection, and closer proximity of the injection site to the levator muscle. It is also possible that the Botulinum toxin enters the superior orbit and reaches the levator muscle through a periosteal opening from the tract of the supraorbital nerve. Compression of the supraorbital neurovascular bundle with the nondominant hand at the time of injection may help to limit diffusion.

29-7 HORIZONTAL FOREHEAD WRINKLES

Contraction of the frontalis muscle leads to a pattern of horizontal forehead furrows and wrinkles. The goal of treatment in this region is to attenuate wrinkles while maintaining facial animation and brow position. The frontalis is a broad, vertically oriented muscle that originates superiorly at the galea aponeurotica; its inferior fibers interdigitate with the procerus, corrugator, and orbicularis muscles. It is typically depicted in two sections superiorly to reflect the more fibrous tissue located medially.

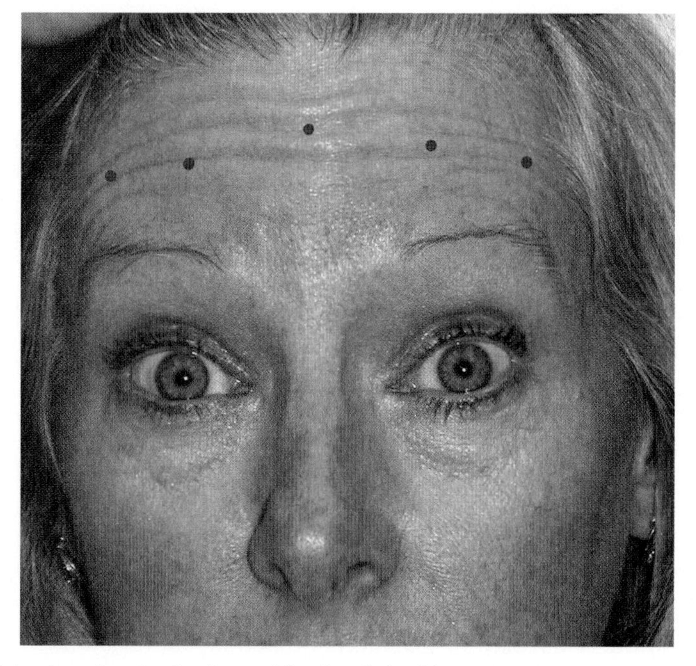

Figure 29-2 Injection sites for horizontal forehead rhytides.

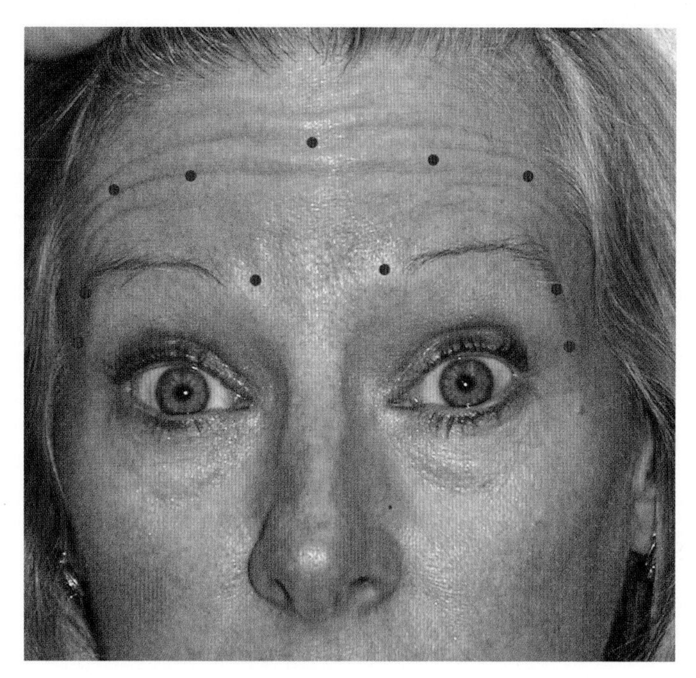

Figure 29-3 Injection sites for balancing forehead and brow position.

This variation in structure may explain why lower doses are needed to treat the central forehead. Contraction of this muscle elevates the eyebrows and wrinkles the forehead.

29-7-1 *Treatment Technique*. A thorough understanding of structure and function is necessary to achieve aesthetic goals in this region. Treatment patterns can vary widely, although a typical injection plan involves four to six sites (Fig. 29-2). Regardless of the pattern, all injections should be evaluated for the potential of creating excessive relaxation of the frontalis muscle, which may result in undesirable brow ptosis. While complete effacement of the horizontal wrinkles may be desirable to some patients, attention to balancing the weakening of the brow elevators and depressors is advised. The loss of frontalis function may be somewhat ameliorated by simultaneously weakening the depressors of the brow (Fig. 29-3).

29-7-2 *Dose*. The Botox Consensus Group suggests a total starting dose of 10 to 20 U.[18] While higher doses may be more effective, fewer doses are associated with lower adverse effects. In thin-skinned women, 5 to 10 U in the frontalis may be adequate. The total dose is divided by the number of injection sites, and a typical concentration is 2.5 to 5 U per 0.1 cc, with a volume of injection of 0.025 cc per site.

29-7-3 *Special Considerations*. Occasionally, avoidance of one of the more laterally placed injections (to prevent brow ptosis) will result in a temporal peaking of the brow position upon contraction of the frontalis, the "Spock effect" (Fig. 29-4). The resting position is satisfactory, but the patient will be displeased with his or her appearance on animation. This may be balanced by adding more lateral injections. The patient should be aware that this can limit the voluntary elevation of the brows.

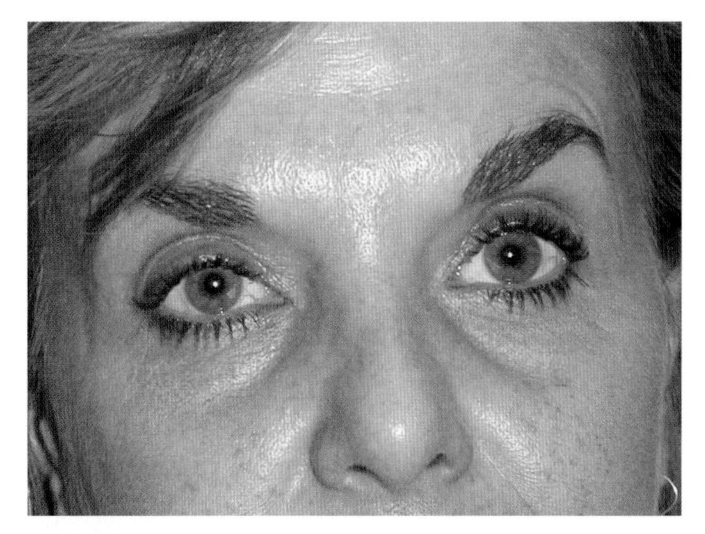

Figure 29-4 "Spock effect." Temporal peaking of the brow position upon contraction of the frontalis.

29-8 LATERAL PERIOCULAR RHYTIDES

Lateral periocular rhytides, or "crow's feet," are augmented by the contraction of the orbicularis oculi, whose fibers run vertically under the skin at the lateral angle of the eyelid. While the orbicularis closes the eyelids, it also functions as a depressor of the brow. Decreased strength of contraction and decreased resting tone will flatten the lateral periocular rhytides and also serve to elevate the temporal brow.

29-8-1 *Anatomy*. The orbicularis oculi muscle is the sphincter muscle of the eyelids. Anatomically it is separated into three divisions: preorbital, preseptal, and pretarsal. Contraction of the lateral portions of the preorbital and preseptal orbicularis is primarily responsible for these wrinkles.

29-8-2 *Treatment Technique*. The injections for the crow's feet lines are fanned along the lateral orbital rim. Typically, three to six sites per side are injected (Fig. 29-5). The injections are placed along but not inside the orbital rim. If the toxin diffuses into the area behind the septum, ectropion of the lower eyelid, epiphora, or upper eyelid ptosis may result.[19]

29-8-3 *Dose*. Depending on gender and treatment goals, total treatment dose ranges from 8 to 16 U per side in women and 10 to 16 U per side in men.[18] Total dose is once again divided by the number of treatment sites. For the lateral periocular rhytides, typically a total of 0.3 to 0.5 cc of 2.5U/0.1 cc solution, given in injections of 0.05 to 0.1 cc per site, are used on each side of the face.

29-8-4 *Special Considerations*. The thin skin in the lateral canthal area is occasionally complicated by troublesome postinjection bruising. Large vessels are visible through

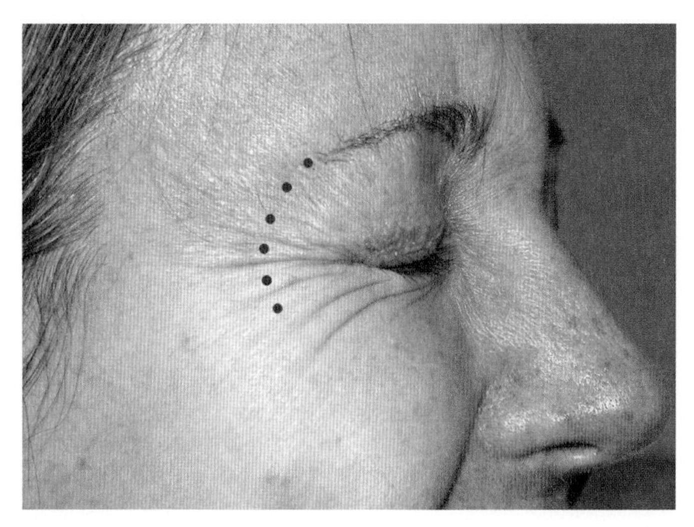

Figure 29-5 Injection sites for lateral canthus.

the skin and can be avoided, but smaller invisible capillaries will create localized ecchymosis. Gentle postinjection pressure along the lateral orbital rim may help to minimize bruising. Complete paresis of the orbicularis is not a desired outcome of treatment as this could result in decreased blink function. Epiphora, irritation of the eyes, ectropion, and redness of the eyes may develop. With subsequent treatments, additional injections may be added inside the lateral orbital rim to address the creases that come out from the lower eyelid to the lateral rim. This requires acceptance of a higher risk/benefit ratio than the injection sites along the superior lateral rim. Diffusion from the lower lid into the zygomaticus major/minor complex may result in alteration of the symmetry of the smile, a very undesirable side effect. Particularly troublesome would be spread across the orbital septum into the extraocular muscles, resulting in diplopia. Although these side effects resolve, cosmetic patients will find them difficult to tolerate. A more common but less troublesome side effect of the lower eyelid orbicularis treatment is subsequent lower eyelid edema. This may occur from decreased muscle contraction and transient lymphedema, or may be the result of herniated postseptal fat that protrudes more readily when the orbicularis is weakened.

29-9 BROW REPOSITIONING

Elevation of the brow and alteration in contour are also possible effects of treatment with Botulinum toxin. While the frontalis serves to elevate the brow, the procerus, depressor supercilii, and lateral orbital orbicularis oculi muscles serve as antagonists, depressing the brow. Isolated treatment of these muscles will result in elevation of the brow (Fig. 29-6). Contour can be affected by treating only particular depressor muscles, such as the lateral orbital orbicularis, to raise the lateral brow. This technique is also used as a balance when treating the horizontal forehead lines and one needs to counteract the weakening of the frontalis.

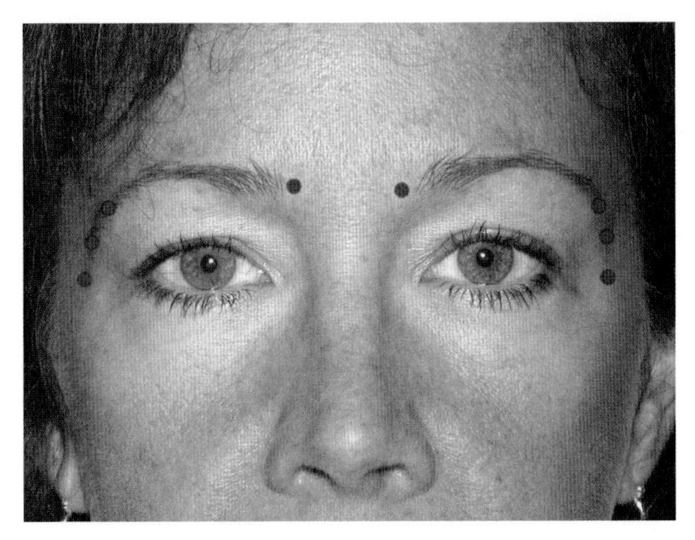

Figure 29-6 Injection sites for brow elevation.

The concentration of the Botox solution is 2.5 to 5 U/0.1 cc. The volume of the injection is 0.025 to 0.05 cc per site, and it is given into three to five sites per side.

29-10 "HYPERTROPHIC" ORBICULARIS

Contraction of the orbicularis oculi may result in a bulging of the eyelid that is exaggerated with activation of the muscle. Treatment of the lower eyelid orbicularis ridge may diminish this phenomenon (Fig. 29-7). In fact, enlargement of the palpebral aperture may also result with strategically placed injections. The concentration used in the lower eyelid is 1 to 2.5 U/0.1 cc. The volume injected is less than 0.025 cc per site. The injection in the lower eyelid is placed subcutaneously to try to avoid spread beyond the orbital septum to the extraocular muscles. This is a danger in this area for creation of extraocular muscle paresis and diplopia. The zygomaticus major/minor complex on the prominence of the maxilla should also be avoided to prevent lateral mouth droop.

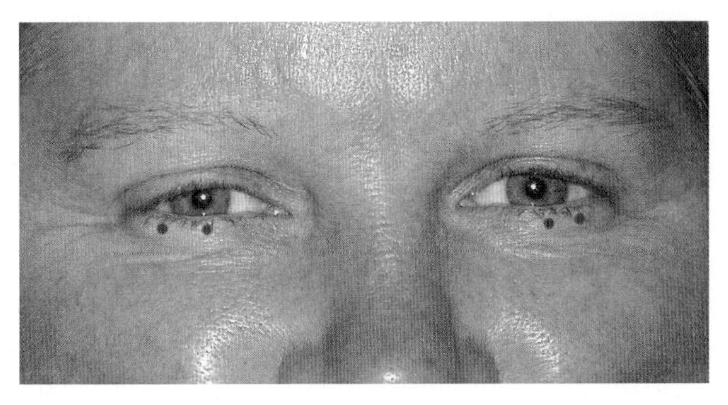

Figure 29-7 Injection sites for hypertophic orbicularis.

29-11 PERIORAL WRINKLES

In the perioral region, vertical ridges can extend above and below the vermillion border on the upper and lower lips. Often referred to as smokers' lines, they can result in significant dissatisfaction in a patient's perception of appearance. These rhytides develop from contraction of the orbicularis oris, a sphincter-like muscle that encircles the mouth. Smoking and sun exposure can accentuate the depth of these wrinkles.

Treatment to this region should be given symmetrically and in low doses. Treatment can be individualized by asking the patient to contract the lips as if kissing, while noting the vertical lines. The injections are then given just above the vermillion border on either side of the crease. The solution is diluted to 1 to 2.5 U per 0.1 cc and less than 0.025 cc is injected per site. The volume given should be just enough to create a bleb in the skin. Care should be taken to avoid the corners of the lips in order to prevent droop. Potential injection sites are demonstrated in Figure 29-8. Adjunctive treatment with soft tissue fillers may also be used. Weakening of the orbicularis alone may result in fuller lips as a result of a mild eversion of the upper lip.[20] In patients with a significant history of oral herpes, pre-injection antiviral medications may be given.

29-12 MELOLABIAL FOLDS

Lower face treatment with Botulinum toxin is more technique-dependent and carries more risk for inadvertent spread to adjacent muscles. The melolabial folds in the perioral region may be effaced with Botox treatment to the depressor anguli oris (Fig. 29-9); however, care must be taken not to overtreat this area. The total dose is 2.5 to 5 U per side. The concentration in this area should be in the range of 1 to 2.5 U/0.1 cc, and 0.05 cc may be injected at two sites per side.

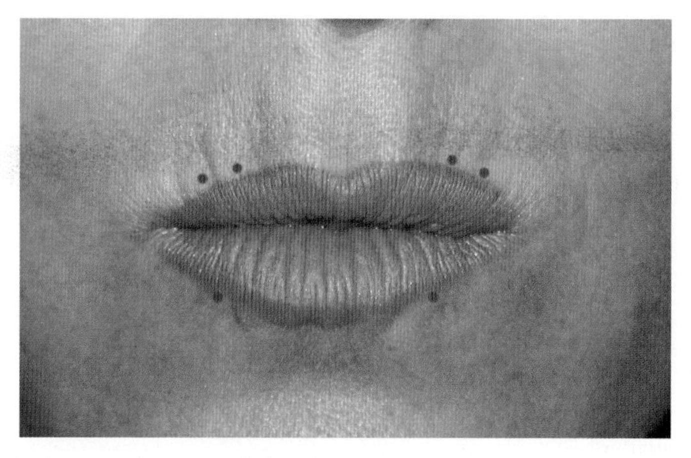

Figure 29-8 Injection sites for perioral rhytides.

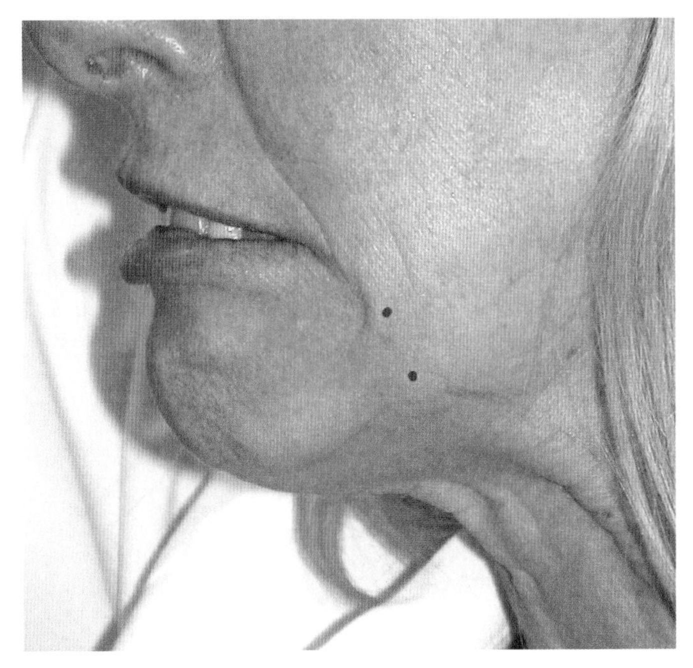

Figure 29-9 Injection for melolabial region.

29-13 PLATYSMAL BANDS

Prominence of platysmal bands is a feature of the aging neck. Loss of skin elasticity and changes of the fat tissue in the submental space result in vertical banding that may be amenable to treatment with botulinum toxin type A.

The platysma muscle is a thin, broad muscle sheet that originates in the subcutaneous layer and fascia covering the pectoralis major and deltoid. It inserts in the skin at the lower border of the mandible. Its action depresses the lower lip and jaw and can form ridges in the cervical skin when the jaw is clenched. High doses are used to soften these bands. Typically a total of 40 to 100 U is needed. The concentration of the solution is 2.5 to 10 U/0.1 cc, and 0.05 to 0.1 cc is injected per site. Three or four sites are chosen along each band (Fig. 29-10). The band is grasped between the thumb and the forefinger and the solution is injected into the platysma muscle or at the subdermal level. Some patients will notice the platysmal weakening when they attempt to elevate their head while in a reclining position.

29-14 ADJUNCTIVE USES FOR BOTULINUM TOXIN

The adjunctive use of Botulinum toxin type A in combination with various other aesthetic techniques continues to grow. Numerous combinations of botulinum toxin type A with other cosmetic surgical procedures have been described. As discussed previously in this chapter, Botox can be combined with injectable soft tissue agents in a synergistic manner to augment the results of treatment for facial rhytides.

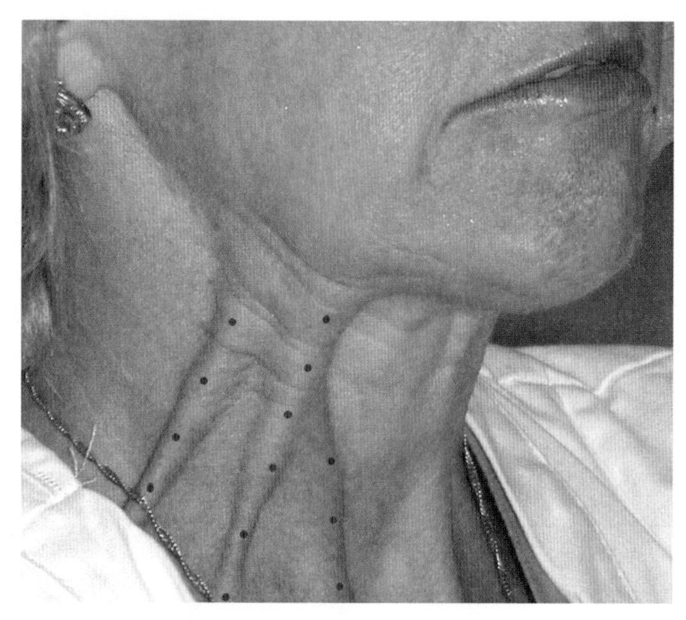

Figure 29-10 Injection for platysmal bands.

It has been reported to prolong the duration of results when combined with laser applications. It has even been used to immobilize lacerations of the face to improve scar formation.[21]

29-15 SUMMARY

The safety and efficacy of Botulinum toxin for various cosmetic techniques has been well documented over the past few decades. The evolution of treatment strategies continues to expand the role of this material once characterized as a poison and now seen as the liquid gold of cosmetic surgery.

REFERENCES

1. American Society for Aesthetic Plastic Surgery. *ASAPS 2009 Statistics on Cosmetic Surgery*. New York: American Society for Aesthetic Plastic Surgery, 2010.
2. Niemann H. Molecular biology of clostridial neurotoxins. In: Alouf JH, Freer JH, eds. *A Sourcebook of Bacterial Protein Toxins*. London: Academic Press, 1991:303–348.
3. Shone CC. *Clostridium botulinum* neurotoxins, their structures and modes of action. In: Watson, ed. *Natural Toxicants in Foods*. Chichester: Ellis Harwood Ltd., 1986:11–57.
4. Coffield JA, Bakry N, Zhang RD, Carlson J, Gomella LG, Simpson LL. In vitro characterization of Botulinum toxin types A, C and D action on human tissues: combined electrophysiologic, pharmacologic and molecular biologic approaches. *J Pharmacol Exp Ther*. 1997;280(3):1489–1498.
5. Poewe W, Schelosky L, Kleedorfer B, Heinen F, Wagner M, Deuschl G. Treatment of spasmodic torticollis with local injections of Botulinum toxin. One-year follow-up in 37 patients. *J Neurol*. 1992;239(1):21–25.

6. Aoki KR. Preclinical update on BOTOX® (Botulinum toxin type A) purified neurotoxin complex relative to other Botulinum neurotoxin preparations. *Eur J Neurol.* 1999;6:S3–S10.
7. Kautter DA, Solomon HM. Collaborative study of a method for the detection of *Clostridium botulinum* and its toxins in foods. *J Assoc Anal Chem.* 1976;60:541–545.
8. Schantz EJ, Kautter DA. Standardized assay for Clostridium botulinum toxins. *J Assoc Anal Chem.* 1978;61:96–99.
9. Schantz EJ, Johnson EA. Dose standardisation of Botulinum toxin. *Lancet.* 1990;335(8686):421.
10. Klein AW. Dilution and storage of Botulinum toxin. *Dermatol Surg.* 1998;11:1179–1180.
11. Alam M, Dover JS, Arndt KA. Pain associated with injection of Botulinum A exotoxin reconstituted using isotonic sodium chloride with and without preservative: a double-blind, randomized controlled trial. *Arch Dermatol.* 2002;138(4):510–514.
12. Kwiat DM, Bersani TA, Bersani A. Increased patient comfort utilizing Botulinum toxin type a reconstituted with preserved versus nonpreserved saline. *Ophthal Plast Reconstr Surg.* 2004;20(3):186–189.
13. Allergan Inc. Botox Cosmetic (Botulinum toxin type-A) purified neurotoxin complex (Package Insert). Irvine, CA: Allergan, Inc.
14. Sloop RR, Cole BA, Excutin RO. Reconstituted Botulinum toxin type A does not lose potency in humans if it is refrozen or refrigerated for 2 weeks before use. *Neurology.* 1997;48:249–251.
15. Gartlan MG, Hoffman HT. Crystalline preparation of Botulinum toxin type A (BTX): degradation in potency with storage. *Otolaryngol Head Neck Surg.* 1993;108:135–140.
16. Paik NJ, Seo K, Eun HC. Reduced potency after refrigerated storage of Botulinum toxin A: human extensor digitorum brevis muscle study. *Mov Disord.* 2006;21(10):1759–1763.
17. Klein AW. Dilution and storage of Botulinum toxin. *Dermatol Surg.* 1998;11:1179–1180.
18. Carruthers J, Fagien S, Matarasso SL, and the Botox Consensus Group. Consensus recommendations on the use of Botulinum toxin type A in facial aesthetics. *Plast Reconstr Surg.* 2004;114:6(suppl):1S–22S.
19. Lipham W. *Cosmetic and Clinical Applications of Botulinum Toxin.* 1st ed. Thorofare, NJ: SLACK Incorporated, 2004:11–20.
20. Fagien S. Botox for the treatment of dynamic and hyperkinetic facial lines and furrows: Adjunctive use in facial aesthetic surgery. *Plast Reconstructr Surg.* 1999;103:701.
21. Gassner HG, Brissett AE, Otely CC, Boahen DK, Boggust AJ, Weaver AL, Sherris DA. Botulinum toxin to improve facial wound healing: A prospective, blinded, placebo-controlled study. *Mayo Clin Proc.* 2006;81(8):1023–1028.

30

Soft Tissue Fillers for Facial Aesthetics

DAVID R. JORDAN, MD, AND
STEPHEN R. KLAPPER, MD

30-1 INTRODUCTION

The search for an ideal soft tissue filler to correct facial folds and wrinkles has gone on for at least 100 years. Many products have been tried, including mineral oil, paraffin, and liquid silicone, in an effort to improve soft tissue imperfections. Most of the early substances were abandoned due to a high incidence of complications, including chronic edema, granuloma formation, scarring, and ulceration.[1–3] The ideal tissue filler should be biocompatible, noncarcinogenic, nonteratogenic, nonmigratory, and free of adverse reaction. The ideal filler should also be inexpensive and easy to use, require little preparation, and provide long-lasting, natural, and predictable results with minimal recovery time.[4–14] Although no currently available injectable substance possesses all of these ideal attributes, many currently available products provide more-than-satisfactory results and have excellent safety profiles.

The indications for injectable filler agents have largely evolved through a better understanding of facial aging, specifically soft tissue deflation typically noted between youth and middle age. The limitations of surgical procedures to correct soft tissue atrophy, as well as the possibility of delaying surgical procedures by early intervention with injectable fillers, have made these agents very valuable in improving the appearance of the aging face.[15] With the continued improvement in products and techniques during recent years, the clinical results with fillers have become more predictable. As a result of this improvement, an increasing number of patients are seeking nonsurgical methods for correcting age-related changes to their facial skin and soft tissue.

There are essentially two types of natural facial wrinkles (or rhytides): dynamic and static.[14] They may occur separately or in combination. Dynamic wrinkles appear within the skin due to repeated contracture by the underlying muscles of facial expression. Static wrinkles are present regardless of facial dynamics and result from intrinsic changes in the components of the dermal ground substance and from extrinsic factors such as smoking, gravity, and sun exposure. The formation of both dynamic and static wrinkles is influenced by the quality of the natural collagen matrix within the dermal layers of the skin. For the most part, dynamic wrinkles are best treated with Botulinum toxin injections, particularly in the upper face. For some areas (e.g., deep glabellar lines), a soft filler in combination with Botulinum toxin may enhance the overall outcome. In the lower face, injectable fillers often serve as the treatment of choice for dynamic and static wrinkles or folds (furrows), as Botulinum toxin around the mouth can easily disrupt the perioral muscular contraction, with resultant speech difficulties, drooling, and problems with mastication.

Table 30-1 Comparison of Common Fillers

Filler	Source	Material	Duration	Placement	Overcorrection
Zyderm 1	bovine	collagen	2–4 mos	Superficial pap dermis	150–200x
Zyderm 2	bovine	collagen	2–4 mos	Mid-dermis	100–150x
Zyplast	bovine	collagen	2–4 mos	deep-dermis	none
CosmoDerm 1	human	collagen	2–4 mos	superficial pap dermis	150–200x
CosmoDerm 2	human	collagen	2–4 mos	mid-dermis	100–150x
CosmoPlast	human	collagen	2–4 mos	deep-dermis	none
Restylane	bacteria	hyaluronic acid	6–9 mos	mid dermis	none
Perlane	bacteria	hyaluronic acid	6–9 mos	deep dermis	none
Restylane Fine Lines	bacteria	hyaluronic acid	4–6 mos	superficial dermis	none
Hylaform	cockscomb	hyaluronic acid	4–5 mos	mid-dermis	none
Hylaform Plus	cockscomb	hyaluronic acid	4–5 mos	deep-dermis	none
Captique	bacteria	hyaluronic acid	4 mos	mid-dermis	none
Juvéderm Ultra	bacteria	hyaluronic acid	6–9 mos	Mid-dermis	none
Juvéderm Ultra Plus	bacteria	hyaluronic acid	6–9 mos	deep-dermis	
Radiesse	synthetic	calcium hydroxylapaptite	>1 year	deep-dermis	none
Sculptra	synthetic	poly-l-lactic acid	>1 year	deep-dermis	none
Artefill	synthetic	Collagen and PMMA beads	permanent	deep-dermis	none
Silicone	synthetic	silicone	permanent	deep-dermis	none
Fat	autologous	fat	permanent	subcutaneous	none

Modified from Dover JS. *Plast Reconstr Surg*. 2006;112(suppl):38s-40s.

That said, botulinum toxin can be very helpful in reducing dynamic vertical lip lines in some individuals when used in small doses (1-4 units in the upper lip, 1-4 units in the lower lip). It may also be beneficial in those with a down turned mouth by injecting the posterior margin of the depressor angulis oris muscle along the jaw line (1 finger breath in front of the masseter (4-6 units), or in those with an "orange peel like" chin skin as a result of the mentalis contractions (1-2 units each side).

Hundreds of filling agents are available worldwide, and the enormity of options has led to confusion about which agents work best, where they should be applied, and their underlying mechanism of action. The vast array of available soft tissue fillers can be arbitrarily divided into three main basic categories: short-term absorbable agents (duration less than 1 year), intermediate-term absorbable agents (duration 1 to 2 years), and long-term absorbable agents (several years duration) (Table 30-1).

30-2 SHORT-TERM ABSORBABLE FILLERS

30-2-1 *Collagen.* In the 1970s, after extensive trials, injectable bovine collagen was introduced and became the gold standard against which other injectables were assessed.[4,5,16–19] They were easily administered and effective in short-term (about 3 months) soft tissue augmentation. The possibility of allergic reactions and their limited duration of effect stimulated the continued search for better fillers.[4,20]

In the United States, injectable bovine collagen is manufactured under the trade names Zyderm® and Zyplast® (Inamed Aesthetics, a division of Allergan Inc., Santa Barbara, CA). Bovine collagen is derived from the skin of a secluded American herd of Angus/Hereford cattle that has lived in the same location in California for 30 years, thus minimizing the possibility of contamination with the bovine spongiform encephalopathy (BSE) prion.[20] Zyderm 1, Zyderm 2, and Zyplast collagen implants are sterile, purified fibrillar suspensions of bovine dermal collagen. Zyderm 1 and Zyderm 2 differ only in concentration: Zyderm 1 has 3.5% by weight bovine collagen, whereas Zyderm 2 is 6.5% by weight collagen. Zyplast also contains 3.5% by weight bovine collagen; however, the collagen is lightly cross-linked by the addition of 0.0075% glutaraldehyde. This cross-linking allows Zyplast to be more resistant to proteolytic degradation. The more substantive nature of Zyplast makes it applicable for deeper contour defects, which are often not improved with Zyderm 1 or Zyderm 2.[21–24] Following injection into the dermis, Zyderm and Zyplast are incorporated into the host tissue without discernable encapsulation and reproduce the texture, consistency, and structural integrity of the host tissues.[25]

Individuals who have a history of an anaphylactic event or previous sensitivity to bovine collagen or a known dietary allergy to beef should be excluded from testing and treatment. Because these products also contain lidocaine, patients with a known sensitivity to lidocaine should also be excluded. For patients without a known history of sensitivity to bovine collagen, potential allergenicity to collagen must be determined by skin testing.[26] A positive reaction to skin testing is an absolute contraindication to treatment. A skin test syringe is provided by the manufacturer and contains 0.3 mL Zyderm 1. For skin testing, a 0.1-mL dose should be administered (similar to a tuberculin skin test) into the dermis of the forearm.[26] A positive skin test is defined as swelling, induration, tenderness, or erythema that persists for 6 hours or longer within 4 weeks after the test injection. Since most reactions (70% of patients) occur within 3 days of testing, the test site should be evaluated at 48 to 72 hours and then again at 4 weeks. A positive skin test response has been estimated to occur in 3.0% to 3.5% of individuals undergoing first-time skin testing.[20] Two percent of patients receiving a collagen injection develop an allergic reaction to the treatment site despite an initial negative skin test. For this reason most authorities recommend a second test as an additional precaution.[27–29] This second test injection can be done in the contralateral arm or in the face near the hairline. The second test is done 4 weeks after the initial testing, with treatment commencing 2 weeks later if both test sites are negative for an allergic reaction.

Concerns regarding the allergenicity of the bovine products led to the concept of creating a nonallergenic human collagen. Autologen (Autogenous Technologies, Acton, MA) was made of human dermis from skin obtained during any surgical procedure.[3] While there was no need for skin testing, a relatively laborious process was required for skin harvesting. Dermologen (Collagenessis Inc., Beverly, MA) was subsequently developed and was identical to Autologen in structure and substance; however, rather than using autologous skin, a cadeveric source was used from approved tissue banks.[3] The widespread use of these agents was limited as many cosmetic surgeons awaited the introduction of newer agents that were simpler to produce and easier to use.

In response to the antigenic limitations of bovine collagen, Inamed Aesthetics (a division of Allergan) developed two bioengineered human-derived collagen products, CosmoDerm® and CosmoPlast®.[29] These human collagen products have the same consistency and injection properties as their Zyderm and Zyplast counterparts but are grown from a single human fibroblast cell culture, and unlike other human-derived products (i.e., Dermologen) they are not cadaveric in origin. CosmoDerm and CosmoPlast are the result of tissue engineering and have undergone extensive pathogen screening for viral and bacterial contamination to minimize the possibility of disease transmission.[4] Unlike bovine collagen, CosmoDerm and CosmoPlast do not require skin testing prior to clinical use since the incidence of allergic reaction in controlled studies was 1.3%.[29] This allows for same-day evaluation and treatment of rhytides, which is advantageous for both physician and patient.

CosmoDerm is available in two forms, CosmoDerm 1 and CosmoDerm 2; these are analogous to Zyderm 1 and Zyderm 2 in terms of the percentage of collagen and indicated usage. Similarly, CosmoPlast is analogous to Zyplast collagen filler and like Zyplast is cross-linked with glutaraldehyde to delay its proteolysis. Both CosmoDerm 1 and 2 and CosmoPlast contain collagen purified from human fibroblast cell cultures. The cell line used for collagen production is extensively screened by testing for viruses, retroviruses, cell morphology, karyology, isoenzymes, and tumorigenicity. CosmoDerm 1 and 2 and CosmoPlast are supplied in individual sterile syringes with needles and are packaged for single use. In addition to collagen, the syringe contains lidocaine (0.3%) as well as saline, which disperses into the soft tissue within 48 hours of injection, with the collagen filler remaining. CosmoDerm and CosmoPlast should be stored at standard refrigerator temperatures (2° to 10°C).

Other collagen-based products are also available, including Cymetra (micronized human cadaveric dermis) and Alloderm (acellular cadaveric dermal matrix) (Life Cell Corporation, Branchburg, NJ).[3] Fascian® is injectable human cadaveric fascia (Fascia Biosystems LLC, Beverly Hills, CA).[3] Both Cymetra and Fascian are relatively more difficult to use than the Zyderm or CosmoDerm products. Because of their large particle size, larger-bore needles are required, which makes precise intradermal injection difficult. Syringes are easily clogged by the product and the result can be an irregular and lumpy appearance.[3] Cymetra and Fascian have also not proven superior with regard to persistence within the tissue. A new cross-linked porcine collagen, Evolence® (Colbar LifeScience Ltd, Herzliya, Israel, a Johnson & Johnson Company), has shown promise as there appears to be a renewed interest in collagen-based products with greater persistence due to cross-linking and other methods.[3] Porcine collagen is less immunogenic than its bovine counterpart. No allergic responses have been reported to date and allergy testing is uneccessary.[4] Each syringe contains 30 mg/mL of product without anesthetic. Its longevity in the tissue is felt to be similar to Zyplast (about 4 months).[4] At the time of this writing, Evolence is not yet available in the United States but undergoing investigation (Dermicol-P35 27G).

30-2-2 *Hyaluronic Acid Products.* The advent of hyaluronic acid (HA) as a viable tissue filler launched a new era in the cosmetic treatment of facial wrinkles and folds.[9,30–32] HA products have become the leading tissue-filling agents worldwide and have immensely popularized the use of injectable soft tissue augmentation and increased the acceptability of tissue fillers in facial rejuvenation. The basis for this increased acceptance includes lack of preprocedure skin testing requirement, a duration of effect 3 to 6 months longer (or more) than most collagen products, a reduced side effect profile, and the ability to manipulate areas of overfill or lumps if they occur.[15,33–36]

HA is a basic building block of the dermis. It is a naturally occurring glycosaminoglycan that is a major component of all connective tissue and exhibits no species or tissue specificity, as the chemical structure of this polysaccharide is uniform throughout nature. There is little potential for hypersensitivity or immunologic reactions to HA in humans (1 in 5,000), so skin testing is not indicated.[37,38] HA molecules in the skin bind water and create volume. The amount of HA in the skin decreases with age and its loss results in reduced dermal hydration and increased skin wrinkling and folding.

HA fillers act by binding water molecules, which leads to increased skin hydration and tissue turgor. HA is manufactured as a polymer that is composed of multiple monomers bound together like a string of beads. In its non–cross-linked form, HA is essentially a liquid since the molecules are suspended individually in solution. Cross-linking HA increases the cohesiveness of the product and transforms its liquid configuration into a gel. It becomes more viscous and water-insoluble. The cross-linking also helps the product resist enzymatic degradation, prolonging its presence within the tissue. Without cross-linking the tissue half-life would be only 1 to 2 days.[39] Other parameters that affect the thickness of the product include the concentration of HA as well as the size of gel particles within the product. To make a product thinner (for injecting finer wrinkle lines) non–cross-linked HA can be added to cross-linked HA and/or smaller HA gel particles can be used. The goal of bioengineered HA is to improve its stabilization via increased tissue residency, viscosity, and elasticity while preserving its innate biocompatibility. Several HA agents are currently available worldwide with slight variations in their chemical composition that define their unique individual characteristics. These differences include the source of HA (animal vs. bacterial), cross-linking (both chemical method and degree), concentration of HA, amount of free HA (non–cross-linked), and particle size/uniformity (structure).[34] With appropriate and precise injection protocols, highly satisfactory treatment of facial furrows and volume depletion can be achieved with a variety of HA products.

30-2-2-1 *Restylane*. Restylane® (Q-Med, Uppsala, Sweden) is a HA-containing soft tissue filler that is composed of HA biosynthetically produced through a bacterial fermentation process. The introduction of Restylane in the marketplace has led to a resurgence in the use of dermal filler agents. Restylane is currently the leading dermal filler in the United States, where it is marketed by Medicis Aesthetics, Inc., of Scottsdale, Arizona. Since it is produced in the laboratory by a bacterial fermentation process, Restylane is referred to as a non–animal-stabilized hyaluronic acid (NASHA) product.[40–42] The concentration of HA in Restylane is 20 mg/mL. Eighty percent of the HA exists in the cross-linked form, while 20% is non–cross-linked to increase the ease of injection. Upon injection into tissue, the Restylane gel dissipates, binds water, and increases the volume. The volume is maintained until the HA is degraded and disappears completely over time.

Three forms of the product are marketed by Medicis: Restylane Touch® (also known as Restylane Fine Lines®), Restylane, and Perlane®. Each product is designed to be injected at different layers in the skin (Fig. 30-1). They may be ordered with or without the addition of lidocaine. The clinical difference between the products is the size of the gel particle. Restylane Touch (not yet available in the United States) has 200,000 gel particles per mL and is used for fine superficial

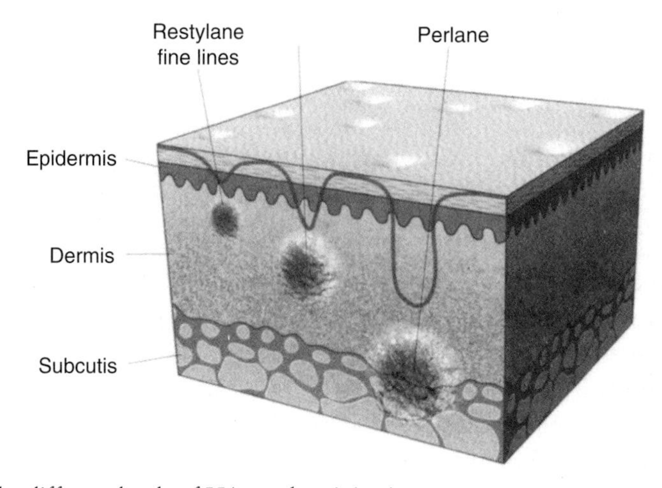

Figure 30-1 The different levels of HA product injection.

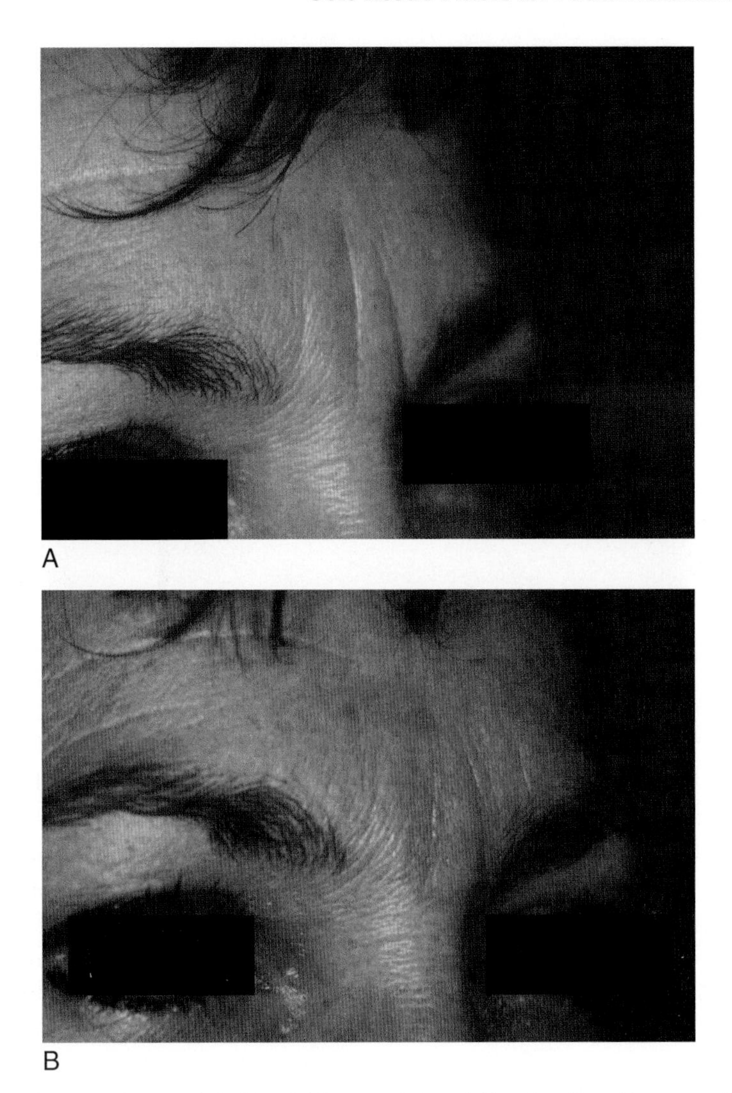

Figure 30-2 (A) Prominent glabellar folds remaining following Botulinum toxin injection. (B) Two weeks following Restylane injection.

wrinkles (e.g., vertical lip lines on the upper lip). Restylane has 100,000 gel particles per mL and is used for larger wrinkles (e.g., glabellar furrows, nasolabial lines, lip augmentation) (Figs. 30-2, 30-3, and 30-4). Perlane (8,000 gel particles per mL) is used for deeper folds (nasolabial folds), volume augmentation (lips), and facial recontouring (e.g., along the jawline). Perlane can also be injected below the dermis to correct deeper volume deficits. Restylane SubQ has 1,000 gel particles per mL and is the thickest product to date (not yet available in the United States). Restylane SubQ is primarily indicated for deeper contour or volume deficits (cheek, submental area, superior eyelid sulcus, orbit).

Restylane and Perlane last approximately 6 to 9 months, while Restylane Touch lasts 4 to 6 months. In some individuals the product lasts a shorter length of time (fast absorbers), and in others it may last beyond a year (slow absorbers). There is

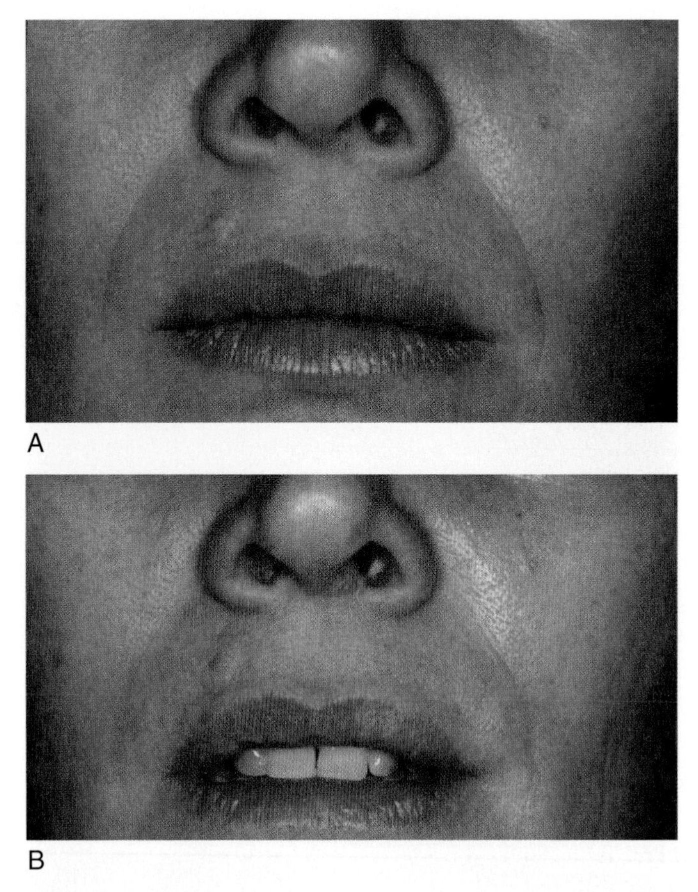

Figure 30-3 (A) Preinjection appearance of nasolabial folds. (B) Three weeks following injection with Restylane (nasolabial folds are much shallower).

no way of knowing who will be a fast absorber and who will be a slow absorber. The duration of effect is influenced by the mobility of the tissue surrounding the injection site. Injection into dynamic areas associated with a great deal of movement, such as the perioral region, may lead to less satisfactory results, as motion will encourage absorption and redistribution. All patients should be informed prior to treatment of the inherent variability in the duration of effect.

30-2-2-2 *Hylaform*®. Hylaform® and Hylaform Plus® (Inamed, a division of Allergan) are HA-based soft tissue fillers and are similar to Restylane. The concentration of HA is 6 mg/mL and it is extracted from rooster combs.[42,43] To date, there have been no reported instances of immunologic reactions to any residual avian products.[31,34] Hylaform is used in the same areas as Restylane (e.g., glabella, nasolabial folds, marionette lines, lip augmentation). Hylaform also comes in a thicker formulation (Hylaform Plus®) and a thinner formulation (Hylaform Fine Lines®). The duration of effect is believed to be 4 to 5 months, which is slightly less than Restylane.[41] While no skin test is required for either HA product, the current trend among physicians is to avoid animal-sourced HA.[39]

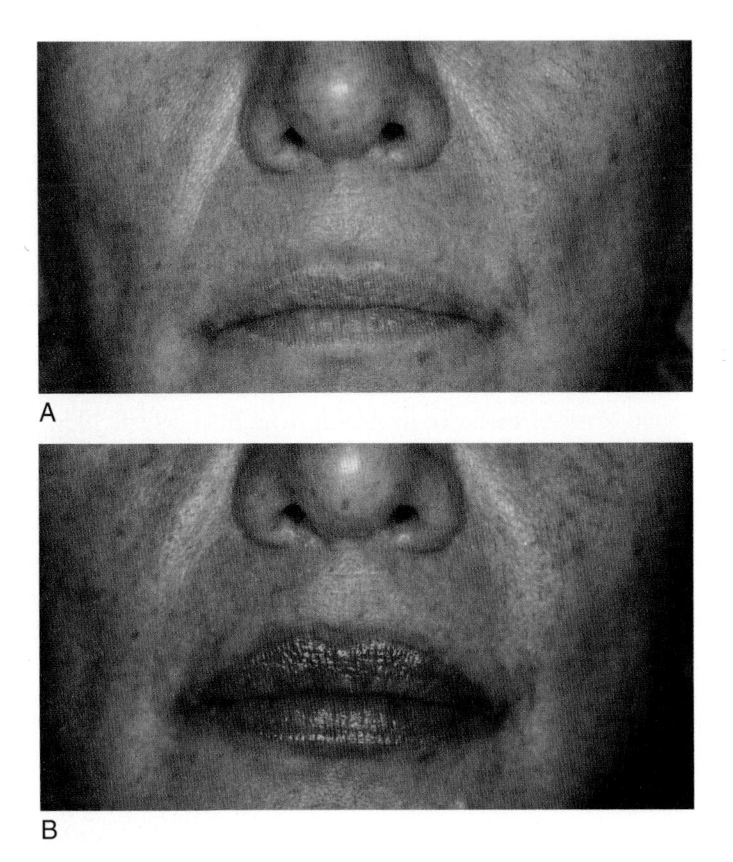

Figure 30-4 (A) Preinjection appearance of lips. (B) Four weeks following lip injection (increase in volume of lips apparent).

30-2-2-3 *Captique®*. To circumvent the aversion to animal-based HA products, Captique® (Inamed, a division of Allergan) was introduced. Captique is a NASHA compound with a concentration of HA of 5.5 mg/mL. It is indicated for moderate facial folds, similar to Restylane, but the duration of action is believed to be less than that of Restylane (4 to 5 months vs. 6 to 9 months). At the time of this publication, it has not significantly penetrated Restylane's market share.

30-2-2-4 *Juvéderm™*. Juvéderm is exported from France (LEA Derm Laboratories, a subsidiary of Corneal Industries SAS, Paris) and is also a HA filler of non-animal origin. It is marketed in the United States by Allergan, Inc. (Irvine CA).[44] The concentration of HA is 24 mg/mL. While 90% of the HA is in cross-linked form, 10% of it is not cross-linked to facilitate smoothness and consistency. Another difference between Juvéderm and Restylane relates to particle size: Restylane is composed of equal-sized gel particles, while Juvéderm has variable-sized particles—some are larger than Restylane and some are smaller. This particle size heterogeneity provides a smoother consistency to the product. Juvéderm can be used in the same areas as the other HA products mentioned and comes in several versions: Juvéderm 18 for fine lines, Juvéderm 24 (also known as Juvéderm Ultra®) for mild to moderate wrinkles (glabella, marionette lines, nasolabial folds, lips), and Juvéderm 30 for lips and deeper folds and for sculpting the cheek area. Juvéderm also comes in a high-viscosity (HV) form (Juvéderm 24 HV, marketed as Juvéderm Ultra Plus®, and Juvéderm 30 HV). The HV products have a slightly greater degree of cross-linking than their non-HV counterparts as well as the presence of some non–cross-linked HA as a lubricant. These products are also available with or without the addition of lidocaine. The duration of action is similar to the Restylane product line (6 to 9 months), but like the other HA products this depends on the site of injection and varies among patients. Like other currently available HA products, Juvéderm does not require skin testing.

30-2-2-5 *Selecting a Hyaluronic Acid Product for Injection*. With so many HA products to choose from, it is often difficult to decide which to select. New products are continuously being introduced, often with great excitement, but they all too frequently fail to fulfill the industry promise of providing an improved injectable filler. The subtle differences in HA concentration, cross-linking, and particle size are difficult to detect clinically, and after trying many of the new HA products plus additional products not yet available in the United States, we typically use one of the Restylane or Juvederm products described for most clinical situations. They are very effective, last as long as or longer than other short-term absobable fillers, and have few side effects. In our view, a product line that allows one to inject fine, medium, and thick lines is ideal.

Recently there has been a renewed interest in the use of collagen for superficial/papillary dermis injections. The medium-thickness HA agents (Restylane, Juvéderm 24) have not worked as well as expected in this area.[3] Visible and palpable nodularities are a manifestation of attempting to place a viscous, clear amorphous gel into the superficial dermis. Restylane Touch (Restylane Fine Lines) and Juvéderm 18 are much better and are more desirable for these fine-line areas. Collagen from any source (bovine, human, porcine) that can be administered through a fine needle is more forgiving in the very superficial plane than HA products and is effective for fine-line injections. On the other hand, for volume augmentation, the collagens that were once more commonly used for this purpose due to the "lack of options" have proven to be dramatically less effective than the HA fillers.[3] A combination of agents is often necessary to optimize results (e.g., Restylane Touch in the superficial dermis and Restylane or Perlane in the middle to deep dermis, or a "collagen" product in the superficial dermis and the HA product in the middle to deep dermis).

30-3 GENERAL INJECTION TIPS AND TECHNIQUES FOR SOFT TISSUE FILLER INJECTION

30-3-1 *Preinjection Considerations*. The use of anticoagulants, aspirin, and nonsteroidal medication as well as several other herbal products and vitamins (e.g., vitamin E, gingko biloba) increases the risk of bruising and bleeding at the injection site with any filler. While some physicians recommend stopping these medications prior to injecting, most simply advise their patients of the increased risk of bruising. If active inflammatory skin conditions are present in the area to be injected (e.g., herpetic lesions, acne, dermatitis, hives) it is best to postpone the injection. Informed consent and a thorough discussion of the expected benefits and limitations of the planned procedure are critical factors in achieving results that are satisfactory to the patient.

Preinjection photographic documentation is important but often limited by the subtle nature of wrinkles being treated or by the loss of three dimensionality in standard photography. Makeup should be removed from the treatment area. The patient should be placed in an upright position in a comfortable chair. Loupe magnification is beneficial for the fine wrinkles as it helps with the accuracy and precision of injection.

As with any procedure, the ability to properly inject soft tissue fillers has a certain learning curve, and proper placement of the different types of fillers within the dermal and subdermal tissue will improve with experience. Although topical anesthesia (e.g., EMLA™, ELA-MAX™, or a variety of others) may be used alone in some areas (crow's feet, glabella, tear trough, nasolabial fold), the majority of patients receive a combination of topical, local, and regional anesthesia (e.g., supraorbital, infraorbital, mental nerve blocks). Even when an agent is premixed with lidocaine injection of some of the filler agents can be uncomfortable. If the patient is not comfortable the injection will be more stressful for the patient and physician, perhaps resulting in incomplete treatment. Obviously, this will affect the patient's motivation for repeat injections. It is important to outline the areas to be injected prior to administering the local anesthesia because the volume of the local anesthesia may distort the area to be injected.

30-3-2 *Standard Injection Techniques*. There are several techniques for injecting soft tissue fillers. Familiarity with these techniques is important as techniques vary depending on the filler used and the area of injection.

30-3-2-1 *Serial Puncture*. The serial puncture technique (Fig. 30-5) is ideal for fine wrinkles. Multiple injections are made serially along the fine wrinkle or fold.

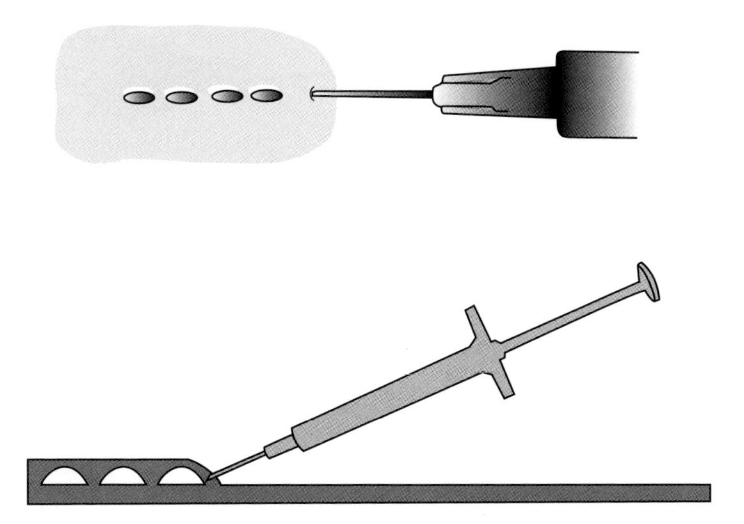

Figure 30-5 Serial puncture technique.

The needle position is fixed; it does not move or track from the entry site. The injection sites should be close together so that the injected material merges into a smooth, continuous line that ultimately lifts the fine wrinkle. No spaces should remain between the serially injected materials. It is helpful to try and stabilize the skin with the adjacent thumb and index finger while injecting. If some minimal gaps are present, postinjection molding and massage can be used to blend the material into a smooth layer. The serial puncture technique is commonly used for collagen injections; it minimizes the risk of overfill in any particular area and provides maximum control over product delivery. However, it is more time-consuming and there is an increased risk of bruising, as many more needle punctures are required to complete any given area when compared to the threading or fanning technique.

30-3-2-2 *Linear Threading*. With the linear threading technique (Fig. 30-6), the needle is advanced along the line or fold to be treated at the appropriate depth and the injection is made with constant pressure on the syringe plunger as the needle is withdrawn. In this fashion a thread of filler is deposited beneath the wrinkle or fold. The needle is re-entered further down the line or fold in a similar fashion. Successive threads may be laid down below, above, or beside previous injections until the entire line or fold has been treated. Once the filler is injected, the material is gently massaged along the line of injection to ensure the skin contour is smooth. If there are small depressions between the linear threads, isolated serial puncture injections are used to fill in these depressions. The goal is to smooth out the wrinkle or fold as much as possible. Linear threading works well for glabellar lines, nasolabial folds, marionette lines, philtral column enhancement, and the vermilion–cutaneous border. In some areas (e.g., lateral brow), one can also inject while advancing the needle (push ahead technique of linear threading), which may push blood vessels out of the way. This method is not frequently employed.

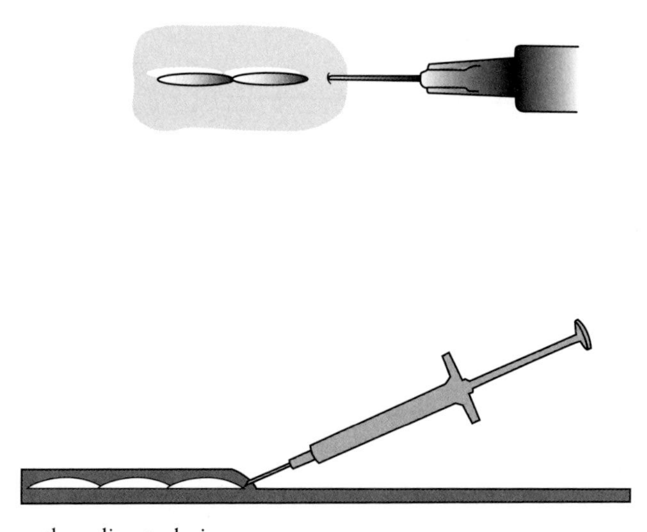

Figure 30-6 Linear threading technique.

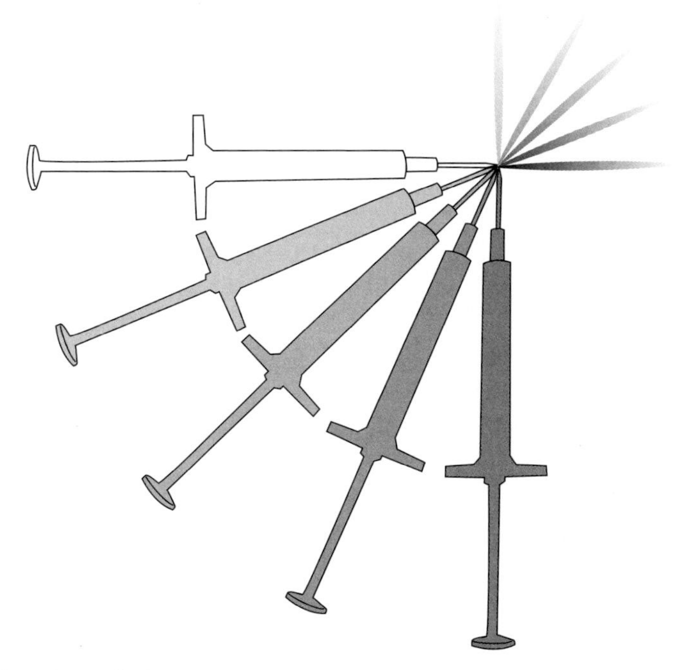

Figure 30-7 Fanning technique.

30-3-2-3 *Fanning*. In the fanning technique (Fig. 30-7), the needle is inserted in a fashion similar to that used in the linear threading technique, but just prior to withdrawing the needle from the skin, the needle's direction is changed and an adjacent area is injected. The fanning pattern of lines should be evenly spaced in a progressive clockwise or counterclockwise direction so that the contour is evenly filled and shaped. This technique is used commonly for the superior end of the nasolabial fold adjacent to the ala of the nose, where a triangular depression often requires filling. It is also useful in the malar and zygomatic area.

30-3-2-4 *Cross-Hatching*. Prior to beginning the procedure cross-hatching lines are carefully demarcated in a grid pattern so that the volume-deficient area will be evenly filled and contoured (Fig. 30-8). A series of linear threading injections are made in the treatment region. The pattern of lines should be evenly spaced. The cross-hatching technique is intended to give a structural augmentation effect, which is thought to provide greater tissue stability. This technique is used when relatively large areas require correction (i.e., facial contours) to maximize filler coverage of the treatment area.

30-3-3 *Injecting Collagen Products*. Zyderm 1 and 2 and CosmoDerm 1 and 2 are designed for the correction of superficial facial wrinkles. Zyderm 1 and CosmoDerm 1 (30% to 35% collagen) are considered the most versatile of all forms of collagen. They are designed for use in the superficial dermis by serial punctures or linear threading using a 30-gauge needle. Because they are not cross-linked they

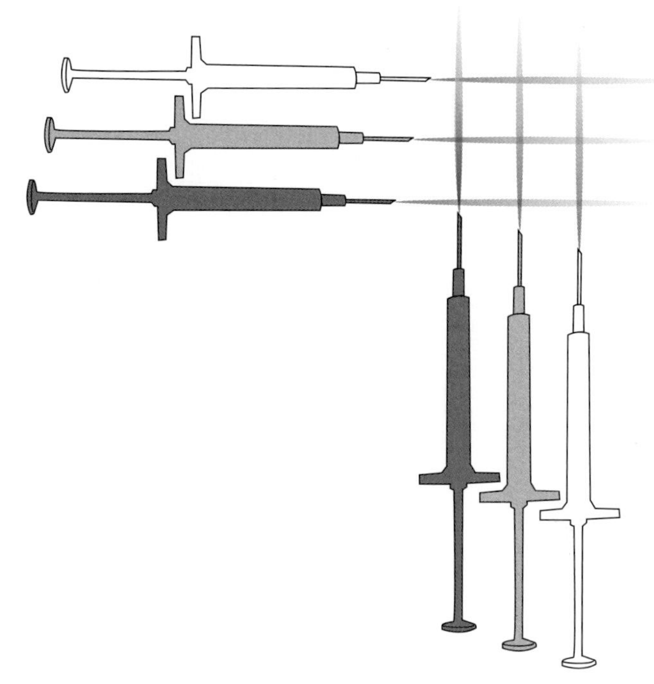

Figure 30-8 Cross-hatching technique.

flow easily within the dermis. When injecting Zyderm 1 or CosmoDerm 1, the syringe is held nearly parallel to the skin surface while stabilizing the treatment area between the thumb and forefinger of the noninjecting hand. The material should flow evenly into the superficial dermis, causing a flat yellow blanch of the skin. A pronounced wheal should appear following blanching, indicating adequate overcorrection. Each subsequent injection should be placed at the advancing edge of the previously injected area, generating a continuum of material that smoothly fills the defect. When placed correctly, the collagen should smoothly fill superficial defects. Although persistent beading and overcorrection can be problematic with superficial placement of CosmoDerm 1 in the periocular area and eyelid skin, beading is not much of a problem elsewhere. In general, up to 200% correction is indicated, except in the periorbital area, where correction should be limited to 100%.[29] Zyderm 1 and CosmoDerm 1 are effective for fine vertical lip lines, superficial periorbital wrinkles, smoothing residual glabellar frown lines following Botulinum toxin treatment, fine horizontal forehead wrinkles, marionette lines, perioral smile lines, and shallow scars.

Techniques for injecting Zyderm 2 and CosmoDerm 2 are almost identical to those outlined for Zyderm 1 and CosmoDerm 1. Zyderm 2 and CosmoDerm 2 contain nearly twice the amount of collagen (65% to 70% collagen) as Zyderm 1 and CosmoDerm 1 and as a result require greater force to inject, and they undergo less condensation upon implantation.[9] Only modest overcorrection (110% to 120%) is recommended to avoid persistent whiteness at the injection site. Zyderm 2 and CosmoDerm 2 are effective for smoothing deeper forehead furrows, glabellar wrinkles, nasolabial folds, marionette lines, and shallow scars as well. These thicker agents should not be used in the delicate eyelid skin (crow's feet) or for treatment of radial lip lines, as lumping and whitish discoloration within the treated skin may occur because of its more viscous nature.

Zyplast and CosmoPlast are cross-linked, thicker, and more resistant to even injection within the dermis. They were designed for placement into the middle to deep dermis (2 mm below the skin surface). One hundred percent correction (with no overcorrection) is recommended when using Zyplast and CosmoPlast. They are used for more pronounced contour problems (deeper scars, lines, and furrows) and for areas where greater muscular activity is going to cause dissolution and breakdown of the compound (i.e., the lip and periorbital region). They are also useful in the oral commissures, vermilion borders, marionette lines, and nasolabial folds. Injection in the superficial dermis will result in persistent overcorrection with beading. Increased longevity of correction and improved aesthetic results can often be achieved by layering, where Zyderm 2 or CosmoDerm 2 is immediately injected over Zyplast or CosmoPlast injection sites. This layering technique is especially useful in the treatment of deep nasolabial folds and marionette lines.

Correction with Zyderm or CosmoDerm and Zyplast or CosmoPlast is short-lived (3 to 4 months), and most patients (70%) require quarterly touchups to maintain the desired results. Correction is lost because the material is slowly displaced from its site of implantation within the dermis into the subcutaneous space.

30-3-4 *Injecting Hyaluronic Acid Products.* All of the HA fillers are supplied as clear colorless transparent gels packaged in a disposable syringe and stored at room temperature. Selection of the appropriate filler will vary according to the depth of the defect to be treated (see Fig. 30-1). Fine superficial wrinkles (e.g., vertical lip lines) will respond better to finer fillers (e.g., Restylane Fine Lines or Restylane Touch) injected in the superficial dermis. Deeper, more substantial folds benefit from volume enhancement in the middle to deep dermis and require a thicker (more viscous) product (e.g., Restylane, Perlane, Juvéderm Ultra, Juvéderm UltraPlus), depending upon the depth of the fold or furrow. In some areas, a wrinkle or fold may have both superficial and deep components. To optimize treatment in these areas, thicker (more viscous) gels may be injected deeply, followed by thinner (less viscous) gels placed more superficially in a layering technique. Injection too superficially can cause the appearance of nodules or other irregularities; conversely, injections too deep may be ineffective. Subperiosteal injections are not recommended because injection in this plane is difficult to achieve and painful. Injections into dynamic areas associated with a great amount of movement, such as the perioral region, may lead to less satisfactory results as the motion will encourage absorption. Care must be taken to avoid injection into a blood vessel, especially in the periocular area.[45] Unlike collagen injections, which require overcorrection to attain a desirable outcome, the endpoint for HA filler injection is 100% of the desired appearance. Once the product is injected, the material should be gently massaged along the line of injection to ensure the material is smooth. The HA products attract water, and patients should be informed they may appear slightly swollen on the day of injection, not only as a result of the anesthesia volume injected (if used) but also due to this uptake of water. Most of the edema improves within 12 to 18 hours, although the filler continues to settle during the first week following injection.

The amount of filler supplied per syringe varies slightly, as do the costs of the fillers. How much filler is required depends on the depth of the wrinkle or fold and how many syringes the patient is willing to purchase. Generally, one syringe (0.8 to 1.2 mL) of Restylane, Juvéderm Ultra, Hylaform, or Captique is adequate for mild nasolabial folds or lip augmentation. For deeper nasolabial folds a thicker product (Perlane, Hylaform Plus, or Juvéderm Ultra Plus) is preferred. A half syringe (0.5 to 0.7mL) of Restylane, Juvéderm Ultra, Captique, or Hylaform is adequate for most glabellar frown lines, marionette lines, vermilion border augmentation, and the vertical upper and lower lip lines.

30-4 THE APPROACH TO SPECIFIC AESTHETIC AREAS

30-4-1 *Correction of Nasolabial Folds.* The nasolabial fold area is the simplest area to inject and a good place to begin for novice injectors. The fold will never fully correct and patients should be informed that the goal is to make it softer and less deep. A 50% or more correction is attainable with proper technique and patient selection.[39] Marking out the area to fill is helpful prior to injecting any local anesthesia or applying topical anesthetic creams. For mild nasolabial folds moderately viscous products (e.g., Restylane, Juvéderm Ultra, Captique, Hylaform) work well. For deeper folds, thicker (more viscous) products (Perlane, Juvéderm Ultra Plus) are recommended. Layering a thinner product above a thicker, more viscous one may be beneficial in some instances. A linear threading technique in the middle to deep dermis is employed for most nasolabial fold corrections. At the upper end of the nasolabial fold adjacent to the ala there is often a triangular depression, requiring two or three injections of filler in a fanlike array (fanning technique). Once the filler has been injected, it is gently massaged for a more even distribution along the nasolabial fold. This is done with a fingertip or by gently rolling a cotton-tipped applicator over the area. Ultrasound gel on the skin may be used as a lubricant to allow one's finger or cotton-tipped applicator to move smoothly over the area. Any gaps or depressions may be treated with a serial puncture technique.

30-4-2 *Marionette Lines or Melomental Folds.* Moderately viscous HA fillers such as Restylane, Juvéderm Ultra, Hylaform, or Captique can be used to fill the marionette lines and areas near the oral commissure. While the perioral area is stabilized and placed on tension with the noninjecting thumb and forefinger, a linear threading injection technique is used in the depths of the marionette line and melomental fold. A fanning injection technique in the triangular area adjacent to the oral commissure is useful to fill this broader area. A linear thread of filler along the vermilion border of the lateral lip (adjacent to the marionette line) is worthwhile to complete the correction in this area. Careful digital massage may be performed in this area with one finger in the mouth and the thumb externally or with both fingers externally along the line of injection.

30-4-3 *Periocular Lines (Crow's Lines).* The only HA product currently available for this area is one of the finer products such as Restylane Touch (or Restylane Fine Lines). The injection can be done under topical anesthetic creams but it is time-consuming and it can be difficult to get great results. The dynamic wrinkles in this area cannot be completely eliminated and lumpiness is common. Without the addition of Botulinum toxin, the high movement in this area decreases the longevity of the filler. Botulinum toxin without the concomitant use of dermal filler is usually adequate to decrease the wrinkles in this region.

30-4-4 *Tear Trough Deformity.* Moderate-viscosity HA fillers such as Restylane, Juvéderm Ultra, Hylaform, or Captique work best to restore volume to the tear trough area. Any injection of local anesthesia into this area may distort the tear trough depression, so either no anesthesia or topical anesthesia is the preferred technique. Serial and linear threading is used in this area, starting medially and working laterally (although some prefer to start laterally and work medially). Entering and re-entering the tissue risks bleeding and should be kept to a minimum. The filler should be placed slowly in the deepest orbicularis fibers immediately adjacent to the periosteum (supraperiosteal space). It cannot be injected subperiosteally because the periosteum is securely attached to the bone. Injection more superficially may leave the patient with a bluish discolored mass within the eyelid. Following injection, massage with a cotton-tipped applicator should be used to smooth the fill along the tear trough.

30-4-5 *Glabellar Frown Lines.* Botulinum toxin works best in this area to decrease the vertical frown lines. In some individuals, despite corrugator and procerus muscle paresis, only a partial resolution of the frown lines has been obtained, and the HA fillers are a nice adjunct to gain additional improvement. Moderate-viscosity fillers such as Restylane, Juvéderm Ultra, Hylaform, or Captique can be used to fill this area under topical creams or regional nerve block (supraorbital, supratrochlear); a linear threading technique with injection in the middle dermis is recommended. Injection along the rhytid is performed while the needle is being withdrawn. Thicker products like Perlane carry an increased risk of vascular disruption and necrosis and probably should not be used in the glabellar region.[42]

30-4-6 *Horizontal Forehead Lines.* Satisfactory treatment of horizontal forehead lines is difficult with fillers. The forehead skin is greatly influenced by the continuous action of the underlying frontalis muscle. Because of this tissue mobility, filler dissolution is common. Botulinum toxin (in small doses) is very effective in diminishing forehead furrows. If there are fine residual lines following Botulinum chemodenervation that bother the patient, then one of the small-particle-sized HA fillers injected with the linear threading technique at the dermal–epidermal junction (i.e., superficial) may be helpful.

30-4-7 *Aging Lips.* The lips and perioral region are the central aesthetic component of the lower face, just as the eyes, eyelids, and brows are the central aesthetic component of the upper face. Lips express emotion, sensuality, and vitality.[39] Some of the

Table 30-2 Features of the Aesthetic and Aging Lip

Aesthetic Lip Features	Aging Lip Features
Upper lip height to lower lip height = 1/3:2/3	Upper and lower lip equal out and become thin
Distinct cupid's bow	Loss of cupid's bow
Central fullness of the upper lip	Thin, uniform, contoured upper lip
Concave sloping of the upper and lower lips	Convex, straight, ill-defined sloping
Lower lip projects 1–2 mm beyond upper lip	Equalized projection of upper and lower lip
Vermilion–cutaneous borders well defined with a pout	Loss of vermilion–cutaneous border, no pout
Philtral columns prominent and full	Philtral columns flattened
Commissures slightly upturned	Commissures downturned

Modified from Rohrich, RJ, Ghavami A, Crosby MA. *Plast Reconstr Surg*. 2007;120(suppl):41s–54s.

characteristics of an aesthetic and youthful lip are listed in Table 30-2.[39] Over time the lips lose their central fullness (become thinner) and the definition of the vermilion–cutaneous junction decreases (loss of pout). In addition, the cupid's bow becomes less defined, the philtral columns flatten, and the commissures become downturned. The aging process of the mouth is also associated with the development of circumoral radial lines and grooves.

The aesthetic correction of lips must be done only after careful evaluation and discussion of the patient's treatment goals and availability options. The treatment approach is not the same in all patients and must be individualized. For lip enhancement or restoration it is important to have some lip structure to build upon. Patients who require subtle refinements in lip fullness, projection, and degree of eversion are ideal candidates for augmentation with a HA product.[39] It is extremely difficult, if not impossible, to make thin atrophic lips appear plump and full. Under-promising and ideally over-delivering is an important adage in treating the lip area. Examination of adjacent areas in the lower face, including the melomental lines and prejowl sulcus, is important as volume loss in these areas may also contribute negatively to the lower facial frame.

Although there are many techniques for lip augmentation, the following approach will provide some basic concepts and guidelines. It is important to ask the patient what he or she is trying to achieve and have the patient show you what he or she would like to achieve. The patient may be able to show you by rolling the lip upward with a finger in the mirror. The lips should be full and well defined (see Table 30-2). Optimal lip rejuvenation involves two main components: volume enhancement and definition (vermilion–cutaneous border enhancement).[39] Older patients often require filler injected into the body of their lips for volume correction as well as filler injected along the vermilion–cutaneous junction for increased lip definition. Younger patients who usually have enough volume may need only vermilion–cutaneous enhancement. The treating physician should also focus on restoration of the lateral aspect of the lips (youthful lips have a slight upward turn to the commissures). Correction of the marionette lines is also a key element in overall lip and perioral enhancement, as volume added in these areas acts like a buttress to support the lateral downturning of the aging lip.[39,46] Careful Botulinum toxin injections into the depressor anguli oris can enhance the lifting effect of filler in this area.

Regional nerve blocks (infraorbital, mental) in addition to direct injection into the gingival sulcus superiorly and inferiorly will typically provide adequate anesthesia for lip augmentation. For those with vertical lip lines to be injected, topical anesthetic creams are also beneficial. For definition of the lip, injecting soft tissue filler (e.g., Restylane, Juvéderm Ultra, Hylaform, Captique) along the vermilion border as well as the philtral columns brings more definition to these areas without making the lip look bigger. There is a potential space within the lip tissue at the vermilion border. When the vermilion–cutaneous junction is injected, the physician should stretch the lip laterally and enter the needle at the lateral end of the lip. With the lip stretched, it is slightly more firm and stable against the dentition. The stretched lip will allow better flow of the filler. The injection technique along the vermilion border is a linear threading technique, and the patient is injected from lateral to medial (Fig. 30-9A). Once the needle enters the potential space at the vermilion–cutaneous junction, injection should be slow but steady to ensure the material stays uniform. Injecting in a smooth and even fashion will help avoid lumping and surface irregularities. Flow out of the channel above the vermilion border can create a visible lump. Flow below the channel is also to be avoided for similar reason. The preservation of the cupid's bow is critical because it is the defining aesthetic unit of the upper lip. If it is injected, the needle should be removed and re-entered along the direction of the bow. Minimal filling of the philtral columns can further enrich the lip augmentation in those who have lost definition in this area.

To make the lips look bigger, one has to add volume to the lip by injecting into the body of the lip (Fig. 30-9B). This can be accomplished at the submucosal level, within the superficial orbicularis oris muscle mass. Placing the HA filler in this deeper level decreases its visibility and augments lip volume. For lip volume augmentation, either the standard products (Restylane, Juvéderm Ultra, Captique, Hylaform) or the more viscous products (Perlane, Juvéderm Ultra Plus) can be used. The filler is injected into the lip at the junction of the dry and wet lip, for the entire length of the lip (again working from lateral to medial). During slow, steady injection, a spreading effect is noted as the material spreads through the plane of injection. In the upper lip, the filler is usually injected along the entire lip, whereas in the lower lip, it is usually injected into the central third to produce central rollout, which enhances the pout effect. Once the injection is complete, the lips should be gently massaged by rolling the lip (upper then lower) between the thumb and index finger to even the product out and correct any lumpy areas. Digital massage can be repeated the next day if lumpiness is noticed. Vertical lip lines (lipstick bleeding lines) are very simple to inject using one of the finer products such as Restylane Touch (Restylane Fine Lines). The injection should be as superficial as possible; a linear threading injection technique is used.

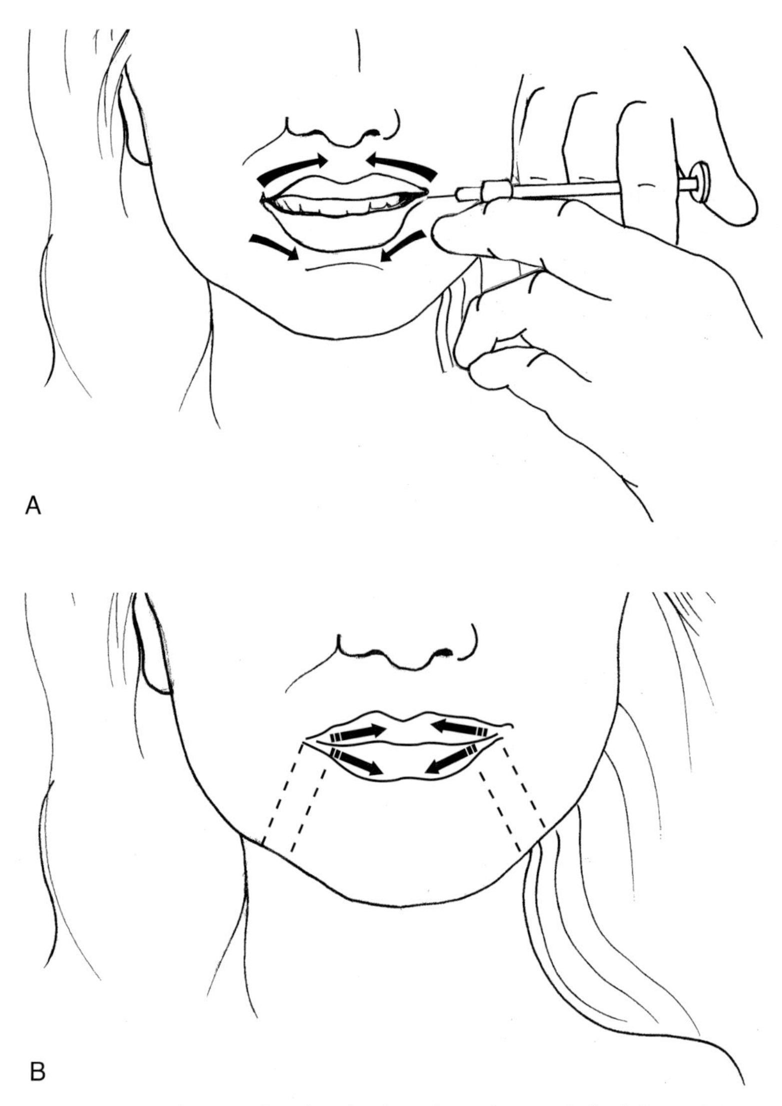

Figure 30-9 (A) Injecting the vermilion border from lateral to medial while applying some lateral tension on the lips. (B) Injecting the body of the lip from lateral side to medial. Dotted lines indicate additional support that may come from injecting the marionette lines.

30-4-8 *Facial Contouring*. The HA fillers are ideal agents to replace volume lost naturally through the aging process. As time goes on and more experience is gained, new facial areas that might benefit from volume augmentation will come to light. Currently, common facial areas to contour and sculpt include the lateral brow, zygomatic prominence, cheek/malar area and jaw line. When filling these regions, thicker products such as Perlane or Juvéderm Ultra Plus are often used, but any of the medium-thickness fillers can be used as well (e.g., Restylane, Juvéderm Ultra, Captique). The injection technique may include a fanning technique (zygoma, malar area), cross-hatching technique (cheek area), or linear threading technique (lateral brow or jaw line).

30-4-8-1 *Lateral Brow Ptosis.* The lateral brow becomes ptotic with age as a result of the downward gravitational effects on lax tissue and a loss of volume in the lateral brow fat pad. HA soft tissue filler can be injected at the subdermal plane (just above the periosteum) over the lateral third of the brow using a 30-gauge needle in a "push-ahead" technique, allowing the forward movement of the filler to elevate the tissue rather than the tip of the needle.[6] With this method, bruising is uncommon. Alternatively, the filler can also be injected while withdrawing the needle. Once the filler is in place, gentle massage to mold the filler in place will give the best aesthetic result.

30-4-8-2 *Midface/Zygomatic Prominence.* Hypoplasia of the zygoma and/or midfacial fat descent and atrophy diminish the normal heart-shaped contour of the face. A soft white eyeliner pencil can be used to draw out the area requiring aesthetic enhancement over the zygomatic prominence. HA-based filler is injected into the deep dermal or subdermal space in each marked area and the esthetic benefit is reviewed with the patient. One of the thicker products (Restylane, Juvéderm Ultra Plus, or Hylaform Plus) works well in this area, but any of the medium-viscosity HA fillers in greater volume can also be used. Fanning or cross-hatching and layering of filler in the zygomatic/malar area provides structural support and projection.[10] The fanning/threading pattern in the malar area roughly approximates an inverted triangle. A second pass of injection to create a cross-hatch is usually not required over the zygoma (Fig. 30-10).

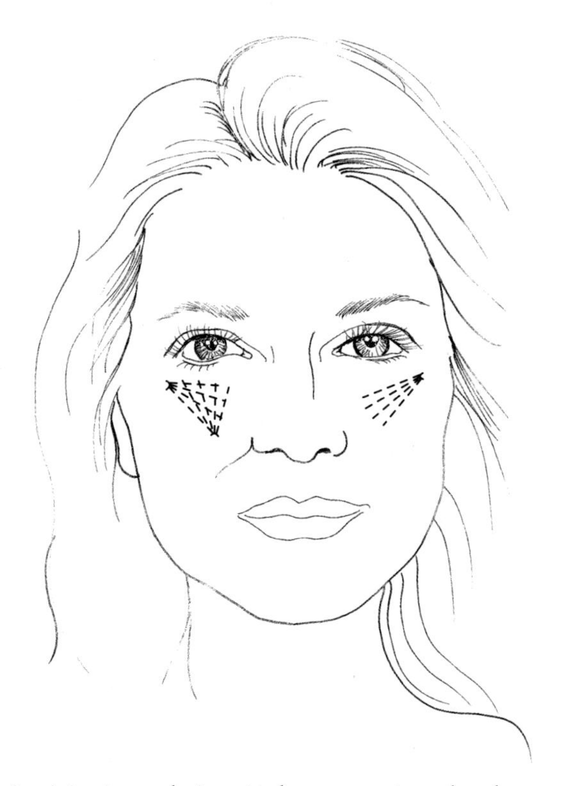

Figure 30-10 A fanning injection technique in the zygomatic and malar area.

Care should be taken not to inject above the orbital rim in either area. Gentle massage after injection is used to smooth the areas.

30-4-8-3 *Prejowl Sulcus.* Gravity's effects on the lower face often lead to a downward sagging of tissue along the jaw line, resulting in a slight depression and shadowing along the jaw line known as the "pre-jowl sulcus." One of the thicker HA fillers (Perlane, Juvéderm Ultra Plus, Hylaform Plus) injected in the subdermal plane along this depression will elevate the area and re-establish the normal contour and provide a more youthful appearance. The key to correction is to recreate the inferior border of the mandible rather than simple volume fill along the body of the mandible. The material should be injected incrementally with a linear threading technique, injecting several rows of filler adjacent and on top of one another.

30-5 HYALURONIC ACID FILLER POSTINJECTION CARE

When using HA fillers, correction to 100% of the desired volume is the goal. Immediately after treatment in any particular area, the physician and patient should examine at the area to see if it looks balanced and smooth. Gentle digital massage using topical ultrasound gel will help smooth any irregularities. Cool compresses (gel packs, frozen peas, crushed ice) are recommended for 10 to 15 minutes at a time on two or three occasions on the day of the injection. Lip enhancement patients, in particular, need to be informed of the potential for substantial edema; the lips may look overcorrected during the first 3 to 5 days as a result of this swelling. If there is any lumpiness or undesirable overfilling, then on the day after the injection, the patient can digitally massage or roll a cotton-tipped applicator over the lump to smooth the area out. Patients are asked to come back to check the overall effect in 2 to 3 weeks. Additional volume can be safely administered at this time if needed. If there is any persistent lumpiness, undesirable volume effect (as a result of too much HA filler placed in the tissue), or even an inflammatory reaction, the HA can be dissolved with a small dose of hyaluronidase. Hyaluronidase (100 units/mL, formulated by a local compounding pharmacist) is infiltrated directly into the affected area(s) using 0.25 to 0.5 mL at each site.[33,47]

30-6 FOLLOW-UP TREATMENTS WITH HYALURONIC ACID FILLERS

In most individuals the effect of the HA filler injection lasts at least 6 to 9 months. Factors influencing the duration of effect include the product used, location of injection, and the concomitant use of Botulinum toxin. Patients are instructed to return when they see the area of correction has begun to diminish to a point that is undesirable to them. Dynamic areas such as the mouth may require more frequent corrections than more static areas such as the tear trough, nasolabial folds, or cheek area. Reinjecting an area that has not returned to its baseline requires less HA filler to re-establish full correction. Most injectors agree that retreatment should be done before full aesthetic correction has disappeared.

30-7 INTERMEDIATE-TERM ABSORBABLE FILLERS (DURATION OF EFFECT 1 TO 2 YEARS)

The advantage of longer-lasting fillers is obvious; however, drawbacks and limitations often include increased expense, difficulty of use, a steeper learning curve for the practitioner, multiple treatment sessions, and a higher incidence of side effects and complications, including granuloma and nodule formation.

30-7-1 *Radiesse®* (*Calcium Hydroxylapatite Microspheres*). Calcium hydroxylapatite is a major mineral component of bone and has been used for bone and craniofacial reconstruction for several decades. Radiesse is a solution of 55.7% calcium hydroxylapatite microspheres (25 to 45 μm in diameter) that are suspended in 36.6% water for injection with 6.4% glycerin and 1.3% carboxymethylcellulose.[48] The uniform microspheres are smooth in shape and are identical in composition to the mineral component of human bone. Radiesse is premixed in 1-mL syringes with a 27-gauge needle. It is biocompatible, nontoxic, and nonirritating and no antigenicity tests are required. In 2006, Radiesse was approved by the FDA for correction of moderate to severe wrinkles and folds and restoration of the signs of facial fat loss (lipoatrophy).[48] It has been proven useful for nasolabial folds, malar/submalar/zygomatic augmentation, marionette lines, prejowl sulcus augmentation, chin projection, and facial volume correction in human immunodeficiency (HIV)-associated lipoatrophy. The injection plane should be in the deep dermis or subdermis. The injection technique depends on the area of treatment. Overcorrection is not necessary, and following injection, gentle massage is required to smooth the injected area. In the nasolabial folds, a linear injection technique with several threads adjacent to one another and on top of one another (depending upon the depth of the fold) is suggested. In the zygoma and malar area, a cross-hatching or fanning/threading pattern with layering technique is helpful. In lipoatrophy associated with HIV, calcium hydroxylapatite is deposited into the deep dermis of the submalar region using a fanning technique with layering. To provide adequate volume, additional threads may be layered into a deeper plane (Fig. 30-11). Radiesse is not intended for superficial lines (crow's feet, perioral lip lines) or lip injection as unwanted lumps may occur. Since it is rather thick and deep injection is required, treatment of glabellar furrows should be avoided to prevent ischemic necrosis secondary to occlusion or compression of the supraorbital/supratrochlear artery.

When placed into the soft tissues, Radiesse provides immediate correction. With time the carrier gel is gradually absorbed and the calcium hydroxylapatite particles remain. Local histiocytic and fibroblastic response at the site appears to result in the production of new collagen (i.e., Radiesse may have some bioactive effect).[49] Eventually the calcium hydroxylapatite particles are broken down into calcium and phosphate ions via normal metabolic processes and eliminated through the body's normal excretory mechanisms. Its duration of effect is felt to be 12 to18 months, but as with other nonpermanent fillers there are those who absorb the product faster and those who absorb the product more slowly than others.

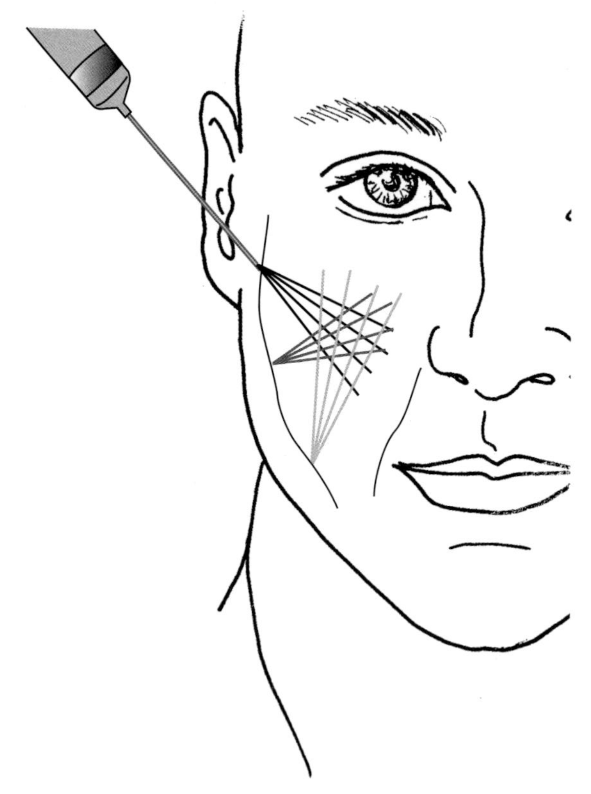

Figure 30-11 A fanning and layering technique for the correction of lipoatrophy.

30-7-2 *Sculptra® (Polylactic Acid Microspheres)*. Sculptra (also known as Newfill in Europe) is another intermediate duration absorbable filler currently FDA approved for HIV facial lipoatrophy.[33,50] Its duration of effect is about 1 to 2 years. Sculptra is supplied in a dry powder and is reconstituted with sterile water, sterile saline, or lidocaine prior to injection. Once reconstituted it should be allowed to sit for 2 hours prior to use and should be used within 72 hours of mixing. Sculptra should be injected with a 26-gauge needle or larger and injections are reserved for the deep dermis or subcutaneous plane.[33,50] It may be useful in deep nasolabial folds, marionette lines, jaw line contouring, cheek augmentation, and areas of severe fat loss in patients with HIV facial lipodystrophy. A 2- to 3-minute sculpting massage of the injected area helps to evenly distribute the product and allows more exact facial contouring in the target area. Only a limited correction should be made during the first injection session. Complete treatment usually requires a series of several injections, with intervals between injections of approximately 4 to 6 weeks. Supplemental treatment sessions might be required to maintain an optimal treatment effect. Anesthesia is best obtained by combining topical, local, and regional nerve blocks as previously described.

After injection of the product, the polylactic acid microspheres gradually degrade with tissue metabolism. The mechanism of action is a foreign body reaction that stimulates neocollagenesis, resulting in a volume expansion (i.e., a bioactive effect).[50] The collagen production that occurs in response to the implant provides the long-term correction of soft tissue defects, with a gradual increase in the volume of depressed areas over the first few months. It is very important to avoid overcorrection, particularly during the initial injection.

30-8 INJECTION-RELATED PROBLEMS AND ADVERSE EVENTS (COMPLICATIONS) ASSOCIATED WITH THE BIODEGRADABLE SOFT TISSUE FILLERS

Common injection-related problems as well as adverse events (complications) may occur during or after placement of any of the biodegradable fillers (Table 30-3). Problems such as swelling or bruising are related to the actual injection and are expected but unwanted. Adverse events are complications that may occur as a result of the filler placement but are not normally expected.

Common injection-related reactions that may occur following any injection include needle marks, erythema, edema, bruising, pain, and tenderness at the injection site; they are a result of the local effects of puncture trauma with the needle.[51,52] These reactions are generally mild and resolve spontaneously in a few days. Overcorrection, undercorrection, and asymmetry are other undesirable side effects related to the injection technique. With the exception of the least viscous forms of collagen (e.g., CosmoDerm, Zyderm), significant overcorrection is not necessary with the other available injectable fillers and should be avoided. Immediate massage can be performed if there appears to be some overfill or asymmetry with any filler. If the overfill persists with the HA products, a small dose of hyaluronidase can be injected to dissolve the HA in the overfilled area. Undercorrection is less serious, as patients can always return for a touchup procedure.

Implanted material that remains visible near the surface of the skin is an aesthetically problematic undesired outcome that is also related to the injection technique or incorrect filler selection for the area being treated. Typically manifesting as a blanched or white papule or a palpable lump, visible injectant is usually the result of injections that are too superficial.[53,54] Thin collagen products (CosmoDerm, Zyderm)

Table 30-3 Injection-Related Problems and Adverse Events (Complications) Associated with the Biodegradable Soft Tissue Fillers

Injection-Related Problems	Adverse Events (Complications)
Needle marks, erythema, edema, bruising	Inflammatory nodules and hypersensitivity reactions
Pain, tenderness	Granuloma formation
Undercorrection, overcorrection, asymmetry	Injection site necrosis
Visible filler (white or blue papule)	Retinal artery thrombosis
Lumps (due to overfill)	Cutaneous infection

can be placed high in the dermis without problems and postinjection yellowish blanching is a good sign, confirming the appropriate superficial fill. For all other fillers, superficial placement can create a problem. When injections are placed using the serial puncture technique or linear threading, the physician should ensure the needle tip is in the dermis before the syringe plunger is depressed and that the injection ceases as the needle is withdrawn. It is important to observe the skin near the needle tip to ensure the absence of blanching (indicative of superficial placement). If an injection is too superficial, firm massage with a cotton-tipped applicator can be used to smooth the affected area. If HA fillers are placed too superficially in the papillary dermis, a bluish papule or blue line (Tyndall effect) may become visible, sometimes immediately, or within a few days.[54,55] These can easily be dissolved with a small dose of hyaluronidase.[33]

An uncommon but troublesome outcome of injectable augmentation is lumps or nodule formation in the area of fill. Lumps or nodules may appear either immediately after treatment with HA fillers, likely a result of superficial injection or excessive injection into a given area, or several weeks later as a result of a local inflammatory reaction or foreign body granulomatous reaction.[4,51,52,56] They are uncommon. Nodules have also been reported after the use of collagen products, polylactic acid, and calcium hydroxylapatite.[33,51–53] Conservative management of nodules entails gentle massage by the patient, reassurance, and close follow-up. Steroid injections are most useful for nodules with an inflammatory component. When the nodules are composed of HA, they can be dissolved with a small injection of hyaluronidase.[33] Rarely nodules may need to be punctured and aspirated or surgically removed.[53]

Hypersensitivity responses and allergic response can occasionally occur with the use of nonpermanent fillers.[33,52,57,58] Most significantly, injectable bovine collagen can cause cutaneous allergy, and patients must be skin-tested twice, one month apart, prior to injection to reduce the likelihood of this complication. With bovine collagen, there are two forms of true classic type IV hypersensitivity to the filler. These reactions develop in about 1% of those with two negative skin tests and who subsequently receive treatment.[4] They occur primarily with Zyderm 1, and approximately 2 weeks after treatment. The most common reaction is manifested by a swollen, indurated bump at both the treatment and test sites. Although these areas typically resolve spontaneously and without permanent scarring, they can take up to 1 year to completely dissipate. In addition to reassurance, treatment may include nonsteroidal anti-inflammatory medications and intralesional injections of corticosteroids (triamcinolone).[4] Sterile abscesses are the second form of delayed hypersensitivity reaction that has been associated with bovine collagen. The incidence is low, approximately one to four in 10,000 treatments, and it is usually associated with Zyplast. This reaction is characterized by the sudden onset of pain, usually a few weeks after injection, followed by tense edema and erythema with fluctuant nodules. These lesions are treated by incision and drainage, intralesional steroids, and oral antibiotics, and scarring can occur. The circulating anti-bovine collagen antibodies that occur in these two allergic scenarios do not cross-react with human collagen.[3] Although skin testing before the use of human collagen (CosmoDerm, CosmoPlast) is not necessary, the package insert continues to note that use in people with a known allergy to bovine collagen has not been studied.[4,53] The HA fillers are much less likely to induce immune responses as they are believed to be highly biocompatible. Adverse reactions thought to be of a hypersensitive nature have been reported in about 1 in 5,000 treated patients.[37,57] Several authors have questioned the purported lack of immunogenicity to HA products, based on reported inflammatory reactions[34,57] and foreign body granuloma development[59–64] that occurred following HA injections. There has been one case of an angioedema-like hypersensitivity response following treatment of the upper lip.[65] Whether these inflammatory reactions are a result of allergy to the HA or a reaction to the impurities in the product has been debated.[38,56–66] An antibody response to HA itself has not been reported, and any immunologic response to these products is most likely due to protein contaminants rather than the HA.[57] The reformation of Restylane in 1999 resulted in a sixfold reduction in protein load in the final product. This reduction resulted in a concomitant reduction in the reported occurrences of suspected hypersensitivity reactions.[37,38,57] It is often difficult to ascertain whether such reactions are attributable to true allergic reaction or local irritation associated with the quantity and location of a bolus of injectant. Whatever the cause, there are several reports of red indurated bumps over areas of treated with HA that appear up to 6 months after treatment (Fig. 30-12).[38,47,53,58–64] Granulomas and inflammatory reactions have also been reported with Radiesse and Sculptra 14 days to 2 years after injection.[51,52,56,61]

An uncommon but significant undesired effect that may rarely occur with filler material (HA, CosmoPlast) is injection-site necrosis.[38,45,55,67,68] These potential complications can result from inaccurate needle placement or applying too much pressure during injection. Inadvertent injection of the angular artery (nasolabial fold area) or supratrochlear artery (glabellar area) with viscous fillers induces an ischemic response with violaceous bluish discoloration, pain, erosion, and ulceration.[45,53,55,67,68]

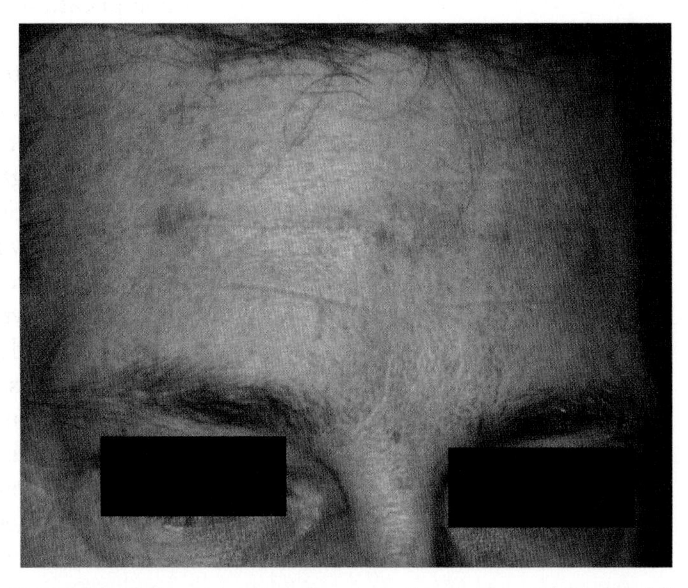

Figure 30-12 Six months following a Restylane injection in the mid-forehead lines, the patient presented with an inflammatory reaction in the area of injection that resolved on its own over 3 days.

Eventual resolution without pain is routine except when a large bolus of material is injected, with ensuing full-thickness necrosis. Once recognized, digital massage, warm compresses, and the application of topical nitroglycerin paste may reduce the size and extent of the area affected by ischemia. The value of massage, warm compresses, or nitroglycerin gel in this situation is as yet unsubstantiated, but any or all of these therapies may be used in an attempt to limit the loss of tissue. Vascular interruption caused by injection is much more likely to occur with more viscous agents (e.g., Perlane, CosmoPlast) because they are intended to be injected deeper in the tissue adjacent to the vascular supply of the dermis. Because 50% of all reported necrotic events occur in the glabellar area, physicians are cautioned against using thick products (e.g., Perlane, CosmoPlast) at this site. The increased incidence of ischemia in the glabellar area is believed to be due to the lack of collateral circulation in this area when the supratrochlear artery is temporarily occluded.[45,68]

Injections in the glabella with the newer injectable HA fillers have not been reported to cause retinal artery thrombosis, an embolic phenomenon reported in the distant past following the use of Zyplast collagen and fat.[45,55,68–70] However, it is just a matter of time since embolization of the dorsal nasal artery has been reported.[45] Caution should be exercised when injecting any filler into the glabellar area.

Itch, acneiform eruptions, and herpes simplex virus reactivation (e.g., cold sores) have been reported in a few instances and may be associated with inadvertent skin irritation during the injection process.[52,53] It is not known whether these effects are related or coincidentally reported by patients around the time of injection. Those undergoing lip injection who have a known history of recurrent cold sores may benefit from prophylactic acyclovir (800 mg BID for 10 days) beginning the morning of the injection. Cutaneous bacterial infection and sterile abscesses may rarely be associated with biodegradable filler.[53,57,33] Management of suspected implant-related infection entails the use of topical and oral antibiotics.

Lastly, it is important to stress that there has been no statistical association between bovine collagen injections and the subsequent development of autoimmune connective tissue diseases.[53] In addition, bovine collagens are derived from the hides of a closed herd of American cattle; therefore, these animals are not believed to be exposed to prions that can cause bovine spongiform encephalopathy.[3,53,71]

30-9 LONG-TERM NONABSORBABLE FILLERS (DURATION >2 YEARS)

Although permanent filler sounds appealing, it is important to appreciate that an individual's soft tissue volume and appearance change with time. One concern with administering permanent fillers is what will happen to the filler material and injected area over the lifespan of the patient. For this reason, many physicians avoid permanent fillers while recommending them in only very selected areas.

30-9-1 *Artefill®*. Artefill (Artes Medical, San Diego, CA) is a long-term (permanent) injectable soft tissue filler that consists of homogenous polymethylmethacrylate (PMMA) microspheres (20% by volume) evenly suspended in a solution of partially denatured 3.5% bovine collagen (80% by volume).[72,73] All microspheres are in the range of 30 to 50 microns in size, are completely round, and have a smooth surface. Artefill also contains an average 0.3% lidocaine hydrochloride. Artefill should be injected into the deep dermis. Following its injection, the collagen vehicle is degraded within 1 to 3 months. The microspheres subsequently become encapsulated with a fine fibrous capsule, a process that is completed within 2 to 4 months after injection. Since the PMMA spheres are nonbiodegradable and too large to be phagocytosed or taken up by the vasculature, the resulting tissue augmentation should be long-lasting.

Artefill has been FDA approved as a filling agent for the reduction of nasolabial folds. Artefill has also been suggested for glabellar frown lines, perioral lines, lip augmentation, and acne scars. It is not designed for fine wrinkle lines, as it must be placed deep within the dermis. The lip area is an area of controversy, as lumpiness is common and extremely difficult to correct because the product is permanent and would have to be surgically removed if lumpy lips occur.

Artefill should be stored in a refrigerator and allowed to warm to room temperature over 4 hours prior to injection. Rapid warming (holding it over a heater or rubbing it between your hands) leads to clumping of the beads at one end. Experienced injectors have found that allowing the product to warm to room temperature for 1 to 2 hours actually works the best. Just prior to injections, the plunger on the syringe should be advanced until some of the product is seen at the needle tip. Occasionally it is difficult to advance the plunger due to clogging of the needle with the product. A change in needle usually remedies the problem but also leads to a loss of some of the Artefill. The volume to be injected depends on the depth and size of the wrinkle. A linear threading technique and/or a serial puncture technique is used to deposit the material into the tissue. Gentle massage immediately postinjection helps smooth the filler area. It is strongly advised to inform the patient that at least two injection sessions are required. Since the product is permanent, one does not want to overcorrect the defect. It is best to aim for a partial correction, wait until the product solidifies over the next few months, and then reinject to augment the area of concern. This gradual correction of skin defects is safest and allows for a more natural, smoother, balanced result. Caution is advised as overly aggressive injections may lead to irregularity or lumpiness, while too-superficial placement can result in permanent "beading" or "ridging."

As with other injectables, postinjection swelling, bruising, and erythema are not unusual. Late side effects include persistent redness, visibility of Artefill through the skin, beading, and contour unevenness, but these are infrequent and seem to be technique-related.[73–75] There have been reports of nodules or small lumps in the lips with this product, which can be a source of discomfort and annoyance to the patient.[74,75] In some instances lip surgery is required to remove the Artefill. If significant beading or ridging occurs at the injection site, an injection of triamcinolone (2 mg/mL) may be of some help to soften and shrink the beading. Surgical excision with potential scarring is occasionally the only answer to correct the problem.

An acute allergic reaction to the collagen component is rare. The reported allergic rate with Artefill collagen is 0.78%, compared with approximately 3% with Zyderm or Zyplast. It is not known whether the FDA will require preinjection skin testing prior to administration, as this agent is currently in its final stages of approval in the United States. The distributors of Artefill recommend a single skin test to the collagen component of Artefill. If no reaction occurs by 1 month, Artefill treatment can be administered.

A significant complication occasionally reported with PMMA microspheres is granuloma formation, with a reported incidence of 1 in 1,000.[73–75] In this situation, rather than normal encapsulation of the PMMA beads occurring, a granulomatous response to the material ensues, with redness, inflammation, and swelling. Intralesional triamcinolone or betamethasone is required to settle the reaction.

30-9-2 *Silicone-Containing Soft Tissue Fillers.* There is renewed interest in high-viscosity silicone for soft tissue filling.[76–82] Two products, ADATO™ SIL-ol 5000 (Bausch & Lomb, Rochester, NY), which is 50 times thicker than water, and SILIKON® 1000 (Alcon Laboratories Inc., Fort Worth, TX), which is 10 times thicker than water, are being used for lip augmentation or nasolabial fold treatment with success.[76–78] SILIKON 1000 is a highly purified injectable silicone oil. It is sterile, nonpyrogenic, clear, and colorless. SILIKON 1000 is approved by the FDA for use as a postoperative retinal tamponade during vitreoretinal surgery. SILICON 1000 is relatively inert, with little potential for biologic toxicity.[81] Silicone has proven not to be easily contaminated with bacteria and may remain sterile indefinitely.[82] The water-like specific gravities of ADATO SIL-ol 5000 (0.98 g/cm) and its insolubility in aqueous fluid impart unique properties of tissue interaction. Silicone is considered a permanent soft tissue filler.

The recommended technique for injection of silicone is to use a small amount (0.5 to 1.0 cc) during each treatment session, let it settle for a few weeks, and then reinject additional amounts, depending on the desired effect. A lump occasionally occurs in the injected area and reportedly responds well to a Kenalog® (Bristol-Meyers Squibb, New York, NY) injection. ADATO SIL-ol 5000 has also been useful in HIV-AIDS patients with areas of lipodystrophy.[83]

30-10 AUTOLOGOUS FAT INJECTION

Autologous fat injections are an advanced technique for tissue augmentation. The use of autologous fat has been advocated for over a century.[84] With the introduction of tumescent liposuction in the 1970s, there has been an increased interest in using the aspirated fat to augment the soft tissues of the face.[85] Unfortunately, many of the reported techniques of autologous fat harvest and injections have given variable results. The most popular current method of soft tissue augmentation through fat transplantation is known as microlipoinjection. Microlipoinjection involves the use of small aspirated fat globules to augment the soft tissues of the face.[86]

Microlipoinjection is intended to correct deeper lines and furrows by injecting harvested fat into subcutaneous tissue. Autologous fat injections are not intended for intradermal injection and are contraindicated in the treatment of fine lines and wrinkles. Clinical experience suggests that fat grafting is most successful when the fat is placed in areas already occupied with adipocytes. Sites most amenable for correction with fat include depressed temples, hollow cheeks, deep nasolabial folds, tear trough abnormalities, hollowed nasojugal folds, atrophic lips, and marionette lines.[86] Fat injections tend to survive best in areas with minimal movement. Several complications have been described.[70,87]

REFERENCES

1. Heidingsfeld ML. Histopathology of paraffin prosthesis. *J Cutan Dis.* 1906;24:513–521.
2. Duffy D. Injectable liquid silicone: new perspectives. In: Klein AW, ed. *Tissue Augmentation in Clinical Practice: Procedures and Techniques.* New York: Marcel Dekker, 1998:235–267.
3. Fagien S, Klein AW. A brief overview and history of temporary fillers: evolution, advantages and limitations. *Plast Reconst Surg.* 2007;120(suppl):6s:8s–15s.
4. Metarasso SL. Injectable collagen: lost but not forgotten—a review of products, indications and injection techniques. *Plast Reconstr Surg.* 2007;120(suppl):17s–26s.
5. Klein AW. Skin filling: collagen and other injectables of the skin. *Dermatol Clin.* 2001;19(3):491–508.
6. Carruthers JD, Carruthers A. Facial sculpting and tissue augmentation. *Dermatol Surg.* 2005;31(11):1604–1612.
7. De Silva LW. Erasing the years: an overview of dermal fillers. *Adv Nurse Pract.* 2006;14(2):31–33.
8. Gotlieb SK. Soft tissue augmentation: the search for implantation materials and techniques. *Clin Dermatol.* 1987;5(4):128–134.
9. Hotta T. Dermal fillers: the next generation. *Plast Surg Nurs.* 2004;24(1):14–19.
10. Kanchwalla SK, Holloway L, Bucky LP. Reliable soft tissue augmentation: a clinical comparison of injectable soft-tissue fillers for facial-volume augmentation. *Ann Plast Surg.* 2005;55(1):30–35.
11. Nairns RS, Bowman PH. Injectable skin fillers. *Clin Plast Surg.* 2005;32(2):151–162.
12. Oagentas HE, Pindur A, Spira M, et al. A comparison of soft tissue substitutes. *Ann Plast Surg.* 1994;33(2):171–177.
13. Wise JB, Greco T. Injectable treatments for the aging face. *Facial Plast Surg.* 2006;22(2):140–146.
14. Carruthers J, Carruthers A. A prospective, randomized, parallel group study analyzing the effect of BTX-A (Botox) and nonanimal sourced HA (NASHA, Restylane) in combination compared with NASHA (Restylane) alone in severe glabellar rhytides in adult female subjects: treatment of severe glabellar rhytides with hyaluronic acid derivative compared with the derivative and BTX-A. *Dermatol Surg.* 2003;29(8):802–809.
15. Fagien S, Stuzin J. Injectable soft-tissue augmentation: the present and future. *Plast Reconstr Surg.* 2007;120(suppl):5s–7s.
16. Klein AW. Implantation technique for injectable collagen. *Am Dermatol.* 1983;9: 224–228.
17. Burgess LP, Goode RL. Injectable collagens. *Facial Plast Surg.* 1992;8(3):176–182.
18. Karam P, Kibbi AG. Collagen injections. *Int J Dermatol.* 1992;31(7):467–470.
19. Keefe J, Wauk L, Chu S, Delustro F. Clinical use of injectable bovine collagen: a decade of experience. *Clin Mater.* 1992;9(3-4):155–162.
20. Clark DP, Hanke CW, Swanson NA. Dermal implants: safety of products injected for soft tissue augmentation. *J Am Acad Dermatol.* 1989;21(5):992–998.
21. Flaguel G, Halimi L. Injectable collagen: an evaluation after 10 years' use as a complement of plastic surgery. *Ann Chir Plast Esthet.* 1994;39(6):765–771.

22. Matti BA, Nicolle FV. Clinical use of Zyplast in correction of age and disease-related contour deficiencies of the face. *Aesthetic Plast Surg*. 1990;14(3):227–234.
23. Bauman L. CosmoDerm/CosmoPlast (human bioengineered collagen) for the aging face. *Facial Plast Surg*. 2004;20(2):125–128.
24. Stegman SJ, Chu S, Bensch K, Armstrong R. A light and electron microscopic evaluation of Zyderm collagen and Zyplast implants in aging human facial skin: a pilot study. *Arch Dermatol*. 1987;123(12):1644–1649.
25. Kligman AM, Armstrong RC. Histologic response to intradermal Zyderm and Zyplast (glutaraldehyde-cross-linked) collagen in humans. *J Dermatol Surg Oncol*. 1986;12(4): 351–357.
26. Belange G, Elbaz JS. The role of an immunologic survey prior to using collagen implants. Theoretical aspects and practical methods. *Ann Chir Plas Esthet*. 1989;34(1):69–72.
27. Elson ML. The role of skin testing in the use of collagen injectable materials. *J Dermatol Surg Oncol*. 1989;15:301–303.
28. Klein AW. In favor of double testing. *J Dermatol Surg Oncol*. 1989;15:263.
29. Bauman L. CosmoDerm/CosmoPlast (human bioengineered collagen) for the ageing face. *Facial Plast Surg*. 2004;20(2):125–128.
30. Biesman B. Soft tissue augmentation using Restylane. *Facial Plast Surg*. 2004;20(2): 171–177.
31. Duranti F, Salti G, Bovani B, et al. Injectable hyaluronic acid gel for soft tissue augmentation: a clinical and histological study. *Dermatol Surg*. 1998;24(12):1317–1325.
32. Lindqvist C, TvetenS, Bondevik BE, Fagrell D. A randomized, evaluator-blind, multicenter comparison of the efficacy and tolerability of Perlane vs Zyplast in the correction of nasolabial folds. *Plast Reconstr Surg*. 2005;115(1):282–289.
33. Soparkar CNS, Patrinely JR. Erasing Restylane. *Ophthal Plast Reconstruc Surg*. 2004;20:4:317–318.
34. Lowe NJ, Maxwell CA, Lowe P, et al. Hyaluronic acid skin fillers: adverse reactions and skin testing. *J Am Acad Dermatol*. 2001;45(6):930–933.
35. Coleman SR. Cross-linked hyaluronic acid fillers. *Plast Reconstr Surg*. 2006;117(2): 661–665.
36. Brown LH, Frank PJ. What's new in fillers? *J Drugs Dermatol*. 2003;2(3):250–253.
37. Carruthers A, Carruthers J. Non-animal-based hyaluronic acid fillers: scientific and technical considerations. *Plast Reconstr Surg*. 2007;120(Suppl):33s–40s.
38. Friedman PM, Mafong EA, Kauvar ANB. Safety data of injectable stabilized hyaluronic acid gel for soft tissue augmentation. *Dermatol Surg*. 2002;28:491.
39. Rohrich RJ, Ghavami A, Crosby MA. The role of hyaluronic acid fillers (Restylane) in facial correction surgery: review and technical considerations. *Plast Reconstr Surg*. 2007;120(suppl):41s–54s.
40. Niamtu J 3rd. The use of Restylane in cosmetic facial surgery. *J Oral Maxillofac Surg*. 2006;64(2):317–325.
41. Dover JS. The filler revolution has just begun. *Plast Reconst Surg*. 2006;117(suppl): 38s–40s.
42. Pollack SV. Some new injectable dermal filler materials: Hylaform, Restylane and Artecoll. *J Cutan Med Surg*. 1999;3(suppl 4):27–35.
43. Monheit GD. Hylaform: a new hyaluronic acid filler. *Facial Plast Surg*. 2004;20:153–155.
44. Bergeret-Galley C, Latouche X, Illouz YG. The value of a new filler material in corrective and cosmetic surgery: Dermalive and Dermadeep. *Aesthetic Plast Surg*. 2001;25(4):249–255.
45. Schanz S, Schippert W, Ulmer A, et al. Arterial embolization caused by injection of hyaluronic acid (Restylane). *Br J Dermatol*. 2002;146(5):928–929.

46. Klein AW. In search of the perfect lip: 2005. *Dermatol Surg*. 2005;31:1599–1603.
47. Soparkar CNS, Patrinely JR. Managing inflammatory reaction to Restylane. *Ophthal Plast Reconstr Surg*. 2005;21:2:151–153.
48. Gravier MH, Bass LS, Busso M, Jusin ME, Nairins RS, Tzikos TL. Calcium hydoxylapatite (Radiesse) for correction of mid and lower face: consensus recommendations. *Plast Reconstr Surg*. 2007;120(suppl):55s–66s.
49. Marmur ES, Phelps R, Goldberg DI. Clinical histologic and electron microscopic findings after injection of a calcium hydroxyapatite filler. *J Cosmet Laser Ther*. 2007;6:223.
50. Vleggar D. Facial volumetric correction with injectable poly-L-lactic acid. *Dermatol Surg*. 2005;31:1511–1518.
51. Duffy DM. Complications of fillers: overview. *Dermatol Surg*. 2005;31:1626–1633.
52. Andre P, Lowe NJ, Parc A, et al. Adverse reactions to dermal fillers: a review of European experiences. *J Cosmet Laser Ther*. 2005;7(3-4):171–176.
53. Murad A, Dover JS. Management of complications and sequelae with temporary fillers. *Plast Reconstr Surg*. 2007;120(suppl):98s–105s.
54. Hirsch RJ, Narurkar U, Carruthers J. Management of hyaluronic acid-induced Tyndall effects. *Lasers Surg Med*. 2006;38:202.
55. Consensus recommendation for soft tissue augmentation with non-animal stabilized hyaluronic acid (Restylane). *Plast Reconstr Surg*. 2006;117(suppl):3s–34s.
56. Prada MB, Michalany NS, Hassum KM, Bagatini E, Talarico S. A histologic study of adverse effects of different cosmetic fillers. *Skin Med*. 2005;4:345.
57. Jordan DR. Delayed inflammatory reaction to hyaluronic acid (Restylane). *Ophthal Plast Reconstr Surg*. 2005;21(5):401–402.
58. Shafir R, Amir A, Gur E. Long-term complications official injection with Restylane. *Plast Reconstr Surg*. 2000;106:1215–1216.
59. Klein AW. Granulomatous foreign body reaction against hyaluronic acid [letter]. *Dermatol Surg*. 2004;30:1070.
60. Micheels P. Human anti-hyaluronic acid antibody: Is it possible? *Dermatol Surg*. 2001;27:185–191.
61. Sayalan Z. Facial fillers and their complications. *Aesthetic Surg*. 2003;23:221.
62. Honig JF, Brink U, Korabiowska M. Severe granulomatous allergic reaction after hyaluronic acid injection in the treatment of facial lines and its surgical correction. *J Craniofac Surg*. 2003;14:197.
63. Fernadez-Acenero MJ, Zamora E, Borbujo J. Granulomatous foreign body reaction against hyaluronic acid: report of a case after lip augmentation. *Dermatol Surg*. 2003;29:1225.
64. Raulin C, Greve B, Hartschuh W, Soegding K. Exudative granulomatous reaction to hyaluronic acid (Hylaform). *Contact Dermatitis*. 2000;43(3):178–179.
65. Leonhardt JM, Laurence N, Nairns RS. Angioedema acute hypersensitivity reaction to injectable hyaluronic acid. *Dermatol Surg*. 2005;31:577.
66. Lowe NJ, Maxwell CA, Patnaik R. Adverse reactions to dermal fillers: review. *Dermatol Surg*. 2005;31:1616–1625.
67. Glaich AS, Cohen JL, Goldberg LH. Injection necrosis of the glabella: protocol for prevention and treatment after use of dermal fillers. *Dermatol Surg*. 2006;32:276.
68. Hanke CW, Higley HR, Jolivette DM, et al. Abscess formation and local necrosis after treatment with Zyderm or Zyplast collagen implants. *J Am Acad Dermatol*. 1991;25:319–326.
69. Stegman, SJ, Chu S, Armstrong RC. Adverse reactions to bovine collagen implants: clinical and histological features. *J Dermatol Surg Oncol*. 1998; 14:39.

70. Egidio JA, Arryo R, Marcos A. Middle cerebral artery embolism and unilateral visual loss after autologous fat injection into the glabellar area. *Stroke.* 1993;24:615.
71. DeLustro F, Dasch J, Keefe J, Ellingsworth L. Immune response to allogenic and xenogenic implants of collagen and collagen derivatives. *Dermatol Surg.* 2001;27:789.
72. Lemperle G, Hazan-Gauthier N, Lemperle N. PMMA microspheres (Artecoll) for skin and soft tissue augmentation Part II: Clinical investigation. *Plast Reconstr Surg.* 1995;96:627–634.
73. Lemperle G, Hazan-Gauthier N, Lemperle N. PMMA microspheres (Artecoll) for long-term correction of wrinkles: refinements and statistical results. *Aesthetic Plas Surg.* 1998;22:356–365.
74. Carruthers A, Carruthers JDA. Polymethylmethacrylate microspheres/collagen as a tissue augmenting agent: personal experience over 5 years. *Dermatol Surg.* 2005;31:1561–1565.
75. Thaler MP, Ubogy ZI. Artecoll: The Arizona experience and lessons learned. *Dermatol Surg.* 2005;31:1566–1576.
76. Bendetto AV, Lweis AT. Injecting 1000 Centistake liquid silicone with ease and precision. *Dermatol Surg.* 2003;29:211–214.
77. Duffy DM. Liquid silicone for soft tissue augmentation. *Dermatol Surg.* 2005;31:1530–1541.
78. Barnett JG, Barnett CR. Treatment of acne scars with liquid silicone injection: 30-year perspective. *Dermatol Surg.* 2005;31:1542–1549.
79. Jacinto SS. Ten-year experience using injectable silicone oil for soft tissue augmentation in the Philippines. *Dermatol Surg.* 2005;31:1550–1554.
80. Fulton JE, Porumb S, Caruso JC, Shitabata PK. Lip augmentation with liquid silicone. *Dermatol Surg.* 2005;31:1577–1586.
81. Pollack SV. Silicone, fibrel, and collagen implantation for facial lines and wrinkles. *J Dermatol Surg Oncol.* 1990;16(10):957–961.
82. Webster RC, Gaunt JM, Hamden US, et al. Injectable silicone for facial soft tissue augmentation. *Arch Otolaryngol Head Neck Surg.* 1986; 112:290–296.
83. Jones D. HIV facial lipoatrophy: causes and treatment options. *Dermatol Surg.* 2005;31:1519–1529.
84. Sclafani AP, Romo T 3rd. Collagen, human collagen, and fat: search for a three-dimensional soft tissue filler. *Facial Plast Surg.* 2001;17(1):79–85.
85. Philips PK, Pariser DM, Pariser RJ. Cosmetic procedures we all perform. *Cutis.* 1994;53(4):187–191.
86. Pinski KS, Coleman WP. Microlipoinjection and autologous collagen. *Dermatol Clin.* 1995;13(2):339–351.
87. Teimourian B. Blindness following fat injections [letter]. *Plast Reconstr Surg.* 1988;82:361.

31

Face-Lifting Techniques

DAVID E.E. HOLCK, MD, JOEL KOPELMAN, MD,
AND LISA MIHORA, MD

Facial rhytidectomy is a rejuvenative surgical procedure designed to improve the aging changes in the lower third of the face and neck. It can significantly improve jowling, the jaw line, and the portion of the neck from the hyoid bone to the jaw line (the cervicomental angle). It is less successful at improving the midface or nasolabial folds. Rhytidectomy optimizes the age-appropriate aesthetic but does not stop the normal aging progression after surgery. While a well-performed rhytidectomy is extremely gratifying for both patient and surgeon, it is elective and invasive, with prolonged rehabilitation and potential morbidity. Complications are poorly tolerated, and therefore pitfalls should be meticulously avoided.

Fundamental steps in facial rhytidectomy include incision planning, skin flap dissection, addressing the superficial musculo-aponeurotic system (SMAS) and platysma, liposuction or direct lipectomy, skin redraping, and wound closure. These are standard in lower-third facial and neck rejuvenation. Face lifting is an imperfect procedure: the surgeon takes advantage of camouflaged incisions and healing patterns to obtain optimal rejuvenation.

31-1 FACELIFT ANATOMY

The facial anatomy of the lower third of the face and neck is complex but may be best viewed in a layered approach.[1–3] Facial skin varies in thickness, with eyelid skin being the thinnest and cheek skin the thickest. The skin of the face is nourished via a dermal plexus, which must be maintained in rhytidectomy surgery. Beneath the skin lies facial subcutaneous fat. This fat is lobulated and enclosed by fibrous septa, which connect the superficial fascia to the dermis.[4–6] The thickest portion of subcutaneous fat is the malar fat pad, bounded by the infraorbital rim above, the nasolabial fold medially, and the zygomaticus major muscle laterally. Minimal subcutaneous fat is located in the lower eyelid region and in the perioral region.

Below the level of the subcutaneous fat is the SMAS.[7–16] This fibromuscular sheet is continuous with the superficial temporalis fascia and galea cranially and the platysma muscle caudally.[17] The SMAS envelops and connects the superficial mimetic muscles to the dermis, expanding the range of facial expression to the skin via distribution of force. The thickness of the SMAS layer varies: it is well developed in the midface over the parotid but thins medially. The dense attachments between the SMAS and the dermis at the region of the nasolabial and melolabial folds accentuate aging changes as the malar fat pad descends and deepens these folds.[18–20]

The SMAS has bony attachments to the infraorbital rim, zygoma, and mandible. These attachments correlate to corresponding osseocutaneous retaining ligaments.[21,22] These retaining ligaments function to suspend and connect the more mobile superficial SMAS, subcutaneous fat, and skin to the more fixed periosteal, parotid, muscular, and deep fascial layers. A second type of retaining ligament is a coalescence of superficial and deep fascia that extends to the dermis, the fascial-cutaneous ligaments. The zygomatic and orbitomalar osseocutaneous ligaments suspend the soft tissue of the malar region. This firmly adherent area is often difficult to release surgically. It is often a source of bleeding intraoperatively.[23] The mandibular osseocutaneous ligament defines the anterior third of the submental mandible. It inserts into the skin and descends into the symphysis to create the submental crease.

Beneath the SMAS in the midface is a distinct layer, the deep cervical fascia, that envelops the parotid gland and overlying the masseter muscle. Beyond the anterior border of the parotid gland the SMAS becomes thinner and more closely adherent to the deep fascia. Buccal branches of the facial nerve are commonly observed during deep-plane rhytidectomy surgery beneath this "cellophane" translucent deep fascia. Meticulous dissection in this dissection plane is necessary to avoid descending below the deep fascia and injuring buccal branches of the facial nerve. The parotidomasseteric fascia is a fascial-cutaneous ligament that forms a weaker retaining ligament to the overlying dermis.

The thin, flat platysma muscle originates on the thorax anterior to the clavicles. This muscle covers the anterior and lateral neck, inserts on the mandibular border and skin, and is contiguous with the fibrous SMAS overlying the parotid gland and cheek. In the neck midline there is variation in the degree of decussation of the platysma muscles across the midline. This leads to vertical banding and bowing over the cervicomental angle. Also, pseudoherniation of the subplatysmal fat results in a clinical "waddle" as part of the aging process.

The facial nerve provides the main innervation to the facial motor supply. The facial nerve exits the stylomastoid foramen deep to the tympanomastoid suture and enters the parenchyma of the parotid gland. The main trunk usually bifurcates within the parotid gland (pes anserinus).[24] The facial nerve then divides with some variability into five divisions: temporal (or frontal), zygomatic, buccal, mandibular, and cervical branches. The branches emerge medially from the parotid gland within the parotidomasseteric fascia on the surface of the masseter muscle. The temporal branch runs in the superficial temporal fascia (the cranial extension of SMAS), where it divides into multiple branches and innervates the frontalis and corrugator muscles.[25] It is felt to be a terminal branch and is therefore at greater risk for injury. The zygomatic branch often parallels Stensen's duct and innervates the zygomatic major and minor muscles, and the orbicularis oculi muscle on its undersurface. The zygomatic division anastomoses with the buccal division in up to 70% of patients. The buccal division exits the anterior border of the parotid gland on the parotid masseteric fascia on the surface of the masseter muscle and buccal fat.[26]

The marginal mandibular nerve found beneath deep cervical fascia usually courses along the mandibular border but may variably course below the mandibular border as well. This terminal trunk may have one to four branches, and is also at greater risk for injury.[27] The marginal nerve lies deep to the platysma until approximately 2 cm temporal to the oral commissure. Here it enters the lower lip depressors. The mandibular nerve anastomoses with the buccal division of the facial nerve only about 15% of the time. Fortunately, permanent paralysis occurs only rarely. If injury does occur, paresis of the depressors of the lower lip (depressor anguli oris, depressor labii inferiorus, mentalis, part of the orbicularis oris and risorius, and occasionally the anterior platysma muscle) can occur.

The cervical division of the facial nerve innervates the platysma muscle. It penetrates the undersurface of the platysma muscle approximately 2 cm anterior to the posterior border of the muscle and 2 cm below the mandibular border.

Facial sensation is provided by branches of cranial nerve V. The midface is mainly served by the maxillary nerve (V_2) through the infraorbital nerve, while the chin and parts of the jaw and ear are covered by the mandibular nerve (V_3) through the mental nerve. Sensation to the neck and smaller areas of the face is supplied through the cervical plexus (great auricular, lesser occipital [C_2-C_3]; supraclavicular [C_3-C_4]). The most commonly injured nerve in facelift surgery is the great auricular nerve (C_2 and C_3). The great auricular nerve is typically found 6.5 cm inferior to the auditory canal, below the cervical fascia lying superficially over the sternocleidomastoid muscle (Erb's point).[28] It provides sensation to the ear and superolateral portion of the neck. Meticulous superficial dissection over this thin difficult dissection area must be performed to avoid trauma of this nerve.

Aging changes to the face are characterized by volume loss, both bony and soft tissue, which is affected by genetics and lifestyle.[29,30] These changes may be seen as early as the third decade of life. Volume loss and ptosis of the midface soft tissue accentuates the nasolabial fold, creates malar fat pad ptosis, and unmasks the infraorbital rim. This is often best appreciated in an oblique view. Marionette lines present as inferior extensions of the nasolabial fold and oral commissure.

Jowling is a major finding of the aging face as well as a common patient complaint. It is related to bony and soft tissue atrophy of the anterior mandibular groove (demonstrating the prejowl sulcus) and platysmal descent. These findings may be aggravated by microgenia[31] and malar hypoplasia, as well as in edentulous patients. The neck may also demonstrate platysmal banding, submental fat accumulation (both preplatysmal and subplatysmal), skin redundancy, and ptosis of the submandibular glands. A low-lying hyoid bone may accentuate the aging changes and limit the rejuvenation results.[32] Also, the skin loses both thickness and elasticity.[33,34] These lower facial changes result in a squaring off of the face in the anteroposterior view, loss of the cervicomental angle, platysmal banding, a waddle, and a double chin.

31-2 HISTORY OF FACELIFTING

Facial rhytidectomy surgery has been described since the early 20th century.[35] The earliest surgeons performed extended subcutaneous dissection with skin tightening, which offered modest short-term success and a significant risk of complications. The first major breakthrough in this procedure was described in the second half of the last century. This involved manipulation of the superficial musculo-aponeurotic tissue in a plication. In this technique the SMAS was folded over and tightened with sutures. Similarly, the SMAS could be tightened by excising a strip over the parotid gland and suturing the free ends (imbrication).[36,37] Multiple variations of these techniques followed, with each addressing the SMAS using variations of plication, imbrication, or a short SMAS flap from the distal imbricated segment.[38–49]

In the 1970s Skoog described the development of the SMAS flap dissecting over the deep cervical fascia.[50] This deep plane flap was repositioned in a vertical vector, providing further improvement in the lower face. By more aggressive dissection in the sub-SMAS plane, less subcutaneous dissection would be necessary (maintaining the dermal–SMAS attachments). Still more aggressive SMAS dissection was developed by extending the deep plane into the composite lift.[51–54] Most recently, efforts to maximize the vertical vector of soft tissue repositioning, especially in the midface, has been described using the subperiosteal approach.[55–62] Significant debate remains regarding the optimal procedure for lower face rejuvenation.[63–69] However, all techniques involve some manipulation of the SMAS.[70–73]

31-3 CONSULTATION

Patients desiring elective facial rejuvenation surgery should be able to identify specific areas of concern. Aesthetic standards vary by gender, culture, and race, and the desired results should be accurately determined in the preoperative consultation. A mirror of sufficient size is a prerequisite for patients to point out areas of concern. Old photographs are useful, as these demonstrate both a desired look as well as the aging process for that patient.

Standardized preoperative photographs are taken early in the consultation.[74,75] Frontal (or anteroposterior) views (from the clavicles to the occiput), right and left lateral views in the Frankfort plane (a straight horizontal line from the supratragal notch to the infraorbital rim), right and left oblique views (which demonstrate midface aging changes particularly well), aligning the medial canthus with the oral commissure, and raccoon eye views should be routinely taken. Asymmetries are pointed out to patients that they may not have previously appreciated (but often note postoperatively).

The patient's past medical history should be comprehensively reviewed prior to considering surgery. Inquiries into the patient's general health, medications (including supplements), allergies, and previous surgeries are mandatory. Anticoagulant use should be identified and discontinued an appropriate duration preoperatively. A social history, including tobacco, alcohol, other drug use, and socially risky behavior, must be obtained.[76] Significant weight loss should be accomplished well before facial rejuvenative surgery. Also, specific review of cardiovascular, respiratory, rheumatologic, and psychiatric systems should be obtained. A low threshold to delay or defer surgery should be maintained to avoid untoward consequences.[77,78]

Complete ophthalmic and facial examination is necessary and laboratory testing is performed based upon the consultation. The status of the facial nerve and facial muscle tone are documented preoperatively. Thorough analysis of the bony facial and neck structure (including hypoplastic areas, microgenia, the patient's bite and dentition, hyoid position) and aging changes (including asymmetries) are made.[79] Photographs document these issues, as well as hairline position and hairstyle choice. Routine preoperative blood testing includes complete blood count, chemistry panel, prothrombin and partial thromboplastin times, and hepatitis and HIV tests. Urinalysis and a baseline electrocardiogram are obtained. As needed, medical clearance from the patient's primary care physician is obtained.

Mature, realistic goals are mandatory for a positive experience for the patient and surgeon. This should be documented in a detailed informed consent. There is no definitive algorithm on the correct procedure of choice for lower facial rejuvenation. SMAS plication, imbrication, short flap SMAS rhytidectomy, or deep-plane face lifting may all be useful, depending upon the surgeon's preference and experience. Lipomatosis may be managed by liposuction or direct lipectomy (both from a submental approach). Platysmal banding is best addressed with platysmal plication, lateral platysmal tightening, or Giampapa sutures. Supplemental procedures including chin, midface, and malar implants (to augment the bony skeleton), fillers (to augment soft tissue volume loss), as well as midface and brow lifting, blepharoplasty, and skin resurfacing often complement facial rhytidectomy.[80–87]

31-4 TECHNIQUES

Facial rhytidectomy surgery may be safely accomplished under general anesthesia or using monitored anesthesia. In either instance tumescent anesthesia facilitates soft tissue dissection and anesthesia. A modified Klein solution giving a mixture of roughly 0.1% lidocaine with 1:100,000 epinephrine is used.[88]

31-4-1 *Incision Placement.* There are many modifications to rhytidectomy incisions. To minimize the stigmata of face-lifting surgery, many surgeons advocate camouflaged incisions, as well as incisions that minimize hair loss (especially in the temporal region). Incisions begin anteriorly at the inferior border of the temporal tuft across the sideburn to the preauricular cartilage at the pretragal skin crease. Some hair may be sacrificed in order to hide the incision in this area, while maximizing the vertical vector of facial flap elevation. In patients with a minimal temporal tuft, the incision may be limited to the inferior border of the tuft to avoid further loss.

From the root of the helix the incision is carried down along the natural preauricular crease to the superior tragal border. In well-developed preauricular folds, or where the preauricular skin is significantly thicker than the tragal skin, the incision is made along the pretragal crease. Some surgeons prefer intratragal incisions in female patients and pretragal incisions in the hair-bearing skin of men. The incision is then continued in the preauricular crease inferiorly to the ear lobule.

The incision is then carried around the ear lobule onto the posterior auricular surface. The ear normally lies 15 to 20 degrees from the vertical. In approximately 60% of patients, the lobule is unattached. If there is no detached lobe, a small amount of skin is left on the inferior lobule to facilitate closure. The incision rides 3 to 5 mm onto the posterior conchal cartilage (not in the sulcus) to avoid postoperative scar migration into a visible retroauricular location. The incision is continued superiorly to the point where the helical cartilage intersects the posterior hairline. The incision backcuts and follows this intersection to the posterior hairline and continues for approximately 6 cm in a curvilinear fashion into the hairline. This incision bisects the posterior hairline and its tangent at the helical intersection. The length of the temporal tuft and posterior hairline incisions will vary to facilitate redraping of the skin upon rhytidectomy skin closure. The overall rhytidectomy incision mimics an inverted omega shape.

31-4-2 *Skin Flap.* The skin flaps are initially developed in the subdermal plane using sharp dissection. The more aggressive the SMAS flap, the shorter the skin flap needs to be dissected. The skin flap should have hair follicles and a uniform cobblestone pattern of subcutaneous fat on its undersurface. This dissection plane does not bleed significantly if adequate tumescence has been infiltrated and dissection remains in the subdermal plane. Transillumination of the flap helps delineate the uniformity of the skin flap. The dissection limits typically extend 5 to 6 cm in the facial region: medially to the angle of the mandible, body of the zygoma (to the zygomatic osseocutaneous ligament), and the medial surface of the parotid gland (roughly one-third the distance from the tragus to the ala of the nose). In the neck (below the inferior border of the mandible), this dissection plane is longer and is taken to the midline. The retroauricular dissection is continued posteriorly approximately 6 cm or greater to facilitate redraping. The skin overlying the inferior border of the mandible is left intact to avoid aggressive dissection in this area and potential trauma to the marginal mandibular nerve.

Areas of difficult skin flap dissection include the area overlying the mastoid fascia, osseocutaneous ligaments (zygomatic and mandibular), and over the sternocleidomastoid fascia. Deep dissection inferior to the ear lobe may traumatize the greater auricular nerve or the sternocleidomastoid muscle. The subdermal supraplatysmal dissection is usually accomplished without difficulty. Horizontal and vertical spreading of long-handled dissection scissors facilitates the subcutaneous flap creation in the neck.

After dissection of the skin flap, landmarks on the superficial surface of the SMAS are marked to maintain surgical situational awareness. The inferior angle of the mandible is marked to avoid aggressive dissection in this area and inadvertent trauma to the marginal mandibular nerve. The inferior border of the zygomatic arch is marked to avoid sub-SMAS dissection cranially and potential trauma to the frontal branch of the facial nerve. The arch marking is continued medially to the notch at the body of the zygoma. This represents the origin of the zygomaticus major muscle. Cutting down in this area facilitates supramuscular dissection of the SMAS in deep-plane rhytidectomy surgery.

31-4-3 *Addressing the* SMAS *Flap*. Most rhytidectomy surgeons appreciate the importance of SMAS tightening, and multiple techniques have been described. The simplest method of SMAS tightening is to simply plicate the tissue in a vertical vector of pull. The SMAS overlying the angle of the mandible is sutured to proximal SMAS at the inferior tragal border; the SMAS at the oral commissure is sutured to proximal SMAS at the superior tragal border, and the platysmal edge at the neck is sutured to the mastoid fascia.

Imbrication involves excising a strip of SMAS, usually overlying the parotid gland capsule, from the inferior border of the zygomatic arch to the angle of the mandible. The free cut ends are then sutured in a vertical direction similar to plication. Still more aggressive techniques involve dissecting a SMAS flap to the medial edge of the parotid gland and mobilizing the short flap in a similar fashion, with direct closure to the free edge of the pretragal SMAS.

In the deep-plane facelift technique, the SMAS flap is begun at the anterior border of the parotid gland from the junction of the zygomatic arch and body (cranially) to the angle of the mandible (caudally). A uniform thickness is developed between the inferior border of the SMAS and deep masseteric fascia. The glistening areolar tissue between the masseteric fascia and the SMAS undersurface is readily apparent, especially in the lower face. Branches of the facial nerve are frequently apparent under this loose areolar tissue and confirm the appropriate dissection plane. A lighted retractor and countertraction are useful in this situation. Care is taken to avoid SMAS flap dissection at the inferior border of the mandible, which may traumatize the marginal mandibular nerve. Often remnants of the platysma muscle are seen running in a vertical or oblique fashion on the undersurface of the SMAS flap. The dissection is continued toward the jowl. In the lower face the platysma muscle is located within the SMAS flap being elevated, while in the neck the subcutaneous dissection leaves the platysma muscle down. The inferior border of the mandible separates the two dissection cavities.

As the SMAS flap dissection is carried medially, greater care is taken to avoid thinning the flap. The extent of dissection is complete upon reaching 1 to 2 cm from the nasolabial fold and modiolus. Cranially, the dissection is continued over the zygomaticus major muscle. As the dissection progresses medially, the buccal fat pad may be entered.

As with other techniques mentioned above, the mobilized SMAS flap is advanced in a (mainly) superior and (slightly) lateral vector of pull. The portion of the SMAS flap from the angle of the mandible is advanced to the inferior tragal border and sutured to the pretragal SMAS with a 3-0 PDS or Prolene suture. The SMAS from the oral commissure is advanced to the superior tragal border and sutured in a similar fashion. Vest-over-pants sutures bury the knots. Excess SMAS is trimmed to create a smooth transition. A dog-ear of SMAS is frequently draped over the zygomatic arch, and this may be excised. Any dimpling at the SMAS–skin interface is managed by judicious undermining. Further caudally, the platysmal edges may be fixed to the mastoid fascia using a 3-0 suture for additional neck support.

31-4-4 *Skin Redraping.* The excess skin is then redraped to maximize a vertical vector of pull. Key staples provide anchoring for the skin redraping: one at the highest point of the preauricular skin, the postauricular skin, and at the posterior hairline. These key staples are removed at 10 to 14 days postoperatively. In the preauricular area, the skin is elevated under moderate tension in a (mainly) vertical and (slightly) lateral vector. The edge of the skin flap is stapled at the level of the insertion of the superior helix (immediately above the ear). The amount of flap elevated is limited by the dog-ear that is formed. The excess dog-ear skin above the temporal tuft ("bird's-beak") hairline incision is grasped under vertical tension and the wedge is excised to preserve the hairline. The incision at the sideburn is closed with 35R staples. Often additional subcutaneous undermining is required to lay down the flap.

The second key staple is placed by advancing the skin from the inferior lobule superiorly to the postauricular incision as it cuts back towards the posterior hairline. This is also stapled under mild tension. The posterior hairline is then elevated in a vertical direction, with care taken to realign the edge to avoid a step-off. After backcutting the excess hair-bearing scalp, the third key staple is placed at the posterior hairline. Excess skin on the posterior conchal bowl is then excised and loosely sutured. Prior to complete closure of the postauricular area, a drain is placed.

Upon redraping, excess skin overlies the inferior lobule. Sharp scissors are used to cut approximately one half to two thirds of the distance from the overlapped skin to the inferior lobule along the outer helix. The inferior lobule is then rotated over the overlying skin. There should be slight "bunching" of the skin at the inferior lobule to accommodate some mild postoperative inferior scar migration. If no bunching exists, the inferior lobule may be pulled inferiorly, contributing to a "pixie-ear" deformity. The skin is then fixed to the inferior lobule.

The excess skin in the preauricular area is then trimmed using backcuts. Excess skin is trimmed to parallel the incision line. A small gap (approximately 2 mm) allows adequate closure without excess tension. If an intratragal incision was made, the skin is backcut over the superior and inferior tragal borders and excised to cover the cartilage. The skin must be thinned to avoid bulk over the tragus. The preauricular skin is sutured using permanent or absorbable sutures in a running or running-locking technique. These sutures are removed by postoperative day 7.

31-4-5 *Neck Management.* The management of the neck is based upon the preoperative analysis. Many surgeons delay liposuction until the end of rhytidectomy surgery as vertical SMAS flap elevation assists in improving neck contour. Residual lipomatosis may then be more accurately addressed at the end of the procedure through liposuction or direct lipectomy.[89–93] Also, platysmal banding is addressed with platysma plication through a submental incision.[94–99] If significant platysmal bands exist, they are marked preoperatively. At or within 1 to 2 mm of the natural submental crease, a 2- to 2.5-cm incision and subcutaneous dissection is created to the paired platysmal edges. The subcutaneous submental dissection is connected to the previously dissected subcutaneous neck flaps started temporally. If a chin implant is planned, it is performed at this stage.[99] The medial edges of the attenuated platysma muscle are grasped together with an Allis clamp and clamped with a larger curved (Kelly) clamp. A conservative amount of the excess tissue is sharply excised, and buried interrupted sutures (3-0 PDS or Prolene) are placed to bind the platysmal edges from the submental incision to the hyoid bone. This also secures preplatysmal submental fat.

Once the platysmal edges are sutured, analysis of residual subcutaneous lipomatosis is made, and direct lipectomy or liposuction is performed. Conservative excision is the rule, as contour irregularities and adhesions between the skin and platysma muscle from too-aggressive fat removal are extremely difficult to manage. Direct palpation and pinching confirm symmetry of fat removal. The submental incision is then closed with interrupted mattress sutures.

31-4-6 *Postoperative Care.* The face and hair are cleaned, and antibiotic ointment is placed on all suture lines. Telfa dressings are placed around the ears and submentally, and Kling and Kerlex wrappings are generously placed in a circumferential pattern. Coban dressing is placed over the Kerlex for improved compression around the base of the neck. The patient's head is elevated and the patient is sent to recovery for observation. If stable, patients are discharged with oral antibiotics, antiemetics, and pain medications with follow-up in 24 hours.

On the first postoperative day drainage is evaluated, and drains are pulled if insignificant. Prior to pulling the drains, gauze dressings are used to milk any fluid posteriorly to the retroauricular area to verify no fluid collections. All staples and sutures are removed at postoperative day 5 to 7, except for the key staples, which are removed at days 10 to 14. Patients are instructed to use cool compresses for 72 hours postoperatively, keep the head elevated ("three pillows for 3 weeks"), and no turning the neck for the first 2 weeks. Hydrogen peroxide is used to keep the incisions clean, followed by topical antibiotics. Patients may shower after the first postoperative day, but no soaking of wounds. Patients are instructed to replace the Coban dressings circumferentially whenever they are at home, resting, and at night. Light activity may be resumed after 1 week, and patients may go out in public typically by 2 weeks. Strenuous physical activity may be resumed after 1 month. Patients are instructed to report any fluid accumulations, fevers, or discomfort that is increasing rather than decreasing. They are counseled that optimal results are not seen until approximately 3 months postoperatively.

31-5 COMPLICATIONS AND AVOIDANCE

Complications, though inevitable, are generally poorly tolerated in elective rejuvenation surgery.[100-127] Extensive preoperative consultation allows patients to understand the normal postoperative course and risks of surgery. Reviews of facial rhytidectomy complications are confounded by the differing techniques and approaches used, each of which may have its own complication profile. The most common acute postoperative complication is hemorrhage, which has been reported in 0.3% to 15% of cases. Meticulous intraoperative hemostasis, placement of drains, compression dressings, and close postoperative observation with blood pressure, pain, and nausea control may limit this complication. Early recognition and treatment also minimizes untoward sequelae.[113–118] Hematomas may be aspirated if small and localized, or the patient may be taken back to the operating room and the wound opened and explored. In long-duration rejuvenation cases, sequential compression devices also are useful to prevent deep venous thrombosis formation.

Facial nerve injury is perhaps the most feared complication of rhytidectomy surgery. Reviews cite a range of nerve injury from 0.4% to 2.6%, again varying by type of procedure. The majority of these complications are temporary and resolve with time.[119,120] Meticulous technique is required to maintain situational awareness intraoperatively to minimize this complication. Anatomically, the zygomatic and buccal branches have greater cross-innervation and are less at risk than the frontal and marginal mandibular branches. The most commonly injured nerve in rhytidectomy surgery is the greater auricular nerve (a sensory nerve). Reports of up to 7% are presented in the literature. This may relate to the well-described difficult dissection over the sternocleidomastoid muscle and the mastoid fascia.

Other rarer acute complications include infection, seroma formation, wound dehiscence, and necrosis. The risk of skin flap necrosis is greater in smokers and those with connective tissue and vasculopathic disorders. Intraoperative errors of increased wound tension, and creating a too-thin skin flap also increase this complication. Application of nitroglycerin paste may benefit mild cases, but skin necrosis, scarring, and vascular and pigmentary changes may still result. Persistent hypervascularity may be managed using pulse dye laser.

Chronic complications involve sequelae of abnormal wound healing, usually related to technique.[121–126] Excessive tension or incorrect redraping may result in pulldown of the earlobe ("pixie-ear"), pulling of the tragus forward, and hairline abnormalities (step-offs, extensive hair loss). Most of these complications may be avoided by preoperative planning and meticulous operative technique. Management is based upon the specific sequelae. It may not be possible to resolve loss of temporal hair, and this is a complication best avoided by preoperative planning. Hypertrophic scars may be managed by observation, massage, silicon gel dressings, triamcinolone injections, and laser resurfacing. Rarely, alopecia, parotid fistulae, tics, and chronic pain have been described.

Contour irregularities may also involve the neck and are often related to asymmetric fat removal. Excessive residual fat may be easily treated by augmented liposuction or direct lipectomy. Small localized fat collections often respond to local steroid injections. Excessive central fat removal may result in the cobra neck deformity, adhesions between the skin and platysma muscle, accentuation of the submandibular gland ptosis, or facial disproportion in heavier individuals.[127] Excessive fat removal from the jowls, especially when performed early in the procedure, may result in cheek depressions seen when the SMAS is elevated.

REFERENCES

1. Larrabee WF, Makielski KH, Henderson JL. *Surgical Anatomy of the Face*, 2nd ed. Philadelphia: Williams & Wilkins, 2004.
2. Larrabee WF. Facelift anatomy. *Facial Plast Clin North Am.* 1993;1:415–426.

3. Larrabee WF Jr, Makielski KH, Cupp C. Facelift anatomy. *Facial Plast Surg Clin North Am.* 1993;1(2):135.
4. Yousif NJ, Mendelson BC. Anatomy of the midface. *Clin Plast Surg.* 1995;22(2):227.
5. Pessa JE, Garza JR. The malar septum: the anatomic basis of malar mounds and malar edema. *Aesthet Surg J* 1997;17:1.
6. Mendelson BC, Muzaffar AR, Adams WP. Surgical anatomy of the midcheek and malar mounds. *Plast Reconstr Surg.* 2002;110:885.
7. Grodinsky M, Holyoke EA. The fasciae and fascial spaces of the head, neck, and adjacent regions. *Am J Anat.* 1938; 63:367.
8. Mitz V, Peyronie M. The superficial musculo-aponeurotic system (SMAS) in the parotid and cheek area. *Plast Reconstr Surg.* 1976;58:80–88.
9. Jost G, Levet Y. Parotid fascia and face lifting: a critical evaluation of the SMAS concept. *Plast Reconstr Surg.* 1984;74:42–51.
10. Wasset M. Superficial fascial and muscular layers in the face and neck: a histological study. *Aesthet Plast Surg.* 1987;11:171–176.
11. Thaller SR, Kim S, Patterson H, et al. The submuscular aponeurotic system (SMAS): a histologic and comparative anatomy evaluation. *Plast Reconstr Surg.* 1990;86:690.
12. Cardoso de Castro C. Superficial musculoaponeurotic system-platysma: a continuous study. *Ann Plast Surg.* 1991;26:203.
13. Stuzin JM, Baker TJ, Gordon HL. The relationship of the superficial and deep facial fascias: relevance to rhytidectomy and aging. *Plast Reconstr Surg.* 1992;89(3):441.
14. Gosain AK, Yousif NJ, Madiedo G, et al. Surgical anatomy of the SMAS: a reinvestigation. *Plast Reconstr Surg.* 1993;192:1254.
15. Levet Y. Surgical anatomy of the SMAS: a reinvestigation (discussion). *Plast Reconstr Surg.* 1993;92(7):1264.
16. Har-Shai Y, Bodner SR, Egozy-Golan D, et al. Mechanical properties and microstructure of the superficial musculoaponeurotic system. *Plast Reconstr Surg.* 1996;98:59.
17. Gardetto A, Dabernig J, Rainer C, et al. Does a superficial musculoaponeurotic system exist in the face and neck? An anatomical study by the tissue plastination technique. *Plast Reconstr Surg.* 2003;111(2):664.
18. Rubin LR, Mishriki Y, Lee G. Anatomy of the nasolabial fold: the keystone of the smiling mechanism. *Plast Reconstr Surg.* 1989;83:1.
19. Youssif NJ, Gosain A, Matloub HS. The nasolabial fold: an anatomic and histologic reappraisal. *Plast Reconstr Surg.* 1994;93(1):60.
20. Barton FE, Ildiko G. Anatomy of the nasolabial fold. *Plast Reconstr Surg.* 1997; 100(5):1276.
21. Furnas DW. The retaining ligament of the cheek. *Plast Reconstr Surg.* 1989;83:11–16.
22. Ozdemir R, Kiline H, Unlu RE, et al. Anatohistologic study of the retaining ligaments of the face and use in face lift: retaining ligament correction and SMAS placation. *Plast Reconstr Surg.* 2002;110(4):1134.
23. Whetzel TP, Mathes SJ. The arterial supply of the face lift flap. *Plast Reconstr Surg.* 1997;100(2):480.
24. Anson BJ, Donaldson JA, Warpeha RL, et al. Surgical anatomy of the facial nerve. *Arch Otolaryngol.* 1973; 97:201–213.
25. Stuzin JM, Wagstrom L, Kawamoto HK, et al. Anatomy of the frontal branch of the facial, nerve; the significance of the temporal fat pad. *Plast Reconstr Surg.* 1989;83:365–271.
26. Stuzin JM, Wagstrom L, Kawamoto HK, et al. The anatomy and clinical applications of the buccal fat pad. *Plast Reconstr Surg.* 1990;85(1):29.
27. Dingman RO, Grab WC. Surgical anatomy of the mandibular ramus of the facial nerve based on the dissection of 100 facial halves. *Plast Reconstr Surg.* 1962;29:266–272.

28. McKinney P, Gottlieb J. The relationship of the greater auricular nerve to the SMAS. *Ann Plast Surg.* 1985;14:310.
29. Bartlett SP, Grossman R, Whitaker LA. Age-related changes in the craniofacial skeleton: an anthropomorphic and histologic analysis. *Plast Reconstr Surg.* 1992;90(4):592–600.
30. Yousif NJ. Changes in the midface with age. *Clin Plast Surg.* 1995;22(2):213.
31. Gonzales-Ulloa M. Ptosis of the chin: the witch's chin. *Plast Reconstr Surg.* 1972; 50:54.
32. Dedo DD. Preoperative classification of the neck for cervicofacial rhytidectomy. *Laryngoscope.* 1980;40:1894.
33. Glogau RG. Aesthetic and anatomic analysis of the aging skin. *Semin Cutan Med Surg.* 1996;15(3):134.
34. Fitzpatrick TB. The validity and practicality of sun reactive skin types I through VI. *Arch Dermatol.* 1988;124(6):869.
35. Larson DL. An historical glimpse of the evolution of rhytidectomy. *Clin Plast Surg.* 1995;22:207.
36. Webster RC, Smith RC, Smith KF. Plication of the superficial musculoaponeurotic system. *Head Neck Surg.* 1983;6(2):696–701.
37. Webster RC, Smith RC, Papsidero RJ, et al. Comparison of SMAS plication with SMAS imbrication in face lifting. *Laryngoscope.* 1982;92:901.
38. Baker DC. Minimal incision rhytidectomy (short scar facelift) with lateral SMASectomy: evolution and application. *Aesthet Surg J.* 2001;21(1);68–79.
39. Lassus C. Cervicofacial rhytidectomy: the superficial plane. *Aesthet Plast Surg.* 1997; 21:25–31.
40. Fodor PB. Platysma-SMAS rhytidectomy—a personal modification. *Aesthet Plast Surg.* 1982;6(3):173.
41. Kamer FM, Halsey W. The two-layer rhytidectomy. *Arch Otolaryngol.* 1981; 107(7):450.
42. Adamson JE, Todsu AE. Progress in rhytidectomy by platysma-SMAS rotation and elevation. *Plast Reconstr Surg.* 1981;68(1):23.
43. Rees TD, Aston SJ. A clinical evaluation of the results of submusculo-aponeurotic dissection and fixation in face lifts. *Plast Reconstr Surg.* 1977;60(6):851.
44. Krastinova-Lolov D. Mask lift and facial aesthetic sculpturing. *Plast Reconstr Surg.* 1995;95(1):31–36.
45. Saylan Z. Purse string-formed plication of the SMAS with fixation to the zygomatic bone. *Plast Reconstr Surg.* 2002;110(2):667–673.
46. Hoefflin SM. The extended supraplatysmal plane (ESP) facelift. *Plast Reconstr Surg.* 1998;101(2):494.
47. Owsley JQ Jr. SMAS-platysma facelift. *Plast Reconstr Surg.* 1983;71:573.
48. Jost G, Wassef M, Levet Y. Subfascial lifting. *Aesthet Plast Surg.* 1987;11:163.
49. McCollough EG, Perkins SW, Langsdon PR. SMAS suspension rhytidectomy. *Arch Otolaryngol Head Neck Surg.* 1989;115:228.
50. Skoog T. Plastic surgery: the aging face. In Skoog TG. *Plastic Surgery: New Methods and Refinements.* Philadelphia: WB Saunders, 1974:300.
51. Hamra ST. The deep plane rhytidectomy. *Plast Reconstr Surg.* 1990;86(1): 53–62.
52. Hamra ST. Composite rhytidectomy. *Plast Reconstr Surg.* 1992;90(1):1.
53. Hamra ST. Repositioning the orbicularis oculi in composite rhytidectomy. *Plast Reconstr Surg.* 1992;90:14.
54. Hamra ST. The role of the septal reset in creating a youthful eye-lid cheek complex in facial rejuvenation. *Plast Reconstr Surg.* 2004;113:2124.
55. Psillakis JM, Rumley TO, Carmagos A. Subperiosteal approach as an improved concept for correction of the aging face. *Plast Reconstr Surg.* 1988;82:383–392.

56. Ramirez OM. The subperiosteal approach for the correction of the deep nasolabial fold and the central third of the face. *Clin Plast Surg.* 1988;22(2):341.
57. Ramirez OM, Maillard GF, Musolas A. The extended subperiosteal facelift: a definitive soft tissue remodeling for the facial rejuvenation. *Plast Reconstr Surg.* 1991;88:227.
58. Ramirez OM. Endoscopic full facelift. *Aesthet Plast Surg.* 1994;18:363–371.
59. Ramirez OM. Fourth-generation subperiosteal approach to the midface. The tridimensional functional cheeklift. *Aesthet Surg J.* 1998;18:133.
60. Ramirez OM. Extended subperiosteal facelift. *Plast Surg Tech.* 1995;1:223.
61. Ramirez OM. Endoscopic techniques in facial rejuvenation: an overview. I. *Aesthet Plast Surg.* 1994;18:141–147.
62. Ramirez OM. Three-dimensional endoscopic midface enhancement. A personal quest for the ideal cheek rejuvenation. *Plast Reconstr Surg.* 2002;109(1):329–341.
63. Becker FF, Bassichis BA. Deep plane facelift vs. superficial musculoaponeurotic system placation face-lift. *Arch Facial Plast Surg.* 2004;6:8.
64. Ivy EJ, Lorenc ZP, Aston SJ. Is there a difference? A prospective study comparing lateral and standard SMAS face lifts with extended SMAS and composite rhytidectomies. *Plast Reconstr Surg.* 1996;98(7):1135.
65. Becker FF, Bassichis BA. Deep-plane vs. superficial musculoaponeurotic system plication face-lift. *Arch Facial Plast Surg.* 2004;6:8.
66. Hamra ST. A study of the long term effects of malar fat repositioning in face lift surgery: short-term success but long-term failure. *Plast Reconstr Surg.* 1992;89(5):83.
67. Baker DC. Deep dissection rhytidectomy: a plea for caution. *Plast Reconstr Surg.* 1994;93(7):1498–1499.
68. Webster BC, Davidson TM, White MF, et al. Conservative face lift surgery. *Arch Otolaryngol.* 1976;102(11):657.
69. Webster RC, Hamdan U, Fuleihan N, et al. The considered and considerate facelift. *Am J Cosmet Surg.* 1985;2:1.
70. Mendelson BC. Surgery of the superficial musculoaponeurotic system. Principles of release, vectors, and fixations. *Plast Reconstr Surg.* 2001;107(6):1545.
71. Alsarraf R, Johnson CM. The facelift: technical consideration. *Facial Plast Surg.* 2000;16:231–238.
72. Mendelson BC. SMAS fixation to the facial skeleton: rationale and results. *Plast Reconstr Surg.* 1997;100(7):1834–1842.
73. Jost G, Lamouche G. SMAS in rhytidectomy. *Aesthet Plast Surg.* 1982;6:69.
74. Thomas JR, Tardy ME, Przekop H. Uniform photographic documentation in facial plastic surgery. *Otolaryngol Clin North Am.* 1980;13:367.
75. Dickason WL, Hanna DC. Pitfalls of comparative photography in plastic and reconstructive surgery. *Plast Reconstr Surg.* 1976;58:166.
76. Rees TD, Liverett DM, Guy CL. The effect of cigarette smoking on flap survival in the facelift patient. *Plast Reconstr Surg.* 1984;73:911.
77 Lewis M, Lavell S, Simpson M. Patient selection and patient satisfaction. *Clin Plast Surg.* 1983;10:321–332.
78. Baker DC, Aston SJ, Guy CL, Rees TD. The male rhytidectomy. *Plast Reconstr Surg.* 1977;60:514.
79. Dedo DD. "How I do it"—plastic surgery. Practical suggestions on facial plastic surgery. A preoperative classification of the neck for cervicofacial rhytidectomy. *Laryngoscope.* 1980;90(11 Pt 1):1894.
80. Hester TR, Codner MA, McCord CD. The centrofacial approach for correction of facial aging using the transblepharoplasty subperiosteal cheek lift. *Aesthet Surg Q.* 1996;16:51.

81. Hobar PC, Flood J. Subperiosteal rejuvenation of the midface and periorbital area: a simplified approach. *Plast Reconstr Surg.* 1999;104:842.
82. Sasaki GH. Cohen AT. Meloplication of the malar fat pads by percutaneous cable-suture technique for midface rejuvenation: outcome study (392 cases, 6 year's experience). *Plast Reconstr Surg.* 2002;110(2):635.
83. Hamra ST. The zygorbicular dissection in composite rhytidectomy: an ideal midface plane. *Plast Reconstr Surg.* 1998; 102(5):1646.
84. Owsley JQ, Fiala TGS. Update: lifting the malar fat pad for correction of prominent nasolabial folds. *Plast Reconstr Surg.* 1997;100:715.
85. Little JW. Three-dimensional rejuvenation of the midface: volumetric resculpture by malar imbrication. *Plast Reconstr Surg.* 2000;105:267.
86. Williams EF III, Vargas H, Dahiya R, et al. Midfacial rejuvenation via a minimal incision brow-lift approach: critical evaluation of a 5-year experience. *Arch Facial Plast Surg.* 2003;5(6):470.
87. Quatela VC, Choe KS. Endobrow-midface lift. *Facial Plast Surg.* 2004;20(3):199.
88. Klein JA. Anesthesia for liposuction in dermatologic surgery. *Dermatol Surg Oncol.* 1988;14(10):1124–1132.
89. Millard DR Jr, Garst WP, Beck RL, et al. Submental and submandibular lipectomy in conjunction in conjunction with a face lift in the male or female. *Plast Reconstr Surg.* 1972;49:385.
90. Cuzalina LA, Koehler JA. Submentoplasty and facial liposuction. *Oral Maxillofacial Clin North Am* 2005;17:85–98.
91. Kamer FM, Letkoff LA. Submental surgery. *Arch Otolaryngol Head Neck Surg.* 1991;117(1):40.
92. Goddio AS. Skin retraction following suction lipectomy by treatment site: A study of 500 procedures in 458 selected subjects. *Plast Reconstr Surg.* 1991:87;66.
93. Gryskiewicz JM. Submental suction-assisted lipectomy without platysmaplasty. *Plast Reconstr Surg.* 2003;112:1393.
94. Dedo DD. Management of the platysma muscle after open and closed liposuction of the neck in facelift surgery. *Facial Plast Surg.* 1986;4:45–47.
95. Kamer FM. Isolated platysmaplasty: a useful procedure but with important limitations. *Arch Facial Plast Surg.* 2003;5:184.
96. Feldman JJ. Corset platysmoplasty. *Plast Reconstr Surg.* 1990;85(3):333–343.
97. Gonzales-Ulloa M. Ptosis of the chin: the witch's chin. *Plast Reconstr Surg.* 1972;50:54.
98. Giampapa VC, DiBernardo BE. Neck recontouring with suture suspension and liposuction: an alternative for the early rhytidectomy candidate. *Aesthet Plast Surg.* 1995;19(3):217–223.
99. Giampapa V, Bitzos I, Ramirez O, Granick M. Long-term results of suture suspension platysmaplasty for neck rejuvenation: a 13 year follow-up. *Aesthetic Plast Surg.* 2005; 29(5):332–340.
100. Baker TJ, Gordon HL. Complications of rhytidectomy. *Plast Reconstr Surg.* 1967; 40:31.
101. Rees TD, Aston SJ. Complications of rhytidectomy. *Clin Plast Surg.* 1978;5:109.
102. Baker DC. Complications of cervicofacial rhytidectomy. *Clin Plast Surg.* 1983; 10:543.
103. Cohen SR, Webster RC. Primary rhytidectomy—complications of the procedure and anesthetic. *Laryngoscope.* 1983;93:654.
104. Muenker R. Problems and variations in cervicofacial rhytidectomy. *Facial Plast Surg.* 1992;8(1):33.

105. Larrabee WF Jr, Ridenour BD. Rhytidectomy: technique and complications. *Am J Otolaryngol.* 1992;13:1.
106. Adamson P, Moran M. Complications of cervicofacial rhytidectomy. *Facial Plastic Surg Clin North Am.* 1993;1:257.
107. Scheflan M, Mailard GF, Cornette de St. Cyr B, Ramirez OM. Subperiosteal facelifting: complications and the dissatisfied patient. *Aesthet Plast Surg.* 1996;20:33.
108. Owsley JQ. Face lifting: problems, solutions, and an outcome study. *Plast Reconstr Surg.* 2000;105:302.
109. Hamra ST. Correcting the unfavorable outcomes following face lift. *Clin Plast Surg.* 2001;28(4):621.
110. Leist F, Masson J, Erich JB. A review of 324 rhytidectomies, emphasizing complications and patient dissatisfaction. *Plast Reconstr Surg.* 1977;59:535.
111. Hurwitz DJ, Ruskin EM. Reducing eyelid retraction following subperiosteal facelift. *Aesthet Surg J.* 1997;17:149.
112. Hamra ST. Frequent face lift sequelae. Hollow eyes and the lateral sweep: cause and repair. *Plast Reconstr Surg.* 1998;102:1658.
113. Straith R, Raghava R, Hipps C. The study of hematomas in 500 consecutive face lifts. *Plast Reconstr Surg.* 1977;59:694.
114. Perkins SW, Williams JD, Macdonald K, Robinson EB. Prevention of seromas and hematomas after face-lift surgery with the use of postoperative vacuum drains. *Arch Otolaryngol Head Neck Surg.* 1997;123:743.
115. Kamer FM, Song AU. Hematoma formation in deep plane rhytidectomy. *Arch Facial Plast Surg.* 2000;2:240.
116. Rees TD, Barone CM, Valauri FA, et al. Hematomas following face lift surgery. *Plast Reconstr Surg.* 1994;93:1185.
117. Baker DC, Chiu ES. Bedside treatment of early rhytidectomy hematomas. *Plast Reconstr Surg.* 2005;115(7):2119–2222.
118. Baker DC, Stefani WA, Chiu ES. Reducing the incidence of hematomas requiring surgical evacuation following male rhytidectomy: a thirty-year review of 985 cases. *Plast Reconstr Surg.* 2005;116(7):1973–1985.
119. Baker DC, Conley J. Avoiding facial nerve injuries in rhytidectomy. *Plast Reconstr Surg.* 1979;64:781–795.
120. Pitanguy I, Cervello MP, Degand M. Nerve injuries during rhytidectomy: consideration after 3,203 cases. *Aesthet Plast Surg.* 1980;4:257.
121. Ellenbogen R. Avoiding visual tipoffs to face lift surgery. *Clin Plast Surg.* 1992; 19:447.
122. Franco T. Face-lift stigmas. *Ann Plast Surg.* 1985;15:379–385.
123. de Castro CC. Preauricular and sideburn operating procedures for natural looks in facelifts. *Aesthetic Plast Surg.* 1991;15:149.
124. Brennan HG, Toft KM, Dunham BP, et al. Prevention and correction of temporal hair loss in rhytidectomy. *Plast Reconstr Surg.* 1999;104(7):2219.
125. Kridel RW, Liu ES. Techniques for creating inconspicuous face-lift scars: avoiding visible incisions and loss of temporal hair. *Arch Facial Plast Surg.* 2003;5(4):325.
126. Becker FF. The preauricular portion of the rhytidectomy incision. *Arch Otolaryngol Head Neck Surg.* 1994;120:166–171.
127. Kamer FM, Minoli JJ. Postoperative platysmal band deformity: a pitfall of submental liposuction. *Arch Otolaryngol Head Neck Surg.* 1993;119:193.

Index

NOTE: Page numbers followed by '*f*' and '*t*' denote figures and tables, respectively.

About the Editor

Michael T. Yen, MD, specializes in cosmetic and reconstructive surgery of the eyelids and face. He is an associate professor of Ophthalmology at the Cullen Eye Institute, Baylor College of Medicine in Houston, Texas. He completed his residency at the Bascom Palmer Eye Institute in Miami and a fellowship in ophthalmic and facial plastic surgery with Dr. Richard Anderson at the Center for Facial Appearances followed. Dr. Yen is a fellow of the American Society of Ophthalmic Plastic and Reconstructive Surgery (ASOPRS) and of the American Academy of Ophthalmology, from which he received an Achievement Award in 2005.